D1544375

Walter Pagel

William Harvey's Biological Ideas

Selected Aspects and Historical Background

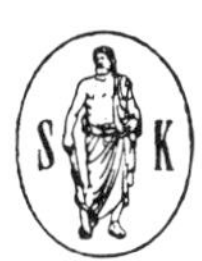

S. Karger Basel/New York 1967

Distributed in North America by
Hafner Publishing Company Inc., New York, N.Y.

Printed in Switzerland by
Basler Druck- und Verlagsanstalt, Basel

To Heinrich Buess and Wilhelm Doerr

Preface

A new book on Harvey? With the multitude of Harveian Orations, biographies, monographs and papers which seem to have appeared in a ceaseless stream almost since the day of Harvey's death in 1657, nothing should have been left over for further discussion. His books are there to be read by everybody in translation and so are now those books of notes which Harvey left in manuscript form. It should be easy to form a true picture of Harvey and what he and his work stood for.

And yet Harvey has remained a problem. His was the light that shone brightest in the new scientific age of the first half of the seventeenth century and it is to his genius that modern biology and medicine owe their foundation. However, he himself entertained thoughts and speculations which remove him far from the modern world of science. It might seem that to appraise him as a man of science we have to forget the body of non-scientific ideas which he made his own, or else to admit defeat in the attempt at understanding him. We can understand some of Harvey, but not all of Harvey.

It is precisely this situation in the history of the biological sciences and medicine which led the present author to Harveian studies, some twenty years ago, and he now ventures to submit the results of his continued research.

Its subject is the world of Harvey as a whole, a world in which the various aspects of his mind are aligned and their relationships with one another are examined against their historical background.

Many of the ideas discussed in this book may admittedly not belong to the History of Science in the general sense. However, they certainly belong to the history of Harvey, and to relegate them to the lumber-room of the "history of human error" would certainly lead to an error in human history.

In this respect Harvey is no different from other savants of the epochs of Reformation and Counter-Reformation: Paracelsus, Servetus and Van Helmont are examples that immediately come to mind. Of these Servetus has been considered in the present book among the contributors to our knowledge of the movement of the blood, prior to Harvey, whilst Paracelsus has formed the subject of earlier books by the present author and a similar work on Van Helmont is now being planned.

As in the preparation of his earlier essays and books the author has enjoyed the support and encouragement of many friends and colleagues to whom he wishes to express his gratitude. This is due in the first place to the Wellcome Trust which, under the auspices of Sir Henry Dale, O. M., F. R. S., promoted the preparation of the present book in its earlier stages. In this respect the author has also to thank Dr F.H.K. Green, C.B.E., F.R.C.P. for continued interest in his work.

Dr F.N.L. Poynter, Director of the Wellcome Historical Medical Institutions and notably of the Wellcome Historical Medical Library has extended to the author his never flagging friendship and guidance in all problems—litterary as well as personal—throughout the years, a help without which the author feels he could not have succeeded in producing a study of a subject which owes so much to Dr Poynter's own research. Dr Poynter also provided most of the illustrations. At the Wellcome Library the author more recently enjoyed the help and cooperation of the Assistant Librarian, Miss Marianne Winder, and was also helped by the Librarian, Mr E. Gaskell, and Mr S.H. Watkins of the Photographic Department.

It has been the author's good fortune to find in Dr Allen G. Debus of the Department of History, University of Chicago, and in Dr Pyarali Rattansi of the Department of Philosophy, University of Leeds, collaborators with whom he could discuss and thereby clarify many problems of mutual interest.

The book could not have been accomplished without the careful revision of the manuscript by Dr Bernard E. J. Pagel who—as on previous occasions—clarified the text in many places.

The author received encouragement, inspiration and valuable suggestions from H. Buess (and his authoritative work on the Harveian tradition in Medicine), O. Kurz, J. O. Leibowitz, Erna Lesky (chiefly through her study on Harvey and Aristotle), J. Needham, G. Scholem, Lloyd Stevenson and O. Temkin. He is also indebted to E. Ackerknecht, F. Arnholz, the late Fred. S. Bodenheimer, P.F. Cranefield, H.A. Feisenberger, Lester S. King, W.P.D. Wightman and Frances A. Yates.

The late Dr Dr h. c. Heinz Karger suggested to the author more than six years ago that a work like the present one should be written and published by him. The author is happy that this has now materialised through the highly efficient and courteous collaboration of his son, Mr Thomas Karger and his brother Dr Fritz Karger.

Table of contents

Appendix

Introduction

In presenting William Harvey's biological thought the author intends to follow the natural division provided by the two grand themes to which his life work was devoted: Circulation of the Blood and Generation of Animals.

Having, by way of introduction, examined his position in the History of European thought and the influences, genuine and reputed, to which he lent himself, we shall attempt to retrace the way which led him to the discovery of circulation. In this task a short analysis of his main work: *De motu cordis et sanguinis* (1628) and of the elements composing it should prove helpful. Such elements include his observations, anatomical and comparative-anatomical, his experiments, his quantification and his non-scientific symbolist speculation. Their role, their mutual relationships and their historical background will thus be examined in the first part of the present book; this accordingly winds up with a new assessment of Harvey's predecessors in the study of the movements of the heart and blood.

No detailed analysis of Harvey's book. *De generatione animalium* (1651) will be attempted. Instead, his leading idea of *Epigenesis* and his related vitalist views will be compared with those of his predecessors and contemporaries. These notably include Aristotle, Peter Severinus and Marcus Marci of Kronland.

A discussion of Harvey's embryological ideas, however, cannot in itself do justice to the strength and wide range of influence which Harvey derived from Aristotle—a subject ever present throughout this book and accorded a special chapter in the introductory part.

From a final review of Harvey's world in all its facets it should become clear that this world is indeed unique and unified in a man who achieved the foundation of modern scientific biology and medicine and yet was neither a modern nor a scientist pure and simple. A child of a pre-rationalist age and a devotee of *philosophia naturalis* he groped for the basic pattern underlying and holding together the greater and the lesser worlds; here it appears as an imitation of eternity in the preservation of individual life through the circular motion of the blood and in that of the species through cycles of generation. To the same mind, then, that observed, experimented and calculated, the results of these activities would appear as the ultimate confirmation of cosmological speculations. This, we believe, was Harvey's world.

Harvey and European thought in the Seventeenth Century

Harvey's life (1578–1657) may be visualised against the background of such varied cultural atmospheres as the Elizabethan, the Jacobean, the first Caroline and the Cromwellian eras in England. Harvey, first and foremost an exponent of the Caroline epoch, was a citizen of London. He must have witnessed its enormous, albeit irregular and unmanageable growth in population, influence and power[1]. Indeed he moved and worked in close proximity to the everyday life of the metropolis. For he was by no means a man of pure research, dedicated to the back-room work of dissection, experiment and natural philosophy. We know of his extensive medical practice which concerned all strata of the population and was not limited to hospital and court service[2]. Moreover it embraced such specialities as obstetrics and neurology. The short chapter which Harvey wrote *On parturition* has been rightly called the first original work on the subject by an Englishman and Harvey himself the "Father of British midwifery[2a]". Again what is most remarkable is that he not only set pregnancy and parturition in alignment with physiology, but also issued a sound warning against "midwives intending to hurry labour by giving medicines with reputed expulsive powers, but really retarding it and making it unnatural, by leaving behind portions of the membranes and even of the placenta, tiring the woman out on the labour stool, and making her in fact run great risks of her life[2b]". Harvey's insight into problems of neurology and the psychological aspects of medicine was of a similar high order[2c]. Indeed, then, Harvey, the physician and medical practitioner, the lecturer and medical administrator, the man of research and medical humanist is unthinkable without the facilities available in a seething and growing metropolis—a centre that was marked, in Harvey's own words, by its "lack of that clean, light, cool and diffusible air which ventilates chest and lungs and thereby promotes life, a lack that causes the filth of multitudes of men, animals and ditches to accumulate, quite apart from the sulphureous fumes that emanate from the carbonised vegetable matter that is used for fuel.[2d]"

Harvey returned from Padua (1602), a newly created doctor of medicine, and he married—one year after the death of Queen Elizabeth (1603)—Elizabeth, the daughter of Dr Lancelot Browne who had been physician in ordinary to the Queen. Harvey may have personally known William Gilbert[3] (1540–1603), the foremost Elizabethan scientist, who, standing in the first rank of early experimentalists, had published his classic *On the magnet* in 1600 and was a friend of Harvey's father in law. Chance may have even made him cross the path of young John Baptist Van Helmont who

1 Mauer, E.F., *Harvey in London. Bullet. Hist.Med.* 1959, XXXIII, 21–36; Clark, G.N., *Jacobean England (1603–1625). Bullet. Hist.Med.* 1957, XXXI, 391–407; Hunter, D., *Harvey and his contemporaries. Lancet,* 1957, II, 811–819 (the state of England about 1650).

2 Keynes, Sir G., *Harvey through John Aubrey's eyes. The 254th Harveian Oration,* reprinted from *Lancet* (17.10.1958), p.9–15 (i.a. Harvey as a surgeon; Harvey and the quacks); see also idem: *The personality of William Harvey. Linacre Lecture,* Cambridge 1949.

2a Johnstone, R.W., *William Harvey—the Father of British midwifery. J.Obstretics and Gyn.Brit.Emp.*, 1948, LV, 293–302.

2b Harvey, W. *Exercitationes de generatione animalium, quibus accedunt quaedam de partu, de membranis ac humoribus uteri et de conceptione,* London, Octav. Pulleyn, 1651, p.265–266; Amstelod. 1662 (Joh. Ravesteynius), p.342–343 (this ed. used and quoted throughout in the present book); *The Works of William Harvey, M.D., translated from the Latin with a life of the author* by Robert Willis. London. Sydenham Soc., 1847, p.533–534. This "standard"-translation is still invaluable; its rendering is beautiful, but free and in not a few places inaccurate. It has been used by the present author after careful collation with the original Latin text which is also given as often as possible. – A new excellent translation of Harvey's writings concerning the circulation of the blood is by K. Franklin: *William Harvey, The circulation of the blood and other writings,* London. Everyman's Library, 1962.

2c Brain, Sir Russell (Lord Brain), *William Harvey, neurologist.* The Harveian Oration, 19th October 1959. *Brit.Med.J.* 1959, II, 899–905 – Hunter, R.A. and Macalpine, I., *William Harvey. Two medical anecdotes, the one related by Sir Kenelm Digby, the other by the Honourable Robert Boyle.* St Barthol.Hosp.J., 1956, LX, 200–206; idem et eadem, *William Harvey: his neurological and psychiatric observations,* J.Hist.Med., 1957, XII, 126–139. – Schurr, P.H., *William Harvey on the nervous system, Guy's Hosp. Rep.*, 1964, CXIII, 79–83.

2d Harvey, W., *Anatomia Thomae Parri, post annos centum quinquaginta duos et menses novem actos, demortui.* In *Opera omnia a Collegio Medicor. Londinensi edita,* London 1766, p.609.

3 The probable influence of Gilbert on Harvey has been rightly pointed out by Buess, H., *Zum 300.Todestag von William*

was Harvey's close contemporary and was a visitor to the Court of Whitehall, quite possibly in the very year of Harvey's return to England[4].

Harvey's admission to the fellowship of the Royal College of Physicians (1607), his appointment as Physician to St Bartholomew's Hospital (1609), as Lumleian Lecturer in Anatomy (1615) and as Physician Extraordinary to the King are the great landmarks of the Jacobean period in Harvey's life. His great book enshrining his discovery of blood circulation was only published three years after the end of King James' reign (1603–1625), but we have it on the best authority, namely Harvey's own, that the idea had been conceived earlier, that is still in Jacobean days[5].

It is well known how close Harvey was to the new king, Charles I[st], whom he accompanied to Scotland when he was crowned at Holyrood in 1633 and to whom he gave regular demonstrations[6]. It is just as well known how much Harvey had to suffer from the lawlessness prevailing in London in the early years of the civil war (1642)—"whilst in attendance on His Majesty the King (and that not only with the permission, but by the command of Parliament) during our late disturbances and more than civil wars, certain rapacious hands not only plundered all my house furniture, but—what is a much more grievous cause of complaint—my notebooks, the fruit of many years of toil, from my museum. Hence most of my observations, notably those on the generation of insects, have been lost, to the detriment, I may venture to say, of the republic of letters.[7]" Harvey left London with the king and was present at the battle of Edgehill near Oxford in October 1642[8]. Moving with the king to Oxford he could hardly have avoided communication with those naturalists of the "Philosophical" or "Invisible College" who were later to found the Royal Society. The turbulence of the civil war and its terrible end left Harvey, then over 70, undaunted. In 1649 his two *Anatomical Exercitations on the Circulation of the Blood* were published in answer to the objections raised by John Riolan, the younger, the most important opponent to Harvey's discovery, and in 1651 his voluminous work *On generation* appeared. These are strong works containing ingenious experiments, subtle observations and a wealth of fertile ideas, all carefully thought out for a long time. Yet the few years which remained of Harvey's life in the Cromwellian era were his declining years, however much encouragement he must have found in the recognition of his discovery—at first almost universally rejected—all over the world and the veneration shown to him by his colleagues.

There is no shred of evidence, direct or circumstantial, that

Harvey. Deut. Med. Wschr. 1957, LXXXII, 1196–1202, p. 1201. Quoting from GILBERT: "Will man Naturgeheimnisse ergründen und die verborgenen Ursachen erforschen, so verdienen sichere Experimente und Beweise mehr Berücksichtigung als Vermutungen und allgemein angenommene Lehrmeinungen", BUESS urges a study of the influence which GILBERT's experimentalism is bound to have exerted on his contemporaries, notably Harvey. – This is borne out, albeit indirectly, by the recent demonstration of GILBERT's influence on ROBERT FLUDD, Harvey's friend, whose role in the history of Harvey's discovery and its reception will be discussed elsewhere in the present book (p. 113). See DEBUS, A.G., *Robert Fludd and the use of Gilbert's De Magnete in the weapon-salve controversy J. Hist. Med.* 1964, XIX, 389–417. – See also on GILBERT, the enlightened experimentalist and "Father of magnetism and electricity" as a figure in the Harveian scene: HUNTER, D., 1957, loc. cit. in note 1.

4 VAN HELMONT, J.B., *De lithiasi* cap. II, 13. *Opuscula medica inaudita. Colon. Agripp.* 1644, p. 39. – *Ortus Medicinae.* vol. II, Amsterod. 1648, p. 19. – *Oriatrike*, tr. by Chandler. London 1662, p. 838. – See the discussion in PAGEL, W., *Paracelsus. An introduction to philosophical medicine in the era of the Renaissance.* Basle and New York 1958, p. 164.

5 Letter dedicatory to Dr ARGENT, President of the Royal College of Physicians, preceding *De motu:* "I have already and repeatedly presented you ... with my new views of the motion and function of the heart and the circuit of the blood, in my anatomical lectures; but having now for nine years and more confirmed these views ... (meam de motu et usu cordis, et circuitu sanguinis sententiam E.D.D. antea saepius in praelectionibus meis Anatomicis aperui novam: sed jam per novem et amplius annos multis ocularibus demonstrationibus in conspectu vestro confirmatam ... Facsimile from the original edition: Franckfort 1628, Canterbury 1894, p. 5, sig. A 3. This facsimile of the first edition is quoted throughout where the citation is from the first edition).

Strangely enough WILLIS translates: "my new views of the motion and function of the heart"—omitting *"and the circuit of the blood"*; it is unlikely that he did so deliberately.

Argent was President of the College between 1625 and 1627. We shall return to the question of the probable date of Harvey's discovery below (p. 213 seq).

6 FRANKLIN, K.J., *King Charles I and Wil-*

Harvey ever made concessions to the new democratic observances[9]. We shall revert to this subject in our final chapter (p. 343) and say something about Harvey's personal appearance and habits when following him on his journey to Prague (p. 286).

The Influence of Padua

However steadfast and true to his loyalties and own convictions Harvey's mind kept aloof from all insularity. Padua left an indelible stamp which we believe we can recognise in his staunch, yet by no means uncritical adherence to Aristotelianism, the basic doctrine of the Paduan school since the late Middle Ages.

For Padua preserved its Aristotelian tradition and allegiance when the main stream of Renaissance thought had turned towards Plato and the Neoplatonists. It was not, however, the scholastic and theologized Aristotle of earlier mediaeval times, but the Aristotle who had created the observational scientific method—an Aristotle who at Padua had always been associated with the Professors of Medicine who had also been commentators on the scientific method, since the days of Pietro d'Abano (1257–1315)[10]. It was at Padua that Jacob Zabarella (1532–1589) developed the theory of scientific induction which proceeds from observation of analysable instances to general principles and from there back to the facts now amenable to synthesis and system[11].

Harvey's critical allegiance to Aristotle forms the keynote of the present book and will be referred to on many occasions under various headings. It will be well to remember that this is one point which far from indicating intellectual backwardness on Harvey's part, shows how open he was to the Aristotelian scientific modernism of a continental school. This equally applied to the Aristotelian methods of comparative anatomical and embryological observation as well as the new Paduan logic of scientific investigation on Peripatetic lines, as we shall see presently (p. 28 seq.).

The Influence of Fabricius of Aquapendente

The first and foremost medium through which the influence of Padua on Harvey becomes palpable is the personality and teaching of the anatomical luminary of the School, Hieronymus Fabricius of Aquapendente (1537–1619). It was in 1603 that he published his treatise on the venous valves[12]. He must have been occupied with it at the very time when Harvey sat at his feet, namely between 1600 and 1602[13]. It was a consideration of the arrangement

liam Harvey. Proc. R. Soc. Med. 1961, LIV, 85–91; Keele, K. D., *William Harvey: the Man and the College of Physicians. Medical History* 1957, I, 265–278 (p. 269).

7 Harvey, *On generation* Exerc. LXVIII, tr. Willis p. 481–482; ed. 1662, p. 294. – Willis' translation is not quite accurate in this place. Harvey mentions expressly his *adversaria*—notebooks—that were lost. Instead Willis has: "my *enemies* abstracted from my museum the fruits of many years of toil". – The translation London 1653, p. 418 has correctly: "... have bereft me of my Notes, which cost me many years industry".

Aubrey's account: "He had made dissections of froggs, toades, and a number of other animals, and had curious observations on them, which papers, together with his goods, in his lodgings at Whitehall, were plundered at the beginning of the Rebellion; he being for the King, and with him at Oxon; but he often sayd, that of all the losses he sustained, no griefe was so crucifying to him as the losse of these papers which for love or money he could never retrieve or obtaine." Aubrey, J., *Letters written by Eminent Persons in the 17th and 18th centuries and Lives of Eminent Men*, London 1813, vol. II, p. 379.

8 Aubrey's famous story of Harvey having the Prince and the Duke of York (i.e. the future Kings Charles II and James II) under his care and having withdrawn with them under a hedge, taking out of his pocket a book, but soon being forced to move to another place by the bullet of a great gun (Aubrey loc. cit. in note 7, p. 379) has been found to be at variance with three eye witness accounts of the happenings of the day and the whereabout of the royal children (Stewart, D., *Harvey and the Battle of Edgehill. Brit. Med. J.* 1946, I, 808). Against this Aubrey has been vindicated by Sir Geoffrey Keynes loc. cit. 1958 in note [2] p. 20–22.

9 In his *Exercitationes duae anatomicae de circulatione sanguinis ad Jo. Riolanum*, Cambridge 1649, i.e. in the year of the King's execution Harvey is still called on the title page: *serenissimae Majestatis Regiae Archiatro*—a position from which he had in fact retired in July 1646—after the surrender of Oxford—at the age of 68 (Franklin, loc. cit. 1961, in note 6, p. 88). – Harvey took no interest in politics. When Ent visited him, at Christmas 1650, he found him "Democritus like, busy with the study of natural things, his countenance cheerful, his mind serene, embracing all within its sphere. Truly (Harvey said) did I not find solace in my studies, and a balm for my

of the venous valves in relation to the heart which, as Harvey told Boyle, touched off the spark of his discovery[14]. The venous valves had been described before Fabricius[15], but the latter gave the first comprehensive anatomical account. He missed, however, the main point—their true function which is bound up with the centripetal direction of the venous blood flow. Fabricius remained an advocate of the Galenic assumption of its centrifugal direction, from the heart towards the periphery and the viscera. To have raised Harvey's criticism would, then, constitute Fabricius' main influence, as it also did with regard to essential questions concerning the generation of animals. It must be remembered, however, that Fabricius, the greatest pupil of the great Falloppio, the man who founded the celebrated Paduan Anatomical Theatre and School, could not have failed to direct his pupil's interest into the proper channels of dynamic anatomy and to the very foci of his lifelong endeavour—the blood vessels on the one hand and the generation of animals on the other. For it is to both of these fields that much of Fabricius' own work had been devoted. In it the Aristotelian lead and especially the spirit of comparative-anatomical enquiry is just as recognisable as in Harvey's work. Indeed the latter nominated Aristotle and Fabricius as his "leaders".

The supposed Influence of Galileo

While it is difficult to overrate the influence of the spirit of Padua in the life and work of Harvey, we must beware of rash conclusions drawn from the simultaneous residence of Harvey, the student, and great luminaries of science, notably Galileo, at the university town. We have no evidence that he attended the lectures of Galileo and the mere juxtaposition of the facts that he was at Padua when Galileo was does not appear to be helpful. Nor does Harvey's "dynamic" view of the motion of the blood as the result of the *impetus* conferred upon it by the contracting heart provide indirect evidence of his familiarity with the person and works of Galileo[15a]. The comparison of the heart with a pump does not seem to belong to the original concept of circulation (p. 213). *Impetus* and *impulsus* are terms that had been used before Harvey by Galen, Vesalius and others with reference to the heart and blood. Galen's "animistic" pulse-making and blood-propelling force of the arteries had come under criticism before Harvey (p. 203, 217). Harvey expressed his discovery and concept in Aristotelian terms. The same applies to Harvey's use of quantitative methods. At Harvey's time J.B. Van Helmont (1579–1644) em-

spirit in the memory of my observations of former years ... this vacation from public business, which causes tedium and disgust to so many, has proved a sovereign remedy to me." (Doctor Ent's Epistle Dedicatory to Harvey, *On generation* transl. by WILLIS, p. 145).

10 RANDALL, J.H. jr., *The development of scientific method in the School of Padua. J. Hist. Ideas* 1940, I, 177–206, passim, p. 182 et seq. and p. 201. – To PIETRO D'ABANO: NORPOTH, L., *Zur Bio-Bibliographie und Wissenschaftslehre des Pietro d'Abano, Mediziners, Philosophen und Astronomen in Padua. Kyklos*, 1930, III, 292–353 (p. 339: *Doctrina resolutiva* and *Doctrina compositiva*).

11 RANDALL, loc. cit. 1940, in note 10.

12 *De venarum ostiolis*, Patav. 1603. Edition used: *Opera omnia cum praefat.* B.S. Albini. Lugd. Bat. 1738, p. 150–160. – The work was translated by K.J. FRANKLIN: *Fabricius ab Aquapendente, De venarum ostiolis, 1603, Facsimile edition with introduction and translation.* Springfield and Baltimore, 1933.

13 "Harvey went in the year 1600, to Padua, and not in 1598": BARLOW, SIR THOMAS, *Harvey the man and the physician. Harveian Oration*, 1916 reprinted in *Brit. M.J.*, 1957, I, 1264–1271 (p. 1265). There are no entries in the Paduan archives mentioning Harvey before 1600. His scholarship at Caius College, Cambridge, lapsed at Christmas, 1599. From 1596 to 1599 the Exit Book shows repeated absences of Harvey on sick leave. – Harvey "finally left Cambridge on October 30th 1599, intending to return in January 1600, but the first part of that year found him instead at Padua where he ... finally on April 25, 1602, graduated as Doctor of Medicine of the University of Padua." Franklin, 1961, loc. cit. in note 6, p. 87. – See also: PAZZINI, A., *William Harvey, disciple of Girolamo Fabrici d'Aquapendente and the Paduan School. J. Hist. Med.* 1957, XII, 197–201.

14 See below p. 209.

15 LEIBOWITZ, J.O., *Early accounts of the valves of the veins. J. Hist. Med.* 1957, XII, 189, with special reference to Canano, Amatus Lusitanus and Sal. Albert (Alberti).

15a See to this: LESKY, E., *Harvey und Aristoteles. Arch. f. Gesch. d. Med.*, 1957, XLI, p. 370, and in particular: SCHMID, M., *Der Weg zu Harvey. Sitzber. d. Physikal.-Medizin. Sozietät Erlangen*, 1958, LXXIX, 66–101 (p. 92–94).

ployed the balance and quantitative methods systematically for the solution of chemical and biological problems—being palpably influenced, not so much by Galileo, but by the older Nicolaus Cusanus (1401–1464)[16].

The quantitative methods of Santorio (1561–1636) who taught at Padua in Galileo's time, his interest in physical apparatus, notably the thermometer and hygrometer, suggest a much closer proximity to Galileo than the observational methods and quantification of Harvey. Though retaining much that is Aristotelian[17], Galileo was by and large against Aristotle whose basic tenets he refuted in physics, astronomy and cosmology. Harvey was a staunch though not uncritical, Aristotelian, and there are hints that he even still subscribed to the geocentric view of the universe[18]. Nor should we forget that Harvey had little patience with astronomy which, he said, has to resort to reason in order to work out facts which cannot be subjected to direct ocular observation, but must be inferred from those mere appearances and phenomena which occur. It is thus that astronomy arrived at the construction of cosmological systems which are to explain all phenomena[19]. It is well known how Galileo's brilliant lectures attracted crowds of students from many countries and we have no proof that Harvey was not among them—this is as far as we can go, but it means very little.

The supposed Influence of Bacon

We are in similar difficulties concerning Harvey's relationship with Sir Francis Bacon (1561–1626), but then, the documentary evidence we have in assessing it is much stronger.

Much has been made of such generalities as Bacon's recommendation of the "subtlety of experiments which is far greater than that of the sense itself", of the examination and dissection of nature and of going to the facts themselves, the progress that is achieved by the study of particulars in preference to syllogism and the "mischievous authority of systems which are founded either on common notions or on a few experiments or on superstition"[20].

In Bacon's case all this is coupled with a strong antagonism to Aristotle and anything Aristotelian and for this reason alone could not have appealed to Harvey. In the light of this the famous passage from Aubrey seems to bear the mark of veracity. He had been "physitian to the Lord Ch. Bacon, whom he esteemed much for his witt and style, but would not allow him to be a great philosopher. Said he to me: He writes philosophy like a Ld. Chancellor, speaking in derision.[21]"

16 PAGEL, W., *Paracelsus* 1958, loc. cit. in note 4, p. 199; 281 and idem, *Das medizinische Weltbild des Paracelsus. Seine Zusammenhänge mit Neuplatonismus und Gnosis.* Wiesbaden 1962, p. 20; in particular see idem, *The position of Harvey and Van Helmont in the History of European Thought. To commemorate H.E. Sigerist's essay on Harvey (1928)* J. Hist. Med. 1958, XIII, 186–199 (p. 193 et seq.).

In Van Helmont's case a certain influence of Galileo may be found in the former's interest in a combined thermo-barometer and his proposal to use the pendulum for time measuring: PAGEL, W. *Van Helmont De Tempore and Biological Time, Osiris,* 1949, VIII, 346–417 (p. 399).

We return to the influence of Nicolaus Cusanus on Van Helmont below, p. 79.

17 RANDALL, loc. cit. 1940 in note 10, p. 199, says that the combination of resolutive and compositive methods and such as were practised by the Aristotelian Zabarella at Padua "were precisely the procedure and the terms of Galileo".

18 The movement of the sun, its accession and recession, and its influence on generation and vegetation is emphasised by Harvey on Aristotelian lines at several places: *On generation,* Exerc. XIV, tr. WILLIS p. 226; L, p. 364; 367; 370—to quote some examples.

19 *Exercit. anatomica ad Joh. Riolanum* II, ed. Roterod. 1649, p. 90–91; tr. WILLIS p. 124. – KEELE, loc. cit. 1957, in note 6, p. 267 says: "In spite of the fact that his demonstration of the circulation of the blood was a mechanical interpretation of events, Harvey persistently ignored Galileo, both the works and the man, even though they were both in Padua, and later Florence, at the same time."

To judge the deep gap by which Harvey is separated from Bacon we should remember the latter's unrestricted banishment of the "final causes" from the domain of natural philosophy—the very frame of thought which, on Harvey's own showing, directly led him to his discovery[22].

When this was published, in 1628, Bacon had been dead for two years. We are ignorant about the actual date when it was conceived, but, as Harvey tells us himself, it had taken shape in his mind and been discussed by him some long time before its publication, and so Bacon may conceivably have known about it. There is one passage in his late work on the *History of Life and Death*, published in 1623, which at first sight appears to be promising in this respect. It occurs in an aphoristic discussion of rapid death following copious loss of blood, experienced sometimes in haemorrhoids, haematemesis, unlocking or rupture of internal veins and from wounds. The aphorism winds up with the reason for the fatal issue of such venous haemorrhages: "for the blood of the veins waits upon the blood of the arteries, the latter upon the spirit" (*cum Sanguis Venarum, Sanguini Arteriarum ministret; Sanguis Arteriarum, Spiritui*)[23]. Taken by itself, this would certainly be a remarkable statement, if it could be interpreted to mean that *venous blood in its entirety* serves the preparation of arterial blood rather than the supply of aliment for the organs. However, it may not have meant any more than the destination of *some of* the venous blood which, since Aristotle and Galen, had been known to be sent from the liver to the heart to serve there for the preparation of the spirit as contained in the arterial blood. What Bacon seems to convey is that the fatal outcome of the copious loss of venous blood is due to a deficiency of the material necessary for the building up of spirit, rather than the loss of nutriment for the peripheral organs—an explanation that is perfectly compatible with and indeed based on the traditional pre-Harveian ideas.

Nor can more be learned from another passage, although here even the term *circuit* is used of the blood. No doubt, Bacon says, blood is cooled and tempered by such "cold" herbs as endives, chicory, liver-wort and purslain, and so is eventually also the spirit. This, however, is by circuit, whereas vapours act immediately, namely on the spirit (*sed hoc fit per Circuitum; At Vapores operantur immediate*)[24]. Obviously what is meant is that substances introduced from outside must take a roundabout way (*circuitus*) through the veins to reach the spirit in the arterial blood, whereas vapours inhaled do so directly and without the "circuit" through the veins. The circuit is not that of the blood, but that of nutriment passing

20 Hale-White, Sir William, *Gilbert, Bacon and Harvey.* Harveian Oration Oct. 18th 1927; Lancet 1927, II, 847 as against Sir Samuel Wilks, quoted from Barlow, 1916, loc. cit. in note 13 who said that Harvey had not read Bacon's works, and owed nothing to Bacon. This Barlow thinks is not correct, as Harvey once quoted a Baconian phrase (see below). Barlow, however, judiciously concludes: "Harvey looked upon him as an academic *litterateur* who had had no claims to eminence in practical investigation, and it may well be that Bacon's deep-rooted antagonism to Aristotle, which dated from the time when he was a student at the university, may have roused Harvey's distrust" (p. 1270).

21 Aubrey, loc. cit. 1813 in note 7 vol. II, p. 381.

22 See on Harvey and Aristotle, below, p. 28 and elsewhere in this book p. 209.

23 Bacon, *Historia vitae et mortis. Atriola mortis ad artic. 15 connexio.* Historia paragr. 25. Francisci Baconi de Verulamio, *Scripta in naturali et universali philosophia.* Amstelod. 1685, p. 170. See below p. 219.

24 Bacon, *Histor. vitae et mortis*, loc. cit. in note 23, *Operatio super spiritus.* Historia paragr. 59, ed. cit. 1685, p. 105.

from the digestive tract into the portal and inferior cava veins towards the heart and arteries.

Indeed, Bacon adhered to the old doctrine. It emerges in his general statement that all aliment moves from the centre to the periphery, from inside to the outer parts, although trees and plants are nourished through the bark and the external parts rather than the medulla and what is inside, and the blood in the veins of animals nourishes the flesh that lies below them no less than that which lies above (*atque Sanguis in Venis animalium, non minus Carnes sub illis sitas nutrit, quam supra illas*)[25]. It follows from this that Bacon still assumed the direct nutritional flow of venous blood to the parts. The motion of the heart and the pulse according to Bacon is one of trembling (*motus trepidationis*), the expression of a twinheaded condition (*status anceps*) resulting from the liberating movement of the dilating spirits and their subsequent reception[26].

Harvey, then, would have had little to learn from Bacon in his own fields of enquiry and indeed he preferred to learn from Aristotle especially in Bacon's main field of interest which was scientific method[27]. Yet Harvey appreciated the Lord Chancellor's "witt and style" and so he adopts at one place the Baconian terms of the "idols" of the speculating mind which must be avoided[28]. At another place he again uses a Baconian term in opening a new discussion. Here he says: it is advisable to review the fruit of our industry and, to use the words of the most learned Verulam, to embark on a second gathering of grapes[29].

Indeed there is little that is Baconian and much that is Aristotelian in Harvey's background, in his leanings and in his choice of subjects and method.

Harvey as an Exponent of his Age

We have mentioned the absence of any insularity in the life and work of Harvey. His lively interest in the customs and natural history of foreign parts is well documented in the reports of fellow travellers on the continent—we shall refer to this elsewhere in the present book[30]. His profound knowledge of contemporary international medical literature and above all of Aristotle and Galen is a prominent feature of his works and particularly noticeable in his—early—lecture notes on anatomy (1616 et seq.)[31]. Indeed Harvey did not live and work in a vacuum, however much he followed his own bent and built up his own world—a world in which it seems futile to look for predecessors and successors, for influences and inspirations.

25 Ibidem, *Alimentatio et via alimentandi*, Hist. ad artic. 4, paragr. 5, p. 48–49.

26 *Novum Organon*, lib. II, cap. 48, paragr. 18 i.f., ed. Th. Fowler, Oxford 1878, p. 552 and Fowler's note 55 with ref. to Bacon, *Hist. densi et rari* containing a similar "vague and fanciful passage".

Here it says: "pulsus cordis et arteriarum in animalibus fit per irrequietam dilatationem spirituum, et receptum ipsorum, per vices". Opp. ed. Ellis and Spedding, vol. II, p. 263; 1857. – Bacon also speaks of the trepidation of the heart in the dying, causing systole and diastole to become confluent: *Hist. vitae et mortis* loc. cit., *atriola mortis* ad artic. 15, paragr. 29, p. 172.

27 See to this Payne, Jos. Fr., *Harvey and Galen. Harveian Oration*, London 1897, p. 13: "Harvey, inspite of Copernicus and Galileo, was still living under an Aristotelian heaven and remained till the close of his life a staunch Peripatetic. This, I suspect, was the main reason for his want of sympathy with Bacon, which has often been remarked. For it was Bacon's avowed aim to destroy the supremacy of Aristotle; and nothing could have been more repugnant to Harvey than this."

28 *Falsa idola* – Harvey, *On generation*, Praef., ed Amstelod. 1662, fol. XI. Tr. Willis, p. 162 (*"false fancies"*).

29 "ut doctissimi Verulamii nostri verbis utar – vindemiatio secunda instituenda est" *On generation*, Exerc. XXV, Amstelod. 1662, p. 95; Tr. Willis, p. 270.

30 Good short accounts of Harvey's continental journeys are found in Barlow, 1916, loc. cit. in note [13] and Guthrie, D., *Harvey in space and time. Brit. Med. J.* 1957, I, 575–579. – In the traditional reports on these journeys no mention is made of Harvey's visit to Prague and his meeting there with Joh. Marcus Marci of Kronland, the "Hippocrates of Prague". See Pagel, W. and Rattansi, P., *Harvey meets the Hippocrates of Prague. Med. Hist.* 1964, VIII, p. 78–84. See our discussion of this journey below, p. 286.

31 See for example: Kilgour, F. G., *Harvey's use of Galen's findings in his discovery of the circulation of the blood. J. Hist. Med.* 1957, XII, 232–240; Whitteridge, G., *The anatomical lectures of William Harvey.* Edinburgh and London 1964, p. XXX and in particular the *Index*, pp. 495–504.

And yet the question of the intellectual climate, of what was shared in common by the giants of the Harveian period is difficult to evade. Francis Bacon (1561–1626), Santorio Santoro (1561–1636), Galileo (1564–1642), Tomaso Campanella (1568–1639) and Johannes Kepler (1571–1630) belonged to a generation that was slightly older than Harvey, Robert Fludd (1574–1637), Jacob Boehme (1575–1624), Peter Paul Rubens (1577–1640), J.B. Van Helmont (1579–1644) and Herbert of Cherbury (1581–1648) were close contemporaries, while Marin Mersenne (1583–1647), Thomas Hobbes (1588–1679), Pierre Gassendi (1592–1655), Jaques Callot (1593–1635), René Descartes (1596–1650), John Laurence Bernini (1598–1680) and Joseph Glanvill (1636–1680) were slightly younger.

To the casual observer it is very simple: all these men, and many more whom we have not named, have one thing in common, the breaking down of "idols"—not only of the bonds by means of which the reasoning of the mediaeval and scholastic mind had enslaved or bypassed the facts, but also of the way in which the thinkers and artists of the Renaissance had built up their own worlds. We are now in the epoch of *Baroque* which emerged with the Counter-Reformation and brought a new orientation in the fine arts. The artist of the *Baroque* period dissolved the straight lines and planes—the "closed forms" of the Renaissance—in favour of movement, chiaroscuro and depth. The *Baroque* master is no longer interested in "Being". He studies "Coming into Being"; in other words he is not concerned with the limitations of objects, but with their infinite possibilities in movement and function. *Renaissance* and *Baroque* thus represent two different ways of looking at nature; they embody two different views of the world. Harvey has been visualised as the true exponent of this new *Baroque* spirit in biology and medicine, for his anatomy is *Anatomia Animata*[32]. Dissatisfied with the mere description of the heart, he integrated it with the functional laws which are obeyed by the pulse and respiration. The same dynamic outlook emerged in his second great work, that on generation. Harvey remains a "dynamist" in all aspects of his creative work, and thus a true master of the *Baroque* period.

It was the employment of computation and the decisive role which it played in Harvey's demonstration of the closed circle described by the whole blood that was to prove the point. Indeed Harvey's quantification was taken as the line which divides him from his predecessors[33]. It was not the break-away from ancient doctrines, as before him all those concerned with the true ways

32 Sigerist, H.E., *William Harvey's Stellung in der Europäischen Geistesgeschichte. Rede gehalten an der Gründungsfeier der Universität Leipzig. Arch.f.Kulturgesch.* 1929, XIX, 158–168. See the discussion of this paper in Pagel, W., *The position of Harvey and Van Helmont in the History of European thought. To commemorate H.E.Sigerist's Essay on Harvey* (1928). *J.Hist.Med.* 1958, XIII 186–199.

33 On this point see below in the present work p. 73.

followed by the blood through the right heart and lungs had implicitly declared war upon the ancient teaching. Nor was experimentalism the decisive step: Harvey's predecessors, Galen, Vesalius and notably Realdus Columbus had performed experiments. Nor was it finally the employment of reasoning on the basis of anatomical and observational data: Caesalpinus, following this way, had formulated and substantiated the "perpetual motion of blood from the veins into the heart and from the heart into the arteries". Yet Caesalpinus remained far short of the true answer and seems to have wavered between truth and error—we refer to a detailed discussion elsewhere in the present book (p. 169 seq.).

Quantification and the discovery which was "demonstrated" through it are not the only modern and scientific features in Harvey's work. We shall return to this when discussing Harvey as a modern in detail (p. 80). Here it may suffice to recall that modern scientific biology and medicine owe indeed their existence and development to the new analytical views introduced by Harvey[33a]. All this seems to fit in well with the idea that it was the age of Harvey in which modern science was born through the work of minds that were thinking along modern lines pure and simple.

However, viewed against his strong Aristotelian background Harvey was not a modern. Aristotelianism meant much more to him than a mere scholarly garb in which he enters the literary stage and in which he appears as an Aristotelian "at first sight"[34]. In fact Harvey was steeped in Aristotle[35].

Nor did Harvey set out to found a new—our modern—biology and medicine, nor even was he solely intent at arriving at a great discovery that was to supersede ancient natural philosophy and medicine and to reform a backward age.

What does appear to be first and foremost in his mind is the problem of *purpose*, namely that of circulation. Indeed, Harvey was the "life-long" thinker on the purpose of circulation[36]. This was the *Leitmotiv* of his investigation and a truly Aristotelian stimulus to natural philosophy at that—a motive that explains much in his life and work.

In Aristotelian philosophy, circular movement occupied a position of high dignity and responsibility. It was the purpose of circular processes to preserve and to regenerate. Thus the cosmos was "held together" by the circular movement of the celestial bodies. The same principle applied in Harvey's opinion to the circular movement of the blood, namely the preservation of the body—the microcosm—through a continual—circular—regenerative movement of the blood. Harvey found the same principle

33a Dale, Sir Henry, *The Harveian Oration on some epochs in medical research.* London 1935, p. 6: Harvey's greatest achievement, not that he made a discovery of such profound and permanent significance, but that he created and displayed for all time the method by which such discovery may be attained and made secure. – Sir Henry Cohen, *Harvey and the scientific method. Brit. M.J.* 1950, II, 1406: Harvey's mind as revealed in his writings "explains why we place Harvey amongst the greatest physicians of all times, not because he *discovered* that the blood circulates but because he *demonstrated* beyond all reasonable doubt that the blood circulates".

34 Sigerist, loc. cit. 1929 in note [32].

35 Pagel, W., *William Harvey and the purpose of circulation. Isis* 1951, XLII, 22–38; idem, *The philosophy of circles—Cesalpino—Harvey. J. Hist. Med.* 1957, XII, 140–157; idem, 1958, loc. cit. note [32]. See also: idem, *The reaction to Aristotle in seventeenth-century biological thought. Campanella—Van Helmont—Glanvill—Charleton—Harvey—Glisson—Descartes. Science, Medicine and History.* Oxford 1953, vol. I, 489–509 (498 seq.); idem, *William Harvey: some neglected aspects of medical history. J. Warburg and Courtauld Inst.* 1944, VII, 144–153. – For a penetrating analysis of Harvey's relationship to Aristotle: Needham, J., *History of Embryology*, Cambridge 1934, p. 19–41 and 112–133, and Lesky, Erna, *Harvey and Aristoteles. Arch. f. Gesch. d. Med.* 1957, XLI, 289–316 and 349–378. – We shall devote a special subchapter to the subject below in the present book; pp. 28 seq.

36 Curtis, J. G., *Harvey's view on the use o the circulation of the blood.* New York 1915 p. 152.

37 See above, p. 21 and below, p. 41.

operative in generation—the ever repeated conversion of a shapeless particle of albumen into an organised body and back again to a shapeless particle, the semen—a cyclic process that serves the regeneration and preservation of the species. With all this we move into the field of "final causes" that are essential in Aristotelianism as well as in the world of Harvey's ideas. As we have seen, it had been such "final causes" that had kindled the spark of discovery in Harvey's mind—the very final causes that had been rejected by Bacon[37].

Yet Harvey's attitude was critical—even towards Aristotle. He made frontal attacks on not a few of the Philosopher's doctrines[38]. It is in this critical attitude towards Aristotle also that Harvey perceptibly advances on his predecessors, notably Caesalpinus. The latter's work is devoted to the defence of the Peripatetic doctrine against Galen and in this naturalistic observation and judicious reasoning are employed as an aid to argument and exegesis.[39] By contrast, Harvey's treatises are predominantly observational, and the support which his findings lend to Aristotelian doctrine is an additional feature, however much satisfaction this provided to the author.

None of this, however, detracts from Harvey's genuine and basic Aristotelianism which is all the more remarkable, as it was actually Galen—whose knowledge of the blood flow by far exceeded that of Aristotle—who really provided the basis for discussion.

Temkin has rightly warned us against purging Harvey of Aristotelian categories to make him appear a modern laboratory man pure and simple"[40]. To-day we easily separate Harvey's scientific discovery from his Aristotelian leanings and speculation. Seen in historical perspective, however, they are inseparable.

What, then, is Harvey's position as an exponent of the *Baroque* era? Here we must first admit the difficulties inherent in any attempt to define this period with reasonable distinctness[41]. It is accepted as coinciding with the Counter-Reformation, from the middle of the sixteenth century onwards. Michelangelo (1474–1563) is often regarded as the master who bridged the eras of Renaissance and Baroque, but is usually claimed to represent the latter rather than the Renaissance. He was active in 1543 when anatomy, as typical product of the Renaissance spirit, reached its climax with the first appearance of Vesalius' *De fabrica*. Michelangelo himself was a dedicated student of human anatomy and was to have illustrated the great anatomical work of Realdus Columbus—which, however, only appeared after the early death

38 See below, p. 42 seq.

39 For a detailed discussion of Caesalpinus' *Quaestiones Peripateticae* (1571) see below p. 169 seq.

40 Temkin, O., *An essay on the usefulness of medical history for medicine. Bullet. Hist. Med.* 1946, XIX, 9–47 (p. 26); idem, *Metaphors of human biology.* In: Stauffer, R. C., *Science and civilisation.* Madison 1949, pp. 167–194 (p. 189 et seq.).

41 The same applies to the Renaissance and for that matter to any cultural age and climate. See the masterly treatment of the subject in Wightman, W. P. D., *Science and the Renaissance. An introduction to the study of the emergence of the sciences in the sixteenth century.* Edinburgh and London 1962, vol. I, p. 1–44 (The Renaissance Problem and Individual and Cosmos). See also idem: *Science and the Renaissance. Hist. Sci.* 1964, III, 1–19.

of the latter, unillustrated. It is true that the Renaissance and notably the sixteenth century meant no more to medicine than a rebirth of ancient classical medicine. Renaissance anatomy was new; not, however, through the introduction of new procedures, but through the true "natural" representation of its substance—again perhaps no more than the fulfilment of ancient aspirations. Indeed the trend towards restitution of a *prisca anatomia* rather than destruction and revolution was expressed by Vesalius—himself a keen humanist[42]. And yet there is more than ancient, static anatomy in Vesalius: looking at his illustrations we soon notice the movement, the dynamic element in many of them. Vesalius himself and to a much greater extent his pupil and successor Columbus performed planned experiments in animals. Moreover, the "modern", "dynamic" methods of measuring and weighing were first recommended in biology and medicine by Nicolaus Cusanus (1401–1464) who died just a century before the end of the Council of Trent (1545–1563) which is usually regarded as the great landmark of Counter-Reformation. If anybody, Nicolaus Cusanus was the typical exponent of Platonism and humanism in the early Renaissance of the fifteenth century.

Only in a very broad sense, then, can the term *Baroque* be made meaningful in medical history and be accepted as a background to Harvey. We are inviting further difficulties when we use it to indicate the departure towards modern science pure and simple—a science that is aloof from all non-scientific speculation, notably philosophical, cosmological and religious.

We have mentioned the speculative—Aristotelian—element that is so closely bound up with the scientific revolution inherent in Harvey's work and we shall have to say more about this anon and indeed throughout the present work.

Seen in this light what was fostered by the *Baroque* spirit was not a simple transition to mechanical science, but a strange coexistence of scientific and non-scientific elements, an attitude in which the latter in no way impeded, but rather supported the enquiring mind.

Perhaps it is this interplay of what the modern regards as opposites that reflects the *Baroque* spirit more faithfully than its identification with modern science pure and simple. The perspective of infinity achieved by the *Baroque* artist through the breaking up of straight lines, the interplay of light and shadow and the representation of depth may indeed find its counterpart in the strange chiaroscuro of speculation and science displayed in the works of natural philosophers in the first half of the seventeenth century.

42 PAGEL, W. and RATTANSI, P., *Vesalius and Paracelsus. Medical Hist.* 1964, VIII, 309–328; p. 323.

43 PAGEL, W., *J. Hist. Med.* loc. cit. 1958, in note [32], p. 192–198.

This is well illustrated by the example of John Baptist Van Helmont (1579–1644), a close contemporary of Harvey. In his case, not Aristotelian, but Neoplatonic and religious-mystical speculation was intimately interwoven with advanced observational and experimental work in science and, most significantly, with determined quantification[43]. The blending of scientific and non-scientific motives, of discovery and speculation, that inspired the early seventeenth century savant is recognisable in all provinces of Van Helmont's work: his proof of the indestructibility of matter by use of the balance, his discovery of gas as the material, but volatile, i.e. "spiritualised", carrier of specificity in every individual object, his discovery of acid gastric digestion which comes very close to the identification of its effective principle with hydrochloric acid, his theory of fermentation and his replacement of such general notions as "occult virtue" by the action of chemically defined substances[44].

Harvey's position in the history of European thought is determined, then, by the peculiar spirit of his age, the age of scientific revolution that is essentially bound up with non-scientific speculation, of the co-existence of to us contradictory tendencies and of a dynamism that seems to burst through the limitations set to the human mind by ancient and Renaissance thought.

Harvey and Aristotle

Harvey's adherence to Aristotle is deeply rooted in his personality: it was avowed by himself in many places and it was sincere though by no means uncritical. It not only concerns comparative anatomy and physiology, but extends into philosophy and epistemology—the question of what can be achieved by the naturalist and by what means. In these fields it would seem as if Harvey made a deliberate attempt at restoring the *old*, i.e. Aristotelian *Organon* in preference to the so-called *new* order imposed by the "Lord Chancellor".

In points of detail we shall discuss the Aristotelian leanings of Harvey and his criticism of the "Philosopher" throughout the present work. It is expedient, however, to review this field now in more general and introductory terms.

Harvey's praise of Aristotle

Already in his early *Lecture notes on Anatomy* which date back to 1616 or earlier, Harvey had called Aristotle "so faithful and diligent an author". In this connexion he was even prepared to allow for a possible change in the anatomy of animals which might have taken place with the passing of time and thus explain Aristotle's

44 Pagel, W., *The religious and philosophical aspects of Van Helmont's Science and medicine.* Baltimore 1944 (on *Gas*, p. 16–26); idem, *J.B. Van Helmont's reformation of the Galenic doctrine of digestion—and Paracelsus. Bullet. Hist. Med.* 1955, XXIX, 563–568; idem, *Van Helmont's ideas on gastric digestion and the gastric acid. Bullet. Hist. Med.* 1956, XXX 524–536; idem, *Paracelsus* 1958, loc. cit. in note [4], p. 95 (gas) and 158 et seq. (gastric digestion).; idem, *Das medizin. Weltbild d. Paracelsus.* 1962, loc. cit. in note [16], p. 49 et seq. (gas); 12, 13, 31, 76, 96 (gastric digestion); idem, *The Wild Spirit (Gas) of Van Helmont and Paracelsus*, *Ambix*, 1962, X, 1–13. – See also in the present work p. 79 and below, p. 266.

description of three—instead of two—ventricles of the heart[45]. In his latest work, that *On generation*, Harvey still confesses: "the authority of Aristotle has always such weight with me that I never think of differing from him inconsiderately.[46]"

This is all the more remarkable as Harvey is fully conscious of the novelty of his own findings and ideas—as he expressed it not only in the famous eighth chapter of *De motu*, but also in his late work *On generation*. In the former he said: "what remains to be said upon the quantity and source of the blood that thus passes (sc. from the veins into the arteries), is of so novel and unheard-of character, that I not only fear injury to myself from the envy of certain individuals, but I fear that I have mankind at large for my enemies: so much does custom and doctrine once imbibed and fixed down by deep roots like a second nature weigh with all, and so much force is exerted by the cult of antiquity. However, the die is cast; my hope lies in the love of truth and the candour of learned minds....[47]" In the same vein Harvey—nearly a quarter of a century later—introduces *On generation:* What I have observed from anatomical dissection ... may be presented for the benefit and use of those who are after the truth—for I found the whole subject to be much different from anything that has been transmitted by philosophers as well as physicians; and later, with reference to traditional opinions: that these are false and carelessly expounded will emerge with ease. Indeed they will vanish like the phantoms of darkness in the light of anatomy[48].

Harvey on scientific method

Harvey makes it quite clear that it is not only the results—the "perspicuous truth"—that are novel, but that "I may propose to the studious a new, and, unless I mistake, a safer way to the attainment of knowledge."

Harvey, then, concerns himself with questions of method. At first sight, the new method which he comes to recommend and to practise looks very simple: it is the examination of objects themselves, as against the acceptance of what others have said in comment on a given subject—the latter being unsafe and ignominious (*intutum, imo vero turpe*), whilst "the *Book of Nature* lies so open and is so easy of consultation (*cum tamen apertus facilisque Naturae liber sit*).[49]"

Harvey's appeal for Empiricism

The mere appeal to Nature and her Book in itself is no new feature emerging only in Harvey's last work. He had given poignant expression to this in reply to those who blamed him for deviating

45 *Praelectiones anat. univers.*, London 1886, fol. 74 verso. See below, p. 227.

46 *On generation*, Exerc. XI, ed. Amsterd. 1662, p. 37; tr. WILLIS, p. 207.

47 *De motu*, cap. VIII, 1628, p. 41; tr. WILLIS, p. 45.

48 *On generat.*, Introduction (*Praefatio*), ed. 1662, fol. V recto: aliter enim multo, quam ab auctoribus, sive Philosophis, sive Medicis tradita est, rem omnem deprehendi; tr. WILLIS, p. 151.

49 *On generat.*, ed. 1662, fol. V verso; tr. WILLIS, p. 152.

from Galen: "The facts cognizable by the senses wait upon no opinions and the works of nature bow to no antiquity; for indeed there is nothing more ancient or of higher antiquity than nature." (*Naturae opera facta manifesta sensui, nullas opiniones, nullamque antiquitatem morari: natura enim nihil antiquius, majorisque auctoritatis*[50].) In favour of *sensus* and *autopsia* as the safest ways of demonstrating the truth Harvey draws a line against astronomy which is left to form indirect conclusions—and "systems" of cosmology which must explain everything—from mere appearances, as he who enquires into the cause of an eclipse must be placed beyond the moon if he would ascertain it by sense, and not by reason. By contrast the observer of things that come under the cognizance of the senses is in a better position: he can rely upon ocular inspection and demonstrate things as they really are[51].

The Significance of Reason

Harvey thus expressed the preference accorded to sensual perception and ocular demonstration in the second letter to Riolan which preceded *On generation*, in print, by no more than two years. At this time Harvey had written much, if not most or all of the latter work and thus must have devoted much thought to scientific method.

Significantly not far from the passage just quoted from the *Second Letter* Harvey goes farther than the mere recommendation of ocular observation. The perception thus gained must be confirmed by reasoning, if we are to arrive at scientific knowledge. Not false reasoning that is utterly opposed to the witness of the senses, not wordy assertions or captious objections (*captiunculis vacuis*), but reasoning that is consistent with the "most certain faith through sense" (*certissima per sensum fides*). This is well shown in geometry where progress is made from things sensible to the rational demonstration of things that are not sensible (*ex sensibilibus de sensibilibus demonstratio rationalis, Geometrica est. Ad cujus exemplar, abstrusa et a sensu remota, ex apparentibus manifestioribus et notioribus, innotescunt*)[52].

Harvey concludes: it is our duty to approve or disapprove, to receive or reject everything only after the most careful examination (*ab examinatione minutim facta*). To examine and to test whether it has been rightly or wrongly brought forward we have to lead it down to the control of the senses and to confirm and stabilise it by the judgment of the senses, also to detect whether some fallacy may be hidden. No kind of science, then, can possibly flow save from some pre-existing knowledge of more obvious things[53].

50 *Exercit. duae* 1649, loc. cit. in notes [9] and [19], ed. Roterod. 1649, p. 87; tr. WILLIS, p. 123.

51 *Exercit. duae* Roterod. 1649, p. 88 ("neque satis factum opinantur [sicut in astronomia] nova systemata ordinare, nisi omnia phenomena solvant"); p. 88–91 tr. WILLIS p. 123–124.

52 *Exercit. duae* Roterod. 1649, p. 110; tr. WILLIS p. 131.

53 *Exercit. duae* ibid. as quoted in note [52].

Harvey thus qualifies the emphasis laid on sensual perception and ocular demonstration: these cannot advance to the realm of science unless they are corroborated by reasoning (*ratiocinatio*). For this Aristotle is invoked as a witness, but in an aside rather than a proper discussion of his theory of knowledge.

Such is found, however, in the long introductory excursus which opens his book *On generation: Of the Manner and order of acquiring Knowledge; of the same Matters according to Aristotle and of the Method to be pursued in studying Generation.*

In the preceding preface Harvey issues a warning against those all too numerous contemporaries who instead of toiling in the field of Nature prefer "going wrong with the many, to becoming wise on their own at the expense of labour and money" (*mallent cum turba errare quam cum laboris aerisque impendio privatim sapere*). It was different in antiquity: then the natural philosophers went the opposite way and, by their indefatigable labours and by their varied experimental inquiries into the nature of things, bore an unfailing torch for our studies. Yet we should extinguish this very light, were we to acquiesce in the discoveries of the ancients and the belief that nothing further can be discovered.

Harvey thus turns the attention of his readers to a *prisca scientia*, to true scientific knowledge as pursued by the ancients and by virtue of the correct methods of experimental probing[54]—in itself a call to continue on this way instead of the customary study of books and the interpretation of traditional texts.

Between this "modern" sounding advice and admonition and the substance of the work, however, Harvey intercalated an epistemological excursus, a free confession to his deeply ingrained leanings towards Aristotle and his theory of knowledge. As Plochmann says: "Harvey's preface to his own treatise on animal generation is virtually a paraphrase of sections of the *Posterior Analytics* and the *Physics* of Aristotle.[55]" If we are to examine Harvey's relationship to Aristotle we cannot avoid analysing these introductory excursuses—however little relation they may bear at first sight to Harvey's discoveries and detailed observations.

Before doing so, however, the main tenets of Aristotle's epistemology as referred to by Harvey should be briefly reviewed.

Aristotle on the Theory of Knowledge

There are things that lie immediately before us, the empirical objects that are grasped by sensual perception (*aisthesis*). They are composite objects, not the simple elements or principles, but

54 See above on Vesalius and Paracelsus in the paper by Pagel and Rattansi as quoted in note [42].

55 PLOCHMANN, G. K., *William Harvey and his methods. Stud. in the Renaissance.* 1963, X, 192–210 (p. 197). – IZQUIERDO, J. J., *Lugar de Harvey en la Historia del metodo cientifico de la Biologia*, Mexico 1944. – On the lead of Fabricius in recognising the biological significance of Aristotelian method: ADELMAN, H.B., *The embryological treatises of Hieron. Fabricius ab Aquapendente*, Ithaca 1942, p. 76 seq.

products of a flowing together of simpler things and finally of the elements (*stoicheia*) and principles (*archai*). They are what is "poured together"—*ta synkechoumena*—and as such the first things of the outside world that are accessible to us; they are "*prior for us*" (*proteron pros hemas*)[56]. They become known to us by *induction* (*epagoge*) which proceeds from the particular, i.e. facts of personal experience, towards the elements, causes and principles—the universals (*ta katholou*). The latter, being the basic constituents of things, are therefore "*prior in Nature*" (*protera physei*), though only a product of "later" reasoning "for us". As such they become known to us by *syllogism*. This represents things as they are in themselves and visualised by the creative mind—and thus proceeds from the universal to the particular, from the abstract to the concrete.

Induction and syllogism, then, correspond to the two great aspects of existence or ways in which things are known[57]. They are "in a way opposed to each other"[58], but really follow and depend upon each other. Induction being of necessity based on sensual perception[59], forms the indispensable first stage, the foundation of knowledge. Indeed there is no direct access for the human mind to the elements and principles, to those that are "prior in the order of nature". Without induction there is no knowledge of universals. It is impossible to come to grasp universals except through induction[60]. Particulars are therefore prior and better known to man[61]. On the other hand, knowledge properly "lies in explaining things by reference to what is absolutely prior, and in seeing that their causes lead necessarily to particular effects". This is also the essence of scientific knowledge (*episteme*), as different from mere opinion (*doxa*); the former appertains to insight into things as universal and in relation to their causes—a knowledge that is productive of absolutely necessary and certain results—whereas the latter relates to particular and unexplained facts[62]. Sense perception, then, is not enough, as it deals with "particular impressions which are now and here", and yet what is perceived has qualities and the perception of these implies gauging by universals[63].

Hence scientific knowledge is arrived at by stages, namely: (a) sense perception, (b) memory, (c) experience or the formation of general conceptions in the mind, (d) science and (e) art[64].

Aristotle made it quite clear that sense, as such, does not give us knowledge[65]. And yet it is from induction through sensual perception that our reasoning intellect (*nous*) forms its earliest conceptions. There are no preformed ideas, there is nothing innate in it. To Aristotle there is "no innate knowledge, and the unfolding

56 ARISTOTLE, *Analyt. Post.* I, 2, 71b 33. – *Physics* I, 1, 184a 16–21; ed. Prantl Leipzig 1854, p. 9 and notes p. 470.

57 WALLACE, E., *Outlines of the philosophy of Aristotle*. 3rd ed. Cambridge 1883, p. 46.

58 *Analyt. Pr.* II, 23, 68b 32.

59 *Post. Analyt.* I, 18; 81a 38 to 81b 1–9: "he d'epagoge ek ton kata meros"; "ton gar kath hekaston aisthesis"; "epachthenai de me echontas aisthesin adynaton".

60 *Post. Analyt.* I, 18; 81a 38 to 81b 1–9: "adynaton de ta katholou theoresai me di' epagoges".

See to this: PRANTL, C., *Geschichte der Logik im Abendlande*. Vol. I, Leipzig 1855, p. 109: "Ja es ist überhaupt schlechterdings unmöglich, ohne Wahrnehmung zum Wissen zu gelangen, und das kath'holou kann ohne Induktion gar nicht erreicht werden, die Induktion aber fußt auf der Wahrnehmung. Der Nous in unserer Seele kann wegen seiner Verflechtung mit den Sinnen gerade dasjenige nicht sogleich oder schon zu Anfang seiner Tätigkeit erblicken, was in den inneren Wesen der objektiven Natur das Hellste und Glänzendste ist, er ist vergleichbar den Augen der nächtlichen Tiere, welche nicht in das Tageslicht blicken können (Metaph. A, 1; 993b9). Für den Menschen ist eben das Sinnfällige und das Einzelwesen das kenntlichere, insofern die Kenntnis desselben früher eintritt."

61 *Anal. Post.* I, 2; 71b33: "objects nearer to sense are prior and better known to man ... the most universal causes are furthest from sense and particular causes are nearest to sense, and they are thus exactly opposed to one another" (pros hemas men protera kai gnorimotera ta engyteron tes aistheseos ... esti de porrotato men ta katholou malista, engytato de ta kath'hekasta). Tr. G.R.G. MURE. Oxford 1928 (ed. W.D. Ross).

62 *Analyt. Post.* I, 33; 88b 30; Metaph. A, 1; 981a 29; *Analyt. Post.* I, 13; 79a 15. Wallace, 1883, loc. cit. in note [57], p. 49–51.

63 *Analyt. Post.* I, 31; 87b 19; II, 19, 100a 16; *Metaph.* A, 1; 981b 10.

64 *Metaph.* A 1; 980a 28; *Analyt. Post.* II, 19; 100b 10; *Ethica Nicom.* VI, 3, 3; 1139b 30. Wallace, 1883, loc. cit. in note [57], p. 57.

65 *Analyt. Post.* I, 31; 87b 28: "Oude di'aistheseos estin epistasthai".

of truth is not the progressive rediscovery of knowledge already contained in the mind by a process of recollection"[66], as Plato had visualised it with reference to the process of learning[67]. Accordingly Aristotle warns against the danger by which the complete and correct knowledge of particulars is threatened through a onesided upholding of the notion of universals[68]. With this Aristotle opposes the Platonic view and seems to justify the Thomistic summary of his epistemology: *nihil est in intellectu, quod non antea fuerit in sensu*[69].

On the other hand Aristotle's theory of knowledge is no mere empiricism or sensualism. In order to gain knowledge we must proceed from sense perception of the particular to the universal.

Induction, though beginning with sensual perception, does not end with the particular, but leads up to the universal. The latter is expressed in terms of classes and species which embrace individuals that are similar to one another and emerges from the consideration of what element they have in common. The same process is applied first to one, then "to another set of individuals which belong to one species and are generically, but not specifically, identical with the former set. When we have established what the common element is in all members of this second species, and likewise in members of further species, we should again consider whether the results established possess any identity, and persevere until we reach a single formula (*logos*), since this will be the definition of the thing.[70]"

All this calls for close cooperation and indeed for harmony between induction leading from the complex objects known to us first to the simple and elementary notions which are of a more extensive validity, on one hand, and knowledge proceeding from the universal to the particular, from abstract to concrete, on the other. The latter—the synthetic or compositive way—should thus correspond to the former—the analytic or resolutive one[71].

It would be wrong to place one-sided emphasis on the sensualist aspects of Aristotle's epistemology. In it, no doubt, all cognition is made to have its *beginning* in sense perception (*a sensibus exordium habet primum*), but this does not preclude its first *origin* in the mind (*a mente primam originem*), for no sense perception will lead to con ception without the universals that are in and from the mind[72]. In fact, the latter is the "implied content" of the former—we cannot recognise an individual man without the universal notion of man in general.

It is true to say, however, that Aristotle saved the right of the particular and accorded to the senses a position of responsibility

66 Plochmann, 1963, loc. cit. in note [55], p. 199.

67 Plochmann with ref. to Plato, Meno 80e.

68 *Analyt. Post.* I, 13; 79a 3: "... for the latter (sc. the mathematicians) are in possession of the demonstrations giving the causes, and are often ignorant of the fact: just as we have often a clear insight into a universal, but through lack of observation are ignorant of some of its particular instances" (hoi to katholou theorountes pollakis enia ton kath'hekaston ouk isasi di' anepiskepsian). To this: Prantl, 1855, loc. cit. in note [60], p. 110: "sowie hingegen anderseits vor der Gefahr gewarnt wird, welche durch einseitiges Festhalten einer aufgefaßten Allgemeinheit dem richtigen oder vollständigen Wissen des Einzelnen droht".

69 Wallace loc. cit. 1883, in note [57], p. 56.

70 *Post. Analyt.* lib. II, cap. 13; 97b; to this: Plochmann, 1963, loc. cit. in note [55], p. 199.

71 Plochmann, ibid. p. 200. – See above note [10] with reference to the School of Padua and Pietro d'Abano on the *Doctrina resolutiva* and *compositiva*.

72 Wallace, 1883, loc. cit. in note [57], p. 56.

which meant a decided break-away from Platonic idealism and the theory of innate though latent and unconscious knowledge. A similar situation prevails with regard to the existence and origin of individual objects. It is the latter that are the bearers of the ideas. These do not dwell in ethereal or celestial spheres that are inaccessible to us, as Plato thought, but are now visualised as immanent in the individual objects on which they confer form, function and final perfection. This is expressed in Aristotle's doctrine of the four principles or "causes" (*archai*, *aitiai*) which enter into "the existence or origination or cognition of any object"[73]. They are (a) the material cause, i.e. the material out of which an object is created, (b) the efficient cause or means by which it is created, (c) the formal cause which makes it what it is and (d) the final end of perfection for the achievement of which it exists. In this the emphasis lies on the latter: the final perfection of the object, its *entelecheia*, the unfolding of its immanent tendencies expressed in form, growth or function. In fact the formal and efficient causes are subject to the final cause—the "last" being the cause of "first".

73 WALLACE, ibidem, p. 71 et seq.

This teleological pattern of Aristotelian thinking shows its particular influence in biology where the question is of the type to which an individual conforms, of the class and species to which he belongs and of the purpose for which a part was formed by nature in an organic whole.

This selection of concepts from Aristotle's theory of knowledge, however brief and inadequate, may serve as a platform from which Harvey's ideas on method—the *Introduction* to his work *On generation*—may be coherently reviewed.

Harvey on the Manner and Order of acquiring Knowledge following from Aristotelian Principles

Harvey sets out with a meditation on a passage from the *Physics* of Aristotle which he confronts with one from the *Posterior Analytics*.

In the former it says that we must endeavour to know the first principles of nature and that the natural way is to proceed from things that are more obvious *to us* to those that are more obvious *by nature*. These are not the same, for to us the concrete or complex object is more obvious—the object that results from the mixture or composition of simple elements, but it is these latter that are "earlier" or more obvious "by nature". As, however, the universal is a whole and wholes are easier for us to perceive, one must proceed from the more general to the particular.

By contrast we are told in the *Posterior Analytics* that "singulars are more known to us, and are the first to exist according to the information of the sense, for indeed there is nothing in the understanding which was not first in the sense. And although that reasoning is naturally prior and more known which proceeds by syllogism, still is that more perspicuous to us which is based on induction. And therefore do we more readily define singulars than universals, for there is more of equivocation in universals: whence it is advisable from singulars to pass to universals.[74]"

74 HARVEY, *On generation*, Praefatio: *De modo et ordine acquirendae cognitionis* ed. 1662, fol. VI verso; tr. Willis p. 154.

This is a résumé, a digest formed from passages occurring in the *Posterior Analytics* rather than the citation of a single passage. Moreover Harvey appears to have given it a sensualist twist—inserting the famous Thomistic summary of Aristotle's epistemology—"*nihil est in intellectu quod non antea fuerit in sensu*", there is nothing in the mind that had not previously been in the sense. Nevertheless he realises the twofold aspect of knowledge, the interdependence of the empirical and logical approaches to it and thus pronounces that both of Aristotle's propositions are very true (*ut verissimum sit utrumque Aristotelis pronunciatum; tum illud in Physicis ... tum etiam illud in Analyticis*). Yet at first sight he seems to place the emphasis on the empirical approach, on induction. However, from what follows this is not really so. The same sensual perception, Harvey continues, derived from the same object at the same time, leads to different mental pictures in different people—which is particularly obvious in the creative artist and the poet. *Ipsa tamen sensatio est universalis*—for what we perceive as a particular, say the yellow colour of an eye, becomes a universal, when it is judged and understood by the internal sensorium. Hence the same object may elicit different *species*, i.e. mental images or impressions in the retaining minds (*phantasia*) of different observers, or even in the same observer who repeatedly tries to place his sensual impression on record, for example a painter "having a certain portrait to delineate, if he draw the outline a thousand times, he will still give a different face, and each not only differing from the other, but from the original *exemplar*". The particular—the picture received in the very moment of seeing it—has become an abstract *in phantasia;* what had been a clear and distinct *singulare* in the very act of vision, appears obscure and indistinct immediately the object is removed (or merely by shutting the eyes). If art consists in the sum total of impressions preserved in the memory of the artist, in the same way all cognition and science is arrived at, for both operate by the reception of a sensual image, the former of a type (*exemplar*, *idea*, *forma informans*) that is imitated by the mind of the artist (*imitamentum*, *idos*, *species abstracta*), the latter of something real, a natural object (*res naturalis*, *ens reale*) that is represented to the mind as something similar and becomes an object of reason (*representatio*, *similitudo*, *ens rationis*). Obviously, then, the object and its perception (*sensibilia*) are first and what happens in the mind (*intellegibilia*) is second and cannot be in us without the help of the former.

There is a moral to this: we can do nothing other than judge falsely from phantoms and appearances, unless we are aided by the senses, i.e. by frequently repeated observation and certain experience. This should be experience gained by ourselves as against reliance on the experiences of others. This will be requisite for passing an opinion in any branch of natural philosophy, and experience in anatomy will be absolutely necessary to judge what Harvey himself is going to advance on generation. He thus appeals not to the credence, but to the eyes of the reader. The principles on which all science rests and which take their origin from sense experience should become clear and certain to him through the frequent dissection of animals. This will prevent such false images as are formed from the perusal of tables and drawings designed for the knowledge of distant countries or of the internal parts of the body—whence the abundance of writers and pretenders to knowledge (*sophistae*) and the scarcity of the real philosopher and naturalist in Harvey's own wanton age (*luxuriante hoc aevo*). If this is heeded, not only a just appraisal of Aristotle and Galen, but the discovery of very many things yet unknown and of still greater value will follow when argumentative niceties and inferences from apparent probabilities are replaced by original observation (*autopsia*).

This again can be supported by the "same matters, according to Aristotle" (*ad mentem Aristotelis*). Here Harvey refers to Aristotle's developmental idea concerning the order and method by which any art or science is acquired: the thing perceived by sense remains; from the permanence of the thing perceived there results memory, from multiplied memory experience, from experience reason generally, definitions, maxims or common axioms, the most certain principles of knowledge from which every demonstrative syllogism, the marrow of all certain knowledge, is derived.

Again, then, there is no perfect knowledge which can be entitled ours, that is in us; none that does not proceed from experience obtained by us or our sense perception, or is at least tested and approved by these and firmly based on knowledge acquired before. For there is no experience without memory—indeed it is nothing but multiplied memory; nor can there be memory without permanence of the things perceived, and the thing perceived cannot remain where it never was. Aristotle was consistent in this: the same developmental concept of experience as based on sense perception and furthered by memory, Harvey recalls from the "most elegant pronouncement of the supreme dictator in philosophy" found in the first chapter of the first book of his *Metaphysics*, where he plainly tells us "that nobody can be called prudent or really possessed of knowledge who has not understood a thing to be as it is by personal experience acquired through reiterated memory, frequent sensation and diligent observation." Therefore the method of investigating truth which Harvey found customary at his own time, when enquiry was made into what others had to say instead of what the things were was inept and erroneous. Thus a whole world of empty visions and fanciful falsehoods (*falsa Idola et phantasmata inania*), of shadows and chimaeras, waking dreams and deliria of a sick mind had been created.

Again Harvey admonishes the reader—"whispering into his ear"—to weigh all that he is going to find in his book in the balance of exact experience and to give credit only to what he finds most firmly established by the testimony of the senses. The same was also the advice of Aristotle who, having dealt with a number of particulars concerning bees, finally says: "generation of bees seems to occur in this way, according to reason as well as to what is seen to happen in their kind. What in fact takes place we have not yet fully explored. When all will be known about it, then more trust will have to be accorded to sense than to reason. Credit will also have to be given to reason, if what is demonstrated concurs with what is perceived by the sense.[75]"

What, then, is the *method* which is finally recommended by Harvey to be applied in the study of generation (*cognitione generationis*)? And how far does Harvey follow the Aristotelian principles in this?

First of all Harvey suggests that one look back from the perfect animal and as it were retrace our steps from the goal (*meta*) to the starting place (*carceres*, sc. in the circus), so that finally when no further regress seems possible we should have arrived at the principles, i.e. the primary matter and the efficient principle and the way in which the plastic force proceeds from these. The way thus leads from grown up man back through boyhood to infancy and the embryo, to what was in the womb before he was an embryo, whether there were three bubbles or a shapeless mass (*rudis indigestaque moles*), or a conceptus consisting of the mixed male and

75 With reference to Aristotle, *De generat. animal.* lib. III, cap. 10; 760b 30.

female semen or a coagulum or anything else, as stated in the literature.

In this we may well recognise the retrograde process of acquiring knowledge which, according to Aristotle, starts with the complex and finished product that is "prior for us" and the first to fall under our sensual perception. We thus follow the embryo back to its earliest stages, that of the "three bullae" or "coagulum" and even further and thus arrive at what is "prior by nature"—the principle that operates as the efficient cause in the plastic force and the prime matter from which the germ emerges.

In the developing chick the reverse order is observed and the changes are recorded day by day in the egg which precede the perfection of the fetus—keeping strictly to what can be seen in a *bona fide* description that avoids opinion and conjecture. An example of the latter had been the idea, unworthy of a prominent anatomist of the rank of Fabricius ab Aquapendente, that the bones are formed before the muscles, the heart, liver and lung and that all the internal organs are built before the external ones[76]. In this Fabricius relied on reasoning from what appeared to be probable and was supported by analogies with the building of a house or a ship rather than on personal observation (*autopsia*); he abandoned the judgment of the senses formed at dissection in favour of petty reasoning from mechanics (*ad ratiunculas e mechanicis petitas confugit*).

When the first stages have been accomplished—namely the study of the order in which the parts develop in all those animals that are available and suitable and of the primary matter out of which and the efficient cause by which generation is achieved—consideration will be given to the more "abstruse" nature of the vegetative soul. It will then also be permitted to understand the mode, order and causes of generation in all animals, i.e. the general laws which are observed by Nature and can be deduced using the analogy that prevails between animals according to genera and species. For "Nature divine and perfect is in the same things harmonious with herself. And as her works either concur or differ (according to genus, species or any other proportional analogy) so is her action (namely generation or formation) either the same or diverse in these." There is no place either for metaphors or for new words in the enormous task lying before the observer, as they would not bring a torch to shed light upon the matter, but rather plunge it into darkness—trying as they do to explain something unknown in terms of something even more unknown and asking the reader to spend more time on the inter-

76 Fabricius, *De formatione ovi et pulli*, cap. II. *Opp. Anat. et Physiol.* ed. Albinus. Lugd. Bat. 1738, p. 18.

pretation of words than on understanding of the things themselves. This is the reason why Aristotle is believed by the inexperienced to be obscure in many places and perhaps why Fabricius preferred pictures to words in his description of the fabric of the chick in the egg.

Harvey thus feels himself driven to a new method and to the occasional use of unusual words, intent not on vain glory (*vanae gloriolae*), but on observations that are true and emerge from the nature of things. And yet he confesses to his following in the footsteps of those who have borne the torch before him and adapts himself to their terminology as far as possible. Among them, Aristotle from the ancients and Fabricius ab Aquapendente from the contemporaries stand in the first rank—the former as his leader and the latter as his guide (*illum tanquam Ducem, hunc ut Praemonstratorem*). As the discoverer of a new land gives it a new name that is preserved by posterity, so also the finder (*inventoribus*) and first describer of things confers names upon them by right.

But at this point, Harvey concludes, I hear Galen reminding us that we should agree about things alone and not quibble about words.

Comment: The Harveian Aristotle

This, then, is the gist of the introductory matter to Harvey's late work *On generation of animals*. It consists of an introduction proper and three excursuses: the first on the manner and order of acquiring knowledge in general, the second on the developmental stages therein as visualised by Aristotle and the third on the moral which should be drawn for the study of generation. At first sight these four introductory chapters may appear to be lengthy and repetitive; given time for a revision of his manuscript, reluctantly delivered at a moment's notice to the editor George Ent, Harvey might have wished to divest them of their discursive tenor and to contract them into a single programmatic preface. Such an inference cannot stand a more thorough examination, however. We have before us variations on a single theme, subtly adapted to its historic mission and importance. Original observation of the natural object versus acceptance of authority is Harvey's theme. To-day there is no question in this matter for the naturalist and scientist. At Harvey's time things were different: original work was still outnumbered by paraphrases and interpretations of ancient works and was indeed rare. The modern observer might say that Harvey could have contented himself with laying his new original findings before the reader who would be bound to see their superiority and novelty and thus could not help accepting them. This was not the case. When the new book on which he must have been busy for many years eventually appeared in 1651, only two years had elapsed after Harvey had at last answered the objections raised by the great French anatomist Jean Riolan against the circulation of the blood. This was still not generally recognised even then. Ancient authority was still required or at least lent much support to any investigation. This is true although Bernardino Telesio (1508–1588) had recommended to treat nature according to her own principles (*juxta propria principia*) as early as in 1565. He had been supported by Tommaso Campanella (1568–1639) at the end of the century (1588–1590) and Harvey seems to reflect their principles when calling for original observation versus acceptance of authority. Nevertheless Harvey had frequently referred to ancient sources, notably to Aristotle and Galen, in his first work on the motion of the heart and blood, although but a few such references occur in its second part which deals with circulation, the great novelty he was submitting to the public. In the present case—his book on generation—we find many quotations from ancient authors throughout the voluminous text. But what the Introduction has to offer is something quite different and new. Harvey here concerns himself with the method of scientific investigation in general terms. It is an attempt at deriving justification for forming experience based on original observation and experiment, from the very ancient sources which to his contemporaries had not conveyed this appeal, but served as a platform for hermeneutic disputation. Harvey's source is Aristotle—the very "dictator" who had been misinterpreted by friend and foe: the former by forcing him into the straitjacket of scholasticism and the latter by representing him as a mere rationalist and logician who was prepared to sacrifice facts to the *entia rationis*, to the *Idols*—the phantoms and spectres—*of the Cave* and of the *Market-place*. A *New Organon* had been created to replace the Aristotelian *Organon* and to secure for observational and experimental Induction its proper place.

Here, then, is Harvey presenting an Aristotle who is quite different from the guise in which he appeared to those great exponents of rising modern science who seemed to have found their main advocate in Bacon. More than that, here are Aristotle's own methodological principles from which Harvey derives with ease his original methods and results. This is not achieved by an un-historical tour de force, a falsification of the historical Aristotle and his mis-representation as a sensualist pure and simple. Harvey rightly emphasises the sensualist approach with which Aristotelian epistemology sets out: there is nothing innate in the mind which is merely awakened, but all knowledge is based in the first place on sense perception which derives from the object outside and newly enters the mind. Harvey realises, however, that this is not true knowledge in itself. To form it a mind is required that repeatedly remembers and classifies sensual impressions, in other words experience. However, between the fact observed by the sense organ and the record made by the mind the picture of necessity becomes blurred—once in the mind, the object, the concrete singular or particular, is judged by an abstract, a universal. It is identified by virtue of mental conceptions that are the result of previous sense impressions. The only means which we have to insure against false impressions is the constant repetition of observations, testing by experiment and proving by experience. This, however, is not enough. Harvey insists in true Aristotelian terms on the harmony between what is observed and reason[77]. It was the failure to preserve this harmony that had led Galen astray, for example about the allegedly cooling purpose of the pulse and the so-called vital spirits[78]. In the same vein Harvey attributes importance to final causes. Different movements and structures are "signs" of different functions and purposes—an example of reasoning from a "thing caused to a final cause"[79]. It had been a teleological consideration of the venous valves, of their purpose, that had led Harvey to the idea of circulation[80]. What was the final cause of circulation? This question occupied Harvey, the "life-long thinker" about its purpose. Yet with all this, Harvey "though he is a teleologist, is one in a limited sense.[81]" Purposes are not the primary causes responsible for structures and movements, "but are used as supporting evidence, so to speak, *after* the heart, arteries and veins have all been mechanically interpreted.... In the same way, Aristotle distinguished between what he called biological necessity and biological reason, the latter working for a definite end, the former not. Both, he thought, were necessary, though in varying proportions, to explain life.[82]"

This is well shown when—following Plochmann—we visualise Harvey's ideas on the physiological function of the heart and blood in terms of Aristotle's four principles and "causes" (p. 34). In this respect Harvey stresses the production and distribution of animal heat as against a cooling action ascribed to the pulse by Galen. In Aristotelian terms, then, the blood can be looked upon as the material cause of the heat, i. e. the fuel that is heated; the heart is the formal cause, i. e. the structure that makes the

77 See the Harveian loci compiled by LESKY, 1957, loc. cit. in note [35], p. 301 et seq. For example: *De motu* cap. II, ed. 1628, p. 22: ex quibus observatis rationi consentaneum; ibid. cap. IX, p. 44: sensui contrarium est et rationi; ibid. cap. XIV: confirmata omnia et rationibus et ocularibus experimentis, and others.

78 Prooemium to *De motu* ed. 1628, p. 15; tr. WILLIS p. 14: nam non solum illud experimentum est in contrarium (quod solvere Galenus nititur).

79 PLOCHMANN, 1963, loc. cit in note [55], p. 202.

80 See above p. 22 and below p. 209.

81 PLOCHMANN, p. 205.

82 ibidem.

heating possible; the heart also acts as its efficient cause, namely the origin of the motion of the blood and the latter as the final cause of the heart, for in it and through it the blood receives its perfection.[83a]

There is an interesting parallel to this in Harvey's ideas on generation which he himself expressed in terms of Aristotelian causes, as Erna Lesky has pointed out[83]. Harvey saw the fecundated egg as the matter, the material cause, of the future chick, the potential chicken. The fecundating agent, that which makes it fruitful by contrast with wind-eggs, is the efficient cause of the chick, i. e. what sets the egg moving and terminating in the formation of a chick. The latter is thus the final cause for the sake of which both the egg and the fertilising agent exist; it is the true reality (*actus*, *energeia*) and reason that causes a chick to be formed, and not something else. This, the final cause, Harvey quotes from Aristotle, is primary, both in nature and in art, to all other causes, since it moves and is not itself moved, whereas the "efficient" moves because it is impelled by the final cause. For there inheres somehow in every "efficient" a final cause (*ratio finis*), and by this the "efficient" is moved, operating through Providence. Harvey adduced further passages which make it quite clear that "the authority of Aristotle supports" him (*Aristotelis autoritas nobis plane suffragatur*). Indeed the final cause, the "reason" for the sake of which (*cuius gratia*) something is done, the "end" (*finis*), is the chief principle among the causes of natural generation. Harvey concludes in syllogistic terms: whenever the "efficient" is in action (moving), the final cause is in action; whenever the matter is in action (being moved), the efficient is; hence whenever the material is in action (being moved and changed), the final cause is (moving, but not moved in itself)[84].

We should finally remember Harvey's distinction between procedures in embryology. Here either a start is made at the finished product—the fully developed individual that is retraced to his "primordia", the fertilised ovum and the structureless albumen preceding it. Or else the reverse way is followed, leading from the "primordia" to the fully developed chick. The former method is that of analysis of the elementary components from a complicated product, corresponding to the search for "universals" in a singular "concrete". The latter method is that of synthesis by which the "concrete" is built up from given "universals". This Harveian distinction of methods sounds like the application to embryology of the distinction between the *doctrina resolutiva* and the *doctrina compositiva* which formed one of the main keys to knowledge used

83 LESKY, 1957, loc. cit. in note [35], p. 315.

83a HARVEY, *On gener.*, Exerc. XIX, ed. 1662, p. 81; tr. WILLIS, p. 255.

84 HARVEY, *De conceptione* (appended to *On generation*) ed. 1662, p. 386 et seq.; tr. Willis p. 583 et seq.

by Pietro d'Abano in the mediaeval Aristotelian school of Padua (see above p. 19).

Harvey's opposition to Aristotle

Harvey opposed Aristotle in many points of detail; we shall discuss this at various places throughout the present book. A few of the major points may be mentioned here.

Aristotle emphatically upheld the heart as the origin and supreme part of the organism, its principle, an *arche*. He rejected the blood as the seat of the vital principle, of the soul[85]. By contrast Harvey subscribed to the latter view and did so already early in his career, for he gave expression to this thesis in the lecture notes on anatomy which date from 1615 onwards[86]. Harvey's motive in opposing Aristotle in this matter was empirical and observational rather than philosophical. His observations in the embryo had taught him that blood was earlier in appearance than the heart. However there is more to the matter than this. Harvey sees in the blood the fountain from which the organs and tissues are continually refreshed and indeed built up, both in embryonic and in later life. Blood therefore can be seen as the final cause for the sake of which the organism at large is made; even the heart would subordinate itself as serving for the perfection of the blood, the latter acting as its final cause rather than the reverse (see above p. 42).

Further important points in which Harvey disagrees with Aristotle concern questions of generation, notably the position of the female part. This, according to Aristotle, was a vegetative "menstrual" coagulum out of which the active male semen forms the embryo[87]. Aristotle had not been quite consistent in this, as already Galen had noticed. For he had observed that certain bastards show maternal characteristics alone, when a certain sequence of generations is completed[88]. Galen, too, had criticised Aristotle's theory of generation for the one-sided attribution of activity to the male partner. We shall discuss this in detail elsewhere in the present book[89]. In this, then, Harvey was not original. He found himself, however, confronted with a different problem: that of fertilisation. For he had failed to detect any trace of male semen shortly after coition; nor was there anything in the uterus that could have been regarded as a female contribution of "matter" on which the male active part could have acted as "form". Harvey was thus driven to assign autonomy to the female part. Indeed he regarded the female, in birds as well as in other animals, as the source from which the first conceptions derive both material and

85 As notably expressed in *De anima*, lib. I, cap. 2; 405 b 14. – HARVEY, *On generation*, Exerc. LII, ed. 1662, p. 197; tr. WILLIS, p. 381.

86 See p. 272 seq.

87 ARISTOTLE, De gener. animal. lib. I, cap. 19; 727b. – As A. L. PECK has pointed out (1953, loc. cit. [on p. 254 in note 13], p. 115) there are many *levels of "matter"*. The menstrual matter as well as the unfertilised egg are in fact informed to a high degree, as they possess the "movements" of nutritive soul. They only lack the movements proper to sentient soul—these are provided by the male.

Nevertheless the *Katamenia* are called *passive matter* (*pathetikon* and *hyle*): *De gen. anim.* I, 20–21; 728a in fine, and the *male* semen the *active* and *moving* (*dynamis* and *kinesis*): ibid. 729b. – Moreover the *ovum* is said to be produced by a stuff analogous to *Katamenia* in birds, or, as Fabricius expresses it: the uterine wall is apt "vitellos expullulare, generare et *ex sanguine producere*."

88 ARISTOTLE, *De gener. animal.* lib. II, cap. 4; 738b 30–35.

89 See below p. 237 and LESKY, 1957, p. 365.

form. For it is the hen which bears the primordial *ova* in a repository[90]. They are *pre*-formed in the ovary of oviparous animals. Nor are they formed from a menstrual discharge of the uterus in viviparous animals, as Aristotle believed. There is no discharge of anything in women during or after fruitful coition; nor is orgasm proof of the emission of female "semen". Indeed the independence of the *ovum* can be demonstrated. It is reflected in the possession by the embryo of its own blood which is entirely responsible for its nourishment. This is not derived, as had been generally assumed, from maternal blood and spirit, either in the ovum which develops separately from the mother, or in the fetus of viviparous animals which dwells in the womb—the latter enjoying its own vital principle, its own powers and its own blood as does the chick in the ovum (*abunde me demonstraturum arbitror viviparorum quoque foetum, dum adhuc in utero continetur, non matris sanguine nutriri, spirituve eius vegetari; sed anima, viribusque suis frui, [ut pullus in ovo solet] proprioque sanguine gaudere*)[91]. Nor would Harvey admit that the male geniture (semen) enters and conjugates with the ovum, since he failed to find any trace of the former after coition. Nor finally could there be any idea of a transference of the vital principle, the soul, by the male geniture to the female—a kind of transmigration of the soul from one body into another (*metempsychosis*)[92]. Instead he believed in a distance action of the male comparable to contagion. This was to touch off a chain of reactions on the part of the ovum which were to lead to the formation of the fetus[93]. As H. Fischer formulated it: there was no *amphimixis*, no coming together of the male and female components, but an almost parthenogenetic generation in which the male has a stimulating effect, but no more[94].

The fertile "conceptus", then, is not the result of a mixture of male and female semen ("genitures")—in this Harvey finds himself at variance with the physicians who followed Galen—nor is it the product of menstrual blood entered into and fashioned by the male semen—in this he challenges Aristotle.

The male cannot therefore claim superiority as the source of semen. Instead, each one, male as well as female, is operative as a parent. The female part is just as much *causa generationis* as the male since it stimulates the latter in various ways[95].

The *ovum*, then, is possessed of innate impulses, the animal virtues of motion, change, rest and preservation[96]. Or, in similar terms, the formative faculty of the developing chick acquires and prepares matter for itself, rather than finding it already prepared, and it seems that it is not made and caused to grow by virtue of

90 HARVEY, *On generation* Exerc. XL, ed. 1662, p. 138; tr. WILLIS, p. 317: "quippe ovorum primordia non fiunt in utero ex sanguine menstruo (qui in gallina neutiquam reperitur), sed in ovario (ubi nullus sanguis praeexistit) ova tam citra galli coitum, quam cum illo progenerantur"; "materia unde cuncta ovorum primordia in ovario nascuntur, et crescunt, videtur eadem illa ex qua reliquae gallinae partes, carnosae nempe, nervosae, et osseae; caput item, ac cetera membra nutriuntur et augentur".

91 *On generation* Exerc. XXXIV, ed. 1662, p. 120; tr. WILLIS p. 298.

92 *On generation*, Exerc. XL, ed. 1662, p. 137; tr. WILLIS p. 315–316; Exerc. XLVII, ed. 1662, p. 167; tr. WILLIS p. 349.

93 *On generation*, Exerc. XLI, ed. 1662, p. 143; tr. WILLIS p. 321; Ex. XL, p. 137 Exerc. XLIX, ed. 1662, p. 176; tr. WILLIS p. 359. – ARISTOTLE, *De gener. animal.* II, 1; 734b 10.

94 FISCHER, HANS, *Die Geschichte der Zeugungs- und Entwickelungstheorien im 17. Jahrhundert.* GESNERUS, 1945, II, 49–80 (p. 58).

95 *On generation*, Exerc. XLI, ed. 1662, p. 140; tr. WILLIS p. 318–319: "quemadmodum autem mas ... ita quoque gallina aliquo modo prima generationis caussa statui potest".

96 *On generation*, Exerc. XXVI, ed. 1662, p. 97; tr. WILLIS, p. 272: "Ovum itaque est corpus naturale, virtute animali praeditum; principio nempe motus, transmutationis, quietis, et conservationis". – See also Exercit. XXXVIII, ed. 1662, p. 130; tr. WILLIS, p. 308: "sunt itaque ambo (sc. tam gallus quam gallina) plasticae virtutis instrumenta, quibus ista species perpetuatur".

somebody else, but by itself (*facultas enim pulli formatrix materiam potius sibi acquirit et parat, quam paratam invenit videturque pullus haud ab alio fieri vel augeri quam a se ipso*)[97].

It is in these terms that Harvey establishes the independence of the *ovum* that is borne by the female partner. This thesis had been prepared by the denial of communications between branches of the umbilical and uterine arteries (Arantius, Spigelius) and by general argument (Nymmanus). It was to arouse criticism by such contemporaries of Harvey as Marcus Marci, as we shall discuss elsewhere in the present book[98].

Again the leading point in Harvey's thesis is observational: his failure to detect the male and female components at an early stage after coition. In addition to this argument from observation, however, there is again a philosophical point: Harvey seems intent on divesting generation of any materialist trace. The action of the male is not by conjugation of material components at all. Nor is it a spiritual impulse imparted by the "active" male entering the female coagulum. Instead Harvey suggests action at a distance on the part of the male comparable with that of a contagium. Even here he finds a connexion with Aristotelian teaching: what is essential for the fertility of the semen is its effervescence, not its emission or material substance and composition[99].

Moreover Harvey's rejection of any material action of the male on the *ovum* strictly follows the vitalist and dynamist principles of Aristotle himself—in this point Harvey appears to be more Aristotelian than the Philosopher. Nor is he in the least drawn away from Aristotle viewing the male as the bearer of spirit and virtue of a divine agent which confers fertility in a moment of time—indeed in this he found the comparison with a contagium.

Even where the autonomy of the *ovum* is concerned and he decides against Aristotle, he collects passages from the latter to support his point: Aristotle had admitted activity of the female, since it produces unfertilised 'wind-eggs' and also believed that in certain fishes an unfertilised ovum can produce an embryo[100]. Similarly Harvey took pains in finding authority from Aristotle for his concept of an *ovum* as the uniform, primordial pattern of everything living (*quodlibet primordium potentia vivens*)[101], or in the popular parlance of the frontispiece to Harvey's book: *Ex ovo omnia*[102].

Harvey endeavours to bridge minor divergencies, for example in the question of the identity of pattern of the *ovum* and the "*worm*" ("*grub*"), as denied by Aristotle and asserted by Harvey[103]. Moreover the autonomy of the *ovum* propounded by Harvey against

97 *On generation* Exercit. XLV, ed. 1662, p. 155; tr. WILLIS p. 336. On the Aristotelian belief in the full development of ova without male fertilisation in certain fishes see: ARISTOTLE, *De gener. anim.* lib. II, 5; 741a30 ad lib. III, 1; 750b25. See also below, note [100].

98 See below p. 318.

99 *On generation*, Exerc. XL, ed. 1662, p. 137; tr. WILLIS, p. 315: "quatenus genitura istaec prolifica est, et vi plastica imbuta; spiritosa nempe, effectiva et analoga elemento stellarum"—with reference to Aristotle, *De generat. animal.* lib. II, cap. 3; 736b 35.

100 *On generation*, Exerc. XXXV, ed. 1662, p. 124; tr. WILLIS, p. 301—with reference to Aristotle, *De generat. animal.* lib. III, cap. 7; 757b15. See above note [97].

101 *On generation*, Exerc. LXII, ed. 1662, p. 271; tr. WILLIS, p. 457–458, with reference to Aristotle, *De gen. anim.*, III, 9; 758a–b.

102 Harvey remained ignorant of the Graafian follicles and the true mammalian egg (discovered by K. E. VON BAER, 1827). He understood by *ovum* in the context referred to above that organic formation which is capable of producing the embryo. In mammals this is the fertilised *conceptus*. He visualised this *primordium* to be of ovoid shape in *all* living beings, including plants. This generalising "analogy" (LESKY, loc. cit. 1957, p. 354) is partly a logical postulate expressing the unity of life in nature, as H. Fischer rightly saw it. – For an exhaustive account of the Empedoclean and Aristotelian roots of Harvey's vision see LESKY, loc. cit. 1957, p. 349–359. – For a survey of some of the literature, especially the widespread misunderstanding of *Ex ovo omnia* see A. W. MEYER, *An analysis of De generatione animal.* Stanford and London 1936, p. 72–83. – We shall revert to the subject and its Aristotelian background in the present book, below, p. 274.

103 HARVEY, *On generation*, Exerc. LXII, ed. 1662, p. 271; tr. WILLIS, p. 458, with ref. to Aristotle, *De generat. animal.*, lib. III, cap. 9; 758b 13: some of the "worms" may be thought to resemble eggs because of their round shape, but we must not judge by shapes nor yet by softness and hardness .. but by the fact that the whole of them is changed into the body of the creature and the animal is not developed from a part of them (tr. A. PLATT, Oxford, 1910); also with ref. to Aristotle, *Hist.*

Aristotle can be set against the background of a fundamental Aristotelian concept[104], namely that of Nature (*physis*)—the force that contains the principle of motion and rest in itself[105].

What is more, Harvey realises in the end that the male as well as his seminal fluid and likewise the female no less than the *ovum* which is borne by her are the efficient instruments of generation. He therefore resorts to a prior, superior and more excellent cause to which all providence, intellect, art and goodness should be attributed and which is as much more excellent than its effect as the architect is more excellent than his work, the king more so than his servants and the workman better than his hands. Male and female, then, are merely the efficient instrument, subservient to the Creator of all things or the highest begetter. In this sense, Harvey continues, it is well said—with the *Summus Philosophus*—that the sun and man generate man, because the approach and recession of the sun are followed by spring and autumn, the seasons in which mostly generation and corruption take place. With this Harvey refers to Aristotle's book *On generation and corruption* from which he reproduces a long passage[106].

Neither divergencies in points of detail nor those in questions of biological principle, then, detract substantially from Harvey's loyalty to Aristotle. The Philosopher remains the "Leader" whom he consults in the first place and follows whenever he can.

Harvey paid no lip service to Aristotelian principles—this is particularly evident in the long introduction on method to his work on generation which we have discussed in detail above (p. 34).

However, Harvey was first and foremost observationalist and experimentalist. Why, then, should he have gone so deeply into matters of the theory of knowledge and method at all? The answer is that he was fully conscious of the pitfalls into which the ancients as well as contemporaries had been trapped, by overstretched and naive observationalism on the one hand and onesided theorising on the other. Harvey, being genuinely concerned with the question of truth and how it can be attained, must have found the guide in his perplexity in Aristotle's careful weighing up of the two approaches to it: induction and logical conclusion. Moreover Harvey sought access to first principles by speculation on Aristotelian lines. Such speculation included the purpose of circulatory patterns in nature at large—in the microcosm as well as the greater world; it also concerned the universal principle, the "same mind or spirit which continually drives about the immense mass of the universe and leads about the same sun from rising to setting

animal., lib. I, cap. 5; 489b 6: What we term an egg is a certain completed result of conception out of which the animal that is to be develops, and in such a way that in respect to its primitive germ it comes from part only of the egg, while the rest serves for food as the germ develops. A grub, on the other hand, is a thing out of which the animal in its entirety develops, by differentiation and growth of the embryo (tr. D'ARCY WENTWORTH THOMPSON, Oxford, 1910).

104 LESKY, 1957, loc. cit. in note [35], p. 370. – Lesky finds in Harvey's thesis a presentiment of modern embryological theory, namely an example of "Konsekutivaetiologie". According to this the various phases of development are represented as causally and not only chronologically dependent upon each other—as against ancient "Executivaetiologie" in which the main role is attributed to an exogenous factor such as the male, as seen by Aristotle. With ref. to MITTERER, A. *Die Zeugung der Organismen nach. d. Weltbild des hl. Thomas v. Aquin und dem d. Gegenwart* Wien 1947 and idem, *Die Entwickelungslehre Augustins im Vergleich mit dem Weltbild d. hl. Thomas u. dem d. Gegenwart* Wien u. Freiburg 1956 (in the latter the "pan-spermatic" theory of Augustine is visualised as foreshadowing modern ideas of immanence of generative impulses and the independence of the ovum of the male generator).

105 ARISTOTLE, *Physics*, lib. II, cap. 1; 192 b 8.

106 HARVEY, *On generation*, Exerc. L, ed. 1662, p. 183; tr. WILLIS, p. 367. – Willis' translation is not quite correct: "it is well said that the sun and moon engender man", instead of "sun and man" (*sol et homo*). – The Aristotelian reference is to: *De generat. et corrupt.* lib. II, cap. 10; 336b.

perpetually through the diverse regions of the lands and acts as the divine principle, working here as the formative, there as the nutritive and again as the auctive force in the gallinaceous tribe, yet always available as the preservative and vegetative virtue, here in the form of a fowl, there in that of an ovum, but remaining the same virtue in eternity.[107]"

Pronouncements like this bear the stamp of sincere and deep-seated beliefs and convictions. Harvey was no orator, no phrase monger. He meant exactly what he said. The time-honoured old *Organon* of Aristotle has thus much more to give him than the "neoteric" *New Organon* of the Lord Chancellor[108]. There is, then, much of the Aristotelian spirit in Harvey's attitude towards the theory and attainment of knowledge, in the speculations in which he engaged, in the methods which he employed and in the observations and discoveries which he made. There is, however, little that is "Baconian" in all this, at all events from Harvey's own point of view, and the introduction to the work on generation may well have been written by its author for the very purpose of leaving contemporaries and posterity in no doubt about just this point.

107 *On generation*, Exerc. XXVIII, ed. 1662, p. 109; tr. WILLIS, p. 285–286.

108 See above on HARVEY and BACON, p. 21–23.

Harvey De Motu

The Hierarchy of Ideas and Facts

Harvey discovered that the blood described a *closed* circle: it is sent from the heart to the organs and returns to it in its *entirety*. It is precisely this unitarian idea about the blood that created a completely new position, rising in sharp contrast to the doctrine that had been accepted and had ruled for a millennium and a half. It had been known since antiquity that *some of the blood* is led to the right heart, through the lungs to the left heart and hence to the periphery. What had not been known was that *all the blood* goes that way *all the time*. It had also been known, since mediaeval times in the East, and for some seventy years before the publication of Harvey's book in the West, that *some of the venous blood*, i.e. that part of it which is sent from the liver to the right heart, passes not through an imaginary interventricular communication, but through the lung into the left heart and hence through the arteries to the periphery. This *pulmonary transit* of venous blood from the right heart to the left is often called: the lesser circulation. There is no justification for this, however; on the contrary, this term would seem to confuse the main issue. For, prior to Harvey, this part of the blood had never been thought to describe a circle, i.e. to revert to its point of departure. The latter is the *right* heart, not the left heart into which it flows after its passage through the lungs. Instead of "reverting" to the right heart it had been thought to be *consumed* by the peripheral organs and to be ever newly formed by the liver from ingested food. In other words it *did not circulate*. There was no idea of a "return" at all, and therefore no idea of circulation, either "lesser" or "systemic". In fact the former is not possible without the latter, and Harvey remains the discoverer of both. This was shown by Max Neuburger in a short and masterly paper[1]. Its effect has so far remained in inverse proportion to its importance.

The salient point in Harvey's discovery, then, lies in the *preservation* of the blood as against its *consumption:* instead of being used up in the peripheral organs and tissues, the blood returns periodically or "cyclically" to the heart—it circulates.

This idea is the master-key; how was it obtained by Harvey? We shall have to say more about this in one of the following sections of the present book (p. 209). What we wish to discuss now is the way in which Harvey marshalled his facts in relation to the idea in *De motu* and what information can be derived from a chapter-by-chapter and, where expedient, a word-by-word survey of its contents.

1 NEUBURGER, MAX, *Zur Entdeckungsgeschichte des Lungenkreislaufes. Arch. f. Gesch. d. Medizin* 1930, XXIII, 7–9.

The student of Harvey cannot fail to be impressed by his conciseness: he means exactly what he says and studying the words he used[2] would seem to be more profitable than inference and circumstantial evidence. What, then, is the hierarchy of facts as revealed in Harvey's own words and arrangement of the presentation?

As the title of *De motu* indicates, the work comprises two separate topics: (a) the motion of the heart and (b) that of the blood. In accordance with this the discovery of circulation forms the subject of the second part, and this begins with chapter VIII. What goes before is a substructure that incorporates observations and arguments that were partly already laid down in the notes prepared by Harvey for his Lumleian Lectures in 1616 and following years and will be discussed elsewhere in the present book (p. 214). The subjects include: movement and function of the heart, arteries and atria and the pulmonary transit of venous blood; in detail: the apical heart beat, its origin and conduction, the muscular nature of the heart and the pulse which is shown to be due to the impulse of the blood that is ejected by the heart as against a wave of contraction running along the arterial wall.

Each of these subjects was enriched by Harvey's new and fundamental observations and sure knowledge of detail. What is more, it was given a new firm basis which is valid to-day. Indeed it is not only the idea of circulation which, through Harvey's genius, superseded all that was known before, but the same is true of much that he had to say in the first part of his book which is *De motu cordis*. This particularly applies to the subject enumerated last: the replacement of Galen's pulse-making "force" of the arterial wall by the entirely new vision of the pulse as the result of the mechanical *impulse* conferred on the blood that is ejected into the relaxed arterial "pipes" by the contracting heart. With this new ground was broken for the modernist and indeed revolutionising abolition of a mysterious "force", fixed in the mind as such and precluding explanation and causative analysis, in favour of a mechanical concept that threw the door open to analysis by the physicist and biologist.

Harvey's *Exercitatio anatomica de motu cordis et sanguinis in animalibus*, as a whole, may not have been the product of a single and sustained literary attempt to treat one single subject, but may have been written, composed and revised on several occasions[3]. It cannot be said, however, that part I: on the motion of the *heart*, and part II: on the motion of the *blood* are merely juxtaposed and presented without expression of their natural coherence. The

2 For a semantic analysis of "zero-level statements", "first-level statements", consequences, definitions and "points" as emerging from each chapter of *De motu*: WOODGER, J.H., *Biology and language*. Cambridge 1952, pp. 75–92 (Appendix A).

For similar analyses see: ROTHSCHUH, K.E., *Über Kreislaufschemata und Kreislaufmodelle seit den Zeiten von William Harvey. Zeitschr. f. Kreislaufforsch.* 1957, XLVI, 241; idem, *Die Entwickelung der Kreislauflehre im Anschluß an William Harvey.* Klin. Wochschr. 1957, XXXV, 605. – RATNER, H., *William Harvey, M.D. modern or ancient scientist? The Thomist* 1964, XXIV, 175–208.

3 KILGOUR, F.G., *William Harvey and his contributions. Circulation,* 1961, XXIII, 286–296, with ref. to Leake, Chauncey, D., *Harvey Exercit. de motu* with an Eng. tr. and annot. Springfield, 1928.

chapters immediately preceding the opening up of the new subject of the blood (ch. VI and VII) treat of the pathways by which the blood is carried from the vena cava into the arteries. Leading up to these topics the fifth chapter contained the statement that the motion and function of the heart pivot around the passage of the blood (*transfusio*) from the veins to the arteries; it concludes with the announcement that a way is to be provided and opened (*via paranda est et aperienda*) whereby all difficulties and any possible objections to Harvey's statement concerning the pulse of the heart and arteries, the transmission of blood from veins to arteries and its distribution to the whole body through the arteries will be removed[4].

It should also be remembered that the pulmonary transit of the blood which forms the topic of chapter VII served as the leading analogy for Harvey's conception of the systemic circuit of the blood (p. 54).

In the closing chapters of the first part of *De motu*, then, we may see the natural transition to the second part, the transition that is from the "lesser" to the "systemic" circulation.

What is novel and unheard-of in what Harvey has now to present is on his own showing (a) the *quantity* and (b) the *source* of the blood that is transmitted from the veins to the arteries by virtue of the action of the heart (*copia et proventus istius pertranseuntis sanguinis*)[5].

Indeed it is in these two words—quantity and source—that the open sesame to the discovery lies and around them the multitude of empirical proofs adduced by Harvey is grouped. Accordingly they reduce themselves to two main groups: (a) those based on the *computation* of the quantity of blood propelled by the heart in a unit of time and (b) those concerned with the fact that the blood in itself forms the *source* of all blood passing through the heart from right to left.

These proofs are based on the facts which Harvey has marshalled. From his own words, however, it would appear that the idea was in his mind first. It occurred to him, he says, when he was seriously and repeatedly considering (a) the quantity of blood that passes, (b) the short time required for its transmission from vein to artery, and (c) the insurmountable difficulties arising when the ingested food was supposed to provide the source for a constantly replenished supply of blood.

From these reflections he had concluded that the veins should be empty whilst the arteries should burst from the excessive intrusion of blood—unless the blood should somehow return from the

4 *De motu*, cap. V, ed. 1628, p. 32; tr. Willis, p. 34.

5 *De motu*, cap. VIII, ed. 1628, p. 41; tr. Willis, p. 45.

arteries anew into the veins and return to the right ventricle of the heart[6].

In the course of these reflections *coepi egomet mecum cogitare*—I for myself began to think, whether there might not be a certain motion, as it were, in a circle (*an motionem quandam quasi in circulo haberet*)[7]. This, namely the motion, or we may infer the idea of its existence, Harvey found to be true *afterwards—quam postea veram esse reperi*.

Indeed this idea seems to have come first, before the proofs were at hand. For it was bound up with the vision of analogy—the analogy, that is, between the passage of blood through the lungs and that through the peripheral organs (*sanguinem ... in habitum corporis...impelli...quem admodum in pulmones...et rursus per venas remeari, quem admodum ex pulmonibus per arteriam venosam*)[8]. In this instance we would seem to be on safe ground using the term "lesser circulation" to indicate the analogy with its systemic counterpart.

Harvey remains in the sphere of analogy for most of the rest of this memorable eighth chapter: the analogy of the circular motion of the blood with that of air and rain and in turn with the circular motion of the celestial bodies emulated by them, also with cyclical generation (sc. of living things) and with cycles of storms and aerial phenomena which are due to the circular motion of the sun, its approach and recession. Still within the realm of the microcosmic analogy, the heart emerges as the true sovereign of the body—restoring as it does fluidity, heat, power and the balm of life to the blood that reaches it from the periphery, cooled, coagulated and effete. *Ita cor principium vitae et sol microcosmi*—thus the heart is the principle of life and the sun of the lesser world, just as the sun deserves to be called the heart of the world[9]. We shall say more about these symbolical aspects of circulation and their background anon (p. 82; 89 seq.).

With the ninth chapter the general position stated thus far begins to be developed into detail. Reflection, ideas and analogy are not enough. Indeed somebody might say that so far mere words and specious assertions have been given without foundation, that an innovation has been proposed without *just cause*. Hence confirmation is required, and this under three headings:

The first two points concern the quantity and speed of blood passing in a unit of time and the third relates to the perpetual return of blood through the veins to the heart. This is the ever recurring theme of the book: the quantity of the blood and its source. The theme has been stated and the proofs that follow are the variations upon it.

6 Ibidem, ed. 1628, p. 41; tr. WILLIS p. 46.

7 Ibidem.

8 Ibidem.

9 Ibidem, ed. 1628, p. 42; tr. WILLIS, p. 47.

1. Blood is transmitted from the veins to the arteries *continuously* and *successively* (*continue et continenter*)[10]. Its quantity is therefore too large and passes too quickly to be suppliable by the ingested food.

2. The amount of arterial blood that is sent to every part *successively, at a constant rate and continuously*[11]. It therefore exceeds by far what is required for its nutrition or what the whole mass (sc. of food) could supply.

3. The veins themselves lead this blood back to the heart and they do so *perpetually*[12].

It should be noted that each of these basic propositions conspicuously reiterates the continuity of the movement of the blood and the equal rate at which it is distributed in a unit of time. Its flow is perpetual without interruption—a fact which by itself excludes the intake of food as a factor instrumental in this.

Still in chapter IX we find the first three *proofs:* (a) by *calculus*, (b) by *experiment* and (c) by *autopsia*[13].

(a) If the actual amount of blood that passes through the ventricles of the heart during half an hour and one hour respectively is computed, the figure obtained is so great as to exclude its supply by the whole of the ingested food. Indeed it exceeds whatever could be contained in the veins at one time. There is no other source for it but the blood itself; in other words the blood perpetually recurs by running in a circuit.

(b) If by way of experiment an artery is opened, the whole system of arteries and veins will be emptied within a short interval of time.

(c) *post mortem* the left heart and the arteries are found empty, because no venous blood is transferred from the right heart to the left owing to cessation of the movement of the lungs whilst the left heart and the arteries continue to send out blood until they are empty.

The tenth chapter briefly resumes the subject of quantity and calculus, but is mainly devoted to the second great theme and its demonstration: *the venous return of the blood.* The new subject requires a new method of research, or at all events new applications of an old method: vascular ligature[13a].

When in fishes and serpents the veins are tied some way below the heart, this is speedily emptied. The stream of venous blood returning to the heart is extinguished—it is death through default (*ob defectum*). When, on the other hand, the arteries are tied, the heart becomes greatly congested—it dies by suffocation from surfeit (*ob copiam*)[14].

In the following—eleventh-chapter, ligature is further exploited

10 *De motu*, cap. IX, ed. 1628, p. 43; tr. WILLIS, p. 48.

11 Ibidem.

12 Ibidem.

13 Ibidem, ed. 1628, p. 44–46; tr. WILLIS, p. 50–52.

13a Ligature in the present context is in the first place Galenic (p. 280), then Cesalpinian (p. 173) and Fabrician (p. 20, note [12]; to Galen, see WILKIE, J.S., *Harvey's immediate debt to Aristotle and Galen, Hist. Sci.* 1965, IV, 118). It is mentioned by Harvey already in the *Lecture notes*, fol. 78 verso. Harvey writes that ligature demonstrates the attraction of humours to the part concerned, comparable to inflammatory swelling and that this is through the arteries. Hence the blueish-gangrenous discoloration after obstruction of the artery. See to this De motu cap. XI where this is corrected, and Whitteridge, G., *The anatomical lectures of William Harvey.* Edinburgh and London 1964, p. 268–269, note [3].

14 *De motu* cap. X, ed. 1628, p. 48; tr. WILLIS p. 54.

to show that blood enters a limb by the artery and returns from it by the vein. The key to this is provided by the intensity with which ligature is applied: if it is moderate, arterial blood still enters, but the venous blood collects (according to common parlance: "is attracted"—*ligaturae attrahant*) below the ligature, causing venous congestion. This is the stratagem used in venaesection. If the ligature is tight, however, no blood will enter by the artery and the latter will be distended above the ligature. This is the practice used in amputation[15].

On this rule events fundamental in practical medicine—so far ill explained—become readily understood. Such are the suppression or cause of haemorrhage, sloughing and gangrene, the assistance derived from ligature in castration and the removal of tumours.

Chapter XII is distinguished by the combination of both basic methods of approach: calculus and ligature. The amount of blood that passes after ligature and phlebotomy is now considered[16].

It remains to show how the blood finds its way back from the extremities by the veins and how the latter form the exclusive path for this purpose. This brings Harvey—in the XIIIth chapter—to a discussion of the *venous valves*. Their true function had so far not been understood. Here again *analogy* has to play its part—the analogy, that is, between the valves in the veins and those found at the roots of the pulmonary artery and the aorta in the heart. Both sets of valves serve to prevent any reflux of the blood that passes by (*hoc ... apparet valvularum officium in venis idem esse cum sigmoidarum illarum trium, quae in orificio aortae et venae arteriosae fabrefactae sunt, videlicet ut ad amussim claudantur, ne retro sanguinem transeuntem remeare sinant*)[17].

The chapter winds up with a consideration of the quantity of blood that passes between two sets of valves, whereby the *rapidity of its flow* and indeed the necessity of its circulation is proved[18].

That circular motion is of necessity ceaseless motion (*circularis motus—perpetuus motus*) and that the ingesta cannot feed it is the theme of the very brief—summarising—chapter XIV[19].

What do the heart and circulating blood achieve for the organism as a whole? This is in the first place *heat*—so we are told in the XVth chapter. The heart is its seat, origin, home and hearth and the blood its vector. Hence the latter has to be in motion, and *motion* is the second achievement—for it is through motion that we see heat and spirits to be engendered and preserved, whereas they evanesce when the matrix is at rest. Were it unmoved it would coagulate when reaching the periphery where it is far remote from

15 *De motu*, cap.XI, ed. 1628, p.48; tr. Willis p.55.

16 *De motu*, cap.XII, ed. 1628, p.54; tr. Willis p.61.

17 *De motu*, cap.XIII, ed. 1628, p.57; tr. Willis p.66.

18 "Tantum sanguinis hoc modo per unius venae partem, in non longo tempore transmissum reperies, ut de circuitu sanguinis, ab eius *celeri motu*, te persuasissimum puto sentires ... observando, *quam cito quam celeriter* sanguis sursum percurrat, et venam ab inferiori parte repleat, illud ipsum exploratum tibi fore non dubito" *De motu*, cap.XIII, in fine, ed. 1628, p.58; tr. Willis p.67.

19 *De motu* cap.XIV, ed. 1628, p.58; tr. Willis p.68.

its source. It is its movement that guarantees its regeneration, its re-charging with heat and spirit—for this is the purpose of its return to the heart. The third point is *nutrition*. Each part receives its aliment carried by the blood and consumes it.

Heart and blood, however, serve the common weal, the heart forming a store (*tanquam in cisternis, et promptuario*) for public use (*publico usui*). It is through the pulse that equality of distribution is achieved to each part and member, however small (*unicuique particulae*), in accordance with the just measure of arterial capacity in the respective part (*secundum iustitiam et proportionem cavitatum arteriarum*). To effect this—and this is the fourth achievement—impulse and force (*impetus et violentia*) are required, and something productive of it, an *impulsor*. This is the heart, and it alone can mete out the force and impulse whereby the blood is forced to leave its source and home in a centrifugal direction towards narrow and cold places, i.e. the periphery of the body. For even if there were no venous valves the blood would follow its natural inclination which is back to its home, the heart, pressed as it is from the venous capillaries (*e venis capillaribus*) into the smaller and then larger branches by the movement of the members and muscular compression[20].

Evidence for the circulation, *a posteriori* as it were, is amply provided by the moral which it carries in practical medicine and pathology, notably the spread of diseases and the distribution of curative medicines (chapter XVI)[21].

The book ends (chapter XVII) with an extensive dissertation on the comparative anatomy of the heart and its muscular function and culminates in the praise of the heart as the sovereign of the body and of Aristotle who rightly appreciated its "principality". Those who, against Aristotle, let the heart receive motion and sense from the brain and blood from the liver (the supposed origin of the veins and the blood), by-pass or do not understand the main argument. This is that the heart is the first to exist and to harbour blood, life, sense and motion before either the brain or the liver was made or became distinctly visible or at least could have functioned. The heart, equipped with its own organs for motion and like an internal animal of its own, is older. It is made first, and from it the whole animal is formed, nourished, preserved and perfected afterwards—as if Nature had intended the whole body to be its work and domicile, comparable to the ruler in a state with whom rests the first and highest power of government. In the same way the heart is the origin and foundation of the animal and from it all power is derived and upon it all power depends in the individual[22].

20 *De motu*, cap. XV, ed. 1628, pp. 58–60; tr. Willis p. 68–71.

The term "*capillary*" is not original Harveian, but Galenic. (See: Prendergast, J., *Galen's view of the vascular system in relation to that of Harvey*, *Proc. R. Soc. Med.*, 1928, XXI, 1840 [79–88]; with ref. tho the Salernitan tradition—Copho—[p. 81, note 4], and more recently Steudel, J., *Beitrag der Schule von Salerno zur anatomischen Nomenklatur. Atti XIV. Congr. Internaz. di Storia di Med.* 1954, II). It was used by Caesalpinus before Harvey. We shall return to this below (p. 183).

21 *De motu*, cap. XVI, ed. 1628, pp. 60–64; tr. Willis, p. 71–75

22 *De motu*, cap. XVII, ed. 1628, p. 70; tr. Willis, p. 83.

The strongly walled big arteries have to sustain the shock of the impelling heart and of the impetuously rushing blood (*sustinent impetum impellentis cordis et prorumpentis sanguinis*). Hence, since there is nothing that nature does in vain, the stronger and more ligamentous the arteries, the nearer they are to the heart and it is here that they differ most from the veins in constitution. The ultimate capillary divisions of the arteries (*ultimae divisiones capillares arteriosae*) impress us as veins—not merely in anatomical structure, but also in function, as they normally do not exhibit any pulse. For similar reasons there is no pulse in the pulmonary vein (*arteria venosa*) which is truly a vein, whereas the pulsating pulmonary artery (*vena arteriosa*) is a true artery. The heart and lungs are full of blood and the lungs are replete with vessels, because the heart and lungs constitute the store-house, source and treasure of the blood and the workshop of its perfection (*in pulmonibus et corde promptuarium fons et thesaurus sanguinis, et officina perfectionis est*)[23].

23 Ibidem, p. 72; tr. WILLIS, p. 85.

All these phenomena, then, which are open to anatomical observation and many others, when considered in the right way, amply illustrate and plainly confirm the truth stated at the outset and at the same time stand against vulgar opinions: for it would be rather difficult to explain why things are thus constituted and made in any way diverging from our own.

With this *De motu* ends. The truth stated has been confirmed and secured. There is no way of explaining the observable phenomnea other than in terms of blood circulation. This is the idea which occurred to Harvey when reflecting upon the quantity and source of the blood that must pass from veins to arteries via the lungs. We shall have to discuss the possible train of thoughts which eventually led Harvey to the idea and its historical background and setting (p. 209). In this not only strictly scientific and rational considerations seem to have been instrumental, but also symbolism.

With this a field of cosmological and metaphysical ideas emerges, a field apparently strange and remote from Harvey, the sober observer and rational thinker. So it appears—at first sight, but not when all facets and aspects of Harvey are taken into account. We are not going to discuss this matter now, however. It may suffice to say here that, on Harvey's own showing, the idea was first in his mind and that "it was found to be true afterwards". The proof of its truth is based on two points: (a) the quantity of blood that passes through the heart in a unit of time and (b) the return of the blood to the heart through the veins. To these two points correspond the two royal methods by which Harvey approached the proof of his idea: (a) *calculus* and (b) *vascular ligature*.

It is as simple as this. The first simple *demonstratio*, then, is afforded by (a) computation of the blood passing through the ventricles of the heart and leading to a figure far exceeding anything that could be supplied by the food ingested, (b) experimental opening of a small artery through which the whole of the blood is emptied out in a very short time and (c) autoptic observation providing the reason why the left heart and the arteries are found empty *post mortem*.

This is the result of a brief analysis of the skeleton of *De motu*, as it impresses the reader to-day. We may ask how it compares with a *similar analysis* made by a *contemporary* of Harvey. It is well known how Harvey was attacked and opposed by exponents of ruling Galenism, notably by Riolan who was really an anatomist of merit, and many smaller men. It would hardly be fair to compare their notes in our present context; nor is this really necessary, since it has been done elsewhere and on many occasions ever since Harvey's discovery has become the beacon that marks the beginning of the modern period in the History of Biology and Medicine.

It would appear to be much more to the point to examine a document to which attention has only recently been drawn: the précis of *De motu* as incorporated in the work of Andrea Argoli. For years Argoli had been a convinced adherent to the new doctrine, and that at a time when partisans were few and the ruling men against it.

Andrea Argoli's Précis of De motu (pl. 2–4)

Argoli was not a physician or biologist, but an astronomer by profession. Harvey's new doctrine did not interest him as a piece that was concerned with circularity as a cosmic principle, obeyed by the sun-like "sovereign" in the living being, the heart, and its messenger, the blood. The mere inclusion of his précis in an astronomical work called *Pandosion sphaericum* would suggest some such motive. But Argoli says nothing of the kind in this work which was published in 1644, although he had used the microcosmic analogy in a preceding work on *Critical days* (1639) in which a brief reference to blood circulation was made. The context in which the précis occurs is an appendix (cap. 41) to a dissertation (cap. 40) on the errors of physicians in working out the "critical days" from the true movements of the moon. Ignorance of circulation, Argoli says, is another source of error.

Who was Argoli? Perhaps his greatest claim to fame rests with his having taught astronomy and astrology to Wallenstein and the latter's court-astrologer Giambattista Zenno (Seni) at Padua.

He was born in Tagliacozzi in the Abruzzi in 1572 and died in 1653[24]. He had studied with Magini and published astronomical tables, ephemerides, a dissertation on the comet of 1652–1653, a treatise on the critical days and the *Pandosion sphaericum*. Of these the two latter works deserve our attention[25].

The two works appeared within those five years (1639–1644) which may be regarded as decisive in the history of the reception of Harvey's discovery, especially in Italy[26]. In 1638 Beverwijk had been the first to publish approval of Harvey's discovery in a medical treatise[27]. In the early forties' Harvey was "strenuously defended" in Rome, by Giovanni Trullio, physician to Pope Urban VIII[28]. In 1643 Claudio Berigardo gave a brief and favourable mention to Harvey's doctrine in a book devoted to Aristotelianism and fittingly called *Circulus Pisanus*[29]. In the same year an edition of Harvey's text with the two supporting letters of Johannes Walaeus had appeared at Padua[30], and only five years later de Back was able to announce the victory of the new order on all fronts[31].

Argoli's *Pandosion* is a sober astronomical treatise, informed by the new spirit of scientific inquiry. It contains for example the contemporary figures for the angle of magnetic dip in the principal cities of Europe and is distinguished by two maps of the moon[32]. However, Argoli rightly figures among the exponents of astrology[33] and especially its application to medical prognosis.

His earlier work on the *Critical days and the laying up of the sick*[34] is largely on the astrological prognosis in disease and adorned with many horoscopic diagrams. Accordingly, one might say, in this work the reference to blood circulation is embedded in an introductory exposition of the astral influence on the sublunar world and the microcosmic analogy. Plants owe their vegetative power to the lower heaven, the firmament, animals their sensitive soul to the higher, crystalline sphere, whilst the most noble rational soul has its origin in the highest of the heavens, the *Empyreum*. From it there emanate the spirits which reach the body of man where they prepare the home for the "divine particle", the soul. Man, Argoli continues, is believed to be similar to the world, the head corresponding to heaven, set with the stars of the eyes and animated with the fire of the rational soul, the arms indicating the tossing and swinging of the air, the abdomen the elementary mixture, the urinary system sea and rain, the feet the earth itself. The veins are rivers, the bones stones and the hair trees. Hence it has been observed by *students of the dissection of bodies* that the *blood*

24 For literature and further detail: PAGEL, W. and POYNTER, F. N. L., *Harvey's doctrine in Italy: Argoli (1644) and Bonaccorsi (1647) on the circulation of the blood, Bullet. Hist. Med.* 1960, XXXIV, 419–429.

For the biographical data: SUDHOFF, K., *Iatromathematiker vornehmlich im 15. und 16. Jahrhundert.* Breslau 1902, p. 79–80; also L. THORNDIKE *History of magic and experimental science* 1958, vol. VII, p. 122. Both Sudhoff and Thorndike concentrate on the treatise on *Critical days* and have not mentioned Argoli's connexion with Harvey's work. This has, however, formed the subject of a paper by MENINI, C., *Il moto circolare del sangue in un' opera astrologica padavano del 1644 (pandosion sphaericum di A. Argoli). Acta medicae historiae Patavina, 1957*–1958, pp. 121–133.

25 ARGOLI, AND., *Medici, philosophi ac in Patavino lyceo mathematicas scientias profitentis, De diebus criticis et de aegrorum decubitu libri duo.* Patavii apud Paulum frambottum 1639. – *Pandosion sphaericum in quo singula in elementaribus regionibus, atque aetherea, mathematice pertractantur.* Patavii typis Pauli Frambotti 1644; *Ed. secunda* emendatior et auctior, ibidem 1653. The number of pages is identical in both editions (354 pp), but there is a portrait and a special folding plate – two charts of the moon—in the first edition, whereas no portrait appears in the second ed. in which the charts of the moon fill one unnumbered page between pp. 22 and 23.

26 POYNTER in Pagel and Poynter, 1960, loc. cit. in note [24], p. 419–420.

27 BEVEROVICII, JOH., *De calculo renum et vesicae liber singularis* Lugd. Batavor. 1638, p. 20–24. See below in the present book pp. 99 seq. It is true that Fludd anticipated approval of Harvey's discovery by nearly a decade, but this was embedded in a cosmosophic argument. See below pp. 114 seq.

28 PAGEL and POYNTER, 1960, loc. cit in note [24], p. 240.

29 *Circulus Pisanus ... de veteri et peripatetica philosophia. In tres libros Aristotelis de anima* Utini Ex typis Nic. Schiratti 1643, circ. V., pp. 28–29 (this part of Berigardo's work may have been inspired by the publication of the Padua edition of Harvey in the same way as was Argoli's). On Berigardo in the context of circular symbolism see PREMUDA, L., *Filosofia de circoli, Aristotelismo Padovano e Guglielmo Harvey.* In: *Guglielmo Harvey—nel tricentario della morte.* Roma 1957 pp. 3–18.

30 *Guilelmi Harveji ... De motu cordis ... cui postrema hac editione accesserunt Cl. V.*

moves in a circle and imitates the stars which appear to irrigate the heavens with their light: for in this most perfect course the blood goes round the spaces in the members. This stands to reason: for were the blood on its slow course through the veins not moved in a circle it would be squeezed and dissipated; nor would it be adapted to ("imitate") the body which, according to Vitruvius, is round when the human figure with outstretched arms is inscribed in a circle[34a]. It is also most evident—for the whole body collapses when a vessel is struck, indicating the circuit of the blood diffusing through the whole circumference of the body. I find, Argoli continues, that this has been noted by some who have confirmed it with the certainty afforded by the art of dissection; they say there are two openings near the heart obvious to the more observant, through which the blood is spread and enters the heart when the veins are congested with great force or are fixed in a reclining posture. There are, then, many things in the body, the power and cause of which nobody can fathom who has not actively worked on them, for only through dissection and observation can we go beyond conjecture and guesswork. Nevertheless it stands out with the greatest clarity that Nature, content with the same small yardstick of her great art, has represented heaven in man, man in the animal and the latter in plants, each of these being somewhat more imperfect than their exemplar. Argoli then goes on to discuss whether heaven is animated and the influx and power of the celestial bodies over the world below[35].

It is thus in a strange mixture of microcosmic symbolism and reasoning based on observation that Argoli presents the circulation of the blood in this early book. There is no mention of Harvey, although an abundance of ancient authors including poets is adduced. There is only the oblique reference to those who found circulation to be established with certainty by anatomical observation.

Five years later, on the other hand, he offers in the *Pandosion* an accurate, extensive and yet succinct exposition of Harvey's doctrine. This time nothing is said about the microcosmic analogy, but again there is no mention of Harvey, although Argoli's text keeps close to *De motu*, even to the extent of repeating Harvey's reference to Fracastor's dictum that the cause of the motion of the heart is known to God alone[35a]. And yet again the number of authors quoted, ancient and contemporary, is considerable. Strangely enough we know of two similar occasions on which the name of Harvey was omitted in discussions of the circulation of the blood, at roughly the same time[36]. There is, however, one citation

Johannis Walaei ... Epistolae duae, quibus Harveji doctrina roboratur Patavii ap. Sebast. Sardum 1643. KEYNES, G., *Bibliography of the writings of Dr William Harvey.* Cambridge 1953, (2nd ed.), No. 4, p. 10 (p. 8 in the first ed. of 1928).

31 BACK, JAC. DE, *Dissertatio de corde, in qua agitur de nullitate spirituum, de haematosi, de viventium calore etc.* Roterod. 1648, p. 2.

32 PAGEL and POYNTER 1960, loc. cit in note [24], p. 421; HELLMAN, C. DORIS, *Was Tycho Brahe as influential as he thought? Brit. J. Hist. Sci.* 1963, I, part IV, 295–324 (p. 315–316).

33 See our note [24] above.

34 See note [25] above.

34a Compare Agrippa of Nettesheym, *De occulta philosophia*, lib. II, cap. 27, ed. Lugduni 1550, p. 266–267: et cum mundi membris atque archetypi mensuris sic convenientes (sc. membrorum commensurationes), ut nullum sit in homine membrum, quod non respondeat alicui signo, alicui stellae, alicui intelligentiae, alicui divino nomini in ipso archetypo deo. Tota autem corporis mensura *tornatilis* est, et *a rotunditate proveniens*, ad ipsam tendere dignoscitur.

35 *De diebus criticis*, 1639, p. 4–5.

35a This alludes to Fracastor, *De sympathia et antipathia rerum*, Venice 1546, cap. XV, fol. 18 recto which deals with alternating constriction and dilatation and mentions as one of their "*beneficia*" the attraction of air that cools the heart and the subsequent expulsion of heated air on the one hand and of soot on the other. It continues: *Quae quidem beneficia cognita Deo et naturae sunt, non autem ipsi cordi....*

36 JAC. FORBERGER in his thesis *De pulsu et eius usu*, defended at Prague under the presidency of Joh. Marcus Marci a Kronland in April 1642. As V. Kruta has shown (*Harvey in Bohemia. Physiol. Bohemo-Slovenica* 1957, VI, 433–439) it incorporates and accepts the main points of Harvey's discovery, but without any mention of Harvey. See also: PAGEL, W. and RATTANSI, P., *Harvey meets the Hippocrates of Prague (Joh.* Marcus Marci of Kronland), Med. Hist. 1964, VIII, 78–84 and below p. 287. A second example is Jean Martet (1652) who "never mentions Harvey by name and seems to draw his knowledge of the circulation from the *Epistolae duae* of Walaeus." LEFANU, W. R., *Jean Martet a French follower of Harvey* In: *Science, Medicine and History*, 1953, vol. II, 34–41 (p. 36).

of a contemporary man with reference to circulation: an otherwise unknown anatomical demonstrator at Padua, Johannes Georgius Verden who does not seem to have published a single line. According to Argoli, he had carried out experiments at Padua "a few months back" designed to measure the volume of arterial blood emitted from each contraction of the left ventricle in small and large dogs.

The appearance, at Padua, of a new edition of *De motu*, just a year prior to the *Pandosion*, may have prompted the inclusion in the latter of a précis of the former. It may also explain the omission of the name of Harvey which, through this very edition, might have been thought to be in everybody's mind in Italy at the time. That this was not the case is shown by Bartholomeo Bonaccorsi's book *On the pulse* of 1647[37]. In this reference is merely made to and an abstract given from Argoli's account, whilst the whole idea of circulation is rejected on orthodox Galenic lines. Strangely enough, however, the milk channels are said to have been "suggested by the Pisan Harvey"[38], although Aselli who first described them and might well have been compared with Harvey by a compatriot was born at Cremona and Professor at Pavia and not at Pisa; he was buried at Milan.

What, then, can we learn from Argoli's précis of *De motu*? He calls it a brief epilogue to the discussion of the errors of physicians in the working out of the critical days in diseases. Their errors due to ignorance of the circular motion of the blood are far worse, however, and for this reason he wants to deal with the circulation of the blood that is the instrument whereby the motion of the heart is communicated to the body and which has remained unknown since antiquity.

1. The heart exists in animals—higher as well as lower species down to insects in which we can feel pulsation in the extreme end of the tail without any doubt. With this Argoli alludes to the fourth chapter of *De motu*[39].

2. He then continues about the movements of the heart in man. Food, converted by the heat of the stomach into chyle, is led to the root of the mesentery from the small as well as the large gut and from here through small milk-ducts conveyed to the liver. This we know by consistent experience as well as by ocular inspection. It is not so conveyed, as erroneously believed throughout antiquity, by the mesenteric veins; for in these even the first rudiment of chyle is never found. Moreover it is the milky ducts which the eye sees filled with chyle, and when they are ligated at the root of the mesentery their central parts near the liver collapse,

37 Bonaccorsi, Barth., *Della natura de polsi*. Bologna, Giacomo Monti, 1647 (dedicated to "alla Serenissima Maria Gonzaga duchessa di Mantova"), p. 42–53. See: Pagel and Poynter, 1960, loc. cit. in note [24], p. 426–429.

38 "Detti condotti lattei furno proposti da l'Arveo Pisano", p. 45.

39 *De motu*, cap. IV, ed. 1628, p. 28; tr. Willis p. 29.

whereas the peripheral parts near the gut swell up, because of the inflow of chyle.

The chyle concocted into blood by the heat of the liver is infused into the vena cava—which is obvious to everybody, because when the vein is ligated above the liver it swells where the blood enters from the latter. Through the vena cava the blood streams into the right ventricle of the heart, as everybody knows. It can also be demonstrated through ligation of the vein—the parts towards the heart being emptied whereas those towards the liver, its origin, are filled. By means of ligation the same thing can be shown to hold with regard to the continuation of the flow through the right heart into the lungs and through the venous artery into the left heart and finally into the arteries large and small.

Argoli's reference to the chyle is not indebted directly to Aselli, the discoverer of the milk ducts (1622), but is clearly based on the first of Walaeus's *Epistolae duae*, *De motu chyli*, published in the Padua edition of Harvey's text. The ligation of the ducts and the vena cava were part of the experiments carried out by Walaeus. Ligation of the vena cava was first mentioned by Harvey in his first letter to Riolan of 1649[40]. Nevertheless it is to the recourse to Harvey's basic method of demonstration and proof, namely vascular ligature, that due prominence is accorded by Argoli.

3. From the arteries the blood is carried down into the veins. That these can be entered through *oscula* is demonstrable in the cadaver. Moreover, when the aorta is tied above the heart and the jugular vein and another artery are opened, every single artery will be found empty and the veins full—a sure indication that the blood had been infused from the arteries into the veins. It is for the same reason that we find the arteries depleted and the veins full *post mortem*. Moreover, in haemorrhage when there is increased pulsation the arteries will empty quickly, whereas in fainting, loss of consciousness, and fear, when there is little pulsation of the heart and arteries, the flow of blood from these is damped down. Here Argoli repeats the argument found at the end of chapter nine of *De motu*[41].

4. If in venaesection the ligature of the arm is very tight above the incision, the blood flow from the vein is diminished because of impaired arterial supply, whereas it will flow freely when the cord is loosened. This comes from Harvey's chapter eleven[42].

5. The motion of the heart—interpreted by the ancients in various ways and thought by Fracastor to be known to God alone —is nothing but a swallowing of blood and its transfusion into

40 Walaeus as quoted in note [30]. – HARVEY, *First letter to Riolan*, Roterod. 1649, p. 44; tr. WILLIS p. 104.

41 *De motu*, cap. IX, ed. 1628, p. 46; tr. WILLIS p. 52.

42 *De motu*, cap. XI, ed. 1628, p. 49; tr. WILLIS p. 55 seq.

the arteries. This is the definition given by Harvey in the fifth chapter[43].

6. It takes place in the following manner: the flowing blood dashes against the auricle of the heart which thereupon contracts and injects it into the ventricle. When the latter is filled the heart erects itself immediately and rises up into a point, contracts sideways, is elongated through tension of the fibres and becomes smaller in width. When it thus moves it beats the chest and pulsates. When touched during its motion it feels somewhat hard—its hardness being due to tension, contraction and motion of the fibres. Hence the motion of the heart is a kind of constriction of all fibres whereby the blood is driven out. For it appears to be erected, hardened, diminished and strengthened by the same mechanism which accounts for the tension, hardening and lifting up of muscles. Pulsating, the heart continually drives the blood received from the auricle through the right ventricle into the lungs and through the left ventricle into the aorta and the rest of the arteries, each time by one contraction and systole. When the heart is moved and constricted, the true systole and coarctation occurs—this phase is wrongly called diastole by the physicians, for in—arterial—diastole the arteries are dilated and produce the pulse, as at this moment of time the arteries are filled and distended like a paunch or bladder.

In this way Argoli summarises Harvey's second and a passage from his third chapter[44].

7. When the right ventricle of the heart discharges and expels the blood which it contains, the arterial vcin pulsates and is dilated from the influx of blood; when the left ventricle ceases to pulsate and to be contracted, the movement of the arteries and the pulse ceases likewise; for the motion of the arteries depends upon immission of blood resulting from the contraction of the ventricle, the blood, that is, by which the arteries are filled and extended; the pulse is nothing but the impulse of the blood driven into the arteries from the left ventricle (abstracted from Harvey's third chapter)[45].

8. This motion of the heart they (!) compare to the drinking of water by a horse, for in each single draught and deglutition a sound is produced through the discharge of the water into the stomach—a sound that is not different from the pulse, as we can see every day; thus when it (sc. the heart) discharges each individual portion of blood into the arteries, this movement and pulse is heard at the chest. Thus we read in a passage from the fifth chapter of *De motu*[46].

43 *De motu*, cap.V, ed. 1628, p.30; tr. WILLIS, p.32.

44 *De motu*, cap.VI, ed. 1628, p.22; tr. WILLIS p.22. – cap.III, ed. 1628, p.24; tr. WILLIS p.25.

45 *De motu*, cap.III, ed. 1628, p.24–25; tr. WILLIS p.24–25.

46 *De motu*, cap.V, ed. 1628, p.30; tr. WILLIS, p.32.

9. Argoli then returns to Harvey's third chapter: Diastole and arterial dilatation are from the impulse of the blood (as we have said) and not from the impact of the same blood that is transferred by the arteries from one part to the other, as some people made out. For in their diastole (i.e. arterial diastole) all parts of the arteries are simultaneously dilated; they cannot[47] be constricted at one and the same time and expel the blood in subsequent parts: for the blood is moved by the pulsation of the heart and not otherwise, as we can observe in the vivisected dog when the heart contracts; for when at that time a hole is made in any of the arteries blood is seen to gush out—the same is seen when the aorta or the arterial vein or the apex or the middle part of the heart are transversely incised: blood is expelled while the heart is contracted in systole and not in diastole[48].

10. In the dying animal the left ventricle is the first to stop pulsating, then follows its auricle, later the right ventricle, and at last the right auricle in which life seems to remain longest, for after two or three motions and contractions of this auricle the heart exerts one sluggish pulse and the animal dies (abstracted from Harvey's fourth chapter)[49].

11. Argoli continues his abstract in the first person: "it seems *to me* that doctors have fallen into a further error about the heart". Really, however, Argoli is contracting several passages from Harvey's Introduction into one paragraph[50]. Whilst doctors concede, Argoli says, that the heart is the spring of vital spirits by which life is communicated to the whole of the body, they contend that spirits are only generated in the left ventricle, but in no way in the right one; the only function of the latter, they say, is to furnish nourishment for the lung. I cannot understand their reasoning (*nec eorum rationem capio*), Argoli continues, for form, pathways, vessels and fabric of auricles, fibres and bands are the same in both, and they are in the same manner and at the same time filled with blood; and it cannot follow that the right ventricle serves a private purpose, namely the alimentation of the lung, the left, however, a public service, the enlivening of the whole body and that by the ministry of the same blood.

12 Repeating Harvey's conclusion from the fourteenth chapter of *De motu*[51] Argoli states: it has been demonstrated that the blood is driven from the liver through the vena cava into the right ventricle of the heart, whence it is conveyed to the lungs by the arterial vein. It returns from there to the left ventricle of the heart by the venous artery; and at last it passes from the left ventricle into the aorta and the remaining arteries from which it is

47 Argoli, *Pandosion*, p. 207 reads in both editions: "nam in diastole omnes arteriarum partes simul dilatantur; possunt eodem tempore constringi, et sanguinem in succedentes partes expellere: sanguis enim pulsione a corde movetur; nec alio modo" —obviously it should read: *non* possunt eodem tempore constringi....

48 *De motu*, cap. III, ed. 1628, p. 24; tr. Willis, p. 24. – Introduction pp. 12 et seq.

49 *De motu*, cap. IV, ed. 1628, p. 26; tr. Willis p. 27.

50 *De motu*, Introd. ed. 1628, p. 15; tr. Willis, p. 14–15

51 *De motu*, cap. XIV, ed. 1628, p. 58; tr. Willis, p. 68.

distributed into the veins and to the whole body for its nutrition. Having completed this course mostly the same blood goes from the small veins to the larger ones and hence the vena cava; from the latter it is again led to the right ventricle of the heart, to the lungs, and from the latter to the left ventricle, the arteries, and finally into the veins, as before, perpetually completing this circulation (*hanc circulationem perpetuo absolvens*); and as the controversy hinges upon a fact, truth is to be confirmed by experience rather than by reasoning (*cumque haec lis consistat in facto; potius experientia, quam rationibus veritas confirmanda*)[52].

13 We have said, and there is no doubt about it, that the heart always transmits in each systole, stress and contraction a certain quantity of blood from the left ventricle into the arteries. The amount is stated differently by different people. John George Verden, the very expert anatomist at Padua, found some months ago that in a small dog about one drachm is expelled at each contraction and in a bigger sheep dog more than two drachms. Supposing that in man the heart transmits at least one scruple of blood to the aorta and arterial system in a single systole and contraction, and contracts at least three thousand times per hour, it will expel in one hour three thousand scruples of blood or one thousand drachms, or one hundred and twenty five ounces or ten pounds five ounces, and in a twenty-four hour day two hundred and fifty pounds of blood, that is more blood than is found in fifteen to twenty men together—and these are not old wives' tales.

Argoli here roughly follows Harvey's computation as laid down in the ninth chapter of *De motu*[53], but with some interesting modifications. These may well express the results obtained by Verden. For the large dog Argoli gives 1–2 drachms per systole as against one third of this (1 scruple) as given by Harvey. Strangely enough, in man Argoli works on a one scruple basis per systole as against Harvey's one drachm per systole, but arrives at the same end result: 10 pounds and five ounces, like the latter, but with the difference that Argoli's is the figure for one hour as against Harvey's half an hour, and Argoli assumed 3000 systoles per hour as against Harvey's 2000. It should be noted that in both cases minimum figures are given, and Harvey enlarges upon the different results that are obtained when different amounts of blood are assumed to be ejected in systole (viz. one and two drachms, half an ounce and one ounce per ½ hour). It is well known that Harvey underestimated the cardiac output considerably and worked on the basis of a pathologically slow pulse rate. Although the latter is somewhat improved in Argoli's account, the latter's figures,

52 Argoli, *Pandosion*, p. 208.

53 *De motu*, Cap. IX, ed. 1628, p. 43 seq.; tr. Willis, p. 49–50.

though tripled in the case of the dog, bring no improvement for man. Obviously Verden had contented himself with a rough estimate on the basis of Harvey's figures and not thought of other confirmatory methods, which he could have employed, such as weighing the amount of blood obtainable from a cut in the aorta in one minute and comparing it with the heart beat[54].

14. If in venaesection, Argoli continues, blood is allowed to flow out for about half an hour, most of the body blood will thus have been evacuated, resulting in collapse of arteries and veins, syncope and fainting. It would be ridiculous to assume that all these pounds of blood are found in the arm locally. Hence it must come from other parts, all the more so as it does not reach the venaesection opening from the parts above, but from those below, such as hand and fingers where such amount of blood cannot possibly be present. Reference is thus made to the twelfth chapter *De motu*[55].

15. That the blood flows in from the inferior parts emerges from experiment, for when an opening is made in the brachial vein and the peripheral part towards the hand is compressed no blood will flow. Hence it must come from the parts below and this is why surgeons (though ignorant of the reason) make their ligature in the upper part of the arm above the venaesection wound, so that the veins swell due to the inflow of blood from the inferior parts of the hands. They relax this ligature somewhat lest no blood be driven from the arteries into the veins because of too tight a constriction.

16. It is also evident from this that when we compress with one hand the inferior part of a visible vein of the arm or hand which has no branches and with the other hand streak the blood upwards, the veins will remain collapsed and bloodless—to be refilled immediately we release the inferior part from the compressing hand.—With these sentences Argoli gives the gist of the thirteenth and partly the eleventh chapter of *De motu*[56].

17. Argoli then interjects with reference to chapter nine[57]: If there were no circulation of the blood, how could butchers remove its whole amount in animals from the jugular veins alone?

18. Moreover, Argoli continues, the mass of blood that is propelled from the arteries into the veins and the parts of the body exceeds that necessary for the nutrition of the latter; nor would it be possible for the liver to furnish, by virtue of its blood production, from nutriment, that quantity of blood that is driven from the heart into the arteries: it is therefore of necessity to be conceded that the blood runs through veins and arteries in a perpetual

54 This alternative method was suggested in the case of Harvey by KILGOUR, F. G., *William Harvey; Scientific American*, 1952, CLXXXVI, 58–62 (p. 61). See below p. 73.

55 *De motu*, cap. XII, ed. 1628, p. 54; tr. WILLIS, p. 61.

56 *De motu*, cap. XI, ed. 1628, p. 50; tr. WILLIS, p. 55–57. – Cap. XIII, ed. 1628, p. 57; tr. WILLIS, p. 67.

57 *De motu*, ed. 1628, p. 45; tr. WILLIS, p. 51.

circular motion: *necessario ergo concedendum est sanguinem circulari motu perpetuo circa venas, et arterias concursantem*. Thus Argoli paraphrases the same passage from the twelfth chapter which he had abstracted before (see above note 55)—the passage that closes with the words: a continual new flow of blood must be suggested, and that from the veins, whence a circuit is necessary, as it cannot be supplied from ingested food and is much greater in quantity than is adequate for nutrition of the parts: *novum continuo sanguinem suggerere debet idque e venis necessarium est, circuitum fieri; cum nec suppeditari ab assumptis possit et longe plus est, quam partium nutritioni congruens erat*[58].

19. In contagious diseases, syphilis, poisoned wounds, the bite of a rabid dog or a snake, and similar lesions, even when the affected part is healed, the whole body is nevertheless damaged; and although the harmful agent is only imprinted into the blood of that small infected part, its virulence and harmfulness is of necessity communicated to the heart and the other parts of the body because of the circuit of the blood. Thus medicines applied externally alter the other parts of the body beyond that to which they have been applied. This is evident in cantharides which, wherever applied, excite the urine at once, and in colocynth and similar herbs that move the belly.

With this Argoli summarises Harvey's chapter sixteen and *concludes:*

The circulation of the blood being thus established disposes of the famous "derivations" and "revulsions" of the physicians and many other things in medicine fall to the ground—just as on the other hand very many problems beset with difficulties meet their solution, on which, with God's help, we will talk some other time[60].

Argoli's, then, is an extensive and factual account of the contents of *De motu* without any resort to argumentation, symbolism or metaphysics. It is on the whole well arranged, although it does not by any means keep to the sequence of the chapters, facts and arguments as arrayed by Harvey. The two main points—quantification and venous return—are accorded due prominence and, being left to the end, so to speak "crown" his narrative. He made a feeble effort to supplement Harvey's figures for the cardiac output of blood, but they are based on vague statements and reference to a completely unknown authority and amount to little more than an ineffectual slight modification of the more precise and still better figures of Harvey (however unsatisfactory the latter may appear today)[61]. Though he went into some detail anatomical as

58 *De motu*, cap.XII, ed. 1628, p.54; tr. WILLIS, p.61.

59 *De motu*, cap.XVI, p.61; tr. WILLIS, p.71–72.

60 ARGOLI, *Pandosion*, p.209.

61 According to Kilgour, loc. cit. in note [54] Harvey obtained a figure for cardiac output which is one 36th of the lowest value accepted to-day. See below, p. 73.

well as experimental, in several places, Argoli omitted to mention the venous valves.

Argoli's précis is well worded and reasoned and his conclusion particularly apt and to the point, referring as it does to the revolutionising role in which Harvey's discovery already made itself felt in Argoli's own time—a time in which still much ink was spilt over the question whether venaesection should be performed on the diseased side, as prescribed by the ancients (by *derivation*), or on the opposite side as advocated by the Arabs (by *revulsion*). Argoli is fully conscious of the fact that the futility of this and similar questions of medical practice had been brought home by the discovery of circulation and that many such "problems" would fall by the wayside in the future.

Harvey's Scientific Approach—
his Quantification—
and Harvey's Circular Symbolism

With the new method of dissection and pictorial representation in Anatomy as introduced by Vesalius (1543), the scientific demonstration of blood circulation by Harvey sometime in the sixteen twenties marks the foundation of modern scientific medicine. The truly scientific element and hallmark of Harvey's discovery is usually found in the *calculus* which he applied[1]. Harvey's quantitative reasoning is said to form the dividing line between him and his predecessors. His discovery—so it is interpreted—pivots around this point; it is its *sine qua non.*

However, this assessment has been criticised in its turn[2]. Harvey's measurements were rough and not accurate, so we are told. There was no need for him to be more precise than he was in demonstrating his great discovery. Moreover he could have resorted to much more elegant quantitative demonstrations than he did; for example he could have measured the amount of blood spurting from an artery and collated it with the number of heart beats in any given period. Instead, he based his conclusions on rough estimates of the volume of the ventricles during systole and diastole, leaving wide margins of error.

A tendency to overemphasise the significance of calculation has thus been said to prevail in the modern appraisal of Harvey's discovery—an endeavour to present Harvey as a modern scientist à *tout prix*. For—it has been inferred—Harvey's discovery loses little when his calculus is not taken into account, its weakness is fully appreciated and emphasis is shifted to his sure reasoning, based as it is on correct interpretation of anatomical, physiological and experimental data.

We are inclined to question at least the historical justification of this point of view. For Harvey himself regarded his calculations as decisive. This emerges from his statements and their frequent repetition to the effect that it is the calculus which makes the circulation of the blood inevitable.

However much time it takes the whole mass of blood to go round, "it is still manifest that more blood passes through the heart continually through its pulsation, than can either be supplied by the ingested food or be contained in the veins at the same time.[3]" And not far below in the same chapter: "Supposing even the smallest quantity of blood to be passed through the lungs and the heart, a much more plentiful amount is taken through the arteries and the whole body than could be possibly supplied by the ingestion of food—which can only be achieved by the return through a circuit" ("*longe uberiori proventu, in arterias et totum corpus deducitur, quam ab alimentorum ingestione suppeditari possibile sit, nisi regressu per*

1 Notably Sigerist, H.E., *William Harvey's Stellung in der europäischen Geistesgeschichte. Arch.f.Kulturgesch.* 1929, XIX, 158–168. To this: Pagel, W., *The position of Harvey and Van Helmont in the History of European thought, J.Hist.Med.* 1958, XIII, 186–199; Peller, S., *Harvey's and Cesalpino's role in the History of Medicine, Bullet. Hist.Med.* 1949, XXIII, 213–235. To this: Pagel, W., *Harvey's role in the History of Medicine, Bullet.Hist.Med.*, 1950, XXIV, 70–73; Shryock, R.H., *History of Quantification in Medical Science, Isis*, 1961, LII, 215–237.

2 Kilgour, F.G., *William Harvey's use of the quantitative method. Yale J.Biol.Med.*, 1954, XXVI, 410–421; idem, loc. cit. above p. 67, note [54]: Harvey "finally calculated that the cardiac output must be at least 3.9 g per beat. According to a present-day estimate, it is actually in the neighbourhood of 89 g ... Harvey also missed the mark widely in his other important measurement—the pulse rate. Somehow he counted it to be 33 per minute, about half the actual average rate... With his two estimates—3.9 g for cardiac output and 33 pulse beats per minute—he obtained a figure for the rate of blood flow which is one–36th of the lowest value accepted today". – See also in more general terms: Jevons, F.R., *Harvey's quantitative method. Bullet.Hist.Med.*, 1962, XXXVI, 462–467.

3 *De motu* cap.IX, ed. 1628, p.44. tr. Willis p.49.

circuitum facto")[4]. It can be shown by computation that the heart passes as much and more in the course of an hour or two than the abundant supply of milk—3–7 gallons—which a cow produces in a day and which is manifestly derived from food[5]. If we calculate how much blood flows through one arm, we can estimate how much passes through the other arm and indeed through the lower extremities, the neck and so on; we shall come to the conclusion that the blood must of necessity make a circuit through the veins, for such quantities of blood cannot be supplied by the food and are much more than is suitable for the nutrition of the parts[6]. If argument and ocular demonstration ("ocularibus experimentis") have shown that blood is thrown through the pulse of the ventricles into the whole body and through the veins taken back from the circumference to the centre, in such a quantity and flux and reflux as cannot be supplied by the food and even surpasses all that is suitable for the nutriment of the parts it is necessary to conclude that in animals the blood is by some circular motion driven in a circuit and is in perpetual motion ("*tanta copia, tanto fluxu, refluxu ... ut ab assumptis suppeditari non possit, atque multo quidem, majori* (*quam conveniret nutritioni*) *proventu; necessarium est concludere, circulari quodam motu, in circuitum agitari in animalibus sanguinem et esse in perpetuo motu*")[7].

4 *De motu* cap.IX, ed.1628, p.45; tr. WILLIS p.50.

5 *De motu* cap.X, ed.1628, p.47; tr. WILLIS p.53.

6 *De motu* cap.XII, ed.1628, p.54; tr. WILLIS p.61.

7 *De motu* cap.XIV, ed.1628, p.58; tr. WILLIS p.68.

Quantification emphasized by Harvey's critic Riolan

It was, then, Harvey himself who attributed major significance to quantification and indeed saw in the result of his computation the crowning proof of his ocular and experimental observations. It is therefore not remote posterity which caused Harvey to appear in this light—bent as it is on the true scientific and "modern" character of Harvey's achievement.

This is further supported by the attitude taken by Harvey's *immediate successors*, by friend and foe alike. In the polemical arguments put up against Harvey by Riolan the younger (1580–1657) the same quantitative considerations which we find in Harvey are given prominence and even used to prove a limited "circulatory" movement of blood. Riolan believed in a consumption of the blood in the periphery and thus denied any circulation through the smaller arterial branches into the smaller veins. He was prepared, however, to admit and to offer as a substitute to true circulation—Harvey's closed circuit of the whole blood—a kind of circle completed by some of the blood from the liver, using the traditional Galenic routes through the vena cava, septal pores, aorta and through direct anastomoses of the latter back to the vena cava. He also admitted that in a state of agitation a "violent circulation" occurs whereby blood is transferred from the right ventricle via the lungs to the left whence it reaches the veins through arterio-venous anastomoses and returns to the right ventricle of the heart—*atque ita perficitur circulatio, continuo fluxu et refluxu sanguinis*. It is thus that venous blood perpetually and naturally ascends and returns to the heart, whilst arterial blood descends and recedes from it. Indeed the continuity of the motion of the heart postulates a "circulation" of the blood which, in Riolan's scheme, could be upheld without "confusion and perturbation of the humours and the destruction of ancient medicine."

Obviously this alternative theory was brought about by the impact of Harvey's discovery—and so was a quantitative consideration which we find in Riolan's earlier work directed against Harvey: the *Enchiridium Anatomicum et Pathologicum* of 1648. Here it says: if in each individual pulsation the heart admits one or the other drop of blood which it ejects into the aorta and within the hour two thousand pulsations occur, a large portion of the whole of the blood will of necessity pass the heart within twelve to fifteen hours, a quantity which can equal fifteen or twenty pounds of blood as contained in the vessels. Hence within twenty four hours the blood is rolled back through the heart twice or three times, according to the greater or lesser rate of velocity of the heart beat[8]. Harvey himself quoted this passage from Riolan as an argument inadvertently put forward by the latter against himself[9].

The same Riolanus gives even more space to "quantification" in his extensive *Great Restitution of Physic and Medicine through the New Doctrine concerning the Circulatory Motion of Blood in the Heart* as contained in his *Opuscula Anatomica Nova* and published in London in 1649. Here he says: It remains to show that the circulation of the blood according to Harvey's scheme cannot possibly take place three times or more often within a day. First it is assumed that more blood is transmitted from the Vena cava to the heart than the liver can supply. This Harvey proves by finding—*experimento*—two ounces of blood in the cavity of the left ventricle, an amount which should be propelled by the ventricle in a single systole. If, then, the heart within an hour pulsates three thousand times or more, the whole venous blood should pass through within six or seven hours, i.e. up to twenty four pounds in a well nourished and sanguine body (as estimated by Avicenna). But, Riolanus continues, Harvey did not take into account that he over-estimated the amount, as he found

8 RIOLANUS, Jo. (fil.), *Encheiridium anatomicum et pathologicum*. Paris 1648, Lib. III, cap. 8: de corde, p. 295. – For a general appraisal of Riolan's position in the history of the reception of Harvey's discovery: ROTHSCHUH, K.E., *Jean Riolan jun. (1580–1657) im Streit mit Paul Marquart Schlegel (1605–1653) um die Blutbewegungslehre Harveys. Ein Beitrag z. Geschichte und Psychologie des wissenschaftlichen Irrtums Gesnerus*, 1964, XXI, 72–82. – On *advanced anti-Galenic views* held by RIOLAN see below: p. 216 and note [31], p. 217.

9 HARVEY, *Exercit. anatom. de circulatione sanguinis I ad Jo. Riolanum*. Roterodami 1649, p. 10; tr. WILLIS, p. 92.

it in hearts that were dying or slowing down and therefore harbouring a quantity which it would have taken twenty systoles and more to eject. Instead even one drop of blood passing through the interventricular septum would in Riolanus' opinion become inflated, foamy, spirituous and thereby prone to escape impetuously. A similar argument had been put forward before by Primrose—so Riolanus says[10]. Farther below Riolanus admits that the consideration of quantities (of blood passing through the heart) is the foundation of circulation (*atque hoc est praecipuum fundamentum circulationis sanguinis*)[11]. There must be a return of blood to the heart in order to keep up its function—which it could not do otherwise in view of the loss of fluid incurred by transpiration and excretion through the gut, the lungs and the brain. Such quantitative considerations are also shown to have a decisive bearing on venaesection and many other provinces of theoretical and practical medicine[12].

Quantification in early accounts of De motu: Argoli, Martet, Micraelius

The high historical significance which Harvey's calculus can really claim also emerges from its inclusion in summary accounts of circulation already in the early forties and fifties of the century. We quote three examples: one is the compendious chapter on the circulation of the blood given by the astronomer Andrea Argoli in his *Pandosion sphaericum* of 1644[13]—the work which we discussed in the preceding chapter[14].

The second example is Jean Martet who, like Argoli, nowhere names Harvey in his *Abbrégé des nouvelles expériences Anatomiques sur la circulation du sang* of 1652. He gives as the first and foremost of the "raisons par lesquelles on prouve la circulation du sang" the known quantity of blood drawn from the veins at each diastole —"judge how much is drawn up in a day, and that if the blood does not return into the veins they would soon be emptied; conversely the same quantity of blood is forced into the arteries and yet they do not burst[15].

As a third example we may cite the short entry *Sanguinis circulatio*, unexpectedly found in the *Philosophical Lexicon* of Micraelius, in 1653. It follows a short note on the blood which is said to be the principal humour of living beings (*animantium*)—rubicund, sweet, warm and analogous to air (*respondens aeri*). It is formed in the liver from the more temperate parts of the chyle by virtue of its innate heat and that derived from the heart for the preservation and nutrition of the parts of the human body. There is on one

10 Riolanus, Jo., *Opuscula Anatomica Nova... Instauratio magna Physicae et Medicinae per novam doctrinam de Motu Circulatorio Sanguinis in Corde.* Londini 1649, cap. VI, p. 40. See also Casp. Hofmann, below p. 197.

11 Riolanus, loc. cit. in note [10] *Opuscula*, cap. XV, p. 63.

12 Riolanus, loc. cit. in note [10] *Opuscula*, cap. XIX, p. 71 et seq.

13 Argoli, And., *Pandosion Sphaericum in quo singula in Elementaribus regionibus, atque Aetherea, mathematica pertractantur.* Patavii 1644. cap. XLI: De motu circulari sanguinis et motu Cordis, pp. 205–209. J. G. Verden mentioned on p. 208 with identical pagination in the second edition, Patav. 1653.

14 See above pp. 59–69.

15 Lefanu, Wm. R., *Jean Martet a French Follower of Harvey. Science, Medicine and History.* Oxford 1953, vol. II, pp. 34–41.

hand the venous blood from the liver which continuously flows in the veins and on the other the arterial blood that is generated in the heart, dispersed through the body by the arteries, warmer than the venous blood, lighter coloured (*flavior*) and spurting forth in a jet (*exeundo saliens*). This brief account of the blood is traditional in the distinction which is made between venous and arterial blood, the former generated in the liver and continually moving in the veins, the latter in the heart, and dispersed through the arteries. However, the entry continues, the *circulation of the blood* has recently started to be demonstrated by Harvey and others. These present it in their writings (*quam fieri scribunt*) in eleven stages: 1. the transmission of chyle through the milky veins from the small gut to the mesenteric lymphnode; 2. from there into the liver; 3. from the liver in the purer form of blood to the vena cava and 4. into the right chamber of the heart; then 5. into the arterial vein, 6. the lungs, 7. through the venous artery into the left chamber of the heart, 8. to the aorta and the remaining arterioles, thence 9. to the smaller veins through anastomoses and openings or even into the flesh itself, 10. from the smaller veins into the larger ones and the vena cava itself and 11. from the vena cava, together with that blood which is newly formed in the liver, back into the right ventricle of the heart etc.

There is only one reason given for the new theory: the argument from quantity. "They" conclude that more than ten pounds of blood pass through the heart per hour. For there are more than 3000 pulses per hour in each of which at least a scruple (20 grains, one third of a dram) leaves the heart. This circulation which is completed in less than an hour, is neither the result of an innate power of the blood nor of spirits, but of the "drive" (*a pulsu*) from the vena cava into the right ventricle and from there into the arterial vein. The author finishes the entry with a short rider concerning the formation of blood from chyle—noting the discovery of the lacteals, but still being ignorant of that of the thoracic duct[16].

16 MICRAELII, JOH., *Lexicon Philosophicum terminorum philosophis usitatorum.* Jenae 1653, p. 979–980.

Quantification ancient (Galen, Erasistratus) and contemporary with Harvey (Santorius, Van Helmont)

Indeed, then, the new teaching of circulation pivoted around the consideration of quantity, not only in the opinion of Harvey, but also in that of his close contemporaries—friend, foe and independent chronicler. The computation as it stood was deemed good enough to demonstrate and secure the principle—whatever "better" proposals present-day scientists may suggest. Harvey obviously had no need for these in "crowning" his demonstration by calculus: "If any transmission of blood occurs in any amount in individual pulsations, let them suppose whatever quantity they wish (I am not referring to how much I saw), immediately convinced on this basis by the computed pulsations, they must agree that the blood goes round."[17]

Nor does it detract from the scientific character and historical significance of Harvey's calculus that he was neither the first nor the only "savant" to set up such a calculus.

As Owsei Temkin has shown[18] Galen had already used quantitative reasoning suggesting "a certain structural similarity with Harvey's calculation in support of the circulation of the blood". The point in question was the rejection of the theory that the urine is residual matter from the nutrition of the kidneys. In Galen's opinion "the amount of urine passed every day shows clearly that it is the whole of the fluid drunk which becomes urine, except for that which comes away with the dejections or passes off as sweat or insensible transpiration." Moreover the larger viscera would have to show much more daily residual matter, and all organs would need bladders to excrete them. Thus it would be quite unreasonable to assume that small organs such as the kidneys "have four whole congii (about 14 quarts) and sometimes even more, of residual matter." This applies even more when one considers the actual amount of fluid as taken in during a drinking bout.

The whole argument was based on Galen's observation that the kidneys "will quickly produce about 10–14 quarts (3–4 congii) of urine from about the same amount of wine ingested"[19]. Galen also had a "quantitative scheme" for food as well as for measuring the potency of drugs, and so had Erasistratus, four hundred years before Galen, for measuring emanations from the body—the latter in fact anticipating the famous experiment made on himself by Santorius and described in his *Medicina statica* of 1614. If, said Erasistratus, one were to weigh an animal (left without food) together with the excrement that has been visibly passed one would find a great loss of weight, because a copious emanation has taken place[20]. Or in the words of Santorius: "If eight pounds of meat and drink are taken in one day, the quantity that usually goes off by insensible perspiration in that time is five pounds.[21]" Since antiquity numerical estimates had always been connected with the observation of the pulse and of the movements of fluid[22].

Santorius preceded Harvey by fourteen years. Van Helmont's quantitative considerations and experiments were contemporary with Harvey, though published only in the year of Van Helmont's

17 WILLIAM HARVEY, *letter to Caspar Hofmann*. Nürnberg, May 20th 1636, as for the first time discussed and completely transcribed by F. N. L. POYNTER in: FERRARIO, E.V., POYNTER, F.N.L. and FRANKLIN, K.J., *William Harvey's debate with Caspar Hofmann on the Circulation of the Blood.* J.Hist.Med. 1960, XV, 7–21.

18 TEMKIN, OWSEI, *A Galenic Model for Quantitative Reasoning? Bullet.Hist.Med.* 1961, XXXV, 470–475 with ref. to GALEN, *On the Natural Faculties* I, cap. 17: Urine is not residual matter from the nutrition of the kidneys.

19 GALEN, *De naturalibus facultatibus* lib. I, cap. 17, ed. Kühn, vol. II, p. 72. – p. 70: hoti men oun auto to pinomenon hapan uron ginetai, plen ei ti kata ton diachorematon hypelthen, e eis hidrotas apechoresen, e kata ten adelon diapnoen, enargos endeiknytai to plethos ton kath' hekasten hemeran ouroumenon. – p. 72: ei gar hoi nephroi tois kothonizomenois treis e tettaras eniote choas poiousi perittomatos, hekastou ton allon splanchnon pollo pleious esontai, kai pithou tinos houto megistou deesei tou dexomenou ta panton perittomata. – See TEMKIN, loc. cit. in note [18], p. 474. To: kata ten adelon diapnoen—insensible transpiration—TEMKIN, O., *Nutrition from Classical Antiquity to the Baroque* in *Human Nutrition historic and scientific.* Monograph III, New York, p. 86 (note): "the Greek word ... may mean respiration as well as transpiration including not only gases but sweat as well."

20 pollen apophoran gegenesthai: *Anonymi Londinensis ex Aristotelis Iatricis Menoniis et aliis medicis Eclogae*, ed. H. Diels. Berol. 1893, *Eclogae physiologicae* XXXIII, 45–55. – See also TEMKIN, loc. cit. in *Human Nutrition* in note [19], p. 87 with ref. to JONES, W.H.S., *Medical Writings of Anonymus Londinensis*, Cambridge 1947, p. 127.

21 Si cibus et potus unius diei sit ponderis octo librarum, transpiratio insensibilis ascendere solet ad quinque libras circiter: *Ars Sanctorii Sanctorii de Statica Medicina* I, aphor. 6 (1614). Venetiis 1634, fol. 2 r.

22 For an example from the Hippocratic Corpus: *De Morbis* lib. IV. Ed. Littré vol. VII, p. 576, paragr. 43–45: estimation of the days needed for the assimilation and excretion of fluid. If the humours stay longer than three days, abnormal heat and obstruction of vessels will ensue. – For the pulse: VESALIUS *De Fabrica* Lib. I, cap. 5. Second ed. Basel 1555, p. 24 concerning the case of de Imersel: the pulse—or more

death (1644) and with the posthumous edition of his collected works four years later (1648).

Van Helmont estimated the quantity of gas that forms when coal is burnt—indeed it was in this way that he arrived at the new concept of "gas" as a volatile substance, different from air and water vapour, but specific to an individual object or a species of objects. "Of 62 pounds of Oaken coal, one pound of ashes is composed: Therefore the 61 remaining pounds are the wild spirit ... this spirit unknown hitherto, I call by the new name of Gas ... bodies do contain this spirit— ... a spirit grown together, coagulated after the manner of a body, and is stirred up by an attained ferment, as in Wine, the juyce of unripe grapes, bread, hydromel, or water and honey ...[23]" Van Helmont also determined the specific gravity of the urine[24] and performed his famous quantitative experiment with the willow tree designed to prove that the substance of the growing tree derived from the water with which it had been sprayed[25]. All these experiments were based on the use of the balance—and so were primitive attempts at a quantitative examination of the urine by Paracelsus and such of his followers as Leonart Thurneisser (1530–1595)[26]. Van Helmont, himself the most outstanding Paracelsian of the second generation, is likely to have been influenced by the earlier Paracelsians whose work he severely criticised and thoroughly reformed[27]. Probably more important in this matter, however, was the influence of Nicolaus Cusanus (1401–1464), as we have mentioned above (p. 20). Indeed it was not one, but several of the ideas and experiments, designed on paper by Cusanus, that were activated by Van Helmont—a fact that almost proves the influence of the former[28]. Systematic weighing and measuring had been recommended by Cusanus, it was put into practice by Van Helmont in the very cases for which it had been specified in Nicolaus Cusanus' Dialogues with the "idiota"—the layman (*mecanicus*) whose empirical wisdom was represented as superior to all the book-learning of the *orator* or *philosophus*, in short of the scholar. This piece of wisdom versus intellect was indeed just as congenial to the world of Paracelsus and Van Helmont as the detailed specification of empirical research which followed from it and was to prove the general philosophical principle. The work was completed on September 13th 1450 and thus antedated Harvey's *De motu* by almost two hundred years[29].

accurately the artery was contracted and remained thus during an interval of 3 to 4 pulsations, or beats ... it was sometimes possible to palpate only three or two beats (*dilatationes*) of the artery at the rate of nine beats of the heart (see: LEIBOWITZ, J.O., *Thromboembolic disease and heart block in Vesalius. Med.Hist.*, 1963, VII, 258–264; ROTH, M., *And. Vesalius Bruxellensis*, Berlin 1892, p. 223 and VESALIUS, *Anatomiae Gabr. Falloppii Observation. Examen*, 1564, p. 154). –The case reported by Vesalius was noted by Harvey in *Praelect. Anat. univers.*, fol. 73 verso: Vesalius found two pounds of gland-like and black flesh in the left heart of a man with strangely unequal pulse.

23 VAN HELMONT, *Complexionum atque mistionum elementalium figmentum* 13–15. *Opp omnia* Amsterodami 1648, p. 106; 1652, p. 86; Hafniae et Francof. 1707, p. 102; Engl. transl. by Chandler 1662, p. 106. PAGEL, W., *The religious and philosophical background of J.B. Van Helmont's science and medicine*, Baltimore, 1944, p. 19; idem, *The debt of science and medicine to a devout belief in God. Illustrated by the work of J.B. Van Helmont, Transact. Victoria Instit.*, 1942, LXXIV, 99–115; idem, *The position of Harvey and Van Helmont in the history of European thought. J. Hist. Med.*, 1958, XIII, 186. – See below, p. 266.

24 VAN HELMONT, *Scholarum humoristarum passiva deceptio*, cap. IV, 31 in: *Febrium doctrina inaudita*, Colon. Agripp. 1644, p. 204; *Ortus medic.*, Amsterod. 1648, vol. II, p. 108; Francof. 1707, II, 193; tr. CHANDLER, 1662, p. 1056. For comment and further detail: PAGEL, W., *Paracelsus. Introduction philosophical medicine in the era of the Renaissance.* Basle and New York 1958, p. 199.

25 VAN HELMONT, *Complexionum atque mist. elemental. figment. Ortus medic.* Amsterod. 1648, cap. 20, p. 109; 1652, p. 88; Francof. 1707, p. 105.

26 For references and detail see PAGEL, W., *Paracelsus* 1958 loc. cit. in note [24], p. 195 and idem, *Das Medizinische Weltbild des Paracelsus. Seine Zusammenhänge mit Neuplatonismus und Gnosis.* Wiesbaden. Steiner. 1962, p. 18–20, notably note [3] on p. 19.

27 PAGEL, W., *Paracelsus* 1958 loc. cit. in note [24], p. 198–200 and idem, Weltbild 1962, loc. cit. in note [26], p. 20; pp. 49–53. – PAGEL, W., *The Wild Spirit (Gas) of John Bapt. Van Helmont and Paracelsus Ambix* 1962, X, 1–13.

Harvey as a Modern

Harvey, then, was not the first to employ quantification. By contrast with his predecessors, however, quantification was in his case associated with the discovery which has opened up the modern period in Biology and Medicine and on which these disciplines have remained firmly grounded.

Quantification is not the only "modern" feature in Harvey's work. There is his whole tendency to see and study movement in structures that before him do not seem to have been visualised as alive. The movement studied by Harvey, being subject to the laws of physics is "given" to the scientist. Moreover there is the model of the *machine*. We mentioned (p. 52) how Harvey demolished Galen's "pulse-making" force, supposedly transmitted from the heart to the arterial wall, in favour of the mechanical impulse of the blood ejected by the ventricle into the passive pipe-like arteries. Indeed he compared the contracting heart muscle and its impetus with a pump or a fire engine (p. 212)—its action can be read from the water jet that emerges at the end of the pipe. The main product of the heart-engine is heat and its transmission. It is in turn sparked off by the blood that becomes ebullient with heat when entering the right auricle. Blood thus forms a source of energy, not, however, like ordinary fuel or nutriment, but by virtue of its own dynamic action of which motion and heat are the most eloquent witnesses. The fabric of the valves, vessels and fibres of the heart assumes with this an entirely new complexion. It calls for the experimental and comparative-anatomical examination of detailed causes that are responsible for local motion of the heart as a whole and each of its parts. In this "modern" programme of research the scientist is liberated from "forces" which have to be accepted as inscrutable in favour of infinite new possibilities that become accessible to human exploration.

However, there is no short-cut through Harvey to the *L'homme machine*.

The concept of the heart as a pump or fire-engine is not conspicuously displayed in Harvey's work—it occurs more as an aside than as an idea of principal importance (p. 213). Quantification, however central in the inventive process leading to his discovery, is not central in his view of nature—it is a method to be applied rather than an aim in itself. It is not the key that would decipher the hieroglyphic script of Nature at large.

Indeed Harvey's vitalistic leanings are so strong that they cannot be easily overlooked even where he seems to be concerned

28 PAGEL, *Paracelsus*, 1958, loc. cit. in note [24], p. 199; pp. 279–284. – Idem, *The position of Harvey and Van Helmont*, *J. Hist. Med.*, loc. cit. 1958, in note [23], p. 192–193.
For a subsequent appraisal concurring with the above: HOFF, H. E., *Nicolaus of Cusa, Van Helmont and Boyle, the first experiment of the Renaissance in quantitative biology and medicine*, *J. Hist. Med.* 1964, XIX, 99–117 (p. 100; 116).

29 NICOLAUS CUSANUS, *De staticis experimentis*, *Opera omnia*, Paris 1514, vol. I, fol. 94 verso; idem, *Der Laie über Versuche mit der Waage*, tr. H. MENZEL-ROGNER, 2nd ed. Leipzig 1944, p. 14 seq. on the instruments used by Cusanus and as to how far he may have carried out his theoretical suggestions.
A new interesting side-line is the discovery of a suggestion of the willow-tree experiment in the *Pseudo-Clementines*—a theological work from early Judaeo-Christian and Ebionitic times.
This work was known to Nicolaus Cusanus who quoted it in quite a different context in his *De pace fidei*. See HOWE, H. M., *On the roots of Van Helmont's tree*. *Isis* 1966. In press. HOWE refers to *Recognitions*, 8, 26–27; MIGNE, *Patrol. Graeca* I, 1384f. It remains to explain how this isolated experimental suggestion should have stimulated Nicolaus Cusanus to draw up a full programme of scientific experiments uniformly employing the balance and quantification and, including such novel ideas as the determination of the specific gravity of urine. Van Helmont took up not only the experiment with the willow tree, but also measured the specific gravity of urine and implemented the idea of quantification in many other ways. From this it is quite clear that he was in the first place dependent upon Nicolaus Cusanus whether he knew the *Pseudo-Clementines* himself or not.

with purely mechanical considerations. The heart is the hydraulic machine that "runs" the body. It owes its rank and responsibility, however, to its position as the *arche* and centre of the body—true to the vitalist teaching of Aristotle.

In all phases of his life Harvey saw the heart and blood as a functional unit in which there is no real room for priority of either partner. Where, however, blood is presented as the first formed and primary driving force of the heart, the vitalistic overtones cannot be ignored. Blood remains a "besonderer Saft" (peculiar juice) enlivened by its inherent "vital" motion and sensation (irritability). Again, its ebullience and immanent heat are regarded as the result of a vital force—that of the Aristotelian *connate pneuma* (p. 254). The latter also provides the denominator that the blood has in common with the semen.

Harvey's idea of the closed circle of the blood, with an automatic pump at the centre that raises fluid above its original level, strikes the present-day observer as an eminently modern "hydraulic" scheme. As we shall see presently, however, it can pass as such only when abstracted from a world of ideas that are quite different in scope and decidedly not modern.

Total Versus Selective Appraisal of Harvey

Harvey as a modern, his quantification and the other eminently modern aspects of his work, will always retain their appeal to the scientist and their exquisite historical significance. However, to recognise this is one thing, to leave matters there another. The Harvey problem confronting the historian is a complex one and it is not exhausted by following up the various stages of the scientific invention that led him to his discovery; it is not enough to find the line that divides him from his predecessors and made him a modern.

Historical research admits of no restriction. There can be no selection from the available facts, nor any limitation to extracts giving what appears "relevant" in the light of present-day standards and leaving out what is not. It is precisely such restrictive practices which have led to an identification of Harvey with the new "quantification" and the discovery finally based upon or at least rationalised by it. He has thus been placed on the level of a modern scientist whose results can be indexed and abstracted from the papers which he has published. A selective approach of this kind may pass as legitimate where not more than the bare history of a certain discovery is at issue or where the student is to be presented with a bird's eye view of the development of a scientific subject or problem, by way of introduction.

Instead of selecting data that "make sense" to the acolyte of modern science, the historian should therefore try to make sense of the philosophical, mystical or religious "side-steps" of otherwise "sound" scientific workers of the past—"side-steps" that are usually excused by the spirit or rather backwardness of the period. It is these that present a challenge to the historian: to uncover the internal reason and justification for their presence in the mind of the savant and their organic coherence with his scientific ideas. In other words it is for the historian to reverse the method of scientific selection and to re-state the thoughts of his hero in their original setting. The two sets of thoughts—the scientific and the non-scientific—will then emerge not as simply juxtaposed or as having been conceived inspite of each other, but as an organic whole in which they support and confirm each other. There is no other way to lay the savant open to our understanding.

Harvey's Circular Symbolism

In the case of Harvey we have to remember that he was a contemporary not only of Galileo and Santorius, but also of J.B. Van Helmont.

We mentioned the latter as one of the early naturalists intent on proving his points by using the balance and computation. At the same time his scientific ideas and discoveries are intimately blended with spiritualist symbolism, metaphysics and religion.

Such a combination is much less conspicuous in Harvey. Yet with his idea of the circle Harvey has recourse to a non-scientific symbol. This was to give the scientific fact of the circuit of the blood its place in Aristotelian cosmology to which Harvey subscribed. It revealed that circular motion, the main driving force in the cosmos at large, was also operative in the living microcosm.

Harvey has been rightly called the life-long thinker on the purpose of circulation and indeed it is here that he is most palpably influenced by Aristotle. The circle is the underlying symbol of the motion of the blood[30].

In Harvey's own words: "I began to think by myself whether it (the blood) has a certain motion, as it were in a circle, which afterwards I found to be true, and that the blood is propelled from the heart through the arteries into the body and all parts ... and back again through the veins ... to the right auricle.... This may thus be called circular motion, in the same way in which, accord-

30 Harvey's position was well summarised by MANI, NIKOLAUS, *Darmresorption und Blutbildung im Lichte der experimentellen Physiologie des 17. Jahrhunderts. Gesnerus*, 1961, XVIII, 85–146, p. 92.

Mani's paper is the best presentation of the immediate repercussions of Harvey's discovery on the physiology of nutrition and haematosis. In it Harvey's new orientation towards the arteries as the nutritional canals, is rightly emphasised. Up to him the veins (and their reputed origin, the liver) had been given this function—the new doctrine being bound up with a reactivation of Aristotle's view in which the heart plays the principal part. This view had also a cosmosophical aspect which was not foreign to Harvey; as MANI says: «Die *kardiozentrale Physiologie* des Aristoteles wird im modernen Gewande der Zirkulationslehre Harveys neu belebt. Die Vorstellung, dass Mikro- und Makrokosmus sich entsprechen, die Bezeichnungen des Herzens als 'Sonne des Mikrokosmus' und die Idee der vollendeten Kreisbahn bezeugen die philosophische und intuitiv-spekulative Seite des Naturforschers Harvey. Aber die philosophischen Leitideen und spekulativen Überlegungen verschmelzen mit den Ergebnissen exakter Untersuchungen. Sie stehen in fruchtbarem Wechselspiel mit der konkreten Forschung am morphologischen Substrat und mit dem exakten Befund der experimentellen Physiologie. Die Harmonie von ideeller Kraft, physiologischer Denkweise und disziplinierter Experimentalforschung verleiht dem Werke Harveys jenen einmaligen köstlichen Zauber, der Jahrhunderte durchstrahlt.» MANI, p. 92. Indeed this is Harvey's real position in the history of science and biology, most aptly and concisely expressed.

In a similar vein F. S. BODENHEIMER said: "Harvey's description of the circulation of the blood starts with anatomy and experimentation, goes over to the calculations, and ends with the philosophical background. Yet the actual progress was the reverse. The philosophical background gave the suggestion which led to the calculations for which proof was sought and found by dissection and experiment." *History of Biology*. London 1958, p. 48. See also: idem, *The transition from classical to new biology. Actes du IXe Congrès International d'Histoire des Sciences*, Barcelona 1959, p. 138–139. See also KING, LESTER S., *The growth of medical thought*, Chicago 1963, p. 154. and NAKAMURA, T., *Will. Harvey and his theories of physiology. Japan. Stud. Hist. Sci.* 1965, IV, 143–161.

ing to Aristotle, air and rain emulate the circular motion of the bodies above. For the moist earth evaporates when heated by the sun; the vapours lifted up are condensed, and condensed into rain come down again, moisten the earth and in this manner generation takes place and similarly tempests and atmospheric phenomena develop through the circular motion of the sun, his approach and recession.

In the same way in all likelihood it should happen in the body through the motion of the blood that all parts are nourished, warmed and quickened by the warmer, more perfect, vaporous, spirituous and so to speak nutritious blood: that by contrast the blood in these parts is cooled down, thickens and as it were becomes effete—whence it returns to its principle, namely the heart, the fountain and hearth of the body in order to recuperate its perfection; here, through the natural, potent, fervent heat, as it were the treasure of life, it is made fluid again and pregnant with spirits and so to speak balsam is dispersed from here again, and all this depends upon the motion and beat of the heart.

Thus the heart is the principle of life and the sun of the microcosm (just as proportionally the sun deserves to be called the heart of the world); it is through its virtue and beat that the blood is moved, perfected, quickened and protected against corruption and clotting. It is this intimate hearth—the fundament of life and author of all—that is devoted to the whole body, nourishing, heating and quickening it.[31]"

The Aristotelian Background

The interpretation of the motion of the blood and of generation as cycles that ever return to their point of departure implies the analogy of the smaller world of organisms with the greater world of cosmic and celestial bodies. This had formed one of the main principles of Aristotelian cosmology. In the latter, phenomena in the sublunary world are seen as imitations of the celestial pattern, notably the circular motion of the stars which, by virtue of its continuity, secures their eternal duration. Aristotle said: "the cause of this perpetuity of coming-to-be ... is circular motion: for that is the only motion which is continuous. That, too, is why all the other things imitate circular motion. For when water is transformed into air, air into fire, and the fire back into water, we say that coming-to-be has completed the circle, because it reverts again to the beginning.[32]" And: "the result is concordant with the eternity of circular motion, i.e. the eternity of the revolution

31 HARVEY, *De motu* cap. VIII, ed. 1628, p. 41; ed. Roterod. 1648, p. 102 ("coepi egomet mecum cogitare, an motionem quandam quasi in circulo haberet"), tr. WILLIS p. 46.

32 ARISTOTLE, *De generatione et corruptione* 337a; lib. II, cap. 10; tr. H. H. JOACHIM, Oxford 1922.

of the heavens.[33]" To have enabled sublunary objects to imitate the rotatory motion of celestial bodies is a feat achieved by nature "in the only way possible, namely by a cyclical arrangement of their serial phenomena.[34]" This is manifest in the periodicity of such phenomena as gestation[35], and above all in the evolution of organisms. Here we see a "circle" formed by the sequence of germ, fetus, infant, man and the germ again, and so on. It is by this "cycle" that the individual is preserved in the species.

Indeed, the use of the symbol found the same wide application in Harvey's speculation. Already in *De motu* of 1628 he says: "Nature in death ... retracing her steps, reverts to whence she has set out ... and so animal generation proceeds from that which is not animal, entity from non-entity, so, by a retrograde course, corruption turns back, from entity into non-entity, whence that in animals which was last created, fails first; and that which was first, fails last.[36]"

Here Harvey refers to one of the passages *On generation* in which Aristotle emphasises the heart as the "first principle" in the sanguineous animals and its analogue in the others—the organ that comes into being first. This, Aristotle says, is plain not only to the senses, but also in view of its end. "For life fails in the heart last of all, and it happens in all cases that what comes into being last fails first, and the first last, Nature running a double course, so to say, and turning back to the point from whence she started. For the process of becoming is from the non-existent to the existent, and that of perishing is back again from the existent to the non-existent.[37]"

When Harvey resumed this theme on a grand scale in *De generatione* (published in 1651) he had been aware of the "circular" character of generation and its identity in principle with the motion of the blood for more than twenty years. Had it perhaps been the expectation of some enlightenment in the vexed problem as to the purpose of blood circulation that had made him turn to a special study of generation? For it was just this which eluded and defied him—a purpose that could be imagined to connect with the purpose of other "circular" processes in the lesser and greater world. In this view the circular motion of the blood ensures the cyclical preservation and regeneration of its virtue (heat) in the heart after its consumption in the organs and tissues. Corresponding with this, generation is interpreted as the preservation and regeneration of the individual in the species, through its cyclical renewal in the male and female geniture.

This circular character of generation is epitomised by the fa-

33 ARISTOTLE, ibidem, 338a; lib.II, cap. 11.

34 W. OGLE in Aristotle, *On the parts of animals*, London 1882 to Lib.I, cap. 1, p. 3; 640a in note [5] on p. 143—with ref. to *De generatione et corrupt.* lib.II, cap. 9 and 10; 336b. *De anima* lib.II, cap. 4; 415b; *De generat. animal.* lib.II, cap. 1; 731b.

35 ARISTOTLE, *De gener. animal.* lib.IV, cap. 10; 777a–b, 33.

36 HARVEY, *De motu*, cap.IV, ed. 1628, p. 28; ed. Roterod. 1648, p. 55: Ita natura in morte, quasi decursione facta, reducem (ut Arist.) agat, motu retrogrado, a calce ad carcerem, eo unde proruit sese recipit, et cum animalis generatio ex non animali procedat in animal, tanquam ex non ente in ens, iisdem retro gradibus corruptio ex ente revolvatur in non ens; unde quod in animalibus ultimo fit deficit primum et quod primo ultimum.
A marginal note to Harvey's text refers to ARISTOTLE, *De motu animal.*, cap. VIII—appertaining not to the retrogression of nature from "entity to non-entity", but to the independence of the semen ("itself a kind of organism"—ARISTOTLE, *De motu animal.* cap. XI, 703b 25), a topic mentioned by Harvey in the same passage just before the sentence quoted above in this note.

37 ARISTOTLE, *De generat. animal.* 741b; lib.II, cap. 6; tr. PLATT, Oxford 1910.

mous conundrum: Which is first, the hen or the egg? The answer to this is: the gallinaceous tribe "describes a *circuit*" which makes the race of the fowl eternal; "now pullet, now ovum, the series is continued in perpetuity, producing from frail and perishable individuals an immortal species. It is in this way that many inferior things emulate the perpetuity of superior things. From this *circuit* it is manifest that there exists some principle governing this rotation (*principium istius revolutionis*) from the hen to the ovum and back from the ovum to the hen whereby eternity is conferred upon them[38]. This is the principle of which Aristotle said that it is analogous to the element of the stars, makes parents engender and imparts fertility on their ova. It is always there, though in a different form in the parents and their ova, changing like Proteus. For as the same mind or spirit continually agitates the prodigious mass (of the universe) and guides the same sun from its rising to its setting over the various parts of the earth, a divine principle, *a vis enthea*, dwells in the tribe of poultry, here as formative, there as nutritive or augmentative virtue, yet always in a preserving and vegetative capacity. Here it assumes the form of the egg, there that of the hen, but remains the same in eternity ... Single individuals, male and female, therefore seem to exist for the sake of hammering out ova so that the species persists the same though the actors perish.[39]"

The *ovum* can thus be seen as the quiescent centre from which the "circular" movement of generation takes its origin and to which it ever recurs. Being the terminus from which all arise and the end to which all their lives tend it confers eternity upon the individual *qua* producer of something similar to himself for the sake of the species. Indeed the *ovum* embodies the circuit implied in this eternity (*est inquam ovum huius eternitatis periodus*): for it would be hard to say whether the *ovum* is the cause of the chick or vice versa, which of these was prior in time or by nature[40].

All this is based on Aristotelian doctrine: "Since it is impossible that such a class of things as animals should be of an eternal nature, therefore that which comes into being is eternal in the only way possible. Now it is impossible to be eternal as an individual (though of course the real essence of things is in the individual)—were it such it would be eternal—but it is possible for it as a species.[41]" Or elsewhere: "Since, then, no living thing is able to partake in what is eternal and divine by uninterrupted continuance ... it tries to achieve that end in the only way possible to it ... continues its existence in something like itself—not numerically, but specifically One.[42]" And finally: In some sequences what re-

38 HARVEY, *De generatione* Exerc. XXVIII, ed. Amstelod. 1662, p. 109; tr. WILLIS p. 285 et seq.

39 HARVEY, ibidem with reference to Aristotle, *De generat, animal.*, lib. II, cap. 3; 736b–737a. – Harvey's text has: pereuntibus licet *actoribus*, not: though their *authors* pass away (WILLIS tr. p. 286).

40 HARVEY, *De generat.* Exercit. XXVI, ed. 1662, p. 96; tr. WILLIS, p. 270–272.

We shall revert to the "circular" character of the *ovum* in the last part of the present book, p. 274.

41 ARISTOTLE, *De gener, animal.* lib. II, cap. 1; 731b (tr. A. PLATT, Oxford 1910) see A. L. PECK's clear translation in his ed. in Loeb's Lib. 1953, p. 131 and *appendix* A, 14, p. 573 seq.

42 ARISTOTLE, *De anima*, lib. II, cap. 4; 415b 3–7 (tr. J. A. SMITH, Oxford 1931).

curs is *numerically* the same, in other sequences it is the same *only in the species.*[43]" Harvey himself refers to yet another passage in which "the law of the universe", namely the cyclical approach and recession of the sun, are invoked as the cause of the perpetuity of animal species[44].

Later, in this book, we shall have to view Harvey as the true follower of the Aristotelian tradition in founding the embryological theory of *Epigenesis* (p. 233). This implies "creation"—the new production of parts in succession—as against *preformation* or *metamorphosis* which consists of the transformation of pre-existing material. The latter is a once-and-for-all process which unwinds and must come to an end. By contrast *epigenesis* is a *cyclical* process which can continue for ever. For preformation serves to supply "fitting material" from which the individual is gradually built up by the addition of part to part—a process in which the whole succeeds the parts. By contrast, in *epigenesis* an operative faculty of divine quality works from the same homogeneous material out of which organs are made which are dissimilar—unfolding a plan, a whole that is earlier than the parts; a process that is repeated cyclically and for ever by the development of a homogeneous particle of matter into an individual and the involution of the latter back to the particle which potentially represents again the whole of the individual to be[45].

43 Aristotle, *De generat. et corrupt.* lib. II, cap. 11; 338b (tr. H.H. Joachim, Oxford 1922).

44 Aristotle, *De generat. et corrupt.*, lib. II, cap. 10; 336b–337a. – Harvey, *On generat.* Exercit. L, ed. 1662, p. 183; tr. Willis, p. 367 (in the first ed., 1651, Exercit. XLIX, p. 144).

45 Harvey, *On generat.* Exercit. XLV, ed. 1662, p. 153–159; tr. Willis, p. 335–339.

Circular Symbolism,
Heart and Blood before Harvey

(*a*) *Plato and the Hippocratic Corpus*

We have dealt with Aristotelian circular symbolism in the first place because it obviously formed the basis of Harvey's speculations. Aristotle, however, was preceded by Plato, and it is from Platonic times that a cyclical pattern was divined in the movements of the heart and blood.

Plato who was the first to formulate the theory of microcosm, was also the first to visualise the blood as imitating the motion of the universe. All the tissues, he thought, as they are irrigated with blood, repair what they have lost by evacuation. This cycle of depletion and repair is basically identical with the movement of the universe through which like joins like and all things move towards their own kind. This is the "circuit of the whole" in which the "mutual attraction of likes and the constant changes of direction of transformed bodies keep the whole together and tend to allow no vacancy to be left unfilled." This movement is reproduced in the microcosm[1]. The ambient elements slowly consume the body, dissolving and distributing its substance and sending each of its parts to join its own kind in the greater world. Such particles carried by the blood throughout the body that is analogous to heaven of necessity reproduce the movement of the universe, the "circuit of the whole". It is thus that each of these particles is set in motion towards its own kind, thereby replenishing the part that has just been depleted[2]. Elsewhere we are told that "the compass of the universe is spherical and tends naturally to return into itself", in other words that its movement is circular[3], and that the flesh—a product of the blood—is loosened and falls back again into the "circulating" blood, or rather into the "current of the blood" (*phoran tou haimatos*). The term used—phora—implies in the present instance a circular movement which is properly called: *periphora* or *periodos*[4].

Moreover it was Plato who had called the heart the "knot of the veins and the fountain of the blood which moves impetuously round throughout all the members.[5]" With this Plato opposed the ruling opinion which made the liver the fountain and source of the blood. He may have done so under the influence of a certain (possibly Sicilian) medical tradition[6], as he himself regarded the brain as the most noble part of the body to which everything is subservient and which arranges and organises all sensation[7]. It is also well known that he attributed much importance to the liver as the "seat" of the "vegetative soul". What he said about the heart, however, connects well with the idea of blood being car-

1 ho de tropos tes pleroseos apochoreseos te gignetai kathaper en to panti pantos he phora gegonen, hên to xyngenes pan pheretai pros heauto ... ta de enaima au, kermatisthenta entos par hemin kai perieilemmena hosper hyp' ouranou xynestotos hekastou tou zoou, ten tou pantos anankazetai mimeisthai phoran. PLATO, *Timaios* 81a–b. ED. STALLBAUM vol. VII, Lips. 1871, p. 84. In A.E. Taylor's translation, London 1929, p. 86: The character of this depletion and repair is the same as that of the movement in the universe whereby all things move towards their own kind ... the contents of the blood in their turn being broken up within our frame into tiny fragments and encompassed by the organism as by a heaven, are forced to imitate the motion of the universe. With little modification: CORNFORD, F.M., *Plato's Cosmology*. London 1937, p. 328.

2 Ibidem 81b—hence each of the fragments within us is carried to its likes and repairs their waste. TAYLOR p. 86; CORNFORD p. 328.

3 He tou pantos periodos, epeide symperielabe ta gene, kykloteres ousa kai pros hauten pephykuia boulesthai xynienai, sphingei panta kai kenen choran oudemian ea leipesthai. Timaios 58a ed. Stallbaum loc. cit. in note [1], p. 52. – tr. TAYLOR p. 58; tr. CORNFORD p. 242: "the circuit of the whole, when once it has comprehended the (four) kinds (i.e. primary bodies), being round and naturally tending to come together upon itself, constricts them all and allows (or tends to allow) no room to be left empty."

4 Ibidem 84b. Ed. Stallbaum p. 88. TAYLOR: "falling itself back again into the circulating blood" p. 89. CORNFORD: "and itself falls back again into the current of the blood" p. 339.

For a compilation of the loci concerning circular movement—*periodos*, *periphora*, *phora*—from Hippocrates and Plato see: KAPFERER, R. and FINGERLE, A., *Platons Timaios oder die Schrift über die Natur.* Stuttgart 1952, p. 97.

5 *Timaios* 70b ed. Stallbaum p. 69: ten de dê kardian archen hama ton phlebon kai pegen tou peripheromenou kata panta ta mele sphodros haimatos eis ten doryphoriken oikesin katestesan ... tr. TAYLOR, p. 73. CORNFORD, p. 283.

6 CORNFORD, p. 283, note [2]. The reference to Hippocrates, *Peri kardies*, 7 is open to criticism, because of the presumable age of the treatise which appears to belong to the Erasistratean period, i.e. the third century b.C. (see below, p. 127 note [1].

ried around (*peripheromenou haimatos*) or "circling throughout the members with *impetus* (*sphodros*)"[8].

These vague analogies between biological phenomena and those occurring in the cosmos outside and between like and like in the components of the body cannot claim any place in the pre-history of the discovery of blood circulation, however often such claims have been raised on behalf of Plato and the Hippocratic writers, since the second half of the seventeenth century up to the present day[9]. On the other hand these speculations do foreshadow the vision of a "circular" motion of the blood as imitating that of the celestial bodies—visions that belong to the era of the Renaissance in which they emerged as the fruit of Neoplatonic ideas concerning the microcosm. We shall return to this below.

(*b*) *St Thomas Aquinas on the Circular Movement of the Heart* (pl. 5, 6)

The *Opusculum* or rather *Letter De motu cordis* of St Thomas Aquinas (1225–1274)[10] has occasionally been looked upon as a work on the motion of the blood—an appraisal that was largely due to a misunderstanding of the term "circular"[11]. The latter does occur in this *Opusculum*, but appertains to the *motion of the heart* and *not of the blood*. It is, however, a work that displays interesting aspects and deserves a short discussion in the present context, if only to show the variety of meanings attaching to "circular" and "circulatio" and for the influence which it exerted in the era of the Renaissance.

It is regarded as a genuine work and has been translated and commented upon in recent times[12].

Ever since the reception of the philosophy of Aristotle and the acceptance of his psycho-physiological ideas in the early thirteenth century, the heart had formed the central focus of biological speculation. This is seen in the role which it played in Alfred of Sareshel's *De motu cordis*, written before the death, in 1217, of Alexander Neckham to whom it is dedicated.[13] Some of St Thomas' statements seem to be directed against Alfred[14]. St Thomas' speculation is mainly concerned with the soul as the vital principle causing and directing the motion of the heart, its character as a "natural" motion and its analogy with the motion of the heavens —its "circularity".

The result is that the movement of the heart is due to the soul as the form of the body and primarily of the heart. With this St Thomas does not mean that the soul resides in the heart. Differing from Alfredus who made it the dwellingplace (*domicilium*) of the

For the possible influence of the Sicilian school (Philistion of Locri) see WELLMANN, M., *Die Fragmente der sikelischen Ärzte Akron, Philistion und des Diokles von Karystos* Berlin 1901, p. 107. – See also ELAUT, L., *Hart en bloedvaten in Platons Timaios. Scientiar. Hist.*, 1959, I, 128–133 and MICHLER, M. *Das Problem der westgriechischen Heilkunde, Arch. Gesch. d. Med.* 1962, XLVI, 137–152.

7 See the loci quoted by Lichtenstädt, I.R., *Platons Lehren auf dem Gebiet der Naturforschung und der Heilkunde.* Leipzig 1826, p. 89 and 97.

8 TAYLOR's translation: "blood that circles so lustily through the members".

9 See our discussion below p. 120 and p. 127 note [1].

10 *De motu cordis ad Magistrum Philippum. Opuscula Omnia.* Antwerp 1612 opusc. XXXV, p. 214. First ed. (folio) Milan. Beninus et Joh. Ant. de Honate. – Edition also used by the present writer: Venetiis 1490 (ed. with a life of St Thomas by Anton. Pizamanus), published in 4° by Herman Liechtenstein Coloniensis. sig. J verso to J 2 verso. – A separate edition with another *opusculum—Libelli doctoris Sancti Thomae aquinatis occultorum naturae effectuum Et proprii cordis motus causas declarantes studentibus phisice summe necessarii* appeared at Leipzig—per Jacobum Thaner of Würzburg—1499.

11 BAYON, H.P., *William Harvey, Physician and Biologist: His precursors, opponents and successors Part III.* Annals of Sci. 1938, III, 445.

12 LARKIN, VINCENT R., *St Thomas Aquinas on the movement of the heart. J. Hist. Med.* 1960, XV, 22–30. See also idem, *Saint Thomas Aquinas on the combining of the elements. Isis* 1960, LI, 67–72—a translation of St Thomas *De mixtione elementorum*, like *De motu cordis* a letter addressed to a Master Philip (ab. 1270).

13 *Excerpta e libro Alfredi Anglici de motu cordis item Costae-ben-Lucae de differentia animae et spiritus liber translatus a Johanne Hispalensi.* ed. C.S. BARACH Innsbruck 1878. – BAEUMKER, C., *Des Alfred von Sareshel (Alfredus Anglicus) Schrift De motu cordis.* Münster 1923. – Idem, *Die Stellung des Alfred von Sareshel (Alfredus Anglicus) und seiner Schrift De motu cordis in der Wissenschaft des beginnenden XIII. Jahrhunderts. Sitzber. Kgl. Bayer. Akad. d. Wiss. Philos-hist. Kl.* 1913, IX, München 1913.

14 See below.

soul[15], St Thomas regarded the latter as the *form* of the body as a whole. In this he followed Plotinus and St Augustine who regarded the soul as "wholly in the whole body, and whole in each of its parts.[16]" The movement of the heart that appears first in the developing organism is the principle of all the movements that exist in the animal, and under this aspect is linked with the soul, the vital principle of the organism as a whole[17].

Secondly the motion of the heart is *natural*. It is so, however, not in the ordinary sense of *motus naturalis*, predicated of a body because it is heavy or light and thus follows one direction, but because movement is immanent to the heart that is animated by a certain kind of soul[18] and not due to an external force causing the so called *motus violentus*[19]. Nor finally is it caused by such external force as heat—for it is the very movement of the heart that engenders heat[20].

In all these points opposition to Alfred's stipulations is recognisable. The latter had denied the intimate connexion of the motion of the heart with the soul: it is not a *motus animalis* as it is independent of *appetitus* and *intelligentia practica*. Alfredus refuted its *natural* character, as the heart does not follow its weight and move to the centre, but remains on its level; moreover it is moved by an outside force, namely the heat which distends air and blood. Its movement, therefore, belongs to the same category as the movement of smoke that moves upwards and that of a burning torch which leads the fire in a downward direction[21].

According to St Thomas the movement of the heart is a rhythmically repeated series of pushing and pulling actions. Though continuous throughout the life of the animal this movement is not strictly circular because there is a rest period inserted midway between the push and the pull. It is a movement not circular, but "like circular movement" (*habuit*—namely cor—*quendam motum non circularem, sed similem circulari compositum*). This circularity comes about because the heart and its movement are the principle and end of all the movements that exist in the animal. It results from the soul, the "form" of the body and primarily of the heart—the noblest form that exists in earthly bodies—and thus resembles the principle of the movement of the heavens. It follows that the movement of the heart must be like that of the heavens. It necessarily falls short of the latter, however, as the effect falls short of the cause. On the other hand it imitates its perfect and uninterrupted —"simple"—circular movement in so far as *it goes from a point back to the same point* (*quem tamen imitatur in quantum est ab eodem in idem*). Though consisting of two parts—systole and diastole[22]—it is

15 Cor igitur animae domicilium est. Alfred, *de motu cordis*, ed. Baeumker loc. cit. in note [13], p. 33, l. 18; p. 43, l. 10; p. 45, l. 20; anima igitur, quae sensus et motus et vitae principium est, arcem corporis, id est cor, inhabitat: p. 86, l. 8 and similar passages as compiled in the index to Baeumker's ed. p. 103. See also Barach loc. cit. in note [13], p. 70: «Auch nach Thomas ist es unmöglich, daß die Seele als eine rein geistige Substanz mit dem Körper in eine solche Verbindung oder Berührung eintrete, wie Diejenigen annehmen, welche ihr einen bestimmten Sitz in einem Körperorgan anweisen ...» p. 71: «Aus dem speziellen Vorstellungskreis der Schrift *de motu cordis* hat Thomas nur einen Gedanken herausgegriffen, um seine Unmöglichkeit insbesondere darzutun: die Ansicht nämlich, daß die Seele das die Herzbewegung unmittelbar bewirkende Princip sei. Thomas findet, daß weder die nutritive Seele, noch die empfindende, noch die Denkseele unmittelbare Ursache der Herzbewegung sein könne. Die erstere darum nicht, weil sie auch den Pflanzen eigen ist, die Herzbewegung aber nur dem Tiere eigentümlich ist; die empfindende und die Denkseele aber deswegen nicht, weil die Herzbewegung *unwillkürlich* sei, der *sensus* und *intellectus* aber nur vermittels des Willens bewegen. Er entscheidet sich dafür, daß die Herzbewegung ein *motus naturalis* sei, *quasi consequens animam, in quantum est forma talis corporis et principaliter cordis*, d. h. die Ursache der Herzbewegung ist eine dem Organ selbst eingepflanzte, angeborene Bewegungsfähigkeit, allerdings bewirkt und hervorgerufen durch die Seele, das bildende Princip des Organismus und besonders des Herzens, keineswegs aber in ihrer fortdauernden Wirksamkeit durch das stets erneuerte, wirkliche Eingreifen der Seele bedingt.»

16 *Hoti hole en pasi kai en hotooun autou hole:* PLOTINUS, *Ennead.* IV, 2, 1. ed. H.F. Mueller Berol. 1880, vol. II, p. 6. – ARISTOTLE, *De anima* lib. I, cap. 5; 411 b. – We return to this in the chapter on Marcus Marci later in this book, see p. 314.

17 Therefore the movement of the heart is natural because it results from the soul, in as much as it is the form of one particular body and primarily of the heart. Thomas Aquinas on the Heart 17 tr. V. R. LARKIN loc. cit. in note [12]. To this LARKIN's long note 23 on Thomas departing from the teaching of his master Albertus Magnus who adopted the opinion of Alfred of Sareshel. See above our footnote [15] with the passage from Barach. The basic ref. to Aristotle is:

really a single movement. Its composite structure does not therefore exclude it from being "natural" although its "naturalness" does not follow from this, but from its animation by a certain kind of soul—the sensitive soul as the form and nature of one particular body[23]. Nor is its going in different directions a point against its circularity, as circular movement also is in some respects like this.

From this short analysis of St Thomas' treatise it emerges, then, that he indeed speaks of a circular movement or at least of one that comes close to the "simple" circular motion of the heavens. It is not the movement of the blood with which he is concerned, however, but that of the heart. In this "circular" means that it starts from one point and returns to it—so does the blood, but in quite a different way. The blood sets out from the heart and returns to it after having travelled for a long distance. St Thomas knows nothing of this or at all events does not mention it. The circularity with which he deals merely indicates the rhythmical repetition of a movement that is uniformly composed of two acts: that of pull and push, of *pulsus* and *tractus*, of systole and diastole.

Perhaps this should be associated with a term used by the—older—Maimonides (1135–1204). The latter speaks of the *circular movement of the arteries*. This is compared with the "moving of a ball, since the palpitation of the artery is explained to the senses by the termination of the circuit (*gemirath ha-sibbub*).[24]"

This seems to allude to the very passage which St Thomas quotes from Aristotle, *De anima:* "that which is the instrument in the production of movement is to be found where a beginning and an end coincide, as for example in a ball and a socket joint; for there the convex and the concave sides are respectively an end and a beginning (that is why one remains at rest while the other is moved): they are separate in definition, but not separable spatially. For everything is moved by pushing and pulling. Hence just as in the case of a wheel, so here there must be a point which remains at rest, and from that point the movement must originate.[25]"

The similar way in which this matter is treated by Maimonides and St Thomas may justify the suggestion that the latter was influenced by Maimonides therein. An additional influence on St Thomas may be found in the use of the terms *systole* and *diastole* with regard to the *arteries* by Alfred of Sareshel. He stipulates that the spirit of life is not moved, but emanates from the left ventricle of the heart by irradiation. He says, the flux of the spirit through the arteries causing them to be repleted and elevated has been called diastole and its cessation systole. Alfred, then, in common with Maimonides speaks of the rhythmically repeated movement

De motu animal. cap. 10; 703a 29 and 703b 1 seq. and 703a 19.

18 Tr. Larkin, 22.

19 Tr. Larkin, 4.

20 Tr. Larkin, 8.

21 Alfredus Anglicus, ed. Baeumker, loc. cit. in note [13], cap. IX: *De specie motus cordis*, p. 35–37.

22 Tr. Larkin, 19–22, referring to Aristotle, *De anima*, III, 10; see below note [25] and text to this note.

23 Tr. Larkin, 22.

24 Leibowitz, J.O. in *Koroth* 1955, I, 7–8 with ref. to the IVth *Particula* of Maimonides, *Aphorismi*, which deals with the pulse. The new translation of the relevant passage suggested by Leibowitz—*termination of the circuit*—is a definite advance over the traditional Latin version—*perfecta rotunditate*—. See the present author in *The philosophy of Circles—Cesalpino—Harvey. J. Hist. Med.* 1957, XII, p. 143, note [8].

25 Aristotle, *De anima* lib. III, cap. 10; 433b 21–22; 25–27 tr. J.A. Smith. Oxford 1931. See also Aristotle, *De motu animal.* cap. 10; 703a 19; see above note [22] and below p. 276, note [115]. Also: Galen, *Defin. med.* cxii, Kühn, XIX, 377.

of the arteries—he does not mention it with reference to the heart. By contrast St Thomas does[26].

(c) *The Circular Movement of the Heart after St Thomas Aquinas Cardan and Leo Hebraeus*

The circular movement of the heart as stipulated by St Thomas Aquinas remained a stock topic for general discussion, especially in the sixteenth and seventeenth centuries.

Jerome Cardan (1501–1576) says that the motion of the heart is similar to that of the heavens, because it is from the soul; it returns, never ceases and is uniform. Yet it is composed of traction and impulse, whereas the celestial movement is simple. It is not circular, but from a centre back to a centre, whereas the latter *is* circular. It is liable to change through emotion, whereas the latter is without such change. It is mediated by the assistance of heat, whereas the celestial movement is from the soul itself. It is mortal, whereas the latter is not.[27]

It is easy to see how St Thomas' doctrine is used and modified by Cardan. The latter was taken up on this point by Scaliger (1484–1558), his adversary who had been a pupil of Pomponazzi[28].

Leo Hebraeus—Don Judah Abarbanel—(ab. 1460– after 1520) is impressed by the similarity of the heart to the eighth sphere of the heavens and to that portion of the whole of the heavens which exists above this sphere and is called *primum mobile*, because it freely bestows uniform, regular and *circular* (*orbicularem*) motion on all the others; it preserves all bodies in the universe through its perpetual and never failing motion. Indeed any other motion in as much as it is continuous in planets or elements derives its origin from it. For the same reason the heart is moved unceasingly in a circle and uniformly, nor does it ever rest, and through its continous and uniform motion it furnishes life to the whole body. It is the first origin of the never failing breathing of the lungs and the continual pulse of all the arteries (''*eadem quoque ratione humanum cor semper in circulum et aequabiliter movetur*, *nec umquam quiescit*, *et sua continua atque aequali motione universo corpori vitam subministrat; et indeficientis pulmonum anhelitus*, *atque assidui omnium arteriarum pulsus prima est origo*'')[29].

Leo Hebraeus' pronouncement can claim our particular attention, as emphasis is laid in it on the life-giving and life-preserving power of circular motion which is achieved by virtue of its continuity, of its primacy in time and dignity in the animal body.

26 ALFREDUS ANGLICUS, *De motu cordis* ed. Baeumker loc. cit in note [13] cap. XI: *Quod spiritus vitae non movetur, sed fit irradiatione virtutis* p. 46: diastolen igitur irradiatio, sistolen spadulatio facit, as against: repleta et elevata arteria per fluentem spiritum diastolen fieri dicunt; sistolen vero, cum arterias egressus fuerit, p. 46–47. See to this: Larkin loc. cit. in note [12], p. 28 note 27 to passage 20 of Thomas' *De motu cordis* on the medical meanings attributed by Alfred to systole and diastole, but used exclusively with reference to the arteries. By contrast Thomas speaks of the rest period inserted midway between push and pull of the heart (paragr. 20) and the increase or decrease in its natural movement in systole and diastole in every emotion. For the latter Larkin quotes from *Summa theolog.* vol. II, pars I–II, q. 24, art. 2, ad 2, p. 850b, ed. Ottawa 1941.

27 CARDAN, *De subtilitate* Lyons 1559, lib. XII, p. 490.

28 SCALIGER, *Exotericar. exercitation. liber de subtilitate ad H. Cardanum* Francof. 1601, exerc. 206, p. 874.

29 LEO, HEBRAEUS, *De amore dialogi tres.* Transl. J.C. Saracenus. Venet. 1564, Dial. II, p. 84 et seq. – For a general appreciation of Leo: ZIMMELS, B., *Leo Hebraeus, ein jüdischer Philosoph der Renaissance; sein Leben, seine Werke und seine Lehren.* Leipzig 1886. – APPEL E., *Leone Medigos Lehre vom Weltall und ihr Verhältnis zu griechischen und zeitgenössischen Anschauungen. Arch. Gesch. d. Philos.* 1907, XX. – The *Dialoghi di amore* were written between 1502 and after 1505, but first published posthumously, Rome 1535, by Mariano Lenzi and dedicated to Madonna Aurelia Petrucci—Zimmels loc. cit. p. 14; 34; 41.

(*d*) *Stephan Rodericus Castro and his citation by Harvey* (pl. 7)

In 1631 Benedict de Castro, a member of the famous family of exiled Portuguese Jewish physicians published his *Flagellum: Scourge of Calumniators*[30]. In this the "malicious charges of an anonymous author are refuted" and a defence is offered of the "legitimate methods of the most famous Portuguese physicians". Castro wrote about his namesake Stephan Roderic de Castro (1559–1627), Professor of Medicine at Pisa and called the "Phoenix of Medicine"[31] as follows: he held the first chair of medicine in Pisa and was a man of outstanding celebrity, an expert in humanities and social sciences; this extraordinary, intelligent man has written works excelling in elegance of speech and in spiritual dignity, and containing very remarkable thoughts, that everyone will be extremely pleased to accept, will enjoy reading and re-reading, and will not hesitate to praise. He became the personal physician of the Grand Duke of Tuscany, and published a book *De meteoris microcosmi*, another *De complexu morborum* and numerous others.

It is of particular interest to us that from the many publications of Stephan Roderic de Castro the author should have selected his book on the atmospheric phenomena in the microcosm: *De meteoris microcosmi*—for this book was cited and recommended by Harvey.

The book is a folio and appeared in 1621[32]. In an introductory allegorical poem Castro refers to the heart which sparkles in the centre like the Sun which cherishes everything through his rays[33].

After a short prelude in which the traditional theory of the elements is refuted the author soon strikes the key-note of his work: It is through recognising the similarity between the greater and the lesser world that the true philosopher becomes the true physician. To search for man in the cosmos and for his temperament and inclination in the conditions prevailing in the cosmos is the aim of the author and in his opinion was the aim of Hippocrates. Many, however, unwilling to go this way and yet wishing not to deviate from Hippocrates make Hippocrates deviate from Hippocrates—by declaring his book *On the winds* to be unauthentic, the very book in which he speaks to the point. Against this Castro wishes to demonstrate its soundness and authenticity[34].

That the world and man belong to the same archetype and that the former is endowed with soul is the subject of the first chapter[35]. The souls of the world as well as that of man are created by God and are not "particles of the divine aura", as Plutarch, Philo

30 Friedenwald, Harry, *Apologetic works of Jewish Physicians* in: *The Jews and Medicine*. Baltimore. Johns Hopkins Press 1944, vol. I, p. 57 on Benedict (Baruch) Nehemias de Castro (1597–1684 at Hamburg).

31 Friedenwald loc. cit. in note [30], p. 62–63. See also Friedenwald, H., *The Doctors de Castro* in *The Jews and Medicine*, vol. II, p. 453–455. Strangely enough in the latter essay Castro's *De meteoris microcosmi* is not mentioned, although a copy was possessed by Friedenwald: *Jewish Luminaries in Medical History and a Catalogue of works bearing on the subject of the Jews and Medicine from the private library of Harry Friedenwald*. Baltimore 1946, p. 55–56 (15 items listed).

32 Stephani Roderici Castrensis Lusitani *De meteoris microcosmi libri quattuor*, Florentiae ap. Junctas, 1621.

33 *Autoris carmen allegoricon de microcosmo* in *De meteoris*, fol. V verso.

34 Ibidem, p. 1–2.

35 Ibidem, p. 3–4.

and even Plato thought—a belief which finally became the Gnostic idea that God is susceptible to infinite change, if He is of the nature of soul, since the latter undergoes changes for better or worse. World soul and human soul are produced by the spirit of God—the former by the spirit that hovered above the surface of the waters and the latter by the *spiraculum vitae* infused by God into man. Both are endowed with twofold power—one that resides in each of his members and the other that is common to all and resides in the heart, the sun of the body and in the Sun proper which is called the heart of the universe (cap. 2)[36]. Just as the greater world falls into two parts, the visible and the invisible, so the lesser world has two aspects, namely body and spirit. Perhaps more appropriately three such aspects should be distinguished, corresponding to the threefold world visualised by the sages of old—the angelical world of intelligences which is emulated by the intellectual soul infused into man; the celestial world represented in man by an abundance of astral signatures and secret motions, and finally the elemental world in which, as in a large book, the nature and disposition of man can be read (*elementalis, in quo, tanquam in magno libro hominis naturam, et conditionem legimus, addiscimus*)[37].

Concerning the elements Castro disagrees with the traditional ancient theories, in Paracelsian and Cardanian terms. Fire, air, water and earth do not deserve the name of elements, for they are neither earlier than the rest of things nor are the latter composed of them. On the contrary the so called elements are composite bodies themselves. Fire has the power to dissolve, but not to compose. Fire—it is said—can be contained and thus enter the composition of objects. But what could be more powerful than fire and thus contain it? Water, earth and air abound with impurities. It may be objected that those which we use in daily life are not the real elements, and that the latter are our "ordinary" elements in a different form and of greater purity—but such do not and cannot exist. The matter assumes a different complexion, however, where "air" has been confused with "spirit", i.e. the efficient cause that moved on the surface of the waters[37a].

Indeed Castro sees in the elements spirits or rather particles each endowed with its own seminal power. Combining to form an organic whole each of these particles retains its own faculty, although the *species* of the whole is different from the multifarious properties of its constituents. When these corpuscles, while remaining together, lose their properties, not mixture, but generation takes place.

36 Ibidem, p. 5.

37 Ibidem, lib. I, cap. 4, p. 8.

37a Ibidem, lib. I, cap. 5, p. 9.

Aristotle "borrowed" the primary and secondary qualities of objects from heaven and its circular motion in preference to making the object itself responsible for them. Moreover all the difficulties arising from the traditional elemental doctrines are due to the fact that the four elements of the ancients as well as their primary qualities cannot possibly exist. If there were humidity, this should be able to alter a body by moistening it—but experience shows that an object only becomes moist by the reception of a moist body and hence not from a quality that alters it. It follows that if by definition air contains humidity no pure air can exist. It also follows that dryness can only obtain by removing moist constituents. Hot and cold are recognised by touch; but touch does not discern whether they are qualities or substances. That it is the latter which cause sensation is shown by smelling—a sensation that is elicited by fine vaporous corpuscles emanating from an object[38]. Nor is there any truth in the ancient idea that all bodies are decomposed into the four "elements" air, water, earth and fire.

Paracelsus thought he could separate sulphur and fatty substances from the elements and distinguish the latter by colour—air having a yellow tinge, water looking like inspissated milk, fire like a ruby, transparent and with all the marks of fire, earth black and burnt. But Castro asks, how can he recognise those elements which are devoid of colour?[39]

Galen professed to believe in Hippocrates' dictum[40] that after death each element returns to its origin—thereby contradicting truth and himself. For Galen had stated[41] that man does not consist of elements, but of substances that are mixed in a ratio corresponding to the elements. If, then, he does not consist of the elements themselves, how can the constituents of his body return to their elemental origins? Nor does Hippocrates really speak of the elements, but of what is cold, hot, humid or dry.

Fire is not an element, but an instrument by means of which the solar virtue operates in objects of nature. It is therefore not contained in the latter as a component or part of a mixture (i.e. as an element), but as a life-giving factor that has been commissioned by something outside itself. Nor could it qualify to enter any mixture, because of its consuming qualities[42]. Thus Aristotle taught that fire cannot generate and is therefore no "principle" of any animal[43]. As "principle" in his philosophy stands for "element" in the philosophy of others, fire cannot be called an element. The true element is what makes the semen fertile—a spirit intrinsic in the foamy body of the semen and endowed with

38 Ibidem, lib. I, cap. 7, p. 16–17.

39 Ibidem, liber I, cap. 8, p. 18.

40 Ibidem.

41 GALEN, *Introductorium*, as quoted by Castro lib. I, cap. 8, p. 18.

42 Ibidem, p. 19.

43 Ibidem, I, cap. 6, p. 13 and I, cap. 9, p. 21.

"astral" power. Such spirits, though of the finest texture, are still bodies and rightly called *prime matter*—the "principles" of bodies that contain in themselves the "*seminaria omnium rerum*". They are informed—"taught"—by the world soul and by gathering things together they are responsible for the composition of things, for their taste, smell, colour and the equilibrium of components, their "*temperamentum*" or "*intemperies*"[44].

Castro's work is concerned with *meteora*—atmospheric phenomena such as rain, hail, snow, frost, storms, comets, arrows, shooting stars etc. It is his contention that there is something corresponding to the *meteora* in the lesser world of man. He believes that these are the diseases and that *meteora* in the greater world are morbid phenomena as well. In the universe they are referable to vapours ascending from water and to exhalations from earth, in the microcosm to the four qualities and humours. But what do they really consist of? Castro—following Hippocrates' work *On winds*—believes them to be spirits and from spirits. In the cosmic as well as the microcosmic *meteora* there is an efficient cause—the heavens—and matter consisting of multifarious spirits. It is the diversity of natural spirits and their seminal virtues derived from the world soul which accounts for the multitude of meteoric phenomena which can be observed. The semina of many things are thus vital for us—we can live without food or drink for some time, but not many seconds without spirit. From this it follows that other spirits are harmful, bringing disease and death. As some *meteora* are very common such as rain, wind and frost, others are very rare such as the newly observed stars—the Novae of 1572 and 1604 for example. Similarly there are common diseases such as tertian, quartan or continual fever and catarrh and on the other hand diseases that had never been observed before such as fever with punctuate spots, syphilis, *plica*, those that are rare such as diabetes and the Falling Sickness and finally phenomena that are unusual or unknown in common diseases. Like the *meteora* of the greater world, diseases have something occult—divine—about them: such as demoniac causes and remedies the action of which defies any rational explanation[45].

The microcosm of man lends itself to the study of its "anatomy" in two ways: (a) ordinary *autopsia* conducted by means of the knife and (b) resolutive analysis that proceeds from the manifest to the occult using physiological reasoning instead of the knife.

The analytical method leads us to distinguish with Hippocrates 1. the parts that contain 2. what is contained and 3. what enters into the parts (*continentia*, *contenta*, *intus permeantia*). The first are

44 Ibidem, I, cap. 9, p. 21–22.

45 Castro, lib. I, cap. 16, p. 36.

the solid parts and organs which correspond to the Paracelsian *salt*. What is contained, the soft and variable semi-fluid flesh, was indicated by Paracelsus as *mercury* and the volatile that can penetrate as *sulphur*. This ternary reduces itself to unity when we bear in mind that owing to continual action of fire a volatile substance is elicited from the solid ("fixed") as well as fluid parts—the continual effluxions which make us old and finally lead us to death. In other words *life is combustion and progressive volatilisation*. It follows that if the volatile is the last in resolution it must also be the first in composition[46].

The anatomy of the *blood* reveals the *superiority of the action of spirits*. The blood itself is rightly called by Greeks and Arabs alike the *dew* that besprinkles everything. It contains acid spirits—an *esurina acetositas*—that it conveys to the stomach from the spleen maintaining appetite and digestion. Indeed Hippocrates was consistent when, in his book *On winds*, he said that all diseases spring from spirits and when, in his work *On ancient medicine*, he attributed the power in the body not to what is dry, humid, cold or warm, but to the sweet, bitter and acid, i. e. to spirits that act in minute quantities and, when cleansed of all bodily residue, are capable of incredible effects. Indeed blood contains such salty, bitter, acid and sweet substances. When they are in equilibrium health is maintained, but disease develops when spirits arise from them and gain superiority—the nature of the disease varying with the nature of the exuberant spirit. Their miraculous effects are shown in an experiment communicated to Castro by Quercetanus: when a golden coin is covered with a heap of salt it is unchanged; when, however, it is immersed in half an ounce of the spirit of the same salt—an acid—it is dissolved into a fluid[47].

Life is fire contained in the blood—its origin is the heart, the microcosmic sun. The blood itself is converted into bodily substance—the *dew* becoming *cambium* (i.e. the substance exchanged) and the latter *gluten* (i. e. glue), as the Arabs (Avicenna) call these final stages. Hence the *blood* as contained in the vessels deserves to be called an element and *part* of the living being[48].

The Circular Motion of the Heart

How is the vital fire preserved? First of all through the perennial *movement of the arteries and the heart*. This is closely related to *circular motion*, though not really circular in nature. For it is interrupted by a double period of rest. This, however, is small and sometimes not perceptible at all. The movement consists of alternating dilatation and constriction[49]. It is *through the pulse of the*

46 Castro, lib.II, cap. 11, p. 77.

47 Ibid. II, 13, p. 82 and II, 11, p. 78.

48 Castro, II, 15, p. 85; see also for "dew" from blood: II, 13, p. 81 and IV, 15, p. 214. For a discussion of these theories and Harvey's position see below: p. 255 (blood as *part*) and p. 257 (*dew*, *cambium*, *gluten*).

49 Sollicitudo naturae in nulla re melius ostenditur, quam in multitudine instrumentorum, quae in eam rem fabricavit. sunt arteriarum myriades, iugiter se moventes, cum corde, quarum motus, quamvis circularis re vera non sit, quia geminam habet quietem, nihilominus ob utriusque quietis exiguitatem, circulari proximus accedit: fit enim perpetuis reversionibus, et aliquando ad tantam devenit crebritatem, ut quies nulla deprehendatur. Castro, lib.II, cap. 17, p. 88. Castro could have referred here to a Paracelsist, namely Severinus, who speaks of the *circular* contraction and dilatation of the heart and its cosmic affiliation (*Idea medicinae philosophicae*, cap. XI, Basil. 1571, p. 175). Instead Castro quotes the source: St Thomas Aquinas; see below p. 99 and note [51].

arteries that the microcosm receives the signature of the celestial world (*pulsatio arteriarum, per quam microcosmum coelestis mundi signaturam habere diximus*)[50]. With this Castro refers to St Thomas Aquinas who in his booklet on the *Movement of the heart* compared the arterial pulse to the *movement of heaven*. For it is produced by the soul—not by any of its faculties, but by the soul itself *qua form* of the organism, just as the heaven is moved by its *form*, i. e. the intrinsic impulses which lead an organism to its specific destination and perfection[51].

We have given more attention to a detailed analysis of the general part of Castro's work than seems to be warranted in the present context, namely circular symbolism in general and St Thomas Aquinas' work on the movement of the heart in particular. However, it is Harvey's quotation of Castro's work that provides the circumstantial evidence for the former's acquaintance with St Thomas Aquinas' tract. In addition Castro has many things to say which also occur in Harvey, for example blood as a genuine part and the stages of *dew*, *cambium and gluten* through which blood goes before it is incorporated into bodily substance, a doctrine expounded by Arabic and Jewish authors of the Middle Ages[52].

The Letters Exchanged by Harvey and John Beverwijck of Dordrecht (pl. 8–14)

What, then, has Harvey to say about Castro and his work? The answer to this is found in the letter which he wrote to John Beverwijck (Beverovicius) of Dordrecht (1594–1647)—one of the first physicians to recognise—in 1638—the truth of Harvey's discovery[53]. Harvey's letter is preceded by one from Beverwijck of the end of 1637 in which he expresses his deep regret at having missed the opportunity of meeting Harvey in person during the latter's continental journey—a man to whom he looks up in admiration for the new inestimable discovery of blood circulation. Those who are alive enjoy the fruit of Harvey's incredible sagacity as much as those who are dead (such as Hippocrates, Aristotle, Galen and similar great "souls") should deplore his late arrival—if the dead were capable of any such sensations. Beverwijck gladly acknowledges his debt to the new doctrine which he embraced with both arms in a little book on the stone of the kidney and bladder, a copy of which he asks Harvey to accept[54].

In reply Harvey assures his correspondent from London on the 20th of April 1638 that the regret was entirely his own, adding his particular satisfaction that his discovery—*sanguinis circulatio inventa*

50 Castro, II, 17, p. 89.

51 Comparatur a D. Thom. in libello de motu cordis motui coelesti, quia hunc motum peragit anima (ut ipse putat) nulla ex quinque facultatibus, sed se sola, ut coelum movetur a sua forma, ita tamen ut talis motus sit ab anima sensitiva prout sensitiva est. Castro II, 17, p. 89.

52 We shall return to this in another part of this book—the discussion of Harvey's embryological speculation p. 257.

53 Reliquum vero sanguinem ab inutili sero jam secretum et a renum nutrimento superfluum, et arteriarum systole in venas expulsum, effluere statuo per venas emulgentes iterum in venam cavam, attractum diastole cordis. Hanc sententiam superstruo doctrinae novae quidem, sed qua veterum nulla elegantior, de circulatione sanguinis, cujus author et inventor Gul. Harveus, magnae Britanniae regis medicus dignissimus. – Joh. Beverovicii *De calculo renum et vesicae liber singularis*. Lugd. Batav. 1638, p. 20–24. The above passage is followed by a short description of the circulation, with a reference to Aristotle, *De partibus animal.* lib. III, cap. 4: *Sanguinem a corde in totum corpus distribui per venas* to which Beverovicius adds: quo nomine etiam arteriae vocantur antiquis. Not far below he continues: Quem motum circularem eo pacto nominare liceat, quo Aristoteles in aere et pluvia circularem superiorum motum aemulatus est. Terra enim madida ab sole calefacta evaporat, vapores sursum elati condensantur, condensati in pluvias rursum descendunt, terram madefaciunt; et hoc pacto fiunt hic generationes, et similiter tempestatum et meteororum ortus, a solis circulari motu, accessu et recessu. Sic verisimiliter contingit in corpore ... – These passages show the acute consciousness of the Aristotelian background of Harvey's discovery in the mind of his first supporters. Beverwijck winds up with the moral drawn from the valves of the veins which in his case refutes the ruling (*communis*) opinion that the kidneys attract blood through them, whereas in truth they are used for the blood sent down by the kidneys into the vena cava. Hoc enim valvularum situs non impedit; uti fluxum a vena cava ad renes. Ibid. p. 24.

54 The book of which he sent a copy to Harvey was *De calculo renum*, 1638, as cited in the previous note. His letter and Harvey's answer, however, were only published three years later in Joh. Beverovicii *Exercitatio in Hippocratis aphorismum de calculo ad N. V. Claudium Salmasium. Accedunt ejusdem argumenti doctorum epistolae.* Lugd. Batav. 1641, p. 190–199.

—does not displease such a learned head as Beverwijck, a fact that makes it more pleasing to himself and greatly encourages him to nourish further and even greater ideas.

Harvey then proceeds to praise Beverwijck's book—a splendid monument of his mind. "Stephanus Rodericus Castrensis, physician to the Grandduke of Toscana and your Sennert—how little they differ from your view, he will best judge who has perused the *Institutions* of the latter and the books on the *Meteora of the microcosm* of the former. Paracelsus in particular and his followers should be pleased with the gem which you unearthed from Paracelsus' mine and polished with the authority of the ancients and illustrated and adorned with the excellent observations and arguments which you have made public. Nor could Hippocrates and Galen be displeased with it, could they be called back to their dwelling on earth—for the reverence with which you have treated their opinions and, without rejecting, have opened them up to better interpretation and understanding. He finally who asserts the liberty of philosophy and wishes to be wise from the bosom of nature rather than to learn from books will derive much help from your work. With the same ingenuity you have followed the correct method and observed the similarities in the production of stones in the greater world and calculus in the smaller. Let us, for the exercise of the mind, look upon what opponents may have to say against this and how we can best meet them.

Hippocrates postulates for the generation of calculus something glutinous in addition to a surplus of earthy matter and dissolved salt—as he observed in the son of Theophorbus in the Vth book of Epidemics; and Galen visualises a product of inspissated juices impacted in the renal cavity—as described in his commentary to the Sixth book of Epidemics I, text. 6. Both these loci have been given by yourself.

Rodericus Castrensis following Paracelsus makes a mucilaginous tartar responsible[55]—that sticky and glutinous material which binds sand together and which you, I and others have often observed in those suffering from stone. You call it aliment of the bladder, the others the material cause of stone. For, exposed to air, it has been observed to be condensed into a sandy, friable and even stony matter within one night or sooner; and I have made the experiment and know a most noble lady, a sufferer from the stone, who from such mucilaginous matter deposited in her urine used to make pills with her own hands and demonstrated them to turn into stones naturally when preserved in a box.

Chemists as well as pure observers of natural things may per-

55 With reference to Castro, Rod. Steph., *De meteoris microcosmi* Florence 1621, loc. cit. in note [32], lib. IV, cap. 16, p. 215–229: mucilaginem seminaria lapidis habentem ... mucilago lapidosa, ut etiam in fundo maris inveniatur ... vegetabilia, ex quibus homo nutritur posse in se habere residuum mucilaginis lapidosae, p. 218–219. All this is on the familiar lines of Paracelsus' doctrine of *tartar* and *tartaric* disease. See PAGEL, W., *Paracelsus. Introduction to Philosophical Medicine in the Era of the Renaissance.* Basle and New York 1958, pp. 153–165; idem, *Das medizinische Weltbild des Paracelsus. Seine Zusammenhänge mit Neuplatonismus und Gnosis.* Wiesbaden 1962, p. 12–14 and 95–98. – The reference to Hippocrates: *Epidem.* V, 17, and to Galen: ed. Kühn, vol. XVII (1), p. 830 seq.

haps dispense with the *stupor of the kidneys* which you elegantly add to the building. For in wells, rivers and almost any water which contains a stone-building matter tartar is seen to condense by itself or through cold air. You yourself agree that such matter adheres to the teeth and all other parts of our body. The observation of a stony fetus in France has been confirmed by others. One is surprised at the concretions of the same material in the joints of the gouty and in the same way a rich crop of very small calculi is known to have broken through the skin of a certain arthritic. A natural disposition inherent in the stony material is sufficient to explain their conglutination—without the *stupor*. Frankly speaking I felt as you did that I should observe the reason why stones in the greater world are growing together. I elaborated and observed what is common and what is rare in order to understand better Aristotle's investigation in the fourth book of the *Meteorology*—the causes of inspissation, exsiccation and concretion; I have done many things, I have seen many things and found that out of anybody's urine calculi or at least sandy concrements can be made, just as salt from any lee. However, being not yet quite satisfied with my own inquiry, I feel that it should be followed up by others. Where I got stuck you will be told hereafter and at leisure. In the meantime fare well, honoured Sir, and live blissfully for the light and splendour of our art and your country, and if you have further thoughts let me enjoy them—as you have started to do so kindly."

Beverwijck answered this letter on the 16th of September of the same year. He mentions a specimen of urine which he is sending to Harvey with the latter's nephew—*juvenis ad omnia magna natus et tali avunculo dignus*. The specimen had been collected from the urine passed by Beverwijck's brother who died shortly afterwards from a big stone of the bladder causing retention of urine. The specimen had been kept for years in order to study its stone-forming qualities—but no sand or stony matter had been formed, only a powder as from decayed wood in which there was nothing hard or solid. He concludes that this fluid cannot have contained the earthy and salty matter constantly deposited on the big stone and converting those "glutinous" humours which do contain it into stones. It is therefore a salty rather than a tenacious and mucinous humour (as commonly believed) which causes the stone. Nor is it the fluid itself that is converted into a stone, but the sandy matter therein. However, what daunted Beverwijck much more was Harvey's criticism of his theory of the *kidney-stupor* as cause of the stone. Quoting Campanella who ascribed sense to every object—animate or inanimate—in nature, Beverwijck explains that he had not meant to regard the stupor as the efficient cause, but merely as an auxiliary one that would prevent the tissue from ridding itself of a noxious substance which would thus find an opportunity of staying and growing by apposition. Beverwijck admits, however, that none of this can really satisfy Harvey's objections—he merely wishes to show by his answer his appreciation of the honour of having received a letter and instruction from Harvey.

In analysing these exchanges between Harvey and Beverwijck we have been guilty of another digression from our subject: circular symbolism. However it is these letters which reveal Harvey's deep interest in the analogies of the greater and lesser world, his knowledge of such a crypto-Paracelsist as Castro, his concern with the latter's speculation and finally Harvey's acquaintance with Paracelsus. It would appear—against expectation—that he by no means dismissed Paracelsus out of hand, but took him quite seriously. We shall return to this in one of the later chapters of this book[56].

Harvey rightly recognised Castro as a follower of Paracelsus—however much Castro had tried to restrict citations from Paracelsus and to take the attitude of the Hippocratic. Castro presents a Hippocrates who believed in the superiority of the spirits rather than in qualities and humours. Hence the Hippocratic treatise *On winds* appears to him as one of the most genuine of the *Corpus* and he rejects those who, like Valleriola and Cardan, cast doubt upon its authenticity. In Castro's opinion it is consistent with other treatises, notably that *On ancient medicine*. For it is here that Hippocrates makes a stand against the qualities and humours in favour of concrete substances that are defined by specific properties such as acidity, bitterness, corrosiveness or sweetness[57]. Indeed the Hippocratic argument is somewhat akin to what Paracelsus had to say against such "qualities" as hot and cold which to his mind were incidental or secondary rather than causal factors in disease in contrast to acid, sour, salty or corrosive agents[58]. In keeping with this Paracelsus holds Hippocrates in high regard—and so did Van Helmont who referred to the same passage from *Ancient Medicine* as did Castro and also like the latter upheld the authenticity of *On Winds* in terms that were almost identical with those used by Castro[59]. It is very likely that he was well acquainted with a provocative—essentially Paracelsian—book such as Castro's *Meteora of the Microcosm* and that he took his argument from there.

The most rewarding part of our digression, however, would seem to lie in the inference which can be made from Harvey's

56 See below p. 270.

57 CASTRO, *De meteoris microcosmi* 1621, loc. cit. in note [32], lib.II, cap.13, p.82 with ref. to the blood (*sanguinis anatomia*); see above note [47], and Castro II, 11, p.78. – In a more general setting concerning the Hippocratic question—authenticity of *De flatibus* versus *De natura hominis*—: lib.I, cap.9, p.20 (*In Hippocratis doctrina de elementis nullam esse discrepantiam, et quid vere elementum sit ostenditur*) and in particular cap.10, p.23 (*Doctrinam quae in libello de flatibus continetur veram esse ostenditur adversus Valleriolam*).

58 PAGEL, W., *Paracelsus* 1958, p.132.

59 VAN HELMONT, J.B., *Blas Humanum* cap.52. In: *Ortus Medicinae* Amsterod. 1648, p.191; ed. M.B.Valentini Francof. et Hafn. 1707, p.182 (not hot and cold, but the acid, bitter etc. is the disease, according to Hippocrates, *Ancient Medicine* XV and seq. Hence, van Helmont says, pus is due to abnormal acidity). – Idem, *Humidum radicale*, ed.1648, p.721; ed. 1707, p.678 (haec igitur est ficta Scholarum de vita doctrina, quam supposita *Hippocratis ficti libelli de natura humana* authoritate stabilire nituntur). – Idem, *Vacuum naturae* cap.2, ed.1648, p.84; ed.1707, p.80 (Hippocrates ... omnes morbos a flatibus esse, suum enhormon recenset inter primarias morborum causas); *De flatibus*, cap.1, 1648, p.413; 1707, p.399 (senex ille omnes omnino morbos sic flatibus consecravit, ut ventos promiscue confuderit cum vitae principiis). In both of these latter passages Van Helmont adds his criticism of a Hippocrates who simplifies matters because of his ignorance of *Gas*, but is in no doubt as to the authenticity of Hippocrates, *De flatibus* as against the treatise *On human nature*.

knowledge of Castro's work—the inference namely that Harvey also knew St Thomas' *De motu cordis* and that he knew and took quite seriously Paracelsus and some of his doctrines.

Lelio della Fonte

A further author who, like St Thomas Aquinas, merely talks about the cyclical movement of the *heart*, but is mentioned among those alluding to the circular movement of the *blood*[60] is Lelio della Fonte. In the 21st book of his *Consultations* he states that the task of diastole is refrigeration which is necessary because of the continual motion of the heart and the conversion of nutritive into vital blood. By contrast systole serves for the expulsion of sooty excrement, the attenuation of blood in the right heart and its dispersion into the lung and through the aorta into all parts of the body respectively. It is through this cyclical movement (*motum in orbem*) of systole and diastole that nutritive blood is converted into vital blood and spirit[61].

(e) Philosophical and allegorical allusions to a circular motion of the blood

Giordano Bruno (pl. 23, 26, 27)

Plato originated the idea of a circular movement in the body comparable with that of the celestial bodies and associated with the constant apposition and consumption of bodily substance carried out by the blood.

The most elaborate form of this idea is found in the cosmological philosophy of Giordano Bruno (1548–1600).

Bruno's ideas are in a large measure based on and illustrated by symbols and "signatures" that are derived from the *Hermetic Corpus* and its spiritual offspring: Renaissance Neoplatonism[62].

One such basic symbol is the *circle*. Indeed, as Kepler in a personal letter epitomised his life and death: "I learnt from Wacker that Bruno was burnt in Rome and that he suffered with fortitude —asserting the vanity of all religions and the *identity of God with the world, the circle and the point.*[63]" God is the sphere whose centre is everywhere and whose periphery is nowhere—this remained one of the basic formulae of Neoplatonic and Hermetic cosmology throughout the centuries and we are reminded of it by the words of Kepler on Bruno. According to the latter—a follower of Plato and Nicolaus Cusanus (1401–1464)—the circle is the first principle and root of all the other geometrical figures. It forms and gauges, embraces and comprises, fills and measures them. The circle is at the same time a whole and a part, a beginning and an

60 Many such pseudo-allusions to a circular movement of the blood can be found scattered in the literature, notably those that have been repeated in the promotional notes of sale-catalogues of antiquarian books through the decades. A well known example is Cecco di Ascoli (1269–1327), the martyred astrologer and naturalist, and his didactic poem *L'Acerba*. Here it is said that the heart is the origin of the arteries, that the latter are accompanied by veins everywhere and that there are two sets of arteries, one that carries blood into the heart and one that is "empty" and conveys the spirit that is comparable to light in its candour and swiftness with which it travels through the air—*artaria in se addoppia ogni via, per l'una al cuore lo sangue se mena, per l'altre uaccio lo spirito corre, come splendore che moue de candela, che senza tempo per l'aiere descorre*—lib. IV, cap. 10. In the emphasis laid on the vein accompanying the artery everywhere a divergence from Galen has been seen (Pazzini, A., *Il dottrinale medico nell'Acerba di Cecco di Ascoli, Bollet. Ist. stor. Ital. Arte sanit.* 1934, XIV, 230–249; 274–292 (p. 242: with reference to Galen, *De usu partium*, lib. XVI, cap. 13). – By contrast with the spirit Cecco speaks of a slow motion of the blood—*e sangue pian se moue con quiete*. His comparison of the spirit with light and its swiftness may well have been influenced by or have a common source with Alfred of Sareshel (see above, p. 90 and note [13]. Nor would the strict separation made between vessels that carry blood and others that convey spirit only justify any idea of an "allusion" to circulation. – Pazzini himself would not concede more to Cecco than the idea of a movement of the blood "de va et vient".

61 Fonte, Lelio della, *De cordis palpitatione. Consultationes medicae in quibus vera vivaque consultandi effigies elucet* Venet. 1608 Ed. used: Francof. 1609, pp. 147–148 (by courtesy of Mr L. M. Payne, Library of the Royal College of Physicians, London). – Fonte is one of the pseudo-allusions adduced by Bertini, Ant. Franc. (1658–1726), *Medicina difesa contro le calunnie degli uomini volgari e dalle opposizioni de dotti, divisa in due dialogi*. Lucca 1699, p. 76 et seq. Bertini also mentions Bernardo Davanzati Bostichi's (1529–1606) book on money. In this money is compared to blood—the juice and substance of food in the body which, *running within minutes* through the broad veins and watering the entire flesh, is made to evaporate by the heat of the latter as raindrops are by the dry and hot earth. In a similar way money runs through large purses within minutes, refreshes everybody and is spent and goes into the things that

end, a central point and a circumference. Any motion that returns to its point of departure of necessity assumes its shape. It is only circular motion that is continual and consistent. Indeed each object of nature constitutes a circle—for its function and activity derives from a centre, the soul. From this the active principle tends to go out into the periphery whence it tends to flow back to the centre[64]. Bruno saw all this to be true in the cosmos at large and in its objects and phenomena. That it also applies to the microcosm of man and in particular to the motion of the blood he asserted in several places. It is in one of his later treatises, however that he gave much space and attention to the movement of animal blood in a circle. This is found in his work *On the principles of things, the elements and causes*—published for the first time some three hundred years after he had vanished into the dungeons of the inquisition[65].

Here Bruno says: "The spiritual life-force is effused from the heart into the whole of the body and (flows back) from the latter to the heart, as it were from the centre to the periphery and from the periphery to the centre, following the pattern of a circle.... The material part of the spirit is a fluid which cannot move on its own account, but moves by means of its innate spirit. Hence there is no circular movement outside the body. For the *blood which in the animal body moves in a circle* in order to distribute its driver, the spirit, lies immovable outside the body, is inert and decays, no longer deserving the name of blood.[66]"

Bruno's primary concern in these passages is not the blood, but the spirit of life, and it is the latter which directs the blood fluid into a circular course. This spirit is a mobile substance which by virtue of its motion communicates life, vegetation and consistency to animate beings. It is alive in itself and so are others through it, for it is the vehicle of all virtue. Being one and the same throughout the Universe, it is multiple according to the multitude of innumerable individuals. In the latter it is comparable to the universal spirit in that it is a particular and unique motion not to one, but to all parts—just as the virtue of life which is called spiritual is effused from the heart to the whole of the body and from the latter back to the heart. In this circular movement from a centre to the periphery and from the periphery to a centre lies the first and foremost hallmark of the spirit which does not seem to differ from the soul.

More commonly the spirit is believed to be a subtle body, just as a flame, an igneous spirit, a watery smoke of spirit or certain imperceptible bodies dispersed through the rarefaction of thicker

life requires, then returns into the large purses and thus circulating maintains the life of the civic body. – A further *pseudo-allusion* is found in: RUDIUS, EUST., *De virtutibus et viciis cordis*, Venet. 1587, lib. I, cap. 6, p. 19 (motion of the *heart*, *not* of the blood).

62 YATES, FRANCES A., *Giordano Bruno and the Hermetic tradition* London 1964. – PAGEL, W., Review of Dr. Yates' book in *Ambix* 1964. XII, 72–74 with *appendix: Hermetic alchemy at Bruno's time*, p. 75–76.

63 Brunum Romae crematum ex domino Wackerio didici; ait, constanter supplicium tulisse. Religionum omnium vanitatem asseruit, deum in mundum, in circulos, in puncta convertit. In Kepler's reply to a letter from Dr Brengger of March 7th 1608. KEPLER, Joh., *Opera omnia* ed. Ch. Frisch Frankf. and Erlangen 1858–1871, vol. II, p. 591–596.

64 BRUNO, JORD., *De monade, numero et figura* cap. II, Francof. 1591, p. 12 et seq. and the notes p. 22 et seq. – See also CLEMENS, F. J., *Giordano Bruno and Nicolaus von Cusa*. Bonn 1847, p. 33.

65 *De rerum principiis et elementis et causis* (1591) in: *Opera latine conscripte* ed. F. Tocco and H. Vitelli. Florence 1891, vol. III, p. 507 et seq (notably pp. 521 seq). – The work belongs to the Abraham Noroff collection, purchased from a Parisian firm of second hand booksellers, described by Noroff in 1868 and copied by Berti. See: LUTOSLAWSKI, W., *Jordani Bruno Nolani opera inedita, manu propria scripta. Arch. f. Gesch. d. Philos.* 1889, II, 526.

66 BRUNO, *De rerum principiis* loc. cit. in note [65]: *sicut a corde virtus, quam spiritalem appelant ad totum corpus vitalis effunditur*, et a toto corpore ad cor, tanquam a centro ad circumferentiam et a circumferentia ad centrum sphaerae progressione facta ... *quod extra corpus illum motum in circulum seu in sphaericum non admittunt.* Sanguis enim, qui in corpore animalis in circulum movetur, *quia vectorem spiritum ibi sortitur, extra corpus jacet immotus, torpet, putrescit et non dicitur amplius sanguis, nisi aequivoce.*

bodies are called spirits by physicians and chemists. All of these have a material base, namely water or a fluid which is not moved by itself, but by the spirit which it contains. Hence such humours are not subject to circular motion outside their proper habitat. Water which has found its way outside its proper place, such as rivers and brooks, is liable to putrefaction. Plants torn from the earth die because they no longer enjoy the communion with its spirit and soul—and so do limbs that are severed from the body. If, then, life and motion are from the spirit, all power and virtue in spirits is a derivative from the primary virtue of spirit—its circular motion from centre to periphery and vice versa.

This is the principle that underlies the circular motion of the blood which, like other fluids in us, is moved *continually* and *most rapidly in a circle*, flows and flows back and is diffused from the centre to extreme parts and takes itself back from the extremes to the centre—a movement that is never interrupted, but continually persevering with the continuity of life (*quod enim in nobis* sanguis *et alii humores* in circulum continue et rapidissime moveatur, fluat et refluat, et a medio ad extremas partes diffundatur et ab extremis ad medium se recipiat, *neque umquam hic motus ad omnes locales differentias intermittitur*, *sed* continuus *cum vitae continuitate perseverat*)[67].

What is it, then, that continually moves the blood in man? Or, looking at the greater world, what makes the sea flow and flow back, what causes springs to break through and emerge from the entrails of the earth and to disappear back into them, what causes warm bodies to ascend and fluid and solid ones to descend, what causes the winds from all directions to blow forth most potent and invisible agents which, with a clear sky, can overthrow mountains and buildings or lift the sea sky-high? Surely no explanation in terms of vapours and fluids as efficient agents can satisfy. For what are the agents that move these vapours and fluids? Nor can any help be provided by such generalities as "action of nature", "natural instinct", "necessity of fate", "providence of God", "nature of the living" or "condition of the soul". Nor finally would motion of the air explain anything. For what moves the air or the spirit? There remains, then, no alternative but to resort to that prime mover and instigator—by some called spirit—which by moving itself moves others. Plato called it soul and defined it as the number which moves itself in a circle. It is the spirit which resides and works individual effects in individuals. The substance, mobile by itself, confers through its motion life, vegetation and consistency on animate beings. The movement of the heavens—should it really exist—would be a universal and single movement

67 Bruno, ibidem, loc. cit. in note [65] following the passage cited in note [66].

in itself; how could it have a bearing on the infinitely diversified effects which are observed in individual objects? By contrast it is to the all powerful spirit that one should attribute all physical and magical effects such as the attraction of like to like—sympathy and antipathy—the selection of special food by individual animals and species, the specific action of remedies and the evocation of watery, airy or fiery spirits or demons by fumigation with certain ingredients. Such include burnt chameleon liver, which can bring down lightning or thunder, and the throat and head of the same animal burnt with oak wood, which can produce rain and thunder. This stands to reason because of the entirely airy and spiritual nature of this animal which lives on spirit and air. Hence its body appears to be most suitable for the alteration of aerial impressions in the presence of certain other circumstances known to magicians. The same applies to the conjuring of demons with the help of burnt coriander, garlic, hyoscyamus and hemlock—the "plants of the spirits" (*herbae spirituum*)[68].

Bruno's treatise *De rerum principiis*, in which the "circular" movement of the blood is given a prominent place, bears the hallmarks of authenticity, although it is not fully elaborated and polished[69]. A marginal note gives the date—March 16th 1590. It is in the handwriting of Bruno's clerk Besler[70]. Moreover it contains a reference to Bruno's *Dialoghi de l'infinito universo et mondi* in which he had demonstrated the existence of a unique infinite space harbouring an infinite substance. This external evidence of authenticity is borne out by internal evidence for the true Brunonian stamp of the passages relevant to our subject—the "circular" motion of the blood. For in his well known works published during his life time the movement of the blood from the heart and back to the heart was referred to, though by far not as clearly and significantly as in *De rerum principiis*. There are two passages which should be chiefly considered[71]. It is significant that they come from treatises that belong to the same period in Bruno's life as the *De rerum principiis*. In the prose notes to the second chapter of *De monade, numero et figura* of 1591 it says that there is one centre in the Microcosm—the heart. From it the vital spirits go out through the whole animal. In it the tree of life for the whole (*arbor universa vitae*) is fixed and rooted. To it finally the spirits are taken back as to the prime custody and preservation of life. What is of particular interest to us is the context: a discussion of the supreme virtues of the *circle*. This is the symbol of Oneness. It is devoid of plurality, as seen in the absence of angles—it is *agonon*. It is the first root, the builder of forms and the principal symbol embracing all the other symbols.

68 Bruno, ibidem loc. cit. in note [65], p. 524 seq.

69 Lutoslawski loc. cit. in note [65], p. 544. See also: Noroff, A., *Bibliothèque de Mr Abraham de Noroff*, St Petersbourg 1868 and Berti, Dom., *Documenti intorno a Giordano Bruno*, Roma 1880. – Frith, I, *Life of Giordano Bruno the Nolan*. London 1887, p. 351. – Spampanato, V., *Vita di Giordano Bruno. Con documenti editi e inediti*. Messina 1921, p. 440. – Guzzo, Augusto, *Giordano Bruno*. (*Scritti di Storia della Filosofia*). Torino 1960, p. 215–217 (under *Gli scritti magici*).

70 Hieronymus Besler was born at Nuremberg in 1566, was a member of the Nuremberg *Collegium Medicum* since 1593 and died in 1632. He defended his thesis *De hydrope* at Basle in 1592. A short *Epistola medica* to S. Schnitzer of Bamberg (March 12th 1607) is printed as No. 184 on p. 359 in Joh. Hornung's *Cista medica* (Nuremberg, 1626)—it deals with pharmaca for the opening of the haemorrhoidal and mesenteric veins, also for the "strengthening of s omach and liver". See on Besler: Will's Nürnberger Gelehrten-Lexicon 1775, pt. I, p. 104 (quoted from: Brunnhöfer, H., *Giordano Brunos Weltanschauung und Verhängnis* Leipzig 1882, p. 324. See also ibidem, p. 96 on Besler's copying for Bruno an old manuscript *De sigillis Hermetis Ptolemei et aliorum* at Padua in autumn 1591, as Bruno stated himself). Besler is said to have written the preface to the famous *Hortus Eystettensis*, a botanical work by his brother Basilius (Nuremberg 1613; 2nd ed. 1640) who, however, signed the preface and may well have been its author.

71 Pagel, W., *Giordano Bruno, the philosophy of circles and the circular movement of the blood. J. Hist. Med.* 1951, VI, 116–124 (p. 119).

It is the all in One; it is without parts. In it the opposites coincide —"cord, arc, spike, point, end, nothing, everything ...., right, left, arriving and returning, movement and rest.[72]" It is *maximum* as well as *minimum*. For it is one circle that comprises the universe which is without bounds. At the same time it is *minimum*, for it can be visualised as a point, the centre of all centres. Hence the circle is the *monad* that first of all develops (*explicat*) all. As a simple centre, however, it implies (*implicat*) all, as it is whatever it can be[73]. Forming a centre of activity and function, the circle sustains everything while dwelling in the fullness of perfection in the innermost centre of objects. Each work of nature is thus after the pattern of the circle and so is all impulse, motion, force, action, passivity, perception, cognition and life[74]. Similarly the soul forms a centre that "pours out" (*fundit*) everywhere in a circle (*per gyrum*) and all things keep to a spherical direction, just as they take themselves back from the sphere to the centre. The soul, by virtue of being a centre, is simple and hence, unlike composite things, not subject to dissolution. It is the immutable substance that generates and into which the individual is involuted after having completed his life span. The soul develops (*explicat*) from the heart which occupies the centre (*a medio cordis*), each member, sending out the warps from the recondite semen and gathering them together again in reversed order in accordance with the fate of each and keeping up a certain succession of things[75]. In Bruno's treatise *On the threefold minimum* published in the same year, the soul is said to act as the *Spiritus architector* which expands when we are born, for 'birth is the expansion of a centre into a sphere, life the maintenance of this sphere in equilibrium, and death its contraction back into the centre'[76].

The second passage which corroborates the authenticity of the relevant pronouncements of *De rerum principiis* comes from the eighth chapter of the sixth book *De immenso et innumerabilibus seu de universo et mundis*—the treatise following *De monade*. Here it says that in our body the blood and all fluids by virtue of the spirit run in circles and run back (*circumcursant et recursant*). In the same way it happens in the whole world, on a star and on earth. For what could be called lower in our body, the feet or the shins? The blood runs here and runs back there nor does it flow to the lower region with power greater than that which makes it flow back to the upper half. For it is poured out throughout the whole uniformly (*aeque*). This applies to all fluids in the world, for there is nothing that could be called heavy or light in the circle (*orbe*) with which it goes forth here and takes itself back there. It follows from this

72 BRUNO, IORD., *De monade*, Francof. 1591, loc. cit. in note [64], cap. 2, p. 13, v. 43; and prose notes, p. 22–23.

73 Ibidem, p. 19 et seq.; vv. 210–220 and p. 21, vv. 281–283.

74 Ibidem, p. 15, vv. 97–100.

75 Ibidem, p. 15, vv. 99–110.

76 BRUNO, *De triplici minimo et mensura ad trium speculativarum scientiarum et multarum activarum artium principia libri V*, Francof. 1591, Lib. I, cap. 3, p. 11–13: "nativitas est expansio centri, vita consistentia sphaerae, mors contractio in centrum."

very circular character of the movement of fluids that all objects of nature are appropriately said to consist of water[77].

It was in this latter passage from *De universo et innumerabilibus* that S.T. Coleridge in 1812 recognised something belonging to the pre-history of the *Circulation of the Blood.* He said: "The ancients attributed to the blood the same motion of ascent and descent which really takes place in the sap of trees. Servetus discovered the minor circulation from the heart to the lungs. Do not the following passages of Giordano Bruno (published, 1591) seem to imply more? We put the question, pauperis formâ, with unfeigned diffidence.

De Immenso et Innumerabili lib. VI, cap. 8
Ut in nostro corpore sanguis per totum *circumcursat*
et recursat, sic in toto mundo, astro, tellure.
Quare non aliter quam nostro in corpore sanguis
Hinc meat, hinc remeat, neque ad inferiora fluit vi
Majore, ad supera a pedibus quam deinde recedat—

and still more plainly, in the ninth chapter of the same book

Quid esset
Quodam ni *gyro* Naturae cuncta redirent
Ortus ad proprios rursum; si sorbeat omnes
Pontus aquas, totum non restituatque perenni
Ordine; qua possit rerum consistere vita?
Tanquam si totus concurrat sanguis in unam
In qua consistat, partem, nec prima revisat
Ordia. et antiquos cursus non inde resumat[78].

Coleridge would have given Bruno his due without any "diffidence", had he lived to see *De rerum principiis* come to light—some fifty years after his death[79].

Certainly there was no place for "confidence" in "rejecting this claim of Coleridge for Bruno" some sixty years after the publication of Bruno's posthumous work with the comment that "the passages quoted are but examples of Bruno's doctrine of cosmic metabolism.[80]" Bruno's clear and unmistakable statement of 1591 must have remained unknown to Coleridge's critic.

It was Bruno, then, who definitely connected the movement of the blood with the circle and its symbolism and did so prominently in a series of writings from the period of his literary maturity. However, geometrical symbolism and the philosophy of circles—

77 BRUNO, *De universo et innumerabilibus* lib. VI, cap. 8 in *De monade* Francof. 1591, loc. cit. in note [64], p. 524–526.

78 [COLERIDGE, S.T. and SOUTHEY, W.], *Omniana or Horae Otiosores* 2 vols, London 1812, vol. I, p. 234–236, essay No. 122 (published anonymously).

The interest of Coleridge in Bruno was evidently stimulated by the Bruno-Renaissance as brought about through the work of FRID. HEINR. JACOBI (*Über die Lehre des Spinoza in Briefen an den Herrn Moses Mendelssohn.* 2nd ed. Breslau 1789 containing translations from Bruno's *De la causa, principio et uno*, pp. 261–306, see also Jacobi's contribution to Rixner, Th.A., and SIBER, TH., *Jordanus Brunus*, vol. V in *Leben und Lehrmeinungen berühmter Physiker am Ende des XVI. und am Anfange des XVII. Jahrhunderts als Beyträge zur Geschichte der Physiologie in engerer und weiterer Bedeutung* Sulzbach 1824, Vorbericht and pp. 51 seq.). SCHELLING's *Bruno oder über das göttliche und natürliche Princip der Dinge. Ein Gespräch.* Berlin 1802 was also influential.

79 Another "allusion" already discussed by Coleridge was the "running and turning" of the blood as found in the work of Francisco de la Reyna, "a farrier who published a work upon his own art at Burgos, in 1564." (Coleridge, loc. cit. in note [78]). – This was recently discussed independently (KEEVIL, J.J. and PAYNE, L.M., *Francisco de la Reyna and the circulation of the blood. Lancet*, 1951, I, 851, with full bibliography of the *Libro de albeyteriá* of Reyna from the first edition, 1546 to that of Alcala, 1647). In this book the veins of the exterior are said to convey blood down and the internal veins to carry blood upward in such a way that the blood turns (*torno*) through the limbs and veins—a movement comparable to a wheel; it has the function of carrying nourishment to the inner parts right up to the emperor of the body which is the heart—inspite of all vagueness an interesting modification of the Galenic doctrine.

80 SINGER, D.W., *Giordano Bruno. His life and thought with annotated translation of his work on the infinite Universe and Worlds*, New York 1950, p. 197 and eadem, *Coleridge suggests two anticipations of the circulation of the blood. Archeion* (Santa Fe, 1943). – Coleridge's citation from Reyna was noted by D.W. Singer.

the *circulationis necessitas in rebus*—is fundamental to the philosophy of Bruno at all periods of his activity as a thinker and writer[81]. Already in *De la causa, principio et uno* of 1584 the soul is praised as the "internal artist", the archeus, i.e. the vital force that forms matter. In plants it elicits and develops stems out of seeds and roots, branches out of stems and out of these buds, leaves, blossoms and fruit. In animals the soul unfolds its work from the original seed and from the centre of the heart in a peripheral direction down to the extremities. Then it draws and collects the unfolded faculties back to the heart as if winding up the stretched-out threads[82].

In a passage quoted above from a later work we met the same concept of the "circular" nature of the heart as the first organ to develop and the last to die—a "circularity" that also applies to the semen from which everything is unfolded and which is the only element to survive by forming semen in the offspring, thereby preserving the species and approaching immortality. All this is based on Aristotelian biological speculation and was revived by Harvey, as we discuss at length elsewhere in this book[83]. Bruno returns to the maintenance and preservation of life by circular motion in yet another of his posthumous treatises: that *On magic*. In this circular motion is extolled as the first and foremost reason for local motion at large. For, it says, life is sustained by virtue of the soul and innate spirit whereby things are moved in their places in a circular direction (*ad vitae consistentiam et conservationem, quae est per motum—virtute enim animae et spiritus nativi res in suo loco circulariter moventur, ut supra dictum est*)[84]. Incidentally, this and other passages bear witness not only to the consistency of Bruno's speculation around the "circularity" of heart, blood and semen, but also to the authenticity of this posthumous tract. Such passages include those on the indestructibility of spirit and matter[85], on the oneness of all spiritual substance, of all soul, of all soul of the universe, of God and mind, and on Life as a way, peregrination and "military service" of the soul and its longest sojourn in the best[86].

Bruno's Ideas and Harvey's Discovery

The "circular" movement of the blood is a genuine Brunonian concept—it fits well into his cosmological and philosophical ideas. What, then, is its significance, if any, in the history of Harvey's discovery?

The present author has no intention of claiming a share for Bruno in this. He believes, however, that Bruno's concept is of considerable importance for the historian of the ideas that form

81 For example in: *Libri physicorum Aristotelis explanati. Opera latine conscripta*, ed. F. Tocco and H. Vitelli, vol. III, Florence 1891, p. 370 concerning reasoning from cause to effect and vice versa.

82 Dialogo II in *Opere di Giordano Bruno*, ed. Ad. Wagner, vol. I, Lipsiae 1830, p. 236: «dal seme primo e dal centro del core a li membri esterni, e da quelli al fine complicando verso il core l'esplicate facultadi, fa, come già venisse a ringlomerare le già distese fila.»

83 «Nempe anima a medio cordis membrum explicat omne Principio, arcano de semine stamina mittens. Inde iterum relegenda suis verso ordine fatis» – Bruno, *De monade*, loc. cit. 1591, cap. II, vv. 102–104, p. 15. See in the present book, p. 84.

84 Bruno, *De magia* In: Opp. latine conscr. loc. cit. in note [81], p. 425.

85 «atqui neque spiritus ullus neque corpus ullum interit, sed complexionum tantum et actuum mutatio est continua» – *De magia*, p. 429.

86 Ibidem, p. 432.

the background of Harvey as the author of biological speculation as well as scientific discovery.

With his concept Bruno gave expression to philosophical truth which was "alive" at his time in which much of Aristotelian philosophy was revived in a Neoplatonic setting. Harvey's discovery and much of his observational work in embryology can be seen as the scientific complement and proof of these contemporary ideas. The supremacy of the heart, its role as the centre from which the prime vital impulse sets out with the blood and to which it continually returns with the blood, its significance as the first to live and to maintain life in the individual as well as the species, in short the "circularity" of the heart and blood are basic speculations which Bruno has in common with Harvey. To Bruno they are a philosophical and cosmological truth which "follows" from the supremacy of the circle, i.e. a thesis of mathematical mysticism, foreshadowed by Plato, Aristotle, the Neoplatonists and Nicolaus Cusanus. So they are to Harvey—with the difference that he had something to give in addition. This addition remains the foundation of modern scientific biology, whereas the speculative background lost all but historical interest. The ideological closeness of Bruno to Harvey is simply explained by the adherence of both to Aristotelian concepts and not necessarily by an acquaintance on the part of Harvey with any of Bruno's works. This also applies to a further interesting coincidence. Bruno discusses at length the circulation of water in the greater world. This is found as an introduction to the thesis of the movement of the blood "in a circle"[87], i.e. in a similar position to that in which it is found in the famous eighth chapter of Harvey's *De motu*[88].

Though devoid of any anatomical or physiological basis, Bruno's concept of the "circular" motion of the blood as such was not basically different in meaning from Harvey's. It did not simply denote a "cyclical" process, i.e. one that is continually repeated. Nor does it stand for "oscillation", i.e. an ever-repeated forward and backward motion in a straight direction. According to Bruno, such an oscillatory movement is displayed by water vapour that ascends and falls back. By contrast, Bruno regards "natural" motion as circular, i.e. as a motion around a centre, in our case the heart—although it need not describe a circle in the geometrical sense. Bruno distinguishes this "natural"—circular—motion of bodies from that observed in secondary products of natural objects, such as exhalations, which may move in straight lines[89].

A further point that secures for Bruno a well deserved place in the pre-history of Harvey's discovery is the emphasis laid by

87 See above p. 105 with reference to Bruno, *De rerum principiis* loc. cit. in note [65].

88 See above p. 83 and note [31].

89 Bruno, *De l'infinito universo e mondi* in *Opp.* ed. Ad. Wagner, loc. cit. in note [82], vol. II, p. 59 in Dialogus III, tr. D. Waley Singer, loc. cit. in note [80], New York 1950, p. 314.

Bruno on the *swiftness* with which the blood is moved throughout the body, down to its extreme parts and back to the centre—*in circulum continue* et rapidissime *moveatur*. The ancient ebb and flood movement of the blood had been conceived in terms of a *sluggish* movement; nor could the Galenic scheme of a venous transport of alimental blood to the periphery make provision for the speed which was to be accorded to the circulating blood by Harvey. Indeed, in this particular point the latter seems to have been foreshadowed by Bruno. Here Bruno's cosmological speculation achieved a major break with the traditional treatment of a fundamental subject of physiology—a correct result on a point of science arrived at by non-scientific speculation.

Bovillus and his Circular Model of the Heart. The "Black Grain"

We may add yet another "circular" model. It was conceived in the spirit of Nicolaus Cusanus, just as was Bruno's idea. Its author is Carolus Bovillus (Charles Bouelles, 1470–1553) who had been brought up in the Cusanian tradition by his teacher Jacques Lefèvre (Jacobus Faber Stapulensis, 1455–1537). He visualised a three-circle scheme for the life of the soul as well as the body. The soul is surrounded by three circles: an inner circle drawn by the soul's own intellectual activity, the circle of contemplative life. This is followed by the circle of the body which contains the soul like a vessel and appertains to the active life of the soul directing and determining the life of the organism. There is finally the outermost circle, that of the visible world of things that are foreign to ourselves and are dealt with in the order of the practical life of the soul. A similar three-circle scheme was devised by Bovillus for the body. Head, heart and abdomen were symbolised, each by one circle. Of these head and abdomen were described as endowed with outlets (*ostia*)—seven in the former and three in the latter. By contrast the heart had no such outlet, but was completely closed in, forming a *closed circle*[90] (pl. 25).

A mediaeval predecessor of the closed circle representing the heart may be found in the *Black Grain*, depicting the origin of the arteries in the heart. It illustrates mediaeval anatomical manuscripts and belongs to the "artery-man" of the so-called *Five-picture series* of anatomical drawings. As Boyd Hill has shown the *Black Grain* also symbolises the origin of the spirit that pulsates in the arteries. In the opinion of the present writer this mediaeval Western tradition is based on oriental mysticism: In Mahmud's didactic poem *Gülschen Ras*—the *Rose Blossom of Secrets*— the seed grain is glorified as the origin of many thousands of

90 Bovillus (Bouelles), Carol., *In hoc opere ... contenta. Liber cordis.* Paris J. Badius Ascensius, 1523, fol. XIII verso (copy used at the Wellcome Library. Catalogue of the latter ed. F.N.L. Poynter vol. I, London 1962, No. 6845, p. 363 in the Supplement). The present author is indebted to Dr F.N.L. Poynter for this.

harvests—just as the whole body is enthroned in one point, the grain of mustard that is called the heart. It is in this corn of the heart that both worlds are joined together, that of the angel and that of Satan. From each point a new circle does develop which turns as circle and stops still as centre.

Paracelsus would seem to continue in this tradition when he says: a bite of bread contains the whole anatomy of man invisibly, for example his brain and heart and also all colours and forms. So does Robert Fludd in his *Philosophicall Key* dealing with wheat, its elemental composition and its "mysticall signification". Wheat, it is said, corresponds to the sun among the planets, to the heart in man's body, and to gold in the mineral kingdom. It is the "only Kinge of all vegetable graines, beinge that in it Nature herselfe the only Queene mother and nurse of this world is most resident", wherefore "nature has indued this graine with an infinite vertue in multiplication" and made it akin to "man's vitall and naturall faculty". Fludd's treatise was incorporated in his *Anatomiae amphitheatrum* of 1623 and fittingly the emblematic frontispice of the latter work correlates the anatomy of "inner man" with the anatomy of the human body and the chemical "anatomy" of wheat—the subject of Fludd's analytical efforts. In the human dissection scene given the demonstrator points to the region of the heart. At the same time his right ear is connected by a horizontal line with the central zone in a furnace in which the elemental components and the quintessence of wheat are separated. This horizontal line forms the basis of a triangle which has its point in the centre of the star-like figure which symbolises inner man and is marked by the monogram of Christ[90a].

The representation of the heart as a "closed circle" by Bovillus is not without Harveian interest. For Harvey compared the heart to the centre of a circle—*ut centro in circulo*—thereby expressing the supremacy of the heart in an original form that had not been anticipated by Aristotle[91]. The latter simply speaks of the situation of the principal part of the body, the heart, in the middle of the chest—the term he uses is *meson*, not *centrum* (*kentron*) or *circle* (*kyklos*)[92]. Nor did Cesalpinus when repeating Aristotle's doctrine—the heart, he says, is in the middle which is the most advantageous position to distribute life to all parts[93].

Bruno seems to extend the scheme of Bovillus—according to him the heart is the centre of the circle from which the blood goes out into the periphery and to which it returns. Bruno thus follows the line that is perceptibly different from the lead given by St Thomas Aquinas. For in Bruno's concept "circularity was emanci-

90a The *Black Grain* in the heart in mediaeval anatomical illustration: Boyd Hill jr., H., *The grain and the spirit in mediaeval anatomy. Speculum*, 1965, XL, 63–73; in Oriental mysticism: Tholuck, F.A.G., *Blüthensammlung aus der morgenländischen Mystik.* Berlin Dümmler. 1825, p.201 (from Mahmud's Lehrgedicht Gülschen Ras – Rosenflor der Geheimnisse, of about 1339).

Paracelsus, *De modo pharmacandi*, tr. IV, ed. Sudhoff vol. IV, p. 460.

Fludd, Robert, *Philosophicall Key* in Josten, C.H., *Robert Fludd's "Philosophicall Key" and his alchemical experiment on wheat Ambix*, 1963, XI, 1–23. With reference to the emblematic frontispiece of the *Amphitheatrum:* p. 22–23. On the Harveian significance of the latter work see in the present work p. 117 seq.

The trend of thought followed by Fludd in the *Key* is *alchemical.* He subjects wheat to putrefaction in the same way as the alchemist putrefies the prime matter of metals and minerals in order to isolate the seed of gold. Indeed the *Lapis philosophorum* is also called *grain of corn* (*granum frumenti*) in the alchemical literature at large: *Theatrum Chemicum*, Argentor. 1613, vol. IV, p. 814; 824; 861: *lapis noster vocatur etiam granum frumenti, quod nisi mortuum fuerit, ipsum solum manet*, in Davidis Lagnei *Harmonia s. consensus Philosophorum Chemicorum*, cap. 1 with ref. to Garlandus cap. 13; *granum incombustibile metallorum, ibid.* with ref. to Vogelius; *philosophi volunt nutrire granum ex humore connaturali, donec vegetetur et fructum afferat talem* with ref. to Aurora, cap. 20, p. 231 (Beati Thomae de Aquino *Aurora* in *Harmoniae Chymico-Philosophicae Decas II*, ed. Joh. Rhenanus, Francof. 1625).

91 Harvey, *Praelectiones Anatomiae universalis* fol. 72r. See below, p. 220.

92 Aristotle, *De partibus animalium* lib. III, cap. 4; 665b 18–666b 7: *en meso keisthai tou anankeiou somatos. On the parts of the animals.* Transl. by W. Ogle. London 1882, p. 67.

93 Cesalpinus, And., *Quaestionum peripateticar.* lib. V, quaest. 3 (1571) Venet. 1593, fol. 115 v: *in medio est, qui locus est commodissimus, ut omnibus partibus vitam impartiatur.*

pated from the scholastic pattern of the systole—diastole "cycle" of the heart and transferred to the spirit and its vector, the blood. He also saw in it one expression of the unity of macrocosm and microcosm rather than the sign of a subordination of the latter to celestial influence. In other words he granted the individual more independence than had been allowed him in previous schemes where he had been subjected to the all powerful direction of a "generality", namely the uniform circular movement of the celestial bodies.

Bruno's concept, then, marked an ideological advance in the direction of Harvey and his speculations on "circularity". We have no evidence that he knew Bruno's works, let alone that they influenced him. It is reasonable to assume, however, that at least he did know about him and the trend of his philosophy and cosmology—for these were well known among all naturalists and philosophers in Europe at the time, as shown for example by Kepler and J.B. Van Helmont. Bruno had been in England and Harvey in Padua—he arrived there in the year of Bruno's spectacular execution at Rome which preceded Harvey's Padovian doctorate and return to England by two years. The circle and its mysteries in the greater and lesser worlds were bound to form a subject of general discussion. Harvey who was steeped in Aristotle cannot have failed to lend his ear to such discussions. He may just have remembered them *after* he had made his discovery, but they are more likely to have been alive in his mind both *before and after*.

(*f*) *Harvey and Robert Fludd (1574–1637; pl. 17)*

Harvey gives ample proof of his belief in the analogies between the greater and the lesser world, between cosmos and man. Circular motion serves the preservation and maintenance of both these worlds—the individual through the circular motion of the blood and the species through the cyclical transition of seed into the developing animal and its involution back into seed again. Had Harvey not given expression to this belief himself we could still have used his friendship with the medical Rosicrucian Fludd as indirect evidence for it. Fludd was Harvey's senior by four years. He came from a family of importance, being the son of Sir Thomas Fludd, paymaster to the forces in France and the Netherlands in the Elisabethan era. A student of St John's, Oxford, Fludd travelled widely on the Continent where he became acquainted with the work of Paracelsus and the Paracelsians. Some two years after Harvey's return from Padua, Fludd came back to England, took his medical degree at Oxford a year later (1605), was finally admitted to the Royal College of Physicians (1609) and settled down to a lucrative practice in London[94]. At the time of the publication of his first defence of the Rosicrucians (1616) he is most likely to have attended the anatomical lectures of Harvey. The evidence for this derives from Fludd's *Clavis*—a reply to the anatomical and physiological arguments assembled by Gassendi against Fludd's ideas on the movement of the blood (p. 117). The former still believed in the percolation of the finer—purer—part of the venous blood from the right heart to the left across the septum. Fludd strenuously denied the existence of such interventricular communications and explained Gassendi's findings in terms of artefacts. Fludd continues: "This inquiry was carried out many times with great diligence by several of my colleagues and particularly by Dr Harvey, most expert anatomist, as he himself put the matter to the test exhaustively for his own sake—the circulation of the blood; however, not in any of many cadavers examined did he find anything like this; neither did I nor others when scrutinising the septum of the heart with sharp and lynx-like eyes." Fludd concludes that Gassendi's observation, in so far as it was not due to an artefact, must have been a solitary instance with no value in normal anatomy[95].

It should be added that Fludd was a keen anatomist. For this we have evidence from Harvey himself (see below and notes 102–103) and Fludd's own words: "Against the time that I was to read my publick Anatomy in the College, I had (as our custom is) a certain body of one that was hanged, to be anatomized at my house privately.[96]"

The first recognition of Harvey's discovery in print Fludd's Medicina catholica of 1629 (pl. 18, 19)

Fludd himself referred to his personal friendship with Harvey in a passage which is of particular significance in our present context. It is found in Fludd's *Medicina catholica* of 1629 and constitutes the first recognition of the truth of Harvey's discovery to appear in print. Fludd discusses here the principle of polarity and its application to the pulse and the movement of the blood. Expansion and contraction of the heart is an instance of that polarity through which the vital spirit achieves the functioning of the organs. This vital polarity inside the animal has its parallel in the greater world. To the cold breath through which the spirit is taken in there is a corresponding contraction of the air, a rise of the water in the thermo-barometer (devised by Fludd) and systole of

94 Craven, F.B., *Robert Fludd, the English Rosicrucian* 1902; Waite, A.E., *The Brotherhood of the Rosy Cross.* London 1924, p. 274; Josten, C.H., *Truth's Golden Harrow.* An unpublished alchemical treatise of Robert Fludd. Ambix, 1949, III, 91–150. – Debus, A.G., *Robert Fludd and the Circulation of the Blood. J. Hist. Med.* 1961, XVI, 374–393.

95 Praeterea ista inquisitio a pluribus collegarum meorum, et praecipue a D. Harueo Anatomico expertissimo, saepius instituta est magna cum diligentia. quatenus ipse ad suam in sanguinis circulationis causam cum fatigatione huius rei experimentum fecit; sed ne in unico quidem ex pluribus cadaveribus invenit ipse tale quidpiam; nec ego nec alii, qui oculis acutissimis et quasi lynceis cordis septum sumus scrutati ... Fludd, Rob., *Clavis Philosophiae et Alchymiae Fluddanae sive Roberti Fluddi Armigeri, et Medicinae Doctoris, ad Epistolicam Petri Gassendi Theologi Exercitationem Responsum.* Francof. 1633, pp. 33 et seq. See Debus, A.G., *Rob. Fludd and the circulation of the blood. J. Hist. Med.* 1961, XVI, loc. cit. in note [94], p. 386–388. Idem, The *English Paracelsians* London 1965, p. 105–136.

96 Robert Fludd, Esq, *Mosaicall Philosophy.* London Humphrey Moseley, 1659, p. 255.

the heart, while conversely we find expansion and diastole. From these parallels Fludd infers the truth of the view that the blood circulates in its vessels, obeying the systole and diastole with a movement resembling the ebb and flood of the tide, and moving in the same way as the world in its orbit. Such considerations confirm, Fludd says, *exacte* the verdict and opinion of his friend, colleague and compatriot, Harvey, who was well versed not only in anatomy, but also in the deepest mysteries of philosophy. The theory which he demonstrated expertly and prudently on many grounds derived from the storehouse of natural philosophy as well as by manifold ocular demonstration is that the movement of the blood is circular. How could it be otherwise, since it is absolutely certain that the spirit of life retains an impression both of the planetary system and of the zodiac? Thus as the moon follows her unchanging path completing her journey in a month, she incites the spirit of the blood, and therefore the blood itself, by virtue of its "imperceptible astra" to follow in a "circular" movement. Every seaman is acquainted with the influence of the moon on wind and tide. Why should she not exercise a similar influence on the microcosm of man?[97]

Fludd and the Publication of Harvey's De motu

Fludd's endorsement of Harvey's discovery on the grounds of its confirmation of the influence of the greater world on the lesser and their basic parallelism cannot have displeased the discoverer. For we have evidence of their long lasting friendship. It was Fludd who had been instrumental in the publication of Harvey's masterpiece, the *De motu*, by a German publisher who was connected with the Rosicrucian circles in which Fludd himself moved[98]. Fludd had his own reasons for having his voluminous and rambling works with their fine allegorical plates published on the Continent—reasons that were largely financial.

As he tells us himself, the Continental publisher not only asked for no subsidy, but even paid royalties[99]. Harvey's reasons are open to speculation—they may have been quite different. It remains strange, however, that he should have sent his small barely illustrated book abroad, in the middle of the Thirty Years' War and to that country where it was raging. Moreover the printing was badly executed and on bad paper.

Personal Contacts and Citation of Fludd by Harvey

Fludd met Harvey on various (and probably not infrequent) occasions[100], mostly on business transacted on behalf of the

97 The first recognition of Fludd in this respect is due to: PAGEL, W., *Religious Motives in the Medical Biology of the XVIIth Century. Bullet. Hist. Med.* 1935, III, p. 277–278 with ref. to Fludd's *Pulsus seu nova et arcana Pulsuum Historia e sacro fonte radicaliter extracta, nec non medicorum ethnicorum dictis et authoritate comprobata. Hoc est portionis tertiae pars tertia, De pulsuum scientia*, p. 11 In: *De Medicina Catholica* Francof. Fitzer. 1629.

98 WILLIAM FITZER at Francfort. – The question was first discussed by A. Malloch, *William Harvey*, New York 1929, p. 99. For further detail see: WEIL, E., *William Fitzer, the publisher of Harvey's De motu cordis. The Library*, 1944, XXIV, 142; also: KEYNES, SIR G., *Bibliography of William Harvey*, Cambridge 1953, p. 3.

99 "because our home-borne printers demanded of me five hundred pounds to Print the first volume, and to find the cuts in copper; but beyond the Seas it was printed at no cost of mine, and that, as I would wish: And I had 16 coppies sent me over with 40 pounds in Gold, as an unexpected gratuite for it" *Fludds Answer unto M. Foster. Or, the squeezing of Parson Fosters Sponge, ordained by him for the wiping away of Weapon-Salve.* London 1631, p. 21 f. Quoted from DEBUS, A.G., *The English Paracelsians.* London Oldbourne Press. 1965 p. 126.

100 "Harvey had many contacts with Fludd beginning in their student days at Padua in 1602...": KEYNES, SIR G., *Bibliography*, loc. cit. in note [98], 1953, p. 3.

It is also of interest that verses in praise of Harvey and Fludd are found in close vicinity to each other in Dr Peter Bowne's *Pseudo-Medicorum Anatomia* of 1624, namely on sig. a 2 verso and a 3 recto respectively: DURLING, A.J., *Some unrecorded verses in praise of Robert Fludd and William Harvey. Medical Hist.* 1964, VIII, 279–281.

Fludd's name appears in a similar close juxtaposition with that of Harvey in Elias Ashmole, *Theatrum Chemicum Britannicum*, London 1652, p. 460: "the *Phisitians Colledge* of *London* ... and though we doe not, yet the World abroad has taken notice of sundry learned Fellowes of that Societie, as *Linacres*, *Gilbert*, *Ridley*, *Dee*, *Flood* etc. and at present *Doctor Harvey*, who deserves for his many and eminent *Discoveries*, to have a *Statue* erected rather of *Gold* then of *Marble*".

College of Physicians in which both Harvey and Fludd served as Censors, such as control-visits to apothecaries and meetings in which the *London Pharmacopoeia* was prepared[101].

Harvey in turn mentions Fludd in his *Lectures on the Whole of Anatomy* as well as in those on the *Local motion of animals*. In the former Fludd is credited with the observation of cartilaginous fungus-like "sugar-icing" on the capsule of a grossly enlarged spleen—excrescences that were comparable to "nails or horn softened in water"[102]. The Fludd citation in the latter is more interesting in the present context. It introduces the chapter: *Of the motive spirit*. Here it says: "According to Aristotle, *De motu animalium* ... the principal organ of movement is the motive spirit for the reason that it is capable of contracting and relaxing. Here: Dr Flud.[103]"

This refers to Aristotle's dictum: "The spirit is well disposed to excite movement and to exert power; and the functions of movement are thrusting and pulling. Accordingly, the organ of movement must be capable of expanding and contracting; and this is precisely the characteristic of spirit. It contracts and expands naturally....[104]"

Harvey's citation of Fludd is apposite as it was he who made contraction and expansion the basic operative principle in the cosmos—a "mysterium" accessible to ocular demonstration by means of a universal instrument that was something between a thermometer and barometer (see above p. 114)[105]. That Harvey mentions Fludd and not the latter's obvious source: Bernardinus Telesius, may be regarded as a token of their friendship—all the more so, as at that very time the Telesian principle of expansion and contraction passed, in the words of Bacon, as "quite fundamental and catholic"[106]. We shall have to revert to related ideas of Fludd elsewhere in the present book[107].

Harvey and John Woodall (pl. 22)

Fludd was not the only unorthodox colleague with whom Harvey maintained a personal relationship. John Woodall (1556?–1643), Paracelsian surgeon, was elected Surgeon of St Bartholomew's Hospital in 1616—a position "which put him constantly in contact with ... William Harvey who had been a physician there since 1609. Indeed, we find some of the earliest printed references to Harvey in the first edition of Woodall's *Surgion's Mate*.[108]" His Paracelsian leanings not only concerned the new chemical remedies, but also medical theory. Woodall was a pioneer in the orange and lemon treatment of scurvy. He also discussed alchemy and

101 In a report drafted by Mayerne and signed by John Argent, president, and seventeen fellows (including Harvey and Fludd) the College demanded that in future all apothecaries be prohibited under heavy penalties from compounding without the prescription of a physician any medicinal substance without exception or administering them—dated May 30th 1632. From: WALL, C. and CAMERON, H.C., *A history of the Worshipful Society of Apothecaries of London*, vol.I, annotated and edited by E.A. Underwood. London. The Wellcome Historical Medical Museum N.S. No 8; 1963, p. 263. See also p. 290 and passim on Fludd's concern with practical pharmacy. There are in addition references to Harvey as a member of the College speaking up against the apothecaries in the various controversies between the latter and the physicians. Harvey appears to have been worried about the apothecaries' improper compounding of medicines and much interested in having the Censors' work enforced. Fludd was a censor on various occasions. Harvey's interest in chemical medicines is shown in his involvement in the Lac sulphuris problem.

102 "Tunicam cum cartilaginibus ut fungi, nayles or horne softened in water, testibus Dr Fludd, Mr Mapes; etiam Bauhinus et Columbus referunt talem vidisse." HARVEY, *Praelectiones Anatomie Universalis* fol. 39 r. Ed. G. Whitteridge. Edinburgh and London 1964, p. 146.

103 HARVEY, W., *De Motu Locali Animalium* (1627) fol. 95 r. ed. G. Whitteridge. Cambridge 1959, p. 94.

104 ARISTOTLE, *De motu animalium* 703 a 20, cap. 10; tr. A.S.L. FARQUHARSON Oxford 1912.

105 PAGEL, W., *Religious Motives* 1935, loc. cit. in note [97], p. 277.

106 TELESIUS, BERNARDINUS, *De rerum natura juxta propria principia*. Neapoli 1586, Prooem. I, 1 seq.; 1,4 p. 7; I, 19, p. 27; III, 34: All natural effects are to be derived from heat and cold; their continual combat causes the different degrees of contraction and expansion by means of which matter emerges. PAGEL, W., *Religious Motives* 1935, loc. cit. in note [97], p. 272. – RITTER, HEINRICH, *Geschichte der Christlichen Philosophie*, vol. V. Hamburg 1850, p. 564. – TENNEMANN, W.G., *Geschichte* der Philosophie, vol. IX, Leipzig 1814, p. 284–286. – CARRIERE, M., *Die philosophische Weltanschauung der Reformationszeit in ihren Beziehungen zur Gegenwart*. Stuttgart und Tübingen 1847, p. 359. – HÖNIGSWALD, R., *Denker der Italienischen Renaissance*. Basel 1938,

such writers as Oswald Croll, Josephus Quercetanus (Duchesne), Leonard Thurneysser and Martin Ruland—all orthodox Paracelsians. His extensive chapters on Salt, Sulphur and Mercury are adorned with the picture of Mercury from Thurneysser's *Quinta Essentia*[109], and the table of alchemical characters occupies some twelve pages in the second edition of the work[110].

These personal contacts, then, reveal facets of Harvey that are quite different from the image of the scientist pure and simple, the "modern" and the founder of something "modern" in terms of which he is usually presented. This multicoloured picture, however, is quite consistent with the body of philosophical thinking and cosmological speculation which is laid down in Harvey's own work and with which his discovery and observational treasure is bound up.

Fludd's Mystical Anatomy as a possible source of the philosophical Idea of Circulation (pl. 20, 21, 24)

It was, then, no rhetorical phrase when Fludd called Harvey his friend, but the token of a close acquaintance that could not have failed to lead to an exchange of ideas, thoughts and experiences. From all the evidence we have this must have gone back far beyond the year in which *De motu* was published. Fludd was the first to stand up for the truth of Harvey's discovery. We know that he attended Harvey's anatomical demonstrations in which the latter, on his own showing, had communicated his ideas on the motion of the heart and blood prior to their publication in 1628. We may well try to find traces of this in those works of Fludd that antedate *De motu*.

What may be regarded as such a trace occurs in a context that is closely akin to that in which Fludd voices his agreement with Harvey after the event, i. e. the appearance of the latter's work in print. This context is mystical cosmology, the parallelism between the greater world and the microcosm of man. The same law of expansion and contraction that governs all realms of the world outside is operative in the living organism and the spirit of life subjected to it. Hence its obedience to the circular motion of the celestial bodies and the imprint of the latter on the blood and its motion, hence the truth conveyed by the comparison of the heart with the sun.

This is the mystical "argument" brought forward in Fludd's *Medicina catholica* of 1629–1631. In 1623 he had published the *Anatomiae amphitheatrum* which contained a chapter on the *mystical anatomy of the blood*[111]. In this the central focus of reference is the

p. 115 seq. (with ref. to Telesius' concept of motion as following from his two principles, especially where certain biological processes are referred to contraction and expansion: "Was Telesio über die Funktion der Blutgefäße lehrt, was er—vielleicht in Verbindung mit Caesalpino und schon ganz im Geiste Harveys—zur Frage des Blutkreislaufes beibringt, gründet sich auf die Idee der wissenschaftlichen Allgegenwart des Bewegungsmotivs.").
BACON, FR., *Phenomena Universi s. Historia Naturalis et Experimentalis de Ventis.* Amstelod. 1695, p. 94 (Historia densi et rari): "nam et Densitates et Raritates Corporum nosse, et multo magis Condensationes et Rarefactiones procurare, et efficere, maxime interest et Contemplativae et Practicae. Cum igitur sit res (si qua alia) plane fundamentalis et Catholica." For further ref. (Sir Kenelm Digby) see PAGEL, *Relig. Motives* 1935, loc. cit. in note [97], p. 272 note [9], with ref. to Jos. NEEDHAM, *Chemical Embryology*, Cambridge 1931, I, p. 130.

107 p. 190.

108 WOODALL, JOHN, *The Surgions Mate.* London 1617, p. 91 and 96 where Harvey is given as the authority for the use of *Pilulae Cambogiae* as a purge. DEBUS, A.G., *John Woodall, Paracelsian Surgeon.* Ambix 1962, X, 108–118; TOTTENHAM, R.E., *Harvey and Woodall, Brit. Med. J.* 1963, I, 752 and KEYNES, SIR G., *ibid.*, p. 680 and 823.

109 The plate was designed by Thurneisser for Sulphur; it is found in the latter's *Quinta Essentia, das ist die höchste subtilitet, krafft und wirckung ... der Medicin und Alchemy.* 2nd ed. quoted Leipzig 1574, p. 79, with the caption: *Spiritus Sulphur*, and the chapter heading: *Vom Geist.* There is a certain justification in Woodall's use of the symbol for Mercurius, as the latter in Paracelsian parlance corresponds to *Geist*, whereas Sulphur stands for *Seele*, i.e. the middle between *Geist* and Body (Salt), the astral *anima vegetativa.*

110 London 1639, pp. 248–260.

111 FLUDD, ROB., *Anatomiae amphitheatrum triplici more et conditione varia* Francof. 1623, p. 33. – See: DEBUS, A.G., loc. cit. 1961, in note [94], p. 376 and 378.

sun, the tabernacle of the great world, paralleled by that of the lesser world, the heart. The breath of life is conveyed from the macrocosm to the living being by the four cardinal winds which in turn follow the dictates of the sun. The latter impresses on the winds its own circular motion—*aeris dispositio a motu solari dependeat*. In fact air owing to the action of the sun moves according to the latter's motion, i.e. in a circle (*non aliter movetur aer naturaliter, quam ad motum solis, cuius actione agitatur motu circulari*). In the same way the spirit of life is seen to blow from the East of the microcosm, that is from the chamber of the heart, as if from a microcosmic ruler of the winds, and through blowing upon it to seize and carry off with it the whole of the aerial spirit of the blood in a circle (*videmus spiritum vitae ab oriente microcosmi, hoc est a cordis Thalamo tanquam Aeoli microcosmici, capsula spirare, atque afflatu omnem sanguinis spiritum aereum secum in gyrum quasi rapere*). This movement Fludd presents as a rhythmically repeated operation: as the sun after setting aspires to return again to the site of his rising in order to perform a new circuit, the life-dispensing sun or vital heat strives to rise again after it has descended to the spermatic region, the south of the body, and quickly travels through the branches of the aorta to the hepatic south and splenic north (*iterum ad novum quasi ortum aspirat, et properat per ramos aortae, ad meridiem hepaticam, et septentrionem lienalem*). As the fire of the heart is the off-shoot and true son of the sun, it follows that it is moved in the same way as the latter moves, for it is its ray which cannot be separated from its source and therefore moves as a part moves with the whole[112].

In these passages a circular motion imitating that of the sun is ascribed to the blood. It is couched in the very general terms of microcosmic analogy. We have examined several such analogical assertions of the circular motion of the blood prior to the time of Fludd and Harvey. The most poignant expression of it had been given by Giordano Bruno when the former were in their youth (p. 103–113). There is nothing in Fludd's passages about reflux of the blood to the heart, as is stipulated for example by Bruno. Nor can we imagine that Fludd learned his mystical visions from Harvey. The latter could not, however, have failed to take cognisance of what his friend Fludd had speculated about the heart and the blood in a book devoted to human anatomy. To the modern this is without any original merit, except the mystical-microcosmic aspects of the subject. Nevertheless Harvey had an extensive knowledge of the literature including minor and quite insignificant books. Fludd's work may well have impressed him—unlike the

112 Fludd, *Anatomiae amphith.*, loc. cit. in note [111], cap. 3, p. 266; Debus, loc. cit. in note [94], p. 379. – For a somewhat kindred passage from Fludd's *Pulsus Historia*, lib. I, cap. 3 (*Medicina catholica*, 1631, loc. cit. in note [97]) see the discussion in: Peters, H. M., *Modell-Beispiele aus der Geschichte der Biologie*, *Stud. gener.* 1965, XVIII, 298–305 (p. 301). There is no allusion to the circle in this passage, however; it belongs more to the Telesian context referred to above, p. 116 note [106].

modern—as an important contribution. For Harvey, too, made use of the microcosmic analogy and did so at a prominent and memorable place. It was at some time in the twenties that the idea of circulation took firm shape in his mind. Fludd's work had appeared in 1623, although the relevant passages were, on Fludd's own showing, completed earlier, i.e. on December 9th 1621[113]. There was admittedly nothing in it about a connexion between the arterial and venous systems. It conspicuously displayed, however, *circulatio* with reference to the blood and the heart: first in the chemical sense of distillation—the right heart "circulating" venous blood, already "distilled" by the liver, into the lungs. We shall return to this meaning of *circulatio* and its significance for Harvey below (p. 188 seq.). Secondly Fludd visualised the sun as impressing his circular motion on the blood—at all events the arterial blood which conveys the spirit, the "flame of the heart". The blood "follows" this motion and continually repeats it in a cycle that parallels the rise and setting of the sun. Again the sun standing as the macrocosmic symbol for the microcosmic ruler and sovereign, the heart, and its messenger, the blood, was used by Harvey. Microcosmic analogy is a standing argument and not merely a rhetorical embellishment in the works of Harvey. It has the ring of seriousness and conviction. Fludd was even not original in bringing forward a "mystical anatomy" of the heart and blood, and Harvey quotes, not Fludd, but Aristotle as authority for this as in so many other topics. So did Fludd, however; and when all circumstances are taken into account it is not unreasonable to assume that Harvey's mind had received a stimulus from Fludd's *Anatomy* that sensitised it to some connexion of the circular movement with the heart and blood. There was nothing that he could use for the demonstration of his idea, but it was the idea that had come first and he only afterwards found that it was true. It occurred to him when he was meditating about the quantity and speed of the blood that passes through the heart and vessels—and not in a vision of microcosmic analogy. But this is there too and conspicuously so in his memorable account in the eighth chapter of *De motu*.

113 Debus, p. 376.

(g) *Circular Symbolism after Harvey*

The circle remained an impressive symbol of biological processes well into the second half of Harvey's century—the era of Iatrochemistry and Iatrophysics, the time of de le Boe (Sylvius, 1614–1672), himself an early supporter of Harvey, and Alphonso Borelli

(1608–1679) and their schools. Indeed the conviction that everything should move in circles led to interesting and scientifically correct observations and experiments concerning the movement of fluids other than blood. It was thus that Maurits van Reverhorst (died 1722) described in an outstanding doctoral thesis the circular motion of the bile (*motus bilis circularis*)—its continual excretion and re-absorption[114] (pl. 29).

Circulation—a "Hippocratic discovery"

Another trend led at the same time to a growing belief in the story that the circular movement of the blood had been known to Hippocrates. It is interesting that this was associated with the high praise accorded to Harvey and his discovery as the key to the Secrets of the Physicians (*Arcana medicorum*) which—largely owing to Harvey's discovery—had no longer remained secrets (*non arcana*). Thus Hermann Grube of Lübeck, municipal physician at Hadersleben (1637–1698), wrote that the circulation of the blood was as it were "called back to light" by Harvey, for Grube was convinced that it had been known to the ancients and in particular to Hippocrates himself (*sanguinis circulatio postliminio velut in lucem ab Harveyo revocata—quamvis veteribus quoque, et ipsi in primis* Hippocrati *eandem innotuisse, mihi persuadeam omnino*)[115]. But, then, Grube was no advocate of symbolism. He had no patience with anything Paracelsian—either with the "universal remedy" or with the "magnetic" forces accounting for the "transplantation" of disease[116]. Strangely enough Grube had Thomas Bartholinus' *Letter on the transplantation of diseases* printed in front of his book on the *Secrets of physicians no longer secrets*—a tract that is deeply imbued with belief in the "magnetic" cure and transmission of diseases[117].

Hippocratic "circular" symbolism is the key-note of the work of Raymond Restaurand (1627–1682) from Pont St-Esprit in Languedoc, Doctor of the Faculty at Montpellier[118], and author of several treatises calling for the renaissance of Hippocratism—Hippocratic physiology and the Hippocratic iron in surgery[119]. Before, in 1675, he had published: *Hippocrates on the circulatory movements in man from which it emerges that the nature of the human body is circular and everything in it is moved in a circle*[120]. In a later edition with altered title of 1684 he passed censure on "the shadows of Harvey, the prince of the new medicine, on Pecquet and Willis, and on the Harveyans.[121]" Such criticism of contemporary luminaries in favour of the ancients had been expressed by him two years before in a treatise on the consensus between the physiology

114 Reverhorst, Mauritius van, *D ssertatio Anatomico-Medica de motu bilis circulari ejusdem morbis quam publice olim habuit* Lugd. Batavor. 1696 (apud Jord. Luchtmans). – The copy in possession of the author has no imprint and seems to be the original form of the dissertation of 1692 (this is the year given by C.E. Daniels in *Biograph. Lexikon herv. Ärzte* ed. Gurlt-Hirsch, vol. IV, 1886, p. 718–the 1696 work being the second edition). The year of Reverhorst's birth, as given by Daniels—1686—is obviously wrong.

115 Grube, Herm., *De arcanis medicorum non arcanis commentatio. Ex inventis recentiorum Harvejanis, Bartholinianis, Sylvianis, Willisianis.* Hafniae 1673, p. 150.

116 Grube, loc. cit. 1673 in note [115], p. 1 et seq.: Agit de vanitate medicamenti universalis; p. 26 agit de unguento armario; p. 45: de transplantatione morborum (see also: idem, *De transplantatione morborum. Analysis nova.* Hamburgi et Amsterod. 1674); p. 52: an in amuletis arcana sint quaerenda?

117 Bartholini, Th., *De transplantatione morborum dissertatio epistolica.* Hafniae 1673.

118 Restaurand is praised by Sprengel for his "very good" work on the Peruvian bark with the significant title: *Hippocrate de l'usage de Kinkina p u l'usage des fièvres.* Lyons 1681 in: *Versuch einer pragmatischen Geschichte der Arzneykunde* 3rd ed. vol. IV, Halle 1827, p. 535. – *Biogr. Lexikon* ed. Gurlt-Hirsch, vol. IV, 1886, p. 710.

119 *Magnus Hippocrates Cous redivivus.* Lyons 1681. – *Hippocrates de inustionibus s. de fonticulis*, Lyons 1681 and others.

120 *Hippocrates de circulationibus humani corporis ... naturam humani corporis circularem esse, omnia in eo moveri circulariter.* Lyons 1675.

121 *Microscopium Hippocraticum sive judicium de umbris Harveyi, novae medicinae principis, Pequeti, Villisii, procerum illius et de motu sanguinis in animalibus.* Ex typogr. regia Principis Elysior. et industria Umbrae Elzevirii, 1684.

We shall mention recent criticism of modern attempts at tracing the circulation of the blood to the *Hippocratic Corpus* (p. 127); see also Grube as quoted in note [115]. The latter expressed an opinion widespread at his time, as shown by the example of Restaurand. It was argued on philological lines by Theodore Janssen ab Almeloveen, Professor of History, Greek and Medicine at Harderwick (1651–1712) in *Inventa Nov-Antiqua id est brevis*

of Aristotle and Epicurus followed by a refutation of Descartes, Gassendi and others[122].

Pitcairn's opposition

The enthusiasm of the partisans of Hippocrates was duly checked by Archibald Pitcairn (1652–1713). He said: "The fabric and motion of the heart were known to Hippocrates and he wrote a book about it. So did Harvey. Those who assert that the circuit of the blood was known to the former, should inspect the books of both with an objective mind (*sedato animo*).[123]" Later in the same text: "To-day after the whole matter has been demonstrated by Harvey, some people say that Hippocrates clearly taught the fabric and use of the heart valves. This does not help, for how many arose who gave better accounts of the fabric and use of the valves than Hippocrates. For all anatomists and physicians who came after Hippocrates were so ignorant of the true circulation of the blood that even some of them to whom Harvey's book was known, wrote against it.[124]" This is the text in the earlier editions of Pitcairn's chapter entitled: *Solutio problematis de inventoribus*— all the laurels are accorded to Harvey. In later editions including the English translation of 1727 Harvey appears either as one "of other moderns" or is cited together with Columbus, Caesalpinus and Servetus[125]. It is possible that this qualification was prompted by William Wotton's *Reflections upon ancient and modern learning* (first published 1694), although Caesalpinus had been appreciated as precursor of Harvey before, namely by Conring, Nardi, Pechlin (Janus Leonicenus), Almeloveen and others (p. 195)[126].

Sachs von Lewenheimb (pl. 28)

Following Aristotle Harvey had referred to the "circular" conversion of water into vapour and back to water again as the basic macrocosmic pattern of the circulation of the blood.[127] This analogy was made the subject of Philip Jacob Sachs von Lewenheimb's *Oceanus macro-microcosmicus* of 1664[128]. He addresses his dissertation to the famous anatomist Thomas Bartholinus, explaining that it deals with the movement of water from the seas and back to it and the analogy between this "circular" motion of water and that of the blood.

The earth, Lewenheimb says, resembles the human body, in that, like the latter, it is pervaded by canals. Moreover it harbours an internal fire. The sea lets water rise by evaporation and return in the form of rain whereby the rivers and subterranean waters are nourished and these finally return the same water to

enarratio ortus et progressus artis medicae ac praecipue de inventis vulgo novis, aut nuperrime in ea repertis. Amstelod. 1684, cap. XXVIII, p. 223–238, also with reference to Caesalpinus and Janus Leonicenus (Joh. Nicol. Pechlin, 1644–1706), *Metamorphosis Aesculapii et Apollinis pancreatici* Gratianopoli 1672 (a satyre directed against de le Boe Sylvius).

122 *L'accord des sentimens d'Aristote et d'Epicure sur les principes des corps naturels et sur les couleurs. Avec la réfutation des sentimens de Messieurs Gassendi, de Descartes, de Rohaut et de Cordemoy* Lyons 1682, in three parts (criticism of Harvey in part II).

123 Pitcairne, *Dissertationes medicae* (from 1693 onwards). Edition used Roterod. 1701, p. 91.

124 Pitcairne, *Dissert.* loc. cit. in note [123], p. 93.

125 Translation by G. Sewell and J.T. Desaguliers, *The works of Dr. Archibald Pitcairne*, London 1727, p. 152–153: "and Harvey and other Moderns have writ upon the same"; p. 156–157: "that some of them who knew *Columbus, Caesalpinus, Servetus* and others, and had read their Books, yet writ against that Doctrine of theirs". In the latter passage Harvey is not even mentioned, but bracketed with "others" who presumably came after Columbus, Caesalpinus and Servetus. – The present author is indebted to Mr R.D. Gurney for drawing his attention to Pitcairne in this context and the restrictions and qualifications in his defence of Harvey.

126 Nardius, I., *Noctes geniales*, Bononiae 1655, p. 743: "si quis a me percunctetur, quid sentiam de nova hac opinione, quam A. Caesalpinus primus inuehexit in campum literarium, et Clarissimus Harueius, et alii complures ad hanc usque diem exco-luere, atque excolunt, dicam cum Plauto, multo nequiores esse quae nunc cuduntur fabulae, quam nummi novi: et vere nequiores essent, si ut hactenus, ut videtur, Medicinam subverterent, quae inde deducuntur conclusiones..." – It is well known that Harvey exchanged friendly letters with Nardi which seem to antedate the publication of Nardi's book, however (Harvei *Opp. omnia* Londoni 1766 p. 619; 627; 639 and translations by Willis, p. 603; 610 and 615). – Pechlin in Janus Leonicenus, *Metamorphosis Aesculapii et Apollinis Pancreatici. Ed. alt.* Lugd. Batav. 1673, p. 74. – Pechlin also refers to Paul Sarpi as the discoverer of circulation and observer of the venous valves which he made known to Fabricius who in turn communicated the "secret" to Harvey. – On Almeloveen see note [121].

the sea. The latter thus acts not unlike the heart from which the blood goes out to the organs, starting on its way attenuated by the influx of heat and "perfected" in the "workshops" of the organs; finally after its absorption and assimilation by the organs, its residue is drawn back to the heart to be attenuated again—just as the waters are diluted when joining the sea. There is not only an active pumping of blood into the organs, but also attraction of the blood by the latter, comparable to that of water into plants. As these depend in their diversity upon the quality of the water which they obtain and the heat of the sun, the structure and constitution of the animal parts vary in accordance with the quality of the blood that forms and nourishes them. It is also the blood that conveys the seeds of disease such as "praeternatural and tartaric" salts. Harvey already had pointed out the significance of blood circulation for the spread of diseases and Grube elaborated on this. Lewenheimb loses himself in further speculation, however. Thus he says that no animal life can subsist, neither in the depth of the sea nor inside the heart, but that it can in extravasated blood which, like stagnant water, gives rise to the birth of worms. As subterranean fire keeps water in motion, so the fire in the heart moves the blood. As the moon moves the sea, the brain cooperates in moving the blood.

Georg Ernst Stahl's Tides of the Microcosmic Sea (pl. 30)

Above we mentioned the concepts of Fludd. These may well have influenced Lewenheimb's comparison of the circular motion of the blood with the circular exchange of water between the sea, the air, the rivers and fountains of the earth.

After Lewenheimb a similar comparison was incorporated into a doctrine designed to limit the power accorded to the central organ—the heart—in the original Harveian teaching. It is Georg Ernst Stahl's (1660–1734) idea of the *Tides of the microcosmic sea*[129]. In this he places emphasis on the role that the *tonus* of the porous parts of the organism has to play in the flux and reflux of the blood—a vindication of the periphery with its own fibrous and neuromuscular equipment as against its subjection to the dictatorial central—pumping—action of the heart. Stahl, as it were, interposed between arteries and veins the porous substance of the organs and tissues which the blood has to traverse. It is possessed of a certain strength and firmness preventing the blood carried into it by the pulse from dilating its pores. On the contrary, it is the latter that by their resistance force the blood to move on. The same pores regulate the amount of blood admitted to a given tissue

127 See above p. 82 and note [31].

128 1627–1672 at Breslau; see Julius Pagel in *Biograph. Lexikon* vol. V, 1887, p. 139–140.

129 Stahl, G.E., *Positiones de aestu maris microcosmici seu fluxu et reflexu sanguinis tam in pluribus aliis luculentis exemplis tum praecipue paroxysmo febrili tertianario ... mediante vero motu tonico partium porosarum ut praecipuo organismo in effectum deduci solito: ad motus sanguinis tonici veritatem et communissimam utilitatem, seu solennem et frequentissimum usum ulterius illustrandum, febrium vero pathologiae fundamentum, digito designandum* (recusa Halae 1716) in: *Dissertationes medicae tum epistolares tum academicae* I. Halae Magdeburgicae 1707.

in a given time. If the *tonus* actively constricts the pores, blood is driven out, if it relaxes blood is admitted—this alternate rhythm corresponds to the ebb and flood of the sea[130] and accounts for such conditions as spastic anemia and its opposite, congestion. These are not caused by the pulse, but by the *tonus* (*congestiones non fiunt a pulsu, sed a tono*)[131].

The analogy of the movement of the blood with the sea and the tides, then, was designed by Stahl to modify rather than to support and illustrate the original scheme of circulation. The blood, according to Stahl, circulates, but it is not simply driven from the arteries into the veins by the "impetus" imparted to it by the central power of the heart. In addition to the circle described by the blood stepping out from the heart and returning to its point of departure, there is the cyclical—tonic—contraction and dilatation of sponge-like peripheral parts, the former accounting for the transference of blood into the veins and the latter for the reception of blood from the arteries. Stahl's interest in this peripheral "cycle" derives in the first place from the role attributed by him to the soul as the origin of movement everywhere in the body as against its explanation in terms of cardiovascular mechanics centralised in the heart. Secondly Stahl's scheme provided an easy interpretation of the multitude of pathological conditions which obviously originated in the peripheral tissues and organs—from goose-flesh, pallor and headache to fever, fatal haemorrhages and gangrene. It is the peripheral "cycle" of tonic action and relaxation of the tissue-pores that greatly supports the working of the heart and relieves it of the strain which it shows in the form of anxiety and palpitations immediately the peripheral "cycle" fails to operate[132].

It would, then, appear that the analogy with the movement of water in the cosmos and notably the tides was applied to the circle described by the blood as well as the cycle of tissue-tone and relaxation acting as it were as a second heart. To Stahl who applied it in the latter sense blood circulation as a whole was nevertheless fundamental in building up his animistic system of life under normal and pathological conditions. Indeed everything in it depended upon the motion of the blood, but equally so upon its correct distribution to all parts, and in this, he thought, the periphery has as much to say as the centre.

To *conclude:* Circular symbolism should be considered under two headings:

(a) the cyclical movement of the heart and
(b) the circular motion of the blood.

130 P. 11; p. 34 and passim.

131 Coschwitius, G.D., *Dissertatio medica de motibus humorum spasmodicis a motu pulsus ordinarii diversis*, p. 35 (ed. used: recusa Halae 1724).

132 Ibidem, p. 17–18.

The main source for the first is St Thomas Aquinas' treatise *De motu cordis*, for the second Giordano Bruno's work *De rerum principiis*. We have reason to assume that Harvey was acquainted with the former—possibly through Stephan Roderic de Castro's *De meteoris microcosmi*. He could not have known Bruno's posthumous treatise, but may have had knowledge of circular symbolism as expressed in other works of Bruno with reference to the movement of the blood. Harvey's own speculations in this field are largely directed by his adherence to Aristotle including the latter's belief in the parallels between macrocosm and microcosm. Nevertheless he could have hardly failed to take notice of contemporary ideas on this subject. For these formed stock topics for cosmological discussion in the philosophy of the Renaissance which in itself may be seen as a broad attempt at reconciling Aristotelian and Platonic philosophies through a revival of Neoplatonism and Hermeticism. In this Bruno played a leading role. He must have been a popular figure at the time of Harvey's studies at Padua—if not through his work, through his tragic end which formed a news item of the first order among the savants of the period.

The Predecessors of Harvey

I. Galen's Ideas on the Heart and the Formation and Movement of the Blood

Among those who methodically studied the movement of the heart and blood before Harvey, Aristotle and Galen remain the outstanding landmarks. The ideas and opinions of the former constituted a gladly acknowledged and cherished source of inspiration for Harvey himself—however much he differed in detail from the Philosopher "so diligent and faithful"[1]. Indeed it is suggestive that the Aristotelian lead actually steered him in the direction of his discovery and can thus claim a legitimate place in its history. For this is bound up with the controversy which had developed in the Renaissance under the heading "*Aristotle versus Galen*". Indeed, Harvey found himself aligned on the Aristotelian front and his discovery has often been presented as a revolutionary break-away from the all powerful Galenic physiology. Although true in its essentials, this view calls for qualification. Galen's observations remained the basis of Harvey's new synthesis and in some respects they were even ahead of it[2]. His merits in the physiology of the cardio-vascular system had been recognised by Harvey. However, it is only recently that Galen has been given his due as a precursor of Harvey[3] and it is pertinent to review his observations and doctrines.

1. The Liver as the Origin of the Veins and of Venous Blood

In Galen's view the liver is (a) the *Arche*, the origin of all veins and (b) the first organ of blood formation (*proton tes haimatoseos*

1 These are Harvey's words in *Praelectiones anatomiae univers.*, London 1886, fol. 74 verso.

Concerning *pre-Aristotelian* sources for the knowledge of the anatomy and physiology of cardio-vascular function and the movement of the blood reference should be made to those studies in which the claim for an anticipation of Harvey's discovery by the Hippocratic writers was examined and refuted: Diepgen, P., *Haben die Hippokratiker den Blutkreislauf gekannt? Klin. Wschr.* 1937, XVI, 1820; Diller, H., *Die Lehre vom Blutkreislauf, eine verschollene Entdeckung der Hippokratiker? Arch. f. Gesch. d. Med.* 1938, XXXI, 201 and more recently Abel, K., *Die Lehre vom Blutkreislauf im Corpus Hippocraticum*, Hermes, 1958, LXXXVI, 192–219 (also in *Gesnerus*, 1958, XV, 71–105). The main points discussed by Abel may be mentioned:

(a) the age of the relevant treatises: *De corde*, *De alimento* and *De ossium natura* are suggested to be younger than the bulk of the Hippocratic Corpus. Hence any cardio-vascular knowledge found in them cannot be claimed for the period around 400 b. C. For example the knowledge of the valvular apparatus shown by the author of *De corde* is indicative of the latter being a contemporary of Erasistratus or even later—for it is Erasistratus (310–250 b. C.) who is credited with the discovery of the heart valves (p. 201). Moreover *De corde* contains traces of Aristotelian, and *De alimento* of Stoic teaching (p. 196; 200; 207).

(b) the divergencies in the cardio-vascular anatomy and physiology of the three treatises: For example, in *De corde* the heart is the fountain of all the blood, whereas in *De alimento* the arteries are derived from the heart and the veins from the liver.

(c) the discrepancy between the presence in these treatises of essential anatomical data and the absence of any correct physiological idea. The result: there was neither an idea of a closed circuit of the blood, nor of its movement in one direction.

2 This partly agrees with the stand taken by Jos. Fr. Payne, *Harvey and Galen. Harveian Oration*, October 19th 1896. London 1897, p. 26: "on this field (sc. the knowledge of physiology) Harvey stands face to face with Galen, nor is there any third figure that can be compared with them except that of the founder of biological science, Aristotle himself", and p. 48: "it is surely evident, then, that the conception of Galen as an ancient philosopher whose errors were exploded by Harvey is totally unjust. He was Harvey's most brilliant model and forerunner in one side of his work—the experimental—just as Aristotle was in another side—that of observation and generalisation." According to Payne, Galen combatted theory and tradition in favour of observaion and experiment, but in vain: the Peripatetics never learnt to dissect, nor the Stoics to use scientific arguments. Payne also finds Galen's methods much more scientific than those of Aristotle—the former leading to actual experimental proof as against the dim adumbrations and analogies presented by the latter. Galen was in fact—so Payne concludes—a modern experimental physiologist and may rightly be regarded as the founder of the physiology of the nervous system (p. 47). The great achievement of Aristotle, on the other hand, and its attraction for Harvey, lay in the derivation of his conceptions from embryology which led to the "indissoluble connexion of the heart, the blood vessels and the blood." He thereby "kept clear of the liver, that great stumbling-block of the medical anatomists. It was this which Harvey so much appreciated and one reason which led him to speak of Aristotle with such generous enthusiasm." (p. 41). See below, p. 135.

3 Temkin, O., *On Galen's Pneumatology. Gesnerus* 1951, VIII, 180–9.

Fleming, D., *Galen on the Motions of the Blood in the Heart and Lungs Isis* 1955, XLVI, 14 and 319.

Wilson, L. G., *Erasistratus, Galen and the Pneuma. Bullet. Hist. Med.* 1959, XXXIII, 293.

Idem, *The Transformation of Ancient Concepts of Respiration in the Seventeenth Century. Isis* 1960, LI, 161.

Idem, *The Problem of the Discovery of the Pulmonary Circulation J. Hist. Med.* 1962, XVII, 229.

Hall, A. R., *Studies on the History of the Cardiovascular System Bullet. Hist. Med.* 1960, XXXIV, 391.

Siegel, R. E., *Galen's Experiments and Observations on Pulmonary Blood Flow and Respiration. Amer. J. Cardiology* 1962, X, p. 738.

Idem, *The Influence of Galen's Doctrine of Pulmonary Bloodflow on the Development of Modern Concepts of Circulation. Arch. Gesch. d. Med.* 1962, XLVI, 311.

organon)[4]. With this Galen set himself up in frontal opposition to the view held by Aristotle and followed by Erasistratus and the Erasistrateans. It was the latter in particular whom Galen singled out as the target of attack[5]. Aristotle had regarded the heart as the central organ—the *Arche*—of all vessels, arteries as well as veins. It had been *Arche* in the anatomical as well as the physiological and embryological sense. The veins, so Aristotle argued, really *come from* the heart, whereas they merely *extend through* (*diechousin*) the organs which hold the veins steady like an anchor[6]. The heart was also *Arche* in the physiological sense, namely as the beginning, source and first receptacle of the blood[7], a point that seemed accessible to embryological proof[8]. There is no evidence, however, that this view implied the distribution of venous blood from the heart to the periphery. It had been Erasistratus himself who had first described the tricuspid as one of the two valves which merely allow of intromission of blood into the heart[9]. In fact, the apparent contradiction between this and the view of the heart as the distributor of venous blood to the periphery—qua *Arche* of the veins and the blood—formed a cornerstone in Galen's argument in favour of the liver as *Arche* of the veins and source of the blood.

Galen says: Not as a servant, but as a master the liver distributes its product. This is not imperfect matter which has to be perfected elsewhere, but it is a finished product, namely blood[10]. Thus all parts that are below the diaphragm doubtless receive their nutritive blood from the liver. And so do the parts above the diaphragm including the lower as well as the upper parts of the heart and neighbouring structures[11]. The blood that is found in the right cavity of the heart is venous blood—for it is as closely similar to the blood of the veins of the whole body as the blood in the left ventricle is to arterial blood[12]. Hence there are two kinds of blood: venous and arterial. It follows that the same—venous—blood that is sent by the liver to the periphery is contained in the right heart. There is only one passage by which the liver is connected with the heart: the inferior vena cava; there should be a further vessel through which a product sent by the liver and supposedly perfected in the right heart could be carried to the periphery. The superior vena cava is not suitable for this, as it does not belong to the heart, but is a straight continuation of the hepatic veins by which the liver conveys its venous blood to the upper half of the body. The second vessel that leads from the right heart—the pulmonary artery—does not transmit venous blood to the periphery, but largely nourishes

4 *De usu partium*, lib. IV, cap. 12, ed. KÜHN, vol. III, p. 297; tr. DAREMBERG, CH. *Œuvres anatomiques, physiologiques et médicales de Galien*, Paris 1854–56, vol. I, p. 304. – GALEN, *De placitis Hippocratis et Platonis*, lib. VI, cap. 3, ed. KÜHN, vol. V, p. 522.

5 WILSON, L. G., *Erasistratus, Galen and the Pneuma*, *Bullet. Hist. Med.* 1959, XXXIII, 293–314, and in particular: LONIE, I. M., *Erasistratus, the Erasistrateans and Aristotle*, *Bullet. Hist. Med.* 1964, XXXVIII, 426–443.

6 ARISTOTLE, *Hist. animal.* lib., III, cap. 2; 511b10 seq; *De partib. animal.* lib. III, cap. 4; 665b27 seq.; 666a30. – On the various meanings of *Arche*, according to GALEN (*De placitis*, lib. VI, ed. KÜHN, vol. V, 505–547): LONIE, 1964 loc. cit. in note [5], p. 433. PECK, A. L., Aristotle, *De gen. anim.* ed. Loeb, 1953, p. XXXVIII seq.

7 ARISTOTLE, *De part. animal.*, lib. III, cap. 4; 666a8.

8 Blood is developed first of all in the heart of animals before the body is differentiated as a whole: ARISTOTLE, *Hist. animal.* lib. III, cap. 19; 521a9; tr. THOMPSON, Oxford 1910. – *De part. anim.* lib. III, cap. 4; 666a10 and 20.

9 WILSON, loc. cit. 1959 in note [5]; LONIE, 1964, loc. cit. in note [5], p. 431, also with ref. to ABEL, K., *Die Lehre vom Blutkreislauf im Corpus Hippocraticum*, *Hermes* 1958, LXXXVI, 201–202: "Erasistratos galt Galen, und nicht nur ihm, als Entdecker der Herzklappen ... In Galens Augen bedeutet Erasistratos' Ansicht einen gewaltigen Fortschritt in der Medizingeschichte. Sie ist wahrhaft epochemachend ... dürfen wir sagen, dass ihm (sc. GALEN) *de corde* (i.e. the treatise from the *Hippocratic corpus* in which the heart valves are mentioned) vorlag. Trotzdem beirrte ihn das nicht in seiner Auffassung, dass Erasistratos das Verdienst zukommt, die Herzklappen gefunden zu haben." *De corde* therefore seems to belong to a post-Erasistratean period. See also ABEL in *Gesnerus* 1958, XV, 71–105 (p. 81 et seq.).

10 *De Placitis* VI, 4; KÜHN V, 535.

11 Ibid. as in note [10].

12 Ibid. *De Placitis* VI, 4; KÜHN V, 537.

the lung. By contrast the left heart is equipped with an inlet admitting preparatory material (air and blood) and an outlet through which the finished product (arterial blood) leaves[13]. Again there is no "fifth opening" (*pempton d'allo stoma*) through which blood arriving from the liver could be sent out to the whole body[14]. All this goes to show that it is not a half elaborated product that is transmitted by the liver to the heart, but blood with its full and perfect nourishing properties. How then could anybody regard the right heart as the origin of the veins in the same way as its left cavity is indeed the origin of the arteries?[15]

2. *The Movement of Blood through Heart and Lung*

The venous blood undergoes a certain change in the right chamber of the heart prior to its filtration through the interventricular pores and its transmission into the pulmonary artery. First of all it is heated up because of the thickness of the walls of the heart chamber. Moreover it is perfectly elaborated and attenuated therein (*apo kardias epipempomenou mono to pneumoni tou haimatos, akribos en ekeine – sc. kardia – kateirgasmenou te kai leleptysmenou*). Galen attaches much importance to this thinning out of that portion of the thick—venous—blood that is sent to the lung. It is the most important of several mechanisms by which nature ensures the appropriate nutrition of the lung (*treis epikourias to pneumati pros euporian trophes he physis eginosken ex anankes esomenas* ... kai he megiste pason ...). The other mechanisms consist in a thorough mincing and vaporising of the aliment by means of the abundant heat in the right chamber and the inspiratory dilatation of the lung which enforces the attraction of nutriment. All this is additional to the thickness of the wall of the pulmonary artery and its branches. It had to be an artery to take the blood through the lung in order to prevent too much and too thick nutriment from flooding the tenuous structure of the lung[16].

Interventricular Pores

It is only a portion of the venous blood transmitted by the liver to the heart that reaches the lung. Another portion passes directly through pores in the interventricular septum.

These Galen believed to be passable for fluid. It had not escaped him, however, that they were not straightforward macroscopical holes through which the blood could simply flow, as it were by its own force. Instead he presented the grooves

13 Ibid. *De Placitis* VI, 5; KÜHN V, 538.

14 Ibid. *De Placitis* VI, 6; KÜHN V, 551.

15 Ibid. *De Placitis* VI, 5; KÜHN V, 539.

16 *De usu part.*, lib. VI, cap. 10 ed. KÜHN, vol. III, p. 452; tr. DAREMBERG, vol. I, p. 412. – It may well have been this Galenic doctrine of the *purification and refinement* of the venous blood in the *right* ventricle which led Haeser to the erroneous location of the separation of soot from the blood in the right ventricle and its discharge via the pulmonary artery into the lungs (instead of the pulmonary veins and the left ventricle, as Galen plainly says). HAESER, H., *Lehrbuch d. Geschichte der Medizin*, 3rd ed., Jena 1875, vol. I, p. 359. Haeser's error was first pointed out by Fleming, 1955, loc. cit. in note [3], p. 14, also its adoption by JUL. PAGEL in *Einführung i. d. Geschichte d. Medizin*, Berlin 1898, p. 124. – Fleming's discovery should be supplemented by the fact that the error was perpetuated by Sudhoff who left it uncorrected in the second edition of PAGEL's work (1915, p. 120) and repeated it in the third edition published under his own name as *Kurzes Handbuch* (1922, p. 118).

It can also be found in NEUBURGER, M., *Geschichte der Medizin*, vol. I, p. 377, Stuttgart 1906, and even in quite recent history books.

as small funnels the terminal parts of which were so small as to be invisible—at all events in the cadaver where all is cooled down and made dense. Indeed it needed a force of attraction to draw the blood through, and only its finer parts are thus drawn[17].

Nevertheless the portion of blood passing through the pores is *not small*, for Galen speaks of *much* that is taken through the pores into the left chamber (poly *kata to meson diaphragma kai tas en auto diatreseis eis ten aristeran metalambanetai koilian*).

Galen is driven to this conclusion from a comparison of the size of the various big vessels leading to and from the heart: the vena cava and the aorta are bigger than the pulmonary artery and the pulmonary veins respectively. The pulmonary artery (*ekphyomene phleps*) is smaller than the inferior vena cava (*emphyomene phleps*) although it receives the blood heated up. But since much of the blood is deviated through the septum the smaller size of the former is well (*eulogôs*) explained. The same obtains on the left side where the aorta is bigger than the pulmonary veins, since it has to carry away not only the *pneuma* that it receives from the pulmonary vein, but also the blood which comes to it from the right chamber. Indeed it is the aorta which forms the origin (*arche*) of all the arteries of the body[18].

The Pulmonary Transit of Blood

From the right ventricle venous blood reaching the lung via the pulmonary artery is pushed forward in its branches and thus finds its way into the ramifications of the pulmonary veins. This intrapulmonary movement of blood is made possible through the closure of the tricuspid valve at the atrio-ventricular border which prevents a back-flow[19]. Were this ostium permanently open and "had not nature invented an opening and closing mechanism the blood could never be transferred into the arterial system through invisible and small openings—a transfer that takes place during contraction of the chest in expiration"[20]. When the chest contracts the pulmonary veins press out the spirit which they contain and receive from the pulmonary arteries a portion of blood which finds its backward path barred. It is a transfer of *fine drops* (*stazei ti dia ton lepton ekeinon stomaton eis tas arterias*)—in other words what percolates is small in quantity. The whole process is "useful for the lung" (*agathon to pneumoni*) which thus receives its nutrition[21].

Entry of Blood and Air into the Left Heart

Galen does not seem to have been definite about the entry of blood and especially that of air from the pulmonary veins into the left auricle[22]. It may be argued, however, that he believed in an

17 Galen, *De natural. facult.* lib. III, cap. 15. Ed. Kühn, vol. II, p. 208 seq. tr. Daremberg loc. cit. vol. II, p. 317. – On the position of the pores in Renaissance anatomy (Berengario, Massa, Vesalius) see below p. 157.

18 *De usu partium* lib. VI, cap. 17; ed. Kühn vol. III, p. 497; tr. Daremberg vol. I, p. 445. – Fleming, loc. cit. in note [3], 1955, p. 18 speaks of "*some* of the blood that passes directly from right to left through the interventricular septum. But *much*, and apparently *most*, of the blood moves into the arterial vein (our pulmonary artery)..." – Against this see Hall, loc. cit. in note [3], 1960, p. 402: "A *great* quantity passes through the interventricular septum into the left ventricle..." The italics are of the present author.

19 The tight closure of the tricuspid valve had been discovered by Erasistratus. See Wilson, loc. cit. in note [3], 1959 and Lonie, loc. cit. in note [5] 1964, and p. 128 and note [9].

20 *De Usu Partium* VI, 10, Kühn III, 455–456; Daremberg I, 414.

21 Ibidem as in note [20] Kühn p. 457.

22 Fleming loc. cit. 1955, p. 17 and 19 says: "Galen does not make clear whether the blood that passes into his "venous artery" (our pulmonary veins) is then transmitted to the left ventricle" (p. 17) and: "Whether Galen's venous artery, corresponding to our pulmonary veins, then carries blood to the left ventricle is in question." (p. 19). Against this: Siegel loc. cit. 1962, p. 740. – See also Wilson loc. cit. 1959, p. 305 seq.

inflow of blood from the lung into the left heart—it had been his main thesis that all vessels, arteries and veins, contain blood and so should the pulmonary vein. Moreover Galen expressly said that when the valves are about to be closed blood and spirit are of necessity drawn into the heart[23]. And even more definitely: the heart can draw from the lung blood mixed with spirit through the mitral valve (*kai mentoi kak tou pneumonos haima kai pneuma memigmenon hoion te estin helkein*)[24].

As to the entry of air the evidence is somewhat contradictory[25]. In some passages Galen denied its direct access to the heart in any appreciable quantity, in favour of its coolness alone which is transmitted (*pantelos oligon e ouden holos tes tou pneumatos ousias eis ten kardian metalambanetai*[26] and *me tes ousias alla tes poiotetos tou pneumatos deisthai ten kardian*[27]). At another place the heart is said to require the substance of the air for the cooling of its effervescent heat (*deomenen kai auten tou aeros tes ousias, to de ti pleiston hypo thermotetos zeouses anapsychesthai pothousan*[28]). Indeed he held this to be in keeping with the whole purpose of respiration which was for the benefit of the heart. L.G.Wilson suggests a solution of the apparent contradiction: Galen, arguing all the time against Erasistratus who had believed in the exclusive transmission of air by the arteries, did not deny the access of air, but its consumption and transmission by the heart into the arterial system[29].

It is not unlikely that by and large this was Galen's intention. It is true that in his book on the *Use of respiration* he says that some of the air drawn in by the heart is transmitted to adjacent arteries. He adds in the same breath, however, that only arteries of the vicinity are involved and that the quantity of air breathed out is therefore no smaller than that breathed in. According to Temkin, the emphasis would not therefore lie on the air as such, but on a product of its digestion in the lung which reaches the heart[31].

Galen seems to have derived his ambivalence in this question from Aristotle. The latter had denied any communication between the tracheal and vascular system in the lungs, but said that the vessels receive the breath by contact (*dia synapsin*) and transmit it to the heart (*dechontai to pneuma kai diapempousi te kardia*[32]). However, as Curtis pointed out[33], no more is said by Aristotle about the function, importance and fate of this part of the breath beyond the heart. It would appear that its function according to Aristotle was the preservation of native heat rather than the production of spirit to be carried by the arterial blood. The point is significant for the relevant ideas of Cesalpinus as well as Harvey and will be discussed elsewhere in the present book (p. 204 seq.).

23 *De Usu Partium* VI, 16; KÜHN III, 490–491; DAREMBERG I, 440.

24 *De Usu Partium* VI, 21; KÜHN III, 509–510; DAREMBERG I, 453.

25 To this see: CURTIS, J.G., *Harvey's views on the use of the Circulation of the Blood.* New York 1915, p. 16–17.

26 GALEN, *An in arteriis natura sanguis contineatur* ed. KÜHN, vol. IV, p. 725.

27 GALEN, *De utilitate respirationis*, cap. 2; ed. KÜHN vol. IV, p. 479. See TEMKIN loc. cit. in note [3], 1951, p. 183.

28 GALEN, *De usu partium* lib. VI, cap. 2; ed. KÜHN vol. III, p. 412; DAREMBERG I, 381.

29 WILSON, loc. cit. in note [3], 1959, p. 306.

30 GALEN, *De utilitate respirat.* cap. 5; ed. KÜHN vol. IV, p. 511.

31 TEMKIN, loc. cit. in note [3], 1951, p. 182.

32 ARISTOTLE, *Hist. animal.* lib. I, cap. 17; 496a 27–32.

33 CURTIS, *Harveys views*, 1915, loc. cit. in note [25], p. 21–34.

Expulsion of Smoky Excrement from the Heart

No doubt attaches to Galen's belief in the expulsion of smoky products of combustion by the heart into the lung in expiration (*he d'ekpnoe tou zeontos en aute kai hoion synkekaumenou kai lignyodous apochysei*[34]).

In other words air enters the heart in order to cool and leaves it again as such taking with it smoky waste products.

Galen made finally provision for abundant arterial—thin, spirituous—blood to flow through the lung[35].

3. Galen's Doctrine and its Significance for Harvey

In conclusion, some basic data concerning the movement of the blood are indeed due to Galen. Such data include the transmission of some of the venous blood from the liver to the heart through the inferior vena cava, and the transfer of a portion of this blood into the lung. Galen probably also indicated the propulsion of some of this blood through the pulmonary veins into the left heart. In addition he was aware of the tight closure of the tricuspid valve which made such a movement of blood through the lungs possible.

However, though conscious of the direction of *some portion* of the venous blood from the liver to the heart and through the lungs, he remained far remote from any idea of the direction of flow of blood in general, i.e. of its "closed" circulation.

In this he was fundamentally encumbered by his dualistic view: to him there were not one, but two centres for the formation and direction of the blood, namely the liver and the heart. From this there followed the distinction between two kinds of blood[36], each with its own origin and particular function: venous blood that was largely nutritional and arterial blood that chiefly transmitted spirit. This admittedly opened up the progressive view of arterial blood as the transmitter of a substance from the air which maintained a process comparable to combustion as engendered by respiration. For it was Galen who asked: what is the substance in the air that is needed to prevent suffocation[37], and furthermore what is it that makes a flame light up and go out—questions which led him to liken the heart to a wick, the blood to oil feeding it and the lung to the instrument fanning it, whilst he supposed blood to be burnt and to leave a smoky waste[38].

It is just this progressive view of the duality of the blood and combustion therein which kept him remote from the idea of circulation, whereas Harvey was led to it ignoring this very view[39].

34 GALEN, *De usu part.* lib.VI, cap.2; ed. KÜHN, vol.III, p.412; tr. DAREMBERG vol. I, p.381.

35 GALEN, *De usu part.* lib.VII, cap.8; ed. KÜHN, vol.III, p.537; tr. DAREMBERG, vol.I, p.473.

36 According to TEMKIN this distinction was one of quantity rather than quality: "whereas blood and pneuma are fine and thin in the arteries they are "crude" and "smoky" in the veins. And whereas the arterial blood has a large pneumatic component, the latter is much smaller in the veins." TEMKIN loc. cit. in note [3] 1951, p.185 with ref. to *De Usu Part.* VI, 16, KÜHN III, 491; DAREMBERG I, 441.

To this should be added the passage from Aulus Gellius, *Noctes Atticae* XVIII, 10 (as quoted by HAESER, H., *Lehrb.d.Geschichte d.Medicin* 3rd Ed. Jena 1875, vol.I, p.363): "Vena conceptaculum sanguinis ... in quo plus sanguinis est, minus spiritus... arteria conceptaculum spiritus in quo plus spiritus est, minus sanguinis".

37 *De Util. Resp.* 3, KÜHN IV, 484: "endeia poiotetos tinos en tais epischesesi tes anapnoes pnigesthai ta zoa. ti goun estin haute, skepteon."

38 *De Util Resp.* 3, KÜHN IV, 488 and 491–492: "kinesin te anankaion echein kato to kapnodes hos an eipoi tis, ekkenoun tes tou haimatos synkauseos."

39 To this LORD COHEN OF BIRKENHEAD, *The Germ of an Idea or what put Harvey on the Scent? J.Hist.Med.* 1957, XII, 102: "If the blood in veins and arteries is the *same* blood, then the Galenic view is untenable and there must be continuity or communication between arteries and veins. And this belief was supported by the overt inconsistencies in earlier hypotheses. The introduction to *De motu cordis* is, in fact, a penetrating critical analysis of past theories." (p.104–105).

In Galen's scheme, the blood which reaches the heart, is not the blood that has taken its course through the arteries and thus returns to its origin, the heart, but it is blood ever freshly formed in the liver from food ingested by the stomach and gut.

Moreover the blood sent to the heart is only a portion of the blood so formed. Most of the latter is conveyed directly to the periphery by the liver through the descending part of the inferior vena cava and the superior vena cava—for it is the task of the venous blood to transmit aliment from the liver to the organs and tissues.

Galen had no real grasp of the pulmonary transit, as he again provided for only a small part of the blood to reach the right ventricle and the lungs from the liver, whilst its major part was made to enter the left ventricle directly through the interventricular pores.

Uncertainties and ambiguity prevail in his ideas concerning the access of blood and air to the left heart from the lungs. It had been one of Galen's main tenets that the arteries contain blood, and not air—as Erasistratus had taught. He had thus to master the difficulty that air should be transmitted to the left heart and hence an airborne substance (*pneuma*) to the whole body through the arteries. Indeed it is in the hypothesis of the pneumatic content of the arteries, i.e. tubes visibly filled with blood and nothing else, that Hall sees the rock on which Galen foundered[40]. Moreover Galen assumed that airy substance (*pneuma*) is drawn into the arteries not only from the lungs via the left heart, but also directly through the skin and that it reaches the brain through the nose and olfactory plate. Some of the waste products of this pneuma were thought to be discharged through the skin[41]. Galen also probably assumed some arterial blood to reach the lung from the left heart through a not tightly closing mitral valve.

Inspite of all this, Galen has been represented as the "*de facto* discoverer of circulation". This view is by no means novel and it has been purchased at the cost of minimising and overlooking some of Galen's difficulties. We refer to the work of J.C.F. Hecker who advanced it between 1817 and 1831[42]. According to him Galen "would have to be regarded as the *de facto* (*der Sache nach*) discoverer of circulation, had he not deprived himself of this honour through the faulty evaluation of his own observations.[43]" And again, ten years later: "There is no doubt that Galen is to be looked upon as the first and true discoverer of circulation.... Except for the knowledge of the valves in the veins he lacked no essential means of proving it; there was no need for him to men-

40 HALL, A.R., loc. cit. in note [3] 1960, p. 410–412.

41 *De Util Resp.* 5, KÜHN IV, 503–504; *De Pulsuum Usu* KÜHN V, 166; *De Placitis Hippocr. et Platonis*, KÜHN V, 263–266. – See also TEMKIN, loc. cit. in note [3] 1951, p. 183 with ref. to *De Usu Part.* VIII, 10, KÜHN III, 663; DAREMBERG I, 557.

42 HECKER, J.F.C., *Sphygmologiae Galenicae Specimen.* Berol. 1817; *Geschichte der Heilkunde* vol. I, Berlin 1822; *Die Lehre vom Kreislauf vor Harvey. Eine historische Abhandlung.* Berlin 1831. See also the Berlin medical thesis: PARISER, BERNH. NATHAN, *Historia Opinionum quae de Sanguinis Circulatione ante Harvaeum viguerint.* Berlin 1830, 46 pp. quoted from JUL. PAGEL, Verzeichnis der Berliner Mediz. Doktordissertationen historischen Inhalts in: *Zum Hundertjährigen Jubilaeum der Universität Berlin. Janus* 1909, XIV, p. 794–817 (p. 812). Hecker was anticipated by Folius of Modena (1615–1650), see TALLMADGE, G.K., *Caecilius Folius on the Circulation, Bullet. Hist. Med.* 1954, XXVIII, 15–31 (p. 21).

43 HECKER, loc. cit. 1822, p. 489.

tion the phenomena which occur when an artery is injured or ligatured and the everyday technique (*alltäglichen Handgriff*) of ligaturing the vein above the site of incision—for knowledge of this trivial nature was common to all physicians and surgeons. Generally speaking it is noticeable that in describing circulation Galen did not put his own discovery to better use and did not raise it to the level of a comprehensive physiological doctrine. His data concerning circulation are scattered so that he does not even seem to have realised their high importance himself.[44]"

Hecker, not surprisingly, comes to this conclusion after having omitted to mention the direct transmission of blood from the liver through the veins to the periphery, as taught by Galen. Nor do we find anything in his account of Galen about the interventricular pores and the direct flow of much blood from the right ventricle to the left through them. Instead this idea is attributed to—Vesalius, of whom Hecker says that he "subscribed to the customary prejudice that the blood entering the heart through the vena cava is rarefied by means of animal heat in the right ventricle and thereby enabled to transfer directly into the left ventricle—a strange and harmful opinion which in this (i.e. Vesalius') century was pretty common"[45].

By a process of abstraction Hecker presents what Galen clearly predicated of a part of the blood as if it had been intended for all of it, i.e. as if *the* blood had been thought by Galen to move in a manner identical in principle with that discovered by Harvey[46].

No such sweeping claims have been raised for Galen in more recent times. Nevertheless the significance of the critical and anti-Galenic part of Harvey's work for his discovery has been greatly restricted if not denied, for, so it was said, Galen's doctrine was in fact nearer the truth than is commonly believed[47]. Moreover it has been stated that Galen knew that "much, if not most, of the blood" passed from the right ventricle through the pulmonary artery into the lung[48]—a statement that calls for reconciliation with Galen's own wording according to which "much of the blood" does not follow this way, but passes directly from the right into the left ventricle through the interventricular septal pores[49].

But for these pores, so it is said, Galen could have demonstrated the unidirectional movement of blood from the right ventricle to the left through the lungs. He is also credited with the description of the transfer of venous into arterial blood—although "what exactly was borne into the left ventricle by the venous artery corresponding to our pulmonary veins Galen failed to make

44 Hecker, loc. cit. 1831, p. 16.

45 Hecker, loc. cit. 1831, p. 21.

46 Hecker loc. cit. 1831, p. 14–15. – Hecker's claims on behalf of Galen have already been rejected by Haeser, loc. cit. 1875, vol. I, p. 363: "Die Meinung Heckers, daß Galen für den Entdecker des Kreislaufs zu halten sey, ist durch nichts zu begründen."

47 Fleming, loc. cit. in note [3] 1955, p. 319.

48 Fleming, loc. cit. 1955, p. 18.

49 See note [18] above.

clear.[50]" It should be added that it was Galen who provided an outlet for smoky waste through an imperfectly closing mitral valve[51].

No doubt, in the history of Harvey's discovery as such the correction of the errors of Galen formed a decisive stepping-stone for a basic revision of physiology. *Subjectively*, i.e. for the discoverer himself, individual points may have been unequal in importance. It has been said, already by Curtis, that Galen's doctrine of the pulmonary transit did not have as much of an awakening effect on Harvey as is often thought[52].

Moreover a comparative indifference on Harvey's part towards the pulmonary transit has been noted on the grounds that his main concern was the common pattern of circulation valid for all animals including those without lungs. This point too was made by Curtis in the first place[53].

Finally Harvey himself was aware of the basic correctness and importance of some of Galen's observations, notably those concerning the anatomy of the heart valves and the anastomoses of veins and arteries in the lungs[54].

On the other hand it will be difficult to overlook the emphasis laid by Harvey on the points that prove the pulmonary transit, and prominently so the impenetrability of the septum. Indeed the analogy with the pulmonary transit was, on Harvey's own showing, one of the leading points in the inventive process that led to his discovery (p. 54).

What is perhaps more, Harvey's attitude is in essentials—and not only in detail—anti-Galenic. It is to the whole field of Galen's vision rather than to individual technical and doctrinal points that Harvey is opposed. His "modern" approach enables him to break through the barrier of Galen's *forces* which had limited and cut short research, notably his "pulse-making" force, and to proceed to a causal analysis of the movements of heart and blood (p. 80).

A further advance which Harvey achieved on Galen shows the close interlocking of his "modern" views with his loyalty to Aristotle. It is the removal of the firm anchorage by which Galen saw the movement of the heart and blood fixed to respiration.

It is of particular interest that Harvey was preceded in this by Cesalpinus and that the latter was actuated by an attempt at vindicating Aristotle against Galen. This very leaning towards the Aristotelian point of view would seem to epitomise Harvey's basic attitude as well. It is hardly accidental that Aristotle formed Harvey's *exemplar*, particularly in his comparative-anatomical approach and in his quest for pattern and type rather than individual properties—a quest which we have just touched upon.

50 FLEMING loc. cit. 1955, p. 319.

51 See note [34] above.

52 CURTIS, *Harvey's views*, loc. cit. in note [25], 1915, p. 39; FLEMING, loc. cit. in note [3], 1955, p. 319.

53 CURTIS loc. cit. p. 39, with ref. to Harvey's letter to Schlegel (March 26th 1651), Opp. omnia London 1766, p. 613; tr. WILLIS, p. 597; FLEMING, p. 322.

54 *De motu cordis*, cap. VIII, ed. 1628, p. 41; tr. WILLIS, p. 45.

Harvey's point of view is unitary. It makes the heart "the foundation of the life of animals, the sovereign of everything, the Sun of the microcosm, on which all growth depends, and from which all vigour and strength emanates"[55].

This indeed is the full profession and programme of Aristotelianism in biology—the piece with which he opens his great work, dedicating it to the King, "the foundation of his dominiums, the Sun of his world, the heart of the state from whom all power and grace emanate." It was this very regal position which Galen had denied to the heart, for he had introduced a second sovereign, the liver, and hence had made no provision for the *return* of blood to the heart, its true and only mother and origin in Aristotelian biology.

Indeed Harvey's attitude towards Galen can only be seen in proper perspective when his "philosophy" is taken into consideration. This was Aristotelian and hence anti-Galenic. Harvey implemented it with a wealth of striking and revolutionary empirical observations and scientific physiological reasoning. It is the latter alone that seems to be of interest to the modern scientist; but the historian cannot help attributing equal significance to Harvey's general ideas.

II. Servetus (pl. 31)

It is not Aristotle and Galen who are customarily treated as *the* precursors of Harvey, but attention is focussed on anatomists and naturalists of the sixteenth century, such as notably Michael Servetus (1511?–1553), Realdus Columbus (1516?–1559) and Andreas Cesalpinus (1525 [1519?]–1603).

It has been said and often repeated that Servetus and Columbus discovered the "lesser circulation" before Harvey. However, as we have pointed out (p. 51), this term is misleading and should be replaced by "pulmonary transit of the blood in the right ventricle of the heart to the left". For there can be no question of a lesser circulation without the systemic circulation: those who described the pulmonary transit of the blood from the right ventricle of the heart to the left knew nothing of its eventual return to its point of departure, the right heart, and therefore of its circulation. William Harvey thus remains the discoverer of the lesser as well as the systemic circulation[1].

It had been Servetus' idea that the venous blood that had entered the right chamber of the heart is not filtered through pores in

55 *De motu cordis*, Dedicatio, ed. 1628, p. 3; tr. Willis p. 3.

1 Neuburger, M., *Zur Entdeckungsgeschichte des Lungenkreislaufes. Arch. Geschichte d. Med.* 1930, XXIII, 7. – Supported later by Izquierdo, J. J., *A new and more correct version of the views of Servetus on the Circulation of the Blood. Bullet. Hist. Med.* 1937, V, 914–932. The author goes farther than Neuburger in denying Servetus' solid empirical knowledge of anatomy. Izquierdo says: On the whole Servetus' work appears rather as a product of imagination and fantasy, than as a conquest by scientific methods which were introduced a century later by Harvey" (p. 931). – A propos Neuburger's paper compare Bainton, R.H., *The Smaller Circulation. Arch. Gesch. d. Med.* 1931, XXIV, 371–374: "the fact remains that Servetus and Colombo retained the generation of the blood in the liver, and so long as they did so it goes without saying that they did not appreciate the full implications of their discovery. At the same time it will not do to overlook the fact that they did make a discovery, whether it be called that of the pulmonary circulation or no. Their advance consisted in the denial of the permeability of the septum and in the location of the aeration of the blood in the lungs rather than in the heart" (p. 371). "One may conclude that they (sc. Servetus and Colombo) were independent" (p. 372). See also: Bainton, R.H., *Michael Servetus and the Pulmonary Transit of the Blood. Bullet. Hist. Med.* 1951, XXV, 1–7. The advanced views held by Lionardo da Vinci (1452–1519) do not concern the pulmonary transit – Keele, K.D., *Leonardo da Vinci on Movement of the Heart and Blood* London 1952.

the interventricular septum into the left ventricle—as Galen had assumed for "much" of this blood—but that it traverses the lung and there receives divine spirit from the air which it leads into the left heart and thence into the arterial system.

This is not found in a treatise devoted to anatomy or medicine, but in his famous *Restitution of Christianity* of 1553—a theological work. In this Servetus developed those heretical views which led to his martyrdom and the destruction of all but three copies of his book, at the instigation of Calvin, the Protestant dictator of Geneva. Servetus here is not primarily concerned with the movement of the blood, but with the origin of the divine spirit in man[2].

How, then, is the one connected with the other and what is the real significance of Servetus' statement in the light of the context in which it is offered?

Servetus on the Movement of Blood and the Seat of the Soul

To answer our question we shall have to introduce the relevant text as such in a new literal translation[3].

The Origin of Life as inherent in Blood and its Generation in the Lung

We are taught in the Scriptures, says Servetus[4], that the blood is the very life itself. How does it acquire this position of dignity and responsibility? *Quomodo sanguis est ipsissima vita*—here lies his main problem, here the reason why he investigated the vital spirit and its generation by the breath and the most subtle part of the blood—the *substantialis generatio ipsius vitalis spiritus, qui ex aere inspirato et subtilissimo sanguine componitur et nutritur*.

The text goes on: "It is formed in the left ventricle of the heart with the eminent help of the lungs—a fine spirit accomplished by the power of heat, bright red (*flavus*—golden) coloured, fiery in vigour, as it were a luminous vapour (*lucens vapor*) from the purer part of the blood, containing the substance of water, air and fire."

It is generated through the mixture of air breathed in with the elaborate subtle blood which the right ventricle communicates to the left. This communication, however, does not take place through the middle wall of the heart—as commonly believed—but through a great artifice the subtle blood is set into motion from the right ventricle of the heart by a long way round through the lung (*fit autem communicatio haec non per parietem cordis medium, ut vulgo creditur, sed magno artificio a dextro cordis ventriculo, longo per pulmones ductu agitatur sanguis subtilis*). It is elaborated by the lungs, made golden coloured and transmitted from the pulmonary artery (*vena arteriosa*) into the pulmonary vein (*arteria venosa*), then mixed

2 For biography and bibliography of Servetus we refer to: *An Impartial History of Michael Servetus burnt alive at Geneva for Heresie*. London 1724, attributed to G. Benson without justification—and to George Hodges (see BAINTON 1932, as quoted below).
ALLWOERDEN, H., *Historia Michaelis Serveti quam praeside Jo. Laur. Moshemio ... exponit*. Helmstadii 1727.
WILLIS, R., *Servetus and Calvin. A Study of an important Epoch in the Early History of the Reformation* London 1877.
TOLLIN, *H., Die Entdeckung des Blutkreislaufes durch Michael Servet* (1511–1553) in *Sammlg. physiolog. Abhandlgn.* her. v. W. PREYER. *Erste Reihe*, vol. VI. Jena 1876 (references of the numerous papers by Tollin on the subject —1874–1894—are given by Bainton 1932, as cited below).
BAINTON, R.H., *The present State of Servetus Studies. J.Modern History* (Chicago) 1932, IV, 72–92. – Idem, *Hunted Heretic. The Life and Death of Michael Servetus* 1511–1553. Boston. The Beacon Press 1953.
O'MALLEY, CH. D., *The Complementary Careers of Michael Servetus: Theologian and Physician*. J.Hist.Med. 1953, VIII, 378–389. – Idem, *Michael Servetus. A Translation of his Geographical, Medical and Astrological Writings with Introd. and Notes. Amer. Philos.Soc.Philadelphia 1953*. – (with ref. to: WILBUR, EARL MORSE, *A History of Unitarianism*. Cambridge Mass. 1945, pp. 49–75 and 113–185 and idem, *A Bibliography of the Pioneers of the Socinian-Unitarian Movement*. Roma 1950, pp. 69–74).
FULTON, J.F., *Michael Servetus. Humanist and Martyr. With a Bibliography of His Works and Census of known Copies, by M.E.Stanton*. New York. H.Reichner. 1953.
For the *religious background* of Servetus the present account is indebted to: TRECHSEL, F., *Michael Servet und seine Vorgänger. Nach Quellen und Urkunden geschichtlich dargestellt*. Mit Vorwort von C.Ullmann. Heidelberg 1839 and Bainton loc.cit. 1953.

3 For *excerpts* of the relevant *text-passages* from Servetus, *Christianismi Restitutio* of 1553: SIGMOND, G., *The Unnoticed Theories of Servetus. A Dissertation addressed to the Medical Society of Stockholm* London 1826, pp. 41–72. – FLOURENS, P., *Histoire de la découverte de la Circulation du Sang*. 2nd ed. Paris 1857, pp. 265–279. – In German translation: Tollin loc.cit. 1876, p. 2–19 (though excellent in general, this translation is occasionally free or not quite in focus, e.g. his designation of the lateral ventricles of the brain as "*Stirnhöhlen*" (frontal sinuses, p. 9; 11; 12), of the quadrigeminal bodies—*glutia*—as "Hinterhirn" (hind-brain, p. 11); nor were Servetus' ideas traced back to the well known tradi-

in the latter with the air breathed and through expiration purged of smoke. And thus finally the whole mixture is attracted by the left ventricle of the heart through diastole—a domestic tool apt to become the vital spirit. (*Atque ita tandem a sinistro cordis ventriculo totum mixtum per diastolen attrahitur, apta suppellex ut fiat spiritus vitalis.*)

That the communication and preparation is thus accomplished by the lungs, is shown by the manifold conjunction and communication between the pulmonary artery and the pulmonary vein. It is confirmed by the extraordinary (*insignis*) size of the pulmonary artery which would not have been made of such quality and so big, nor emit so big a force of the purest blood from the heart to the lungs, were it merely for the nutrition of the latter; nor would the heart serve the lungs in this way, notably since just before, in embryonic life, the lungs derived their aliment from elsewhere, since those small membranes or valves of the heart are not patent until the hour of birth, as Galen teaches. Hence it is for another purpose that the blood is poured out from the heart, at the very time of birth, and in such quantity. Likewise not simply air, but air mixed with blood is sent from the lungs to the heart by the pulmonary vein. Hence it is in the lungs that the mixture takes place. That golden colour is conferred to the spirituous blood by the lungs, not by the heart. In the left ventricle of the heart there is no space capable of such a big and copious mixture nor sufficient elaboration of the golden colour—whilst that middle wall, as it is devoid of vessels and faculties, is not apt to bring about that communication and elaboration, although something may be able to sweat through (*licet aliquid resudare possit*). Through the same artifice by which a transfusion takes place in the liver from the portal vein into the vena cava for the sake of the blood, a transfusion also takes place in the lung from the pulmonary artery to the pulmonary vein for the sake of the spirit. He who compares this with what Galen writes in the sixth and seventh book on the *Use of the parts* will wholly understand the truth not observed by Galen himself (*veritatem penitus intelliget, ab ipso Galeno non animadversam*).

Further Elaboration of the Vital Spirit in the Chorioid Plexuses of the Brain

This vital spirit, then, is transfused from the left ventricle of the heart into the arteries of the whole body so that the finer it is the more it tends upwards where it is still further elaborated, partic-

tional theory of brain localisation—see below pp. 152). – For *short excerpts: Impartial History* loc. cit. 1724 p. 67–69; ALLWOERDEN, loc. cit. 1727 p. 231–234; WILLIS loc. cit. 1877 (in English translation), p. 206–210; O'MALLEY loc. cit. Philadelphia 1953, p. 197 (following large excerpts from other works of Servetus, notably *Syruporum Universa Ratio* of 1537); in English translation); FULTON loc. cit. 1953, p. 37–40. SCHACHT, J., *Ibn al-Nafis, Servetus and Colombo. Al-Andalus,* 1957, XXII, 319–336 (p. 331).

4 *Christianismi Restitutio*, lib. V, pp. 168 et seq. in the original ed. Vienne 1553.

ularly in the retiform plexus under the base of the brain: here psychic (*animal*) spirit begins to be formed from vital spirit, approaching as it does the seat of the rational soul. Again it is further attenuated, elaborated and perfected by the fiery power of the mind, in the most subtle vessels or capillary arteries situated in the chorioid plexus and containing the mind itself. These plexuses penetrate the most intimate parts of the brain and cover the inside of its ventricles—keeping in position (*servantes*)[5] the vessels that are intricately interwoven down to the origin of the nerves so that the sensory and motory faculties are induced in them.

These vessels, through a great miracle interwoven in the most subtle manner, are called arteries, but they are really the terminal parts of arteries tending towards the origin of the nerves by means of the meninges. They constitute a new type of vessels (*est novum quoddam genus vasorum*). For as a new type of vessel is formed when blood is transfused from the veins into the arteries in the lungs, a new type of vessel formed by the arterial coat and the meninx emerges when blood is transfused from the arteries into the nerves: for the meninges themselves keep their coats in the nerves. The sensibility of the nerves does not have its seat in their soft matter any more than it does in the brain[6]. All nerves terminate in filaments of membranes which are possessed of most exquisite sensibility: hence it is to them that spirit is always sent.

These fine vessels of the meninges or chorioid membranes are the source from which the luminous animal spirit is effused like a ray throughout the nerves towards the eyes and other sensual organs. The same route is used in turn by the luminous images of things perceived which approach from outside and are sent to the same source, penetrating as it were through a lucid medium.

Obviously the soft mass of the brain is not really the seat of the rational soul, as it is cold and senseless. It serves, however, like a cushion for the vessels mentioned lest they be broken, and as a watchman for the animal spirit lest it fly away when it is to be communicated to the nerves. Moreover it is cold for the moderation of that fiery heat inside the vessels. Hence the membranous coat which is common to these vessels is preserved by the nerves in their internal cavity for the faithful custody over the spirit—deriving an enveloping coat from the pia mater and an external one from the dura mater. Those empty spaces of the ventricles of the brain—wondered at by naturalists and physicians—contain nothing like the soul[7]. But it is their first purpose to receive, like drains, the impurities of the brain, as evidenced by the excrements there received and the ducts towards the palate and nose from

5 The present translation is in agreement with that of Tollin and at variance with Willis 1878, p. 209: "the arterial plexuses which *subserve* the faculties of sensation and motion"; and with that of FULTON 1953, p. 39: "these plexuses ... *serve* to introduce in these last the faculties of sensation and motion".

6 From the context it is quite clear that the correct reading is: "sicut *nec* in cerebro", as given by Flourens, 1857, p. 269 (as against SIGMOND, 1826, p. 48 and FULTON, 1953, p. 40: "sensibility of the nerves is not in their soft material as in the brain").

7 "Nihil minus continent quam animam" SIGMOND, 1826, p. 49.

which morbid fluxions spring. And when the ventricles are so filled with mucus that the arteries of the vascular plexus are submerged in it, sudden apoplexy is the result. When a noxious humour whose vapour affects the mind obstructs a part epilepsy or another disease develops according to the part in which the expelled vapour is deposited. We shall say that the mind is in the place where we clearly see it affected. From immoderate heat of these vessels or an inflammation of the meninges raving and phrensy result. Hence from the diseases that suddenly arise according to the place and substance affected, from the power of the heat, the artful beauty of the vessels which contain it and from the actions of the soul which there appear, we conclude again and again that those small vessels are to have preference—for all this is subservient to them and the sensory nerves are tied to them in order that they may receive their power from there, and finally because we perceive the intellect working there when in strenuous meditation those arteries pulsate down to the temples. He who has not seen the place will hardly understand this. The second purpose of these ventricles is the refreshing of the animal spirit contained therein and the fanning movement for the soul (*animam ventillet*) through that portion of the inhaled air that penetrates into the empty spaces of the ventricles by way of the ethmoid bone and is attracted by the very vessels of the soul through dilatation (*ab ipsis animae vasis per diastolem attracta*). In those vessels there is mind, soul and fiery spirit that is in need of continual fanning, lest it be suffocated through inclusion, like external fire. It is in need of fanning and blowing like fire, not only in order to take its pabulum from the air, but also to belch its smoke out into it. Just as the external elementary fire is tied to an earthy thick body because it shares with it dryness and the form of light, takes the liquor of the body as its pabulum and is ventilated, maintained and nourished by air, our fiery spirit and soul are similarly tied to the body, form one whole with it, use its blood as pabulum and are ventilated, maintained and nourished by an airy spirit through inspiration and expiration, thus enjoying a double aliment—a spiritual and a corporeal one. The place and spiritual nature of nutriment made it convenient that this luminous lair of our spirit should be breathed upon by another spirit, namely the holy, celestial and lucid spirit through the expiration from the mouth of Christ, in as much as this spirit is attracted to the same place by us through breathing in. It was proper that the same place where our intellect and luminous soul dwell should be illuminated anew by the light of another fire. For God kindles in us the first lamp and converts into light again the darkness that has gathered there, as David says in the 17th psalm and the 22nd chapter of the second book of Samuel. The same is taught by Elihu in Job, chapter 32 and 33, and by Zoroaster, Trismegistus and Pythagoras.

Good formation and quality of the vessels make for a good mind, so that better souls are possessed by those in whom these vessels are better disposed. However, as from a good spirit the innate light is more and more illuminated, it is obscured by a bad one. When, together with our luminous psychic (*animal*) spirit, a dark and mischievous spirit thrusts itself in, you will see demoniac fury—just as luminous revelations are the gift of a good spirit. Those vessels are easily attacked by the bad spirit which has its seat nearby in the abyss of the waters and cavities of the brain ventricles. That bad spirit whose power is that of the air, enters and leaves freely, together with the air which we breathe, in order to fight vigorously against our spirit contained in those vessels as if in a citadel. Indeed it besieges the latter on all sides so that it can hardly breathe, unless the light of divine spirit comes to its succour and drives away the bad spirit. How much, then, is this the place suitable for mind, spirit, revelation and intellect—both inborn and superadded—and for the battle of the higher temptations, to omit now others (sc. temptations). By a similar breathing mechanism (*simili inspirationis ratione*) the love of God is kindled in the heart through the holy spirit. In the heart, besides the principle of life, there is the realm of the will and, following the temptations of the intellect and the sting of the flesh, the first origin of sin to which St Matthew agrees (ch. 15). The actions of the mind vary according to the diversity of those vessels of the brain, just as there are various instruments (*organa*) in the various ventricles of which I will speak now.

A small part of the air breathed in is communicated to that fiery animal spirit which is contained in those choroid vessels through the ethmoid bones, tending towards the two anterior ventricles of the brain that are on the right and left side of the forepart of the head. There the capillary arteries of the chorioid membrane when dilated draw the air for the fanning of the soul. To them also the optic nerves after having been joined together bring down the visual images as well as the auditory and other sensory nerves, with the cover of the common membrane kept always intact, for the most faithful and secure custody of all. For if the images (*species*) and spirits together with the soul were to wander about in these empty spaces, they would all be ejected by snuffing out or at least by sneezing. If the soul were there it would not be in the blood, as there is no blood outside the vessels. Hence the mind is most securely seated in the chorioid vessels. Indeed its cover is most secure, and it is to those vessels which are partly located in the anterior ventricles that the principal sensory nerves tend so that there is the beginning of reception (*initium sensus communis*) and the grasping (*in commune lata apprehensio*) of what the exterior senses have apprehended or of things retained so that the impressions begin to be compared and mixed with each other.

The air breathed into the brain is then taken from the two anterior ventricles to the middle ventricle or rather a common passage where they come together below the lyra[8]; and here is the more lucid and pure part of the mind. The latter sows out its innate divine seeds of ideas and can think out or compose new things from the images already taken up by way of comparison (*similitudine*), can mix up thoughts (*imaginata*), infer one thing from another, discern between them and with the light of God grasp truth itself. The chamber is smaller there and the intellectual power more excellent, for there are more copious chorioid arteries which dilate and refresh the fiery spirit and bring the common sensual perceptions to more and more luminous reasoning, the spiritual light penetrating inside through the vessels where the Deity itself shines. There is not as much empty space as in the other chambers —hence it is more a passage than a ventricle or rather a long and winding path of exploration (*longam et anfractuosam scrutinii viam*). It is made thus with wisdom, because of the difficult intellectual exertion (*ob scrutinii difficultatem*). The chamber is smaller for the reason that not so much excrement should collect where the purer and more lucid part of the mind has its seat. What excrement does collect, straightway sinks down into the underlying funnel (*choana*), lest it might extinguish the lamp or impede it. More copious are the vessels around the pineal; there are more arterial pulses and the action of the mind and the fiery spirit is more potent, there. We too notice the stronger pulsation of the working intellect around the temples outside and inside—leading us by this single experience to the true seat of the mind. Add to this that the sense of hearing is nearer to this place—the sense of learning. Indeed the greatest miracle lies in this constitution of man. Many and long are the windings towards the cerebellum so that through long intellectual exploration any and even the most complicated things can be investigated and darkness illuminated—with the help of those impressions which had been stored away in memory before, by dint of the faculty of remembering. There the worm-like janitor and the sinuous quadrigeminal bodies (*a janitore scoli-*

8 *Commissura hippocampi* s. *Lyra Davidis* or *Psalterium*.

coide et sinuosis glutiis) retain and sometimes strengthen the poultice of the air breathed in, until through the fanning and strong pulsation of all the arteries of the mind the explorative process of thinking has been brought to perfection and everything is clearly elucidated. It is therefore with the mind which is fiery and partakes of the light of God that this fiery place is associated, even after the thought has been conceived—the concept which is also a ray of light and a certain luminous image. The external shapes of things that are perceptible and sent to the eye are also luminous and sent from a luminous object, i.e. from one that has the form of light and through a luminous medium. It is thus that the mind itself becomes more and more enlightened.

Not only from vision, which shows us several distinguishing features of things, is the intellect adorned, but also from the objects perceived by other senses which all have a certain affinity to our lucid spirit. This affinity is derived from the essential form of all things which is light and from its spiritual kind of action in each individual thing. Sound and smell are like spirit, and are perceived and act in us as such. Hearing is due to the external spirit beating the internal spirit at the site of the ear membrane—the internal spirit in which the light of the soul is seated and the spiritual harmony, made concordant through diastole and systole. The same applies to smell. What is tasted and touched, though more corporeal, is endowed with forces that are apt to change the soul, the former through its fluid contents, the latter through resistance: both deriving from the common form of light and its varying action on the spirit. It is by reason of light that this substance as a whole acts on the soul, as it impresses on the latter the idea of the whole. The sophists who used to teach that nothing can be seen, neither in God nor in ourselves but qualities and painted masks, now see the substances. We, however, who see the essential light in Christ, follow the vision of the true light also in other objects.

When all things mentioned have been illuminated in the middle ventricle, the spirit, with the permission of the janitor, tends to the fourth ventricle in the cerebellum, and with it the luminous image that has been kindled ("fused together"—*conflata*[9]) and lies in the light of the soul itself. There, as it were in the bottom of the brain, the vessels tenaciously guard their treasure of memories and hide what has been conceived (*inventa*) by sensual perception and reasoning—not that this is attached to the walls, but it is in the very substance of the soul as if in a kind of matter (*ut in materia quadam*). There the soul has stronger vessels to retain the spirit

9 TOLLIN, p. 12: "und es folgt ihm das *zusammengewehte* lichtvolle Bild, das in dem Licht der Seele selber gelegen ist".

and to prevent memory from being easily dispersed. It may be mentioned in passing only that by this way through the big nerves of the spine the motor faculty of the whole body is sent to the muscles—as it were by radiation of this animal spirit.

There are therefore in the brain four chambers and three internal senses. For the first two ventricles produce one *sensus communis*, the receiver of images. The middle chamber is for cogitation and the last one for memory. So much, then, for the portion of the spirit that reaches the brain, the instruments of the brain and their functions...

The larger portion of the air breathed in is taken through the trachea to the lungs in which it is elaborated and then proceeds to the pulmonary vein in which it is to be mixed with the golden and subtle blood and still further elaborated. The whole mixture is then attracted by the left chamber of the heart through diastole. Here it attains to its destined perfection (*ad suam formam perficitur*) through the very strong and enlivening power of fire that dwells there. It becomes vital spirit, after discharge of the copious smoky excrement which developed in the process of its elaboration. All this constitutes as it were the *matter of the soul* itself. Besides that mixture there are two further elements in the soul: *something alive* that is *generated by breathing* or produced in its (i.e. the soul's) matter, and the *spirit*, *divinity itself* implanted through breathing—all this being One and one soul. That intermediate element which is chiefly called soul is breath and spirit—on both sides and essentially linked to spirit. It is an ethereal substance similar to that which is archetypal and superelemental, but also to this inferior one: a single soul, natural, vital and animal. (*Naturalis anima una, vitalis et animalis.*) This, then, is the whole essence (*ratio*) of the soul and why the soul as a whole is in the blood, and the soul itself is blood, as God says. For through the breath of God that aura of the celestial spirit or spark and idea (*idealis scintilla*) is taken in through the mouth and nostrils into the heart and brain of Adam and his descendants; inside it is joined to the essence of that sanguineous spiritual matter and made soul in his entrails."

Servetus: Religious Ideas and Physiological Insight

We have presented to the reader a larger excerpt from Servetus' book than is normally given: this alone will—we believe—enable us to see where he stood and what his purpose was in enlarging on the blood and its movement through the lungs, heart and brain—in short why he wrote the passages regarded as relevant in the history of circulation. It is obvious that any anatomical or physiological observations which Servetus had to contribute were designed to support his general religious, cosmological and metaphysical ideas. This cannot mean to deny that the former had been the result of genuine anatomical studies. For this we have the testimony of Guntherus of Andernach (1487–1574) who acknowledged his debt to Vesalius and to Michael Villanovanus—Servetus—who succeeded the former in assisting Guntherus in dissections and literary matters where his (Servetus') knowledge of Galenical doctrine proved second to none[10]. Yet this observational matter is subservient to a non-scientific idea which is Servetus' leading concern: the idea of the single and unique divine spirit and its communication to man. What are Servetus' sources?

Servetus was, by upbringing and inclination, first and foremost a theologian and as such a fundamentalist and "simpliste". He strove to restore the simple words and meaning of the Biblical text against the artificial overgrowth of dogma which had obscured it in the course of centuries. There was nothing of the *Trinity* which he could discover in Scripture itself—reason enough to write the *Errors of Trinity* (1531) which duly earned him the reputation of a heretic, forced him to adopt a pseudonym and prepared his cruel end some twenty years later[11].

The clear statement which the Bible[12] gives us on the nature of man is to the effect that the blood is the seat of the soul and indeed is the soul itself and that this was *breathed* into man by God. Hence Servetus' interest in the blood and its relationship with the ambient air. This is the medium through which we receive the divine soul and thus the means of developing our vital and psychic (animal) faculties and above all of achieving personal salvation[13].

Provision had therefore to be made for the broadest possible contact between blood and air. No such provision had been made, however, by Galen—for the latter had merely allowed that small quantity of blood to reach the lungs which was deemed sufficient to nourish them. By contrast the bulk of the blood that is carried from the liver to the right heart had been thought to pass direct from the right ventricle to the left through septal pores.

Servetus' concern was with just this—the contact between blood and air—and not with the movement of the blood as such. It was not his intention to combat any traditional view about the latter. Hence he did not expressly deny the existence of the pores through which he admitted that something might "sweat" through. Nor did he do away with the idea of an ebb and flow movement of the blood as conceived by Aristotle[14]. Nor finally

10 "Qua in re auxiliares habui, primum Andream Vesalium, juvenem Mehercule! in Anatome diligentissimum; post hunc Michael Villanovanus familiariter mihi in consectionibus adhibitus est, vir omni genere literarum ornatissimus, in Galeni doctrina vel ulli secundus. Horum duorum praesidio atque opera, tum artuum tum partium exteriorum, musculos omnes, venas, arterias et nervos in ipsis corporibus examinavi studiosisque ostendi". Jo. Guintheri *Anatomicarum Institutionum a Galeni Sententia libri IV* Basil. 1539, a3b of the preface, as quoted by WILLIS loc. cit. in note [2] 1877, p. 107, note [1].

11 For an account of Servetus' anti-trinitarian arguments: TRECHSEL loc. cit. 1839, p. 67 et seq. Trinity designating not three persons but multifarious divine "dispositions" and the greatness of divine power (p. 73) with ref. to *Trinit. Erroribus* f. 26b. Nor are there three things in God, but there are various forms, grades and modifications of the unique divine substance, by virtue of divine economy. The same divinity which is in the father is communicated to Jesus, the son, as well as to our spirit—"eadem divinitas, quae est in patre, communicatur filio J. Christo et spiritui nostro, qui est templum Dei viventis; sunt enim filius et sanctificatus spiritus noster consortes substantiae Patris, membra, pignora et instrumenta, licet varia sit in eis deitatis species; et hoc est quod distinctae personae dicuntur, i. e. multiformes deitatis aspectus, diversae facies et species" (ibid. fol. 28b, TRECHSEL p. 74). Bainton, loc. cit. 1953, p. 22 et seq.: Jesus is man. If he is also God, then only in the sense in which man is capable of being God. – God can communicate divinity to humanity (*Tr. Error.* 11b). God Himself is our spirit dwelling in us, and this is the Holy Spirit within us. Everyone that is born is of the spirit of God (67a). Yet the difference between Jesus and other men is upheld. He is son in a more excellent way—he is *the* i.e. the natural son of God, whereas others are born and *become* sons of God through His gift and grace (9a). Hence Jesus could be God without ceasing to be man. Before his incarnation Jesus was called the Word, after his union with the man Jesus he was called the Son. The Word, therefore, was eternal, the Son was not (111a; BAINTON p. 48). – The Holy Spirit is accordingly not a distinct Being, but merely God's spirit moving in our hearts (31b). The light sent by God is God Himself (102a).

12 "Flesh with its soul, its blood, shall ye not eat" Gen. 9,4. – "For the soul of all flesh is its blood" Levit. 17,14. – "For the blood is the soul, and thou mayest not eat

did his innovation imply anything that anticipated the idea of circulation—either the lesser or the systemic. That he had nothing of this in mind already follows from the pinpoint limitation of his interest which lay with the spiritualisation of blood in the lung and its further elaboration in the heart and brain.

Servetus' discovery, then, lies in the field of anatomy and physiology only in so far as these were productive of information ancillary to theology.

In addition to the biblical source and authority that was paramount, Servetus seems to have been inspired by *Stoicism*. This would appear from his preoccupation with the air as vector of divine spirit or the world-soul with its unifying and divinising power for all and everything. In the Stoic vision the air was full of immortal souls which reveal truth and confer mantic power on man[15].

At the time of Servetus ideas of this kind had been elaborated by such savants as Agrippa of Nettesheym and Paracelsus[16]. In their philosophies air claims the privileges of a "magic medium". According to Paracelsus it is indissolubly bound up with the *Mysterium magnum*, the immediate divine source of life, the "mother of all things"[17]. Most of the writings of Paracelsus came to light only after Servetus' death, whereas Agrippa's *Occult Philosophy* was accessible in print at the very time of Servetus' literary activity. Like Paracelsus Agrippa had designated the air as the vital spirit which penetrates all and bestows life and durability on all. In it all astral force is concentrated—it is the divine mirror which reflects all, nature, art, language and natural voice. It can do so by virtue of the spirit that binds all, moves all and fills all[18]. It is in this divine medium of air that, according to Agrippa, spiritual images may condense and become visible—as Plotinus had already taught[19]. It is through the air that, according to Paracelsus, spirits communicate with each other[20].

The Stoic view of the world was informed by materialist and pantheist ideas—spirit was identified with matter, however subtle and ethereal. There are traces of this outlook in Servetus as well. For he said that All is One, because all are one in God and consist in one, and each individual is thus a *modus divinus*[21].

Neoplatonism was opposed to this Stoic materialism and pantheism—holding up the original Platonic division between spirit and matter. At the same time, however, Neoplatonists insisted upon cosmic continuity. For this reason a "*tertium quid*"—middle forces —were introduced which may be regarded as a concession to Stoic monism. Indeed there was soul and there was body, but the

the soul with the flesh" Deut. 12,23. – "God breathed into his nostrils the breath of life" Gen. 2,7. – See below, p. 345.

For interpretation and Rabbinical sources (Abraham Ibn-Ezra 1092–1167 and Maimonides 1135–1204) consonant with Servetus' biblical quotations see: Leibowitz, J.O., *Annotations on the Biblical Aspects of Fulton's Servetus. J.Hist.Med.* 1955, X, 233–238.

See also below, note [29a].

13 As Bainton has shown (loc.cit. 1953, p.124) the problem of personal salvation was one of the main religious themes in Servetus' mind. According to the latter it is acquired not by faith alone, as Luther dictated, but by union of man with God i.e. through his becoming a son of God, and, in some sense, divine (see above in note [11]). This is achieved by the soul and spirit "breathed" into us—the divine idea that confers specific and individual existence.

14 This is not infrequently believed to be Galenic in origin. On its Aristotelian origin and revival by Cesalpinus see below p. 177.

15 Wachsmuth, C., *Die Ansichten der Stoiker über Mantik und Dämonen* Berlin 1860, p.20 et seq. – Pagel, W., *Das Medizinische Weltbild des Paracelsus. Seine Zusammenhänge mit Neuplatonismus und Gnosis.* Wiesbaden 1962, pp.43; 113 seq.

16 Pagel, W., *Paracelsus. An Introduction to Philosophical Medicine in the Era of the Renaissance*, Basle and New York, 1958, p. 117; 141; 298. – Pagel, W., 1962, loc.cit. in note [15], p.58; 113.

17 Paracelsus, *Volumen Paramirum*, tract. I *de Ente Astrorum*, cap.6 seq., ed. Sudhoff vol.I, p.182. – *Philosophia ad Athenienses*, I, 1, ed. Sudhoff vol.XIII, p.390 and 395: dan keiner subtiler element ist vom höchsten arcanen beschaffen, dan der luft. – *Liber Azoth*, ed. Sudhoff, vol.XIV, p.558: dann im luft ist die kraft aller leben.

18 Agrippa of Nettesheym, *Occulta Philosophia*, lib.I, cap. 6, ed. Lugduni 1550, p.11 seq.

19 Ibidem p.15.

20 Paracelsus, *Philos.tract.quinque*, Tr. V: von dem schlaf und wachen der leiber und geister, ed. Sudhoff, vol.XIII, p. 353–357: von den luftigen geistern... spiritus humani genennet. – *Philos.sagax.* I, 4; ed. Sudhoff, vol.XII, p.95 (chaomantia).

21 "ultimo ex praemissis comprobatur vetus illa sententia, omnia esse unum: quia omnia sunt unum in Deo, in uno con-

gulf between them was bridged by an *ethereal pneuma* which served as an envelope and carrier (*ochema*) bringing the former to the body and making possible its activity therein. This envelope is acquired by the soul while descending through the spheres of the stars and is returned to the latter when ascending again on leaving the body. Hence it is called the *Astral body*—the "body" of angels and demons without which there is no union of spirit and body, no syncretism of physics and theology[22].

Such Neoplatonic ideas also emerge in the theology of Servetus. He speaks of the element in the soul that is *intermediate* between the *matter of the soul* (*materia ipsius animae*) that consists of air and "fiery" blood and the divine spirit itself. This intermediate element which is chiefly called "soul" (*id medium, quod principaliter anima dicitur*) is a "breath" (*halitus*) and spirit, an ethereal substance (*substantia aetherea*). It is on both sides linked with spirit and thus related to the superelemental (*archetypal*) spirit as well as to the inferior material breath (p. 144). In this we recognise the astral body of the Neoplatonists[23]. Like the latter Servetus saw it as "luminous" or more precisely as a "luminous vapour"[24].

Moreover, as in Neoplatonism, pantheist leanings are tempered in Servetus' theology by emanationism—at all events in his later work, the *Restitution of Christianity* which is of interest in our context. Indeed, according to Servetus, God is everything, but He is everything by virtue of his conferring form, essence and true substance on each individual object. God does not, however, contribute its matter. God is everything and is manifested in everything, in fire, stone, a flower...God in wood is wood, in a stone He is stone—but He is the *form* of stone, its *essence* and true *substance*, and not its matter[25]. God confers being, essence and particularity upon all that is, and it is thus that God sustains all things. God fills all things, even Hell itself[26].

From all this it follows that the objects of the material world are really and merely expressions of ideas and the result of the activity of spirit—another token of more idealistic and Neoplatonic thinking, found side by side with Servetus' pantheism.

In Servetus' view thus each individual object is determined by the "God in it"—i. e. its inherent and specific divine idea which is also designated as *spirit*, *logos* or *light*. As the divine idea is luminous, so all things in the last resort consist of light. It is the formative power of light which is responsible for all generation. Similarly all knowledge is acquired by luminous images that reach the soul. Each seed contains such luminous images—the form and properties of the individual to be.

sistunt. Rerum ideae, in quibus res ipsae in esse uno consistunt, sunt unum in Deo, res alias eo medio unum cum Deo esse facientes in umbra ejus veritatis, qua Christus sine medio est hypostatice unum cum Deo." *De Trinit. div.* IV, p. 161, as cited by TRECHSEL loc. cit. 1839, p. 126.

From Bainton's account loc. cit. 1953, p. 48 seq. it would appear that this view is connected with Servetus' basic antagonism to the "Errors of Trinity". If God is "All in All"—as Servetus sees it—there is no need for a mediator and hence the dogma of Trinity should fall (with ref. to *De trinitatis erroribus* 81b–82a). It was precisely this to which Oecolampadius, the reformer of Basle and host of Servetus, objected and which terminated the latter's welcome (BAINTON p. 51).

22 For the concept of the *Astral Body:* DODDS, E. R. in *Proclus, The Elements of Theology*. Oxford 1933, Appendix II: *The Astral Body in Neo-platonism* p. 313. – VERBEKE, G., *L'Evolution de la Doctrine du Pneuma du Stoicisme à St Augustin.* Paris et Louvain 1945, p. 364. – RÜSCHE, F., *Das Seelenpneuma.* Paderborn 1933, p. 55. – The *Journey of the Soul* (in Gnosticism): BAUR, F. CH., *Die Christliche Gnosis.* Tübingen 1835, p. 214 seq. – BOUSSET, W., *Hauptprobleme der Gnosis.* Göttingen 1907, p. 361 seq. – LEISEGANG, H., *Dante und das Christliche Weltbild. Schriften der Dante-Gesellschaft* vol. VI, Weimar 1941, p. 17; pp. 21–26. – PAGEL, W., *Das Medizinische Weltbild des Paracelsus.* Wiesbaden 1962, p. 35; 38 and passim. See also below note [68] on p. 264.

23 Plato in Timaeo aperte docet substantiam animae esse elementaris et divinae substantiae commixtionem quandam. Esse *tertiam quandam substantiam mediam, utriusque participem.* Nam continet anima symbolum Deitatis et mundi elementorum. *De Trinit. div.* L. V., p. 178. – Est anima una ex elementis seminis et sanguinis elicita et a Deo afflata. Una est anima plures habens vitas. *Dial. II de Trinit.* p. 260. – Dei essentia ... quatenus mundo communicatur, est spiritus. Quemadmodum in verbo erat idea princeps creati hominis, ita in spiritu erat idea princeps creati spiritus. Erat spiritus in archetypo spirationis constitutio certa, sempiterne in Deo constans et inde velut exiens. Prodibat cum sermone spiritus, Deus loquendo spirabat. Sermonis et spiritus erat substantia eadem, sed modus diversus. *De Trin. div.* L. V, p. 163. – TRECHSEL, loc. cit. 1839, p. 132–133.

24 Animae brutorum eliciuntur de potentia lucis creatae, in qua diximus esse endelecheian vivificam. *Dial. II de Trin.* p. 261. – TRECHSEL, p. 132.

With all this the unity of God and His creatures is stipulated—a principle of outstanding significance for the proper appreciation of Christ. Just as is man, but on an exalted level, Christ is one with God, is inseparable from Him, a personal manifestation (*Hypostasis*) of God. The same deity which is in the Father is communicated to Christ as well as to our spirit which is a temple of the living God. When Christ was made man, his generation was essentially the same as the generation of man—though in place of the paternal semen there stood the divine *Logos*, the archetypal idea, the uncreated divine life which vivified and united with the maternal blood. Thus the vital spirit that fills the world, the world-soul, the *Logos* assumed human nature and was joined to the material *breath of life* to form the soul of Christ[27]. There is, then, no mediator between God and Christ, as the whole of God's substance and nature is in Christ and not only a part of Him. In this lies one of the major points which was raised by Servetus in opposition to the dogma of Trinity which in his opinion involved the recognition of three Gods[28].

According to Servetus, then, all action in the material world is spiritual action operating through union of the divine spirit, omnipresent in the "breath" of air, with the elements of the body. This action is recognisable in the *movement* of matter and the body, notably that expressed in respiration and the motion of the blood. Such movement serves the elaboration of matter, its elevation to a higher status, the production of vital spirit in the heart and of psychic (animal) spirit in the brain.

Independence and Originality of Servetus

It is, then, against this theological background that Servetus' account of the movement and transformations of the blood must be examined. Indeed the blood is a divine instrument. God breathes life and soul into it by means of the air that surrounds us. Adhering to the biblical appreciation of the blood as the seat of the soul and indeed as the soul itself, Servetus finds himself in opposition to Aristotle who had opposed the crude materialistic ideas of some Presocratic thinkers who also regarded the blood as the seat of the soul[29]. On the other hand Servetus followed the Aristotelian tradition in several points. On the whole he is independent of Aristotle and Galen. As Servetus saw it, Galen not only had failed to make provision for the broadest possible contact between blood and air, but also had been ambiguous as to the place where and the extent to which air has access to the blood. He had been wrong

Non solum in luce omnia repraesentantur, sed et in luce omnia consistunt, De Trin. div. L. IV, p. 145. – Ejusdem lucis et ideae ratione continet semen quodvis quandam nasciturae rei formalem proprietatem, ibidem.

This also applies to the theory of knowledge, for this is the result of a reviving of the *originale seminarium* of images contained in the light of the soul, by images which reach the soul from external objects. Trechsel p. 128.

See also Bainton loc. cit. 1953, p. 133 with reference to Plotinus (*Ennead. I*, 6,3) where Light *qua* metaphysical principle is separated from material things and identified with *Logos* and *Form*. Proclus made Light the bond between the upper and nether worlds and so did Hermes (*Corpus Hermeticum* I,21: the Father of all things from whom man is generated consists of Light and Life. Ed. Nock and Festugière, *Hermes Trismegistus*, Paris 1960, Tr. I, *Poimandres*, p. 14). – Concerning Light as Form in mediaeval philosophy:

Baeumker, C., *Witelo. Ein Philosoph und Naturforscher des XIII. Jahrhunderts. Beitr. z. Gesch. d. Philos. d. Mittelalters.* vol. III, 2, 1908, pp. 357–421. – On *Pyr Noeron* originating in Stoicism and as precursor of the distinction between the *bright* and *dark Fire* in Gnosticism, the Kabbala, Dionysius Ps.-Areopagita, St. Hildegard of Bermersheim (Bingen), Ficinus, Reuchlin, Agrippa of Nettesheim and Paracelsus—the latter distinguishing between *essential* (bright) and *material* fire—see: Pagel, W., *Paracelsus*. Basle 1958, 212–213 and idem, *Das Medizinische Weltbild des Paracelsus*, Wiesbaden 1962, p. 71. – See below, p. 292.

25 *Christ. Rest.* p. 589. – Bainton loc. cit. 1953, p. 133.

26 *Christ. Rest.* p. 240. – Bainton loc. cit. 1953, p. 133.

27 *Dial. II de Trin.* p. 250. – Trechsel loc. cit. 1839, p. 131; *Trinit. Error.* f. 28b; Trechsel p. 74.

28 Trechsel, p. 80; 96. – Bainton pp. 22 et seq.

29 *De anima* lib. I, cap. 2; 405b. Tr. J.A. Smith. Oxford 1931. On the other hand: *De gen. anim.* III, 11; 762a—animals and plants come into being in earth and in liquid because there is water in earth, and air in water, and *in all air is vital heat*, so that in a sense *all things are full of soul.*

in reserving the large pulmonary artery for the "private" office of nourishing the lungs and had left unanswered the question as to where the conversion of blood into bright-red—golden (*flavus*)—arterial blood takes place. It should be noted in passing that this designation of the arterial blood was not original, but had already been used by Galen (*xanthos*) and by Vesalius (*flavus*)[29a]. It was obvious to Servetus that the elaboration through which vital spirit was conferred upon the blood occurred in the lungs. The interventricular septum was no fit place for this perfection of the blood. What little might "sweat through" this septum after all could not be of any significance in this vital process. By contrast the extensive anastomoses between the pulmonary arteries and veins in the lung provide all the conditions that were necessary for it. Again opposing Galen and anticipating Cesalpinus[30], Servetus invoked the analogy with the broad communication of the branches of the Vena portae with those of the Vena cava in the liver where also an elaboration of blood takes place inside the vascular system.

The Influence of Ibn an-Nafis

In his correct description of the flow of the blood from the right ventricle to the left and the denial of any significance to interventricular pores, Servetus was probably original.

There is still no direct evidence that he knew of Ibn an-Nafis who opposed Galen and Avicenna on this score in the thirteenth century. The question of indirect evidence is still *sub judice*. As Temkin has pointed out[31], Ibn an-Nafis was quite definite about the impenetrability of the interventricular septum, whereas Servetus did not even mention the pores and left it open whether something might "sweat through"—a term used by Vesalius whose probable influence on Servetus we shall discuss in a separate chapter below[32].

Moreover, Ibn an-Nafis visualised the mixture of blood with air as taking place in the air cells of the lung whereas Servetus thought of arterio-venous anastomoses as the site of this process.

On the other hand, if the account of Ibn an-Nafis is formulated in definite propositions, no less than eleven out of sixteen recur in Servetus, as Schacht has shown[33]. These parallels include the following theses: 1. that the blood is refined in the right ventricle of the heart, 2. that its septum is impervious, 3. that the pulmonary artery carries the blood from the right ventricle to the lung where it is mixed with air, 4. that there are passages between the pulmonary artery and vein in the lung, 5. that the mixing of the refined blood with air begins not, as traditionally believed, in the heart,

29a GALEN, *De placitis* lib.VI, cap.4 ed. KÜHN vol.V, p.537: leptoteron t'esti kai xanthoteron (sc. the blood in the left chamber of the heart) – tenuior et flavior: Vesalius, *De corpor. humani fabrica* lib.VI, cap.15; ed. 1543, p.598.

LEIBOWITZ, 1955, loc.cit. in note [12] drew attention to the Hebrew equivalent of *flavus* (yellow, golden, bright-red), used by Servetus for the arterial blood: *zahov*—usually designating yellow colour, but used several times in the meaning of *bright* (translated by Buxtorf *fulgens*, i.e. bright, brilliant). In the present author's opinion Servetus is likely to have followed Galen's terminology (*xanthos*). He was, however, a Hebrew scholar (as also pointed out by Leibowitz) and may therefore have been aware of the parallel with the Hebrew *zahov*. Leibowitz finally refers to small modifications in the Hebrew motto on the title page of the *Christianismi restitutio*, devised as a hint to Servetus' authorship.

30 CESALPINUS, *Quaest. Peripatet.* V, 3; ed. Venet. 1593, fol.118 v. See our discussion of Cesalpinus as a precursor of Harvey below p. 185 and note [56] in the section devoted to Cesalpinus.

31 TEMKIN, O., *Was Servetus influenced by Ibn an-Nafis? Bullet.Hist.Med.* 1940, VIII, 731–734.

32 VESALIUS, *Fabrica*, lib.VI, cap.11; ed. 1543, p.589. – For the full text of the passage see below p.157 note [61].

33 SCHACHT, 1957, loc.cit. in note [3], p.327–328.

but already in the lung, 6. that this is a preparatory stage in the production of vital spirit, 7. that the pulmonary vein carries the mixture to the left ventricle, 8. that the mixture of refined blood and air is apt to become vital spirit, 9. that the vital spirit is produced in the left ventricle, 10. that the unused residue is discharged from the left ventricle through the pulmonary vein into the lung and breathed out and 11. that there is innate heat in the left ventricle.

To this may be added the support given by Servetus to the opinion that the attraction of blood and air by the left ventricle takes place in diastole.

It should be noted, however, that several of the points enumerated are in no way opposed to Galen and Galenic tradition—notably the refinement of the blood in the right ventricle, the passages joining branches of the pulmonary artery and vein, the discharge of smoky waste through the pulmonary vein and lung and the admission of blood to the heart in diastole; as we have seen (p. 131) there are hints that Galen assumed a mixture of air and blood to reach the left heart. The production of vital spirit in the heart is in keeping with Postgalenic tradition, even if Galen himself had not clearly stipulated the existence of vital spirit as such[34].

Moreover, Servetus contradicts one of Ibn an-Nafis' points—the size of the left ventricle which, in Servetus' opinion, is not big enough for the mixture of the blood and air to take place, as Schacht himself has pointed out[35]. The latter author lists four statements in Ibn an-Nafis' account which are not found in Servetus e.g. that the amount of refined blood in the left ventricle is small, but the quantity of spirit is great. We add Servetus' original assessment of the size of the pulmonary artery.

The hypothesis that Ibn an-Nafis' break-away from Galen in the question of the ventricular septum had been made known to the Western world in the Renaissance through the mediation of Andreas Alpago Bellunensis—an industrious collector and translator of Arabic manuscripts including works of Ibn an-Nafis—has always been intriguing and was for a short time breath-takingly promising[36]. So far it has not been possible to implement it.

In giving his account of the movement of the blood Servetus was admittedly actuated by religious and philosophical motives. This in itself does not favour, let alone prove that he had borrowed his anatomical data elsewhere. Indeed the evidence we have for his skill and knowledge in anatomy[37] rests on firmer ground than the nest of assumptions built around the elusive figure of Alpagus Bellunensis.

34 Temkin, 1951, loc. cit. in note [3] on p. 127, p. 184.

35 Schacht, loc. cit. in note [3], 1957, p. 328.
See also: Bittar, E. Edward, *A Study of Ibn Nafis. Bullet. Hist. Med.* 1955, XXIX, 352–447: p. 429 Ibn Nafis Commentary on the Anatomy of the Canon of Avicenna; p. 430 translation of the description of the cardiovascular system.

36 Coppola, Edward D., *The Discovery of the Pulmonary Circulation: A new approach. Bullet. Hist. Med.* 1957, XXXI, 44–77 (p. 67: "A possible way by which Ibn An-Nafis' theory of the pulmonary circulation could have reached the West"): Andrea Alpago knew of Ibn an-Nafis, had read his exposition on the Vth canon of Avicenna, his exposition on the book of Samarcandi and was familiar with certain of Ibn an-Nafis' ideas concerning the cardio-vascular system. But he makes no mention of the latter's account of the pulmonary transit. "It is possible that somewhere among the unpublished manuscripts of Andrea Alpago is to be found a rendering of Ibn an-Nafis' description of the lesser circulation. Certainly such manuscripts are extant" (p. 70). Coppola refers to Paolo Alpago who in the dedicatory letter of Avicenna, *Compendium de Anima*, translated by Andrea Alpago (Venetiis, ap. Juntas, 1546), mentions that since his youth he had been a constant companion of his uncle Andrea. He continues that the latter, at his death left manuscript translations from the Arabic, both of Avicenna and other authors "*pluraque alia*". "It is possible that these and other manuscripts left by Andreas Alpago may yet come to light, and that among them we eventually may find a description of the pulmonary circulation by Ibn an-Nafis" (p. 71). Possibly the latter had not been forgotten in the West and may somehow have reached Valverde and his teacher Columbus (p. 74). O'Malley, C.D., *A Latin translation of Ibn Nafis (1547) related to the problem of the circulation of the blood. J. Hist. Med.* 1957, XII, 248.

37 See above and note [10].

Servetus had an original mind which did not shirk the unpleasantness and danger connected with defiance of authority. With this an original break-away from the Galenic tradition in anatomy is well compatible and indeed consistent, although the difficulties encountered by Vesalius in tracing interventricular communications are not unlikely to have formed a source of inspiration (p. 156 seq.)[38].

38 See above, p. 140 and note [32] and below, p. 164. – The idea that Servetus might have been indebted to Columbus was rejected by SCHACHT, 1957, loc. cit. in note [3], p. 325–326 and 331.

The Significance of Servetus' Views

What, then, is the significance of his anti-traditional view of the blood flow from the right ventricle to the left and its aeration in the lung for the history of the discovery of blood circulation?

His merit is customarily described as the "discovery of the lesser circulation". This term and its use with reference to Servetus and for that matter to all predecessors of Harvey has rightly been rejected (p. 136). The censure thus passed on an unfelicitous slogan takes nothing away from Servetus and his original approach to a matter which indeed became an important stepping stone in the history of the discovery, although Servetus himself did not dream let alone know of its importance in this context. He fully realised that it was significant—but to his mind its significance did not lie in the elucidation of the movement of the blood as such, but in the proposal of a theory that would explain the acquisition of divine spirit by the blood in conformity with the anatomically correct pathways of that portion of the blood which is destined to receive this spirit from the air. To assess the position of Servetus correctly the context in which his various statements are found is therefore all important. This context bears the hallmark of individuality—it would not be surprising if the support which he draws from anatomy for his theological view of man was also original. At all events an account of Servetus' position in the history of Harvey's discovery should not stop short at his statement about the blood flow through the heart, but should include his ideas concerning the soul and its corporeal aspects.

In this connexion Servetus carefully examined the brain. He would not regard it as the "seat" of the soul, but favoured for this role the vascular plexuses which it contains. This is the result of an analogy with the anatomy of the lung. Here it was in arterio-venous plexuses that a new spirit was produced through the mixture of air with blood—the vital spirit. In the brain it is in the chorioid plexuses that a further "new" spirit is formed—the psychic (animal) spirit. In both cases it is a new "third" kind of vessel, of rather the terminal part of the artery that matters. In the brain this terminal artery becomes a part of the nervous substance—an Aristotelian idea, adopted by Cesalpinus to which we shall return below (p. 176). The soft parts of the nervous substance notably in the peripheral nerves are in Servetus' opinion devoid of sensitivity —by contrast with their membranous filaments to which the animal spirit is sent by the terminal chorioid arteries. Similarly the soft parts of the brain are "cold"—again a reminiscence of the ideas of Aristotle[39]—and devoid of sensation. Hence they do not qualify as the seat of the rational soul. They merely act as "cushion" and container of the spirit, preventing its dissipation. Nor can the ventricles claim any higher dignity than that of drains of excremental matter that is led through them to the palate and nose. In this we readily recognise the ancient doctrine of *catarrh*[40]. In this vapours ascending from the stomach to the cold brain are made to condense in the latter as in an alembic and to flow downwards again in liquid condition. According to Galen there are two main ways for this: (a) in a straight downward direction through the floor of the third ventricle and (b) obliquely downwards along the aqueduct. Both these ways join to form a funnel which eventually leads through holes in the base of the skull to the epipharynx[41].

It is the brain plexuses, then, which are the "seat" of the soul. Moreover it is these vessels that attract air from outside through the ethmoid bone—whereby Servetus characteristically modified the ancient doctrine of the "breathing" of air by the brain. According to him the soul substance present in the plexuses is in need of fanning so that smoky excrements can be removed. For just like light so the soul is tied up with burning matter—forming as it does a "luminous ray" or "fiery vapour".

Servetus followed the ancient theory of localisation of the faculties of the mind, as first fully developed by Nemesius of Emesa, the Christian bishop of the middle of the fourth century[42]. Servetus, too, assumed that sensory impressions and the images and associations formed from them—the *sensus communis*—are controlled in the two anterior ventricles. The third ventricle—a narrow passage rather than a chamber—is responsible for the complicated and "winding" exploration which leads the higher faculty of thinking to the grasp of truth, corresponding to the winding and circuitous form of the passage. At the same time it is equipped with a particularly strong and copious vascular plexus. Here Servetus repeats the story of the "worm"—elaborated by Arabic authors, notably Ali Abbas—according to which the chorioid plexus joined to the pineal (*red vermis*) formed a valve[43], called by Servetus *janitor;* this regulates the flow of air and the pulsation of

39 *De partibus animal.* II, 7, 8; 653a: the brain is made of cold elements. Ibid. II,7,5; 652b: of all the parts of the body there is none so cold as the brain ... it is cold even to the touch ... it is the one that has the least blood ... when it is touched no sensation is produced.

40 For a history of traditional catarrh theories: PAGEL, W., *Jo. Bapt. Van Helmont. Einführung in die Philosophische Medizin des Barock. Berlin.* Springer. 1930, pp. 48–62, followed by an account of Van Helmont's refutation of catarrh: pp. 62 et seq. – For the role of catarrh in the history of tuberculosis: PAGEL, W., *Die Krankheitslehre der Phthise in den Phasen ihrer geschichtlichen Entwickelung. Beitr. z. Klin. d. Tuberk.* 1927, LXVI, 66–98; – idem, *Zur Geschichte der Lungensteine und der Obstruktionstheorie der Phthise. Ibidem* 1928, LXIX, 315–323.

41 PAGEL,, *Van Helmont* loc. cit. in note [40], 1930, p. 53–55 with reference to Galen, *De usu partium* lib. VIII, cap. 6 ed. KÜHN vol. III, p. 649; VIII, 14; KÜHN pp. 674 seq.; IX, 1; KÜHN pp. 684 seq (686); IX, 3; KÜHN p. 693 seq.

42 PAGEL, W., *Medieval and Renaissance Contributions to Knowledge of the Brain and its Functions.* In: POYNTER, F.N.L., *The History and Philosophy of Knowledge of the Brain.* Oxford. Blackwell. 1958, pp. 95–114 (98 seq).

43 PAGEL, loc. cit. 1958 in note [42], p. 101 with reference to Costa ben Luca, *De differentia animae et spiritus* ed. C. S. Barach. Innsbruck 1878, p. 125 and Ali Abbas (Haly), *Liber totius medicinae ... a Stephano ... in latinam ... reductus.* Lugd. 1523, fol. 33v. – AVERROES, *Colliget* Lgd. 1531, fol. 33v. – The text of Costa ben Luca is also found in: Constantini Africani *Opera* Basil. H. Petrus 1536, p. 308–317 unter: *Constantini Africani medici de animae et spiritus discrimine liber, ut quidam volunt.* See also THORNDIKE, L., *History of Magic and Experimental Science* vol. I, p. 657 seq. New York 1923. – For a mediaeval text-book representation of the matter: F.S. Bodenheimer's translation and edition of Rabbi Gershon ben Sh'lomoh d'Arles, *The Gate of Heaven* (*Shaar ha-Shamayim*) Jerusalem 1953, p. 76; 246; 299 (in particular) and 312.

the arteries—both of which essentially influence the intensity and clarity of thought. It is through these that the light is generated which is the essence of spirit and soul in heaven as well as on earth. Again following traditional doctrine, Servetus ascribes retentive faculties to the fourth ventricle and cerebellum—the vessels there being strong enough to prevent impressions committed to memory from being dispersed.

Air and blood, then, are the material constituents of the soul and it is in the latter that life is generated by breathing, i.e. the implantation of spirit. The spirit is still a substance, though a most subtle and ethereal one. It corresponds to the *Astral Body*, the starborne material envelope of the divine soul which is "archetypal" and immaterial. Yet all these constituents—from the superelemental divine via the most subtle *astral body* down to the material air and blood—form One and one soul. It is for this reason of unification that it is bound up with the blood and perfected first in the lungs (and heart) and subsequently in the brain-vessels where it unfolds the faculties of the mind. The pathways of the blood through right heart, lung and left heart thus form an essential element for the knowledge of the soul and thereby for the connection of the individual with the world at large and with divinity.

Harvey and Servetus

Harvey knew the work of Columbus and must have been aware of the latter's opposition against the Galenic interventricular communication. However, by Harvey's time, it was still the Galenic doctrine and not Columbus' opinion that was ruling. Caspar Hofmann had rejected the former, following the anti-Galenic Aristotelian lead, not long before Harvey's *De motu* was published[44]. Inspite of this Harvey had to fight his own battle against the interventricular pores and annihilated them on the basis of his long dissecting experience[45]. We return to this topic below (p. 190). Nor is Harvey likely to have known the physiological ideas and the text of Servetus. The latter formed a stock topic in the current histories of religion and heresies[46], but his contributions to physiology had to wait to be discovered by Wotton at the end of the century, perhaps in connexion with the Socinian movement and its influence in seventeenth century England which made itself palpable in its second—post-Harveian—half[47].

44 HOFMANN, CASP., *De thorace*, Francof. 1627, lib. III, cap. 11, p. 94. See below, p. 190.

45 HARVEY, *De motu*, Prooem., ed. 1628, p. 18; tr. WILLIS, p. 17: me hercule porositates nullae sunt, neque demonstrari possunt. – On Harvey's earlier views, see p. 228 below. On Fludd having witnessed Harvey's search for them, above p. 114.

46 See for example: MELCHIOR ADAM, *Decades duae continentes Vitas Theologorum exterorum principum qui Ecclesiam Christi superiori seculo propagarunt*. Francof. 1618, p. 87–90 in *Vita Calvini*. ALEX. ROSS, *Pansebeia: a view of all religions in the world*, London 1653, p. 43.

47 MCLACHLAN, H. J., *Socinianism in 17th century England*, Oxford 1951, p. 291, note [4]: Daniel Mark Szent-Ivani bringing with him a copy of Servetus' *Christ. Restit.* from England to Hungary (June 5th 1668).

III. Realdus Columbus (pl. 32)

In Servetus' case the break-away from traditional Galenic doctrine concerning the passage of blood from the right ventricle to the left was ancillary to a theological and cosmological concept: the introduction of the divine spirit into man and the location of its "seat" in the latter's body. It had nothing to do with the demonstration of a circulatory mechanism and therefore it did not imply the "discovery of the lesser circulation".

In the case of Columbus (and his pupil Valverde), no such non-scientific background is recognisable. The statement about the passage of blood through the heart and lung constitutes a chapter of Anatomy and nothing else. *Yet, in common with Servetus' statement, it is removed from the idea of circulation.* For it merely concerned that portion of the blood which was sent up to the heart from the liver to be converted into and used up as spirituous—arterial—blood[48]. "Lesser circulation" implies continuity in contrast to new formation and using up: it is the same blood that "circulates" through the right heart—lungs—left heart—right heart ever and ever again. This is impossible without the systemic circulation and of necessity concerns the whole of the blood. It is the same blood that is sent out through the arteries and returns to the heart by the only way open to it—namely through the veins—as the same blood, albeit in an effete condition.

By contrast Galen and the Galenic tradition had it that blood was sent out to the periphery from two centres, namely arterial blood from the heart and venous blood from the liver, the latter including that portion which was sent up to the heart in order to be arterialised. This is precisely what Columbus teaches.

Unlike Servetus, Columbus is quite explicit on this point. To start with he upholds—against Aristotle—the liver as the "head, source, origin and root" of the veins. Its substance is nothing but blood clotted and interwoven with many veins and dedicated to the formation of blood, though not of natural spirit. The intestinal veins carry chyle to the liver for the purpose of sanguification; in addition, however—true to Galenic doctrine—, they bring blood from the liver down to the gut, stomach and omentum. Branches of the portal vein extend towards the stomach "so that the latter may be nourished by their blood". Another branch runs to the spleen in order to carry to it melancholic blood from the liver; for the spleen is the only organ that is nourished by black bile—an excremental matter. Branches of the vena cava extend through the whole body in order to convey the blood that is formed in the

48 "... pulmo vero aerem illum una cum *eo sanguine* miscet, qui a dextro cordis ventriculo profectus per arterialem venam deducitur." Columbus, *De re anatomica* (1559) lib. XI, *De visceribus*, cap. 2 (*De pulmone*) Francof. 1593, p. 411 (the italics are of the present author). The meaning of this sentence implies a restriction to a certain portion of the total of the blood. This follows from the further passages from Columbus cited by the present author (p. 155 and 168).

49 "Est igitur jecur omnium venarum caput, fons, origo et radix" Columbus, loc. cit. (in footnote 44) Lib. VI, *de iecore*, ed. 1593 p. 300.

liver, and fully elaborated there, to the individual members; for it is from blood that each part of our body is nourished[50].

Otherwise Columbus shows his independence: first of all with regard to Aristotle. He said: Portius of Naples made himself a slave to Aristotle in stating that the pericardial fat was no proper fat, as it was not liquefiable by heat. When Columbus demonstrated the contrary by means of a candle, he silently absented himself, almost "exploded"[51]. The heart has two ventricles, not three, as Aristotle believed[52]. The vena cava does not originate in the heart; it is merely split at the site of the right auricle to which it "adheres". Nor does the arterial vein (pulmonary artery) stem from the heart, but from the liver; for in the fetus it is continuous with the vena cava. Hence wherever there is a vein, it takes its origin from the liver, and wherever an artery it comes from the heart. Nor finally is the heart the origin of the nerves, as Aristotle said—the latter having mistaken the filaments of valves for nerves[53].

Similarly Columbus opposed Galen and those who regarded his words as gospel which is inevitably true. The pulmonary vein is not designed to emit smoke, nor does it serve as a carrier of air for the refrigeration of the heart which had been looked upon as a stove in which wood is burned and gives off fumes. Indeed the opposite is true—the pulmonary veins carry blood mixed with air to the left ventricle. For whenever the left auricle is examined in the cadaver or in the live animal it is found filled with blood[54].

The pulmonary artery is far too big to serve the mere purpose of taking blood to the lung, and this over such a small distance[55]. Instead it traverses the lungs in order to be attenuated there and mixed with air to be sent down to the left ventricle via the pulmonary vein. This negatives the Galenic opinion shared by nearly everybody that the blood in the right ventricle has direct access to the left through the interventricular septum—*per quod fere omnes existimant sanguini a dextro ventriculo ad sinistrum aditum patefieri: id ut fiat facilius, in transitu ob vitalium spirituum generationem tenuem reddi*. But they all err by a long way—*sed longa errant via*[56]. This again is an anti-Galenic statement of historic significance.

Perhaps Columbus also rejected the *pulse-making force* assumed by Galen to make the arteries contract and thereby move the blood. The artery, Columbus said, is continually moved, not by itself, but because of the *spiritus*[57].

What is more, Columbus had a much clearer insight into the nature of systole and diastole than anybody else before Harvey. This was recognised by the latter as early as in his Lumleian *Lectures on the Whole of Anatomy* dating back to 1616. Here he quoted

50 "Substantia ejus (sc. hepatis) nihil aliud est, quam concretus sanguis venis compluribus, quibusdamque arteriis intertextus" ibid. p. 300. – "Huc vero missi hi venarum rami (sc. venae portae), ut illorum sanguine ventriculus nutriretur" ibid. p. 301. – "Quartus ad lienem se confert, ut sanguinem melancholicum ab hepate ad ipsum deferat, estque ramus satis insignis..." ibid. p. 301. – "Nam venae nihil aliud sunt, quam vasa concava ... ut sanguinem ad singula membra deferant, fabrefacta. nam sanguine alitur omnis pars nostri corporis" ibid. p. 305.

51 "tacitus abiit, ac pene explosus", ibid. p. 324, lib. VII (de corde et arteriis).

52 "Duae insunt cordi cavitates, hoc est ventriculi, duo, non tres, ut Aristoteli visum est", ibid. p. 325.

This statement is obviously observational, and there is no reason why he should have borrowed it from Ibn an-Nafis (as suggested by SCHACHT, loc. cit. in note [3], 1957, p. 331). – The Aristotelian doctrine had already been attacked by Berengarius (see below p. 157), and Vesalius had left no doubt that there are only two ventricles in the heart (*De corp. humani fabrica*, lib. VI, cap. 11: De cordis sinibus s. ventriculis, Basil. 1543, p. 588). – FERNEL, too, clearly describes two cavities of the heart exclusively (*Universa medicina, Physiol.* lib. I, cap. 8, ed. Heurnius, Traj. ad Rh. 1656, p. 25).

53 Neque tamen existimes id, quod multi sunt opinati, venam cavam hinc (i.e. circa cordis basim) exoriri ... illa enim cor non ingreditur, ut falso arbitrantur, sed cum scissa sit eo loco, lataque, dextro ventriculi orificio dumtaxat adhaerescit. Vena item arteriosa non a corde oritur, sed a iecore, quod verum esse facile perspicies, si animadverteris: nam, dum in utero matris faetus latitat, si eius introspiciamus, comperiemus cavam venam cum vena arteriosa continuam esse. Igitur quatenus vena, ab hepate ortum ducit, at quatenus arteriosa, ex corde est. est nam cor arteriarum omnium principium" ibid. p. 326–327. – "deceptus est magnus Aristoteles, qui filamenta haec, quae dixi, nervos esse opinatus est. hincque factum est, ut Aristoteles cor nervorum principium esse scriptum reliquerit, et per consequens sensus motusque" ibid. p. 329.

54 "Scribunt Anatomici in hoc (pace eorum dixerim) parum prudentes harum (sc. arteria venosa, i.e. of the pulmonary veins) usum esse, ut aerem alteratum ad pulmones ferant, qui flabelli instar ventulum cordi faciunt idque refrigerant non cerebrum, ut Aristoteli visum est: existi-

Columbus' statement that the heart is pulled upwards and appears to swell when it is constricted and when relaxing tends downwards and at that time is said to be at rest. Columbus had still called this systole, but nevertheless had warned against those who were convinced that the heart is dilated when in reality it is constricted[58].

On the other hand Columbus agreed with Galen that the valves at the point of entry of the veins close when the heart contracts and the semilunar—arterial—valves open. It is thus that blood is prevented from flowing back into the vena cava—a further indication that the heart is not the origin and primary distributor of the blood[59].

We shall return to Columbus and the question as to how far he was original and independent of Servetus as well as Vesalius below.

IV. The Influence of Vesalius

The anatomical achievement due to Servetus and Columbus can best be assessed in the light of the relevant statements found in the first and second editions of Vesalius' *Fabrica* of 1543 and 1555 respectively.

We mentioned above that in the use of his words Servetus was evidently influenced by Vesalius. Columbus had been Vesalius' assistant and successor—intent on criticising and superseding the greater man. He could not have failed to take notice of any alterations which Vesalius introduced into his text twelve years after its first appearance.

Vesalius on the Interventricular Septum of the Heart and the Pulmonary Transit of Venous Blood

One and perhaps the most important and historic of the alterations introduced by Vesalius into the second edition of the *Fabrica* concerned his doubts on the permeability of the heart septum.

It has often been mentioned that Vesalius voiced grave doubts as to the permeability of the septum, especially in the second edition of the *Fabrica* of 1555. At the same time, it was noted that he failed to suggest an alternative pathway for the blood, and the suspicion arose that when expressing himself more definitely in the second edition he may have had knowledge of Servetus[60] or even of still unprinted observations of Columbus, his collaborator and successor.

mantes iidem eas tunc fumos nescio quos capinosos (ita enim ipsi vocant linguarum ignoratione) excipere a sinistro ventriculo profectos ... existimant in corde ea fieri quae in caminis assolent: quasi in corde viridia ligna existant, quae dum cremantur, fumum edant ... Ego vero oppositum prorsus sentio: hanc scilicet arteriam venalem factam esse ut sanguinem cum aere a pulmonibus mixtum afferant ad sinistrum cordis ventriculum. Quod tam verum est, quam quod verissimum: nam non modi si cadavera inspicis, sed si viva etiam animalia, hanc arteriam in omnibus sanguine refertam invenies: quod nullo pacto eveniret, si ob aerem dumtaxat, et vapores constructa foret" ibid. p. 328.

55 "Vena arteriosa ... magna est satis: immo vero multo maior quam necesse fuerit: si sanguis ad pulmones supra cor exiguo intervallo deferendus dumtaxat erat", ibid. p. 327.

56 Ibidem, p. 325.

57 Movetur enim arteria continuo non per se, sed propter spiritus, ibid. p. 331.

58 HARVEY, *Praelectiones anatom. univers.*, London 1886, fol. 77 recto; ed. G. Whitteridge, Edinburgh 1964, p. 264. The reference is to Columbus, *De re anat.*, lib. XIV, de viva sectione, 4th ed. (as used by Harvey), Francof., LECHLER, 1593, p. 474. See below, p. 215.

59 "duo ex his (of the vessels at the base of the heart) constructa sunt, ut intro ad cor deferent, hoc autem evenit dum cor dilatatur: duo vero alia, ut, dum cor constringitur, foras deferant. Idcirco quando dilatatur, sanguinem a cava vena in dextrum ventriculum suscipit, necnon ab arteria venosa sanguinem paratum, ut diximus, una cum aere in sinistrum: propterea membranae illae demittuntur, ingressuique cedunt: nam dum cor coarctatur, hae clauduntur: ne quod suscepere, per easdam vias retrocedat, eodemque tempore membranae tum magnae arteriae, tum venae arteriosae (pulmonary artery) recluduntur, aditumque praebent spirituoso sanguini exeunti, qui per universum corpus funditur, sanguinique naturali ad pulmones delato... Ex hac doctrina collige, cor nullo pacto id membrum esse, in quo sanguis gignatur, quemadmodum sensit Aristoteles cum a vena cava sanguis distribuatur..." ibid. p. 330.

60 TOLLIN, loc. cit. note [2], p. 26.

At all events a detailed comparative review of what Vesalius actually said in the first and second editions of the *Fabrica* appears to be called for.

Vesalius' Statement in the First Edition of the Fabrica and its reputedly sarcastic Meaning

In the eleventh chapter of the sixth book we read on page 589: ... the septum of the ventricles is very thick; it is formed by heart substance and abounds on both sides with grooves impressed in it, thereby assuming an unequal surface towards the ventricles. Of these grooves none (at least as far as can be perceived by the senses) penetrates from the right ventricle into the left so that we are indeed forced to admire the care of the Creator whereby blood sweats through passages which escape vision from the right ventricle into the left[61].

Vesalius here alludes to Galen's well known doctrine concerning grooves in the heart septum which allow blood to pass from the right ventricle directly to the left. We discussed this doctrine (p. 129) and pointed out that in Galen's opinion the amount of blood thus passing is not small—indeed there is "*much*" (*poly*) that is taken through the septal pores into the left ventricle. We also mentioned that Galen presented the pores not as straight-forwardly and macroscopically patent holes, but as small funnels, manifestly open at the top, but ending almost blindly—at any rate in the cold cadaver. Hence he thought that an attractive force was needed to draw the blood through and that only its finer parts were thus drawn[62].

Berengarius da Carpi and Nic. Massa on the heart septum

This Galenic doctrine remained the ruling opinion up to the time of Vesalius. In it allowance had been made for the difficulty in demonstrating the actual interventricular communication in the dead body. The pointing out of this difficulty by post-Galenic writers—with the exception of Niccolò Massa (1536)—does not, therefore, convey a doubt as to their existence. This also applies to Berengarius da Carpi (1470–1530) whose *Commentaria* to Mundinus' Anatomy have been interpreted in this sense[63]. Berengarius' doubt seems to be concerned, not so much with the Galenic pores—however difficult to demonstrate in man—but with their function as a third ventricle. In Berengarius' opinion, Aristotle could not have meant them to constitute the "third ventricle" which he had postulated. By contrast there are only two proper "ventres" in the heart. The small "concavitates et porositates"

61 "... ventriculorum igitur septum crassissima, ut dixi, cordis substantia efformatum, utrinque foveis ipsi impressis scatet, hac imprimis occasione inaequali superficie qua ventriculos respicit donatum. Ex his foveis nullae (quod sensu saltem comprehendere licet) ex dextro ventriculo in sinistrum penetrant, adeo sane ut rerum Opificis industriam mirari cogamur, qua per meatus visum fugientes ex dextro ventriculo in sinistrum sanguis resudat." VESALIUS, *De humani corporis fabrica libri septem*, Basileae, 1543, lib. VI, cap. 11, p. 589.

62 In Galen's own words: the most subtle part of the blood is drawn from the right cavity to the left, as the septum between them is endowed with small holes which for the most part can be seen like grooves with a broad mouth that becomes much narrower in its course. Their very terminal parts cannot be seen because of their smallness, especially as in the dead animal all is cooled down and condensed—*echontos tina tremata tou mesou diaphragmatos auton ha mechri men pleistou dynaton idein hoion bothynous tinas ex eurytatou stomatos aei kai mallon eis stenoteron proiontas, ou men auta ge ta eschata perata dynaton eti theasasthai dia te smikroteta, kai hoti, tethneotos ede tou zoou, katepsyktai te kai pepyknotai panta;* GALEN, *De natural. facultat.*, lib. III, cap. 15, Kühn ed., vol. II, p. 208; Daremberg trans., *loc. cit.* (note [17] on p. 130), vol. II, p. 317.

63 BAYON, H.P., William Harvey, physician and biologist: his predecessors, opponents and successors. Part II. *Ann. Sci.*, 1938, 3, p. 452 with reference to Berengarius, *Commentaria ... super anatomiam Mundini*, Bonon., 1521, fol. 341: "In homine cum maxima difficultate videntur." Thus the sentence quoted out of context by Bayon. The whole passage reads as follows: "et istae porositates dicuntur ventriculus medius cordis: sicut latius infra dicemus [see the following note]: quae porositates notabiliter videntur in cordibus bovuum et magnorum animalium: sed in homine cum maxima difficultate videntur."

Berengarius therefore had no doubts as to the existence of the pores, but merely comments on the difficulty of their demonstration in man by contrast with quadrupeds. Nearly a century later Bauhin referred to the conspicuousness of the narrow windings of the pores (*spiracula*) in the heart of the ox after it has been cooked for a long time (*Theatrum anatomicum*, Francof., 1605, p. 422 in lib. II, cap. 21)—a finding mentioned in Harvey's *Praelectiones anatomiae* universalis, London, 1886, fol. 76r; see O'MALLEY, C.D., POYNTER, F.N.L., and RUSSEL, K.F., *William Harvey: Lectures on*

which are notable in the hearts of large quadrupeds, but otherwise difficult to demonstrate, as Galen has shown, serve for the passage of blood from the right ventricle to the left with subsequent rarefaction and spiritualisation—yet the smallness and state of condensation owing to the cold of the dead body make it impossible to "consider their extreme endings"[64].

Massa, however, observed the septum to be "thick, dense and hard of substance and devoid of a cavity". On the other hand, he believed he had found a "cavity" above the septum, near the base of the heart and concluded that a third ventricle indeed existed, not only in large animals, as Galen said, but also in man. With this Massa seems to have intended a criticism of Berengario's statement and thus confirms that the latter adhered to the traditional assumption of interventricular pores[65].

The reputed sarcastic note in Vesalius' statement

Seen against the background of the Galenic text the present-day observer may well be tempted to look upon the statement of Vesalius as given above as a sarcastic off-hand dismissal of the Galenic doctrine: only recourse to a divine miracle could save it, and, of course, no such miracle could have claimed serious consideration in the mind of Vesalius, the "modern". Thus, Sir Michael Foster interpreted the passage as follows:

Even in this which he ventured to print the sarcastic note of scepticism makes itself heard, but what he really thought he did not dare to put forward ... he tells us in a later writing that he "accommodated his statements to the dogmas of Galen" not because he thought that these were in all cases consonant with truth, but because in such a new great work he hesitated to lay down his own opinions and did not care to swerve a nail's breadth from the doctrines of the Prince of Medicine[66].

Following Foster, Bayon stated: "We find that the anatomist Andreas Vesalius (1514–1564) in his first edition of *De fabrica humani corporis*, published in 1543, contains a passage which may indicate ironical doubt as to the existence of the Galenical passages which doubt is further reinforced in the edition of 1555[67]. In a subsequent paper the same author commented more carefully on the passage in question: "this is not very assertive, and leaves room for considerable doubt"[68].

By contrast Roth, in his classical monograph on Vesalius, knows nothing about an intended sarcasm on the part of Vesalius, but simply says: "Although he knows the heart septum to be thick

the whole of anatomy, Berkeley and Los Angeles, 1961, p. 183; PAGEL, W., An Harveyan prelude to Harvey. *Hist. Sci.*, 1963, 2, 121; WHITTERIDGE, G., *The anatomical lectures of William Harvey*. Edinburgh, and London, 1964, pp. 260–261.

64 BERENGARIUS, *loc. cit.* (note [63]), fol. 347 recto: "et isti ventriculi ab Avi. XI tertii dicuntur esse tres s duo ventres magni et alter medius quasi venter qui non est iudicio sensibili proprie venter i.e. una concavitas: sed ut infra dicetur est plures concavitates sive porositates ... et ita sensibiliter non sunt nisi duo ventres notabiles in corde ..."—fol. 350 verso: "ad ventriculum medium me converto ... concavitates sive porositates parvas ... notabiles sunt in cordibus magnorum bovuum ... teste Galeno sunt difficilia ad videndum, quae foramina dicuntur a Medicis venter medius cordis: et ista foramina pro medio ventriculo cordis non cognovit Aristoteles ut supra patuit ... ita per talia foramina transit sanguis a ventre dextro ad sinistrum, qui continue in transitu subtiliatur et sic praeparatur ad spirituositatem ... non tamen ipsos demum ultimos fines possibile adhuc considerare propter parvitatem: et quoniam iam mortuo animali infrigidata sunt omnia et densata..."

65 *Anatomiae liber introductorius*. Venet. 1536; edition used: 1559, fol. 56. – On the possible influence of Massa's findings on Jac. Sylvius—Vesalius' teacher—and his reticence about the heart septum, see O'MALLEY, C.D., *Andreas Vesalius of Brussels*, University of California Press 1964, p. 52.

66 FOSTER, SIR M., *Lectures on the history of physiology during the 16th, 17th, and 18th centuries*. Cambridge, 1901, p. 14. With reference to the 2d edition of the *Fabrica*, lib. VI, cap. 15, p. 746 see below p. 162.

67 BAYON, H. P., The study of avian biology in relation to science progress. J. comp. Path. Ther., 1934, 47, 302–329 (p. 313).

68 BAYON, *loc. cit.* note [63], 455–456.

and entirely solid, he merely wonders how blood could pass from the right into the left chamber. Here too he sticks to the Galenic doctrine. In all cases the same reason prevails: isolated facts are not sufficient for him to abandon Galen's physiology.[69]"

It may be argued in support of an intended sarcasm that when the *Fabrica* was first published in 1543, Vesalius enjoyed a comparatively independent position—under the auspices of the liberal Venetian republic and in the "bright academic circles of Padua"[70]. This may have allowed him to make fun of what might have struck less progressive contemporaries as a divine miracle.

When the second edition of the *Fabrica* appeared in 1555 things looked different: Vesalius was now serving as Imperial Court Physician under Charles V, and indeed it may well have been true that in deference to his new loyalties to the Habsburg Court and its strict religious observances he did omit material the mere inclusion of which might have been objectionable to the orthodox.

This applies, for example, to the long passage at the end of chapter 8 of book VI which deals with the pericardium[71]. The omitted passage includes the terminal sentence about the spear wound in the body of Christ. The topic of the paragraph is the postmortal collection of fluid in the tissues of persons that had been hanged in summer time and left overnight on the gallows, as was customary in France and in Germany. But let us leave this rather fatuous discussion, Vesalius ends, and move on to the heart, lest we finally become entangled with the topic discussed by theologians who reverently deal with the fluid in the body of our Saviour Jesus Christ, full of mysteries, and lest we mingle the most veracious gospel of the divine John with our arguments concerning the effects of the sun on the bodies on gallows and instruments of torture.

Moreover, looking at the first chapter heading of the book in which the seemingly "sarcastic" passage occurs, one may notice that it introduces the term "Nature" (as the maker—*fabrefecerit*—of those parts that renew the aereal substance and individually—*privatim*—serve the vital spirit)[72]. This may be said to indicate a vein of enlightenment, especially when compared with the second edition in which at this place "Nature" is replaced by "Creator" (*opifex*)[73].

Was it perhaps for the same motives of loyalty to his new master that Vesalius altered the chapter heading as mentioned and in the text replaced the ironic recourse to a divine miracle by the simple statement of doubt?[74]

However, the terms *Natura* and *Opifex* are used synonymously

69 "Obschon er die Herzscheidewand als dick und durchaus solid kennt, wundert er sich bloß, wie Blut von der rechten in die linke Kammer durchtreten könne (*Fabrica*, 1543, VI, 11, p. 589. Von seiner zunehmenden Sicherheit in dieser Sache späterhin bei der Fabrica 1555); er bleibt auch hier bei der Galenischen Lehre. In allen Fällen wirkt der gleiche Grund: vereinzelte Thatsachen genügen ihm nicht, Galens Physiologie aufzugeben."

70 This phrase is Sir M. Foster's, *loc. cit.* note [66].

71 P. 585 in the 1st edition and pp. 728–729 in the 2d edition.

72 "*Quas partes Natura aereae substantiae reficiendae fabrefecerit, ac quae privatim vitali spiritui subministrent.* Vesalius, *Fabrica*, 1543, lib. VI, cap. 1, p. 569.

73 Ibid., 1555, p. 708.

74 Ibid., lib. VI, cap. 11; 2d ed., p. 734.

in *both* editions[75]. Moreover—and this makes the argument untenable—Vesalius introduced the term *Natura* in one passage of the second edition—speaking of its great care (*magna industria naturae*) where it should have been *Opifex*, if the argument were true[76].

Conversely, the invocation of Deity in the first edition is nothing special suggesting by itself a hint of irony. Speaking, for example, about the tireless action of the heart, independent of will and cerebral innervation, and quite unlike ordinary muscle, Vesalius invokes the inscrutable care (*inscrutabilis industria*) of the Creator in all seriousness and in the same terms in which he speaks about Nature[77].

Finally, Vesalius makes provision for the Galenic doctrine of the interventricular passage at several places in the *Fabrica*[78]. Why should he have resorted to its sarcastic dismissal only at one place in his work and failed to express sarcasm or doubt at others?

We conclude: It is not unlikely, then, that Vesalius intended no sarcastic dismissal in the first edition of the *Fabrica*, but that he followed the Galenic doctrine of the day in mooting the possibility of blood filtration through invisible interventricular communications.

75 For example, in lib.VI, cap. 15; 1st ed., pp. 595, 596; 2d ed., 1555, pp. 742, 743.

76 Ibid., p. 742, line 42 in the 2d ed. as against p. 595 of the 1st; lib.VI, cap. 15, à propos: coronalis venae usus. In the 2d ed.: magnamque Naturae suorum ramorum attestantur industriam.

77 De cordis substantia, lib. VI, cap. 10: 1543, p. 587; 1555, p. 732.

78 Lib.VI, cap. 1, p. 569 *et seq.*; lib.VI, cap. 15, pp. 596, 598.

79 Lib.VI, cap. 11, 2d ed., 1555, p. 734: utcunque interim hae foveae sint conspicuae, nullae tamen, quod sensu comprehendi potest, ex dextro ventriculo in sinistrum per eorundem ventriculorum septum permeant: neque etiam mihi meatus vel obscurissimi occurrunt, quibus ventriculorum septum sit pervium, quamvis illi a dissectionum professoribus enarrentur, quum sanguinem ex dextro ventriculo in sinistrum assumi persuasissimum habent. Unde etiam fit (quemadmodum quoque alicubi monebo apertius) de cordis hac in parte officio, me haud mediocriter ambigere.

The qualified statements and alterations in the Second Edition of 1555

With the publication of the second edition of the *Fabrica*, Vesalius' uneasiness about Galen's doctrine became manifest. As he tells the reader, he has failed to demonstrate even the most obscure passages although such are cited by the professors of dissection in their firm belief in the reception of blood into the left ventricle from the right. It is thus, Vesalius continues, that I am not a little doubtful as to the function of the heart in this part (*me haud mediocriter ambigere*)—a point on which I shall issue a warning in more open terms (*monebo apertius*) elsewhere[79]. Already, in the first edition, Vesalius had drawn attention to the ubiquity of the grooves throughout the whole surface of the ventricles; they are not limited to the site where the right ventricle is adjacent to the left (p. 589)—although, he now added in the second edition, all other professors of anatomy have it differently (p. 734).

In this passage Vesalius promises to return to the subject later on (*monebo*). He cannot therefore have been referring to the remark inserted in the same book, namely, in its first chapter, some twenty-five pages earlier (p. 709). Here he mentions the regeneration of vital spirit and innate heat achieved for the heart by virtue of respiration and the reception by the left ventricle of blood direct from the right ventricle. Vesalius adds the clause: "however much meanwhile this reception appears to us most obscure"[80].

With his promise to return to the subject, as given in the eleventh chapter, Vesalius could not have meant a small alteration that is found some eleven pages later on, in the fifteenth chapter. Here it is said of the left ventricle that it attracts and uses air for the cooling of innate heat, for the nutrition of its substance and for the vital spirit; further that it elaborates this air so that it can be sent to the great artery and thus to the whole body—"together with the blood which in copious amount has sweated from the right ventricle into the left through the septum of the ventricles" (*una cum sanguine, qui ex dextro ventriculo in sinistrum per ventriculorum septum copiosus resudaverit*)[81]. This is the wording in the first edition. In the second it is altered to: "the blood ... which *is believed to* sweat through the septum in quantity (*sanguine, qui ... copiosus resudare* putatur)[82].

Evidently Vesalius here wished to express doubt in the existence of interventricular pores. It is still, however, a cautious approach and an indication of personal doubt and uneasiness in this matter, rather than a flat and definite rejection, as it was expressed, for example, by Columbus.

There is internal support for this appraisal of Vesalius' attitude. For at another place and strangely enough in the same fifteenth chapter, Vesalius left the relevant passage *unaltered.* This occurs nine pages after the promise of a more frank revision and two pages before the slightly altered passage just quoted. The theme is the *Function and Use of the Heart and its Parts so far mentioned and the Reason for their Construction*[83]. In those animals, Vesalius says, which have it, the right ventricle when dilated attracts a large quantity of blood from the vena cava. This blood is elaborated by the right ventricle with the help of its grooves, and thereby attenuated. It is thus made lighter and apt to be carried through the arteries—its greater portion being allowed to sweat through the pores of the septum into the left ventricle, whilst the rest flows off into the lung when the ventricle is contracted. The relevant passage, *his namque ventriculus (sc. dexter) ... magnam sanguinis vim attrahit ... excoquit ... attenuans, leviorem que ... reddens, maxima portione per ventriculorum septi poros in sinistrum ventriculum desudare sinit,* remained unaltered in the second edition[84].

Was this merely an oversight on the part of the author in revising a voluminous text or is it perhaps an indication that Vesalius had not been all too keen on the full expurgation of a matter on which he was still not ready to pronounce final judgment?

80 First ed., p. 570: et quemadmodum respiratio et sanguinis ex dextro cordis ventriculo in sinistrum assumptus, cordi ad vitalis spiritus calorisque nativi repositionem faciunt: sic pari ratione materia a sinistro cordis ventriculo per arterias reliquo deducta, corpori aliarum partium spiritum et nativum calorem recreat.

In the 2d ed., p. 709: et quemadmodum respiratio, et sanguinis a dextro cordis ventriculo in sinistrum *assumptio* (*quantumvis interim haec nobis sit obscurissima*), cordi.... Italics are the present author's.

81 Lib. VI, cap. 15, 1st ed., p. 598.

82 Ibid., 2d ed., p. 745.

83 Cordis ipsiusque hactenus commemoratarum partium functio et usus ipsarumque constructionis ratio—heading to the 15th chapter of the sixth book: 1st ed., p. 594; 2d ed., p. 741 (ipsarumque adeo constructionis....)

84 Lib. VI, cap. 15; 1st ed., p. 596; 2d ed., p. 743. Vesalius' failure to alter this passage in the second edition had been noted by TOLLIN, loc. cit. note [2], p. 26.

The latter alternative seems to be borne out by yet another passage at the very end of the same fifteenth chapter of the sixth book of the *Fabrica*. It is a long paragraph that was newly inserted in the second edition where it is found on p. 746.

This obviously is the passage promised in the eleventh chapter, containing a more frank (*apertius*) "admonition" concerning his grave doubts as to the existence of interventricular pores.

The historical significance of the passage lies not only in the denial of the existence of pores with greater clarity than anywhere else in the book, but also in the association of this observational detail with a statement of general policy of presentation.

Vesalius here confesses to a lack of that self-confidence which could have enabled him to furnish a newly reformed account of the true function and task of the heart as a whole. Hence, he says, he "accommodated" his text to a large extent to the doctrines (*dogmata*) of Galen. He did not do so because he believed them everywhere to be true. It was, however, a feeling of diffidence which made him not dare to deviate as much as a nail's breadth from the opinion of Galen, the Prince of Physicians in this matter (*hic*). For, he continues, the ventricular septum is not a matter lightly to be weighed up for the students—notably the right side of the left ventricle which is as thick, compact, and dense as the rest of the left ventricular wall. Hence I do not know, he says, by what way even the smallest amount of blood could be received by the left ventricle from the right—whatever I can make out about the grooves at this site, and not forgetting the sucking action exerted by the portal vein on the stomach and gut, and all the more so when considering that the vessels of the heart gape open with such patent orifices comprising the whole width of their respective ventricles: *in cordis itaque constructionis ratione, ipsiusque partium usu recensendis, magna ex parte Galeni dogmatibus sermonem accommodavi: non sane, quod undique haec veritati consona existimem, verum quod in novo passim partium usu officioque referendo*, adhuc mihi diffidam, neque ita pridem de medicorum principis Galeni sententia vel latum unguem hic declinare ausus fuerim. Haud enim leviter studiosis expendendum est ventriculorum cordis interstitium, aut septum *ipsum've sinistri ventriculi dextrum latus, quod aeque crassum compactumque ac densum est atque reliqua cordis pars, sinistrum ventriculum complectens.* Adeo ut ignorem (*quicquid etiam de foveis in hac sede commenter, et venae portae ex ventriculo et intestinis suctionis non sim immemor*) quî per septi illius substantiam ex dextro ventriculo in sinistrum vel minimum quid sanguinis assumi possit: praecipue quum tam patentibus orificiis vasa cordis in suorum ventriculorum amplitudinem dehiscant....[85]

Evidently, then, by 1555 Vesalius had made up his mind: there are no interventricular pores. Yet even then he avoided any dogmatic rejection. For he realised that in this lay the crux for a complete reappraisal of the function of the heart and the pathways of the blood. For this he did not feel ready.

His position in 1543 had been different. At this time he had been just as unable to demonstrate the pores as he was twelve years later. But in the earlier days he still tried to "save" the Galenic doctrine pivoting on interventricular communication. He then followed Galen in suggesting invisible pores for the maintenance of a transudation of blood that was apparently inexplicable in scientific terms, bordering as it did on a "divine miracle". He must have meant this quite seriously and not as a satirical dismissal. For it is to such a process of filtration that he refers in the second edition in this connexion, namely, the transfusion of nutritive fluid from the stomach and gut into the branches of the portal vein—an analogy with a possible interventricular transmission of blood which he had ceased to find convincing by 1555[86]. The serious intent of his statement in 1543 is further borne out by his use of the term *resudare*—to "sweat through"—expressing the filtration of fluid through a membrane without visible openings, comparable to an effusion or exudation. Galen, characteristically and by contrast, speaks of no such transfusion, but of "much" blood that is "drawn" or "taken over" (*metalambanetai*) through the septum into the left ventricle, implying a straightforward flow through real pores whose extreme ends became invisible after death[87].

Transudation of blood through invisible pores, resorted to by Vesalius in the first edition of 1543, was thus replaced by a denial of the existence of any pores in the second edition, twelve years later. Yet even here it was a note of grave doubt that prevailed rather than flat rejection. The topic as a whole remained "most obscure". Blood is now "*reputed*" to "sweat through" instead of: it "*sweats through*" and finally there is the confession of ignorance as to how, in the presence of a wall just as dense on the lateral side of the left ventricle as on its medial aspect, any, even the slightest amount of blood could be transmitted directly from the right to the left ventricle.

The Position of Servetus and Columbus

Vesalius, then, had left the matter of the ventricular septum on a negative-critical note in both editions of the *Fabrica*. This partic-

85 Lib.VI, cap. 15; 2d ed., p. 746.

86 See as quoted above from lib.VI, cap. 15; 2d ed., p. 746.

87 Poly kata to meson diaphragma kai tas en auto diatreseis eis ten aristeran metalambanetai koilian: GALEN, loc. cit. note [18], p. 130, vol. III, p. 497; Daremberg trans., note [4], p. 128, vol. I, p. 445.

ularly emerges in his failure to provide an alternative path for the blood. From the insertion which he made at the end of the fifteenth chapter in the second edition, it looks as if he had come close to this, pointing as he did to the discrepancy between the obvious closure of the septum and the wide patency of the arterial orifices adapted in size to the full volume of their respective ventricles. Moreover, he seems to have realised that it was from the anatomy of the septum that a full reform of the physiology of the heart and of our knowledge of the flow of the blood would have to take place.

It is precisely at this point that the next step was achieved by Servetus and Columbus.

Moreover it was Servetus and Columbus who offered the correct description of the alternative route taken by the blood—the essential complement to the progress achieved by the denial of the interventricular pores or their importance. This complement is entirely missing in Vesalius.

But this is not all. Vesalius had been indefinite as to the contents of the pulmonary vein. He thought that it serves in the first place to carry air to the heart for the building up of vital spirit[88]. He also makes provision for the discharge of smoky excrement from the heart to the lung by the pulmonary vein[89] and speaks of foamy blood conveyed by the same route to the lung[90]. Here again both Servetus and Columbus superseded Vesalius. They clearly indicated that the formation of vital spirit takes place in the lungs and that a mixture of air and blood is brought to the left heart by the pulmonary vein which is found full of bright-red (*flavus*) blood. The latter is therefore not formed in the heart, but in the lungs[91].

Servetus and Vesalius

As we pointed out (p. 145) Servetus was a fully trained anatomist and thoroughly acquainted with Galenic anatomy as presented in the *Institutes of Anatomy* by his master Winter of Andernach (1487–1574) with its more accurate teaching that superseded Mundinus and Berengarius (Wilson, 1962)[92].

Indeed, Servetus' criticism of Galen has an anatomical root. It is based on his—probably original and first-hand—appreciation of the size of the pulmonary artery[93] and on the discrepancy between this and the Galenic idea that it merely serves for the nutrition of the lung. Galen had regarded the pulmonary artery as smaller in width than the vena cava[94]. He consequently assumed that only part of the blood admitted to the right ventricle from the

88 The pulmonary vein carrying air: Vesalius lib. III, cap. 15; second ed. p. 503.

89 Smoky excrement—*Fuligo*—sent by the left heart to the lungs: Vesalius lib. VI, cap. 1; first edition p. 569 seq; and cap. 15, p. 598 (unaltered in second edition). – See below note [106].

90 Foamy blood sent to the lung from the heart via the pulmonary vein: Vesalius lib. VI, cap. 15; second ed. p. 743.

91 Flavus ille color a pulmonibus datur sanguini spirituoso, non a corde. In sinistro cordis ventriculo non est locus capax tantae, et tam copiosae mixtionis, nec ad flavum elaboratio illa sufficiens. Demum, paries ille medius, cum sit vasorum et facultatum expers, non est aptus ad communicationem et elaborationem illam, *licet aliquid resudare possit*. Eodem artificio, quo in hepate fit transfusio a vena porta ad venam cavam propter sanguinem, fit etiam in pulmone transfusio a vena arteriosa ad arteriam venosam propter spiritum. (Italics are the present author's.) Servetus, *Christianismi restitutio*, 1553, lib. V, p. 169 seq. See above p. 138.

92 Wilson, L.G., The problem of the discovery of the pulmonary circulation. *J. Hist. Med.*, 1962, 17, 229–244 (pp. 235–237); see above p. 145 and note [10].

93 *Christianismi restitutio*, loc. cit., note 91, and above p. 138.

94 Wilson, loc. cit., note [92], p. 239.

vena cava is sent into the lung and "much" directly into the left ventricle[95].

The criticism levelled by Servetus against Galen also applied to Vesalius who had left Galen's physiology of the heart and blood flow intact. Yet it would seem that Servetus derived his very first inspiration to look out for an alternative passage of the blood from the very inability of Vesalius to demonstrate interventricular communications.

Conversely, it may be asked whether Vesalius had any knowledge of Servetus when he corrected his text for the second edition. This has actually been suggested[96] and its mere possibility cannot be denied. It is true that most copies of Servetus' book had been destroyed two years before the publication of Vesalius' second edition, but the evidence for a dissemination of Servetus' views in Italy and for the existence of manuscripts from 1546 onwards cannot be lightly dismissed[97].

A small verbal alteration introduced by Vesalius in the second edition of the *Fabrica*[98] may perhaps be considered with reference to his possible acquaintance with the "new" doctrine of Servetus. It concerns the pulmonary artery and its function as the nutritional vessel for the lung. In the first edition Vesalius had "*censetur*"—the artery is "*assessed*" as having chiefly been made for the purpose of bringing to the lung nutriment suitable for its substance from the right chamber of the heart—nutriment that has to be light, airy and foamy in order to maintain the ratio between the substance changing the air and the air that has to be changed. Moreover the lung itself has to be kept amenable to compression and extension and follow these movements easily. In the second edition this passage is somewhat shortened. It simply says: the pulmonary artery is *believed*—"*creditur*"—to bring nutriment to the lung—nutriment suitable for its substance that has to be light, airy and foamy considering the necessity for the lung to be easily compressed and expanded again and to follow these movements.

Against the significance of this verbal alteration, however, we may hold the fact that no alteration was provided concerning the belief that the width of the pulmonary artery was much smaller than that of the vena cava—a belief which Vesalius shared with Galen[99].

It may be more significant that Vesalius mentions, in the additional passage to the second edition (as quoted in note 85), the transference of blood in the system of the vena portae in the same setting as did Servetus (note 91). Again this may be mere coincidence. If it is not, are we to believe that Vesalius preferred leav-

95 GALEN, De usu partium, lib. VI, cap. 17, and De natural. facult., lib. III, cap. 15, as cited in notes [18], p. 130 and [62], p. 157.

96 TOLLIN, loc. cit. (note [2]).

97 See the data collected by TOLLIN, note [2], p. 32 seq. and the somewhat tenuous criticism of BAYON, H.P., WM. HARVEY IV Ann. Sci. 1939, IV, 95 et seq. See also below note [101].

98 Lib. VI, cap. 7, 1st ed., p. 583; 2d ed., p. 726.

99 Lib. VI, cap. 12, p. 590 in the first edition and pp. 735–736 in the second.

ing matters with Galen instead of taking the progressive road with the "Prince" of heretics, Servetus, or for that matter, the "upstart" Columbus? At all events, this is a matter for speculation. It should also be noted that Vesalius speaks about the transference of blood from the stomach and gut by suction, whereas Servetus is concerned with the traffic between the vena portae and the vena cava in the liver, and its analogy with the assumption of "spirit" in the vessels of the lung.

By and large, then, the very wording of Vesalius' text, his hesitating and cautious attitude, and his omission of any advanced knowledge which he could have derived from Servetus militate against his having had knowledge of the latter's view. The aggravation of doubts eventually amounting to a denial of the interventricular transit which Vesalius experienced in the interval between the first and second editions of the *Fabrica* appears to have been genuinely his own.

Columbus, Servetus and Vesalius

In arriving at his historic statement concerning the pulmonary transit Columbus may well have been original. On the other hand, he may have had knowledge of Servetus, as suggested by Tollin and Schacht[100]. Servetus' book was printed in 1553, six years before the *Anatomy* of Columbus. However, it was seen by few people, as most of the copies were destroyed before distribution. But there is evidence that at least one manuscript copy was extant before 1550, as has been convincingly shown by Bainton[101]. Moreover the doctrines of Servetus seem to have enjoyed widespread publicity in Italy owing to his personal influence and the impact of his heretical ideas before 1553 as well as after.[102] On the other hand it is difficult to dismiss as irrelevant that Columbus had been in possession of his facts many years prior to the (posthumous) publication of his work in 1559, as we are told by his pupil Valverde de Hamusco[103]. Such facts included observations which are not found either in Servetus or in Vesalius. The same applies to the shadow of Ibn an-Nafis from whom Columbus is suspected to have benefited directly or indirectly, but this remains distinctly conjectural[104].

With regard to Vesalius' *Fabrica* Columbus cannot have failed to take notice of the alterations introduced into the second edition of 1555. But by this time he must have had formed his own conclusions based on original knowledge and interpretation of facts, as reported by Valverde and incorporated in his own *Anatomy*.

100 Tollin, 1876 loc. cit. in note [2], p. 39.
A comparison of certain passages from Servetus and Columbus compiled by Tollin, as the latter says, "läßt keinem Zweifel Raum, daß Colombo des Servet *Restitutio* vor sich hatte wegen der öfters fast wörtlichen Übereinstimmung und auch der Identität beider in ihren Angaben über das Gehirn... so ergibt sich, daß in der That Colombo, der ruhmredige, ein anmaaßender Plagiator ist."
Schacht, 1957, loc. cit in note [3], p. 330, adding to the parallels adduced by Tollin, says, Servetus is "not dependent on Colombo, nor on Valverde, for his theory—he would certainly not have omitted Colombo's and Valverde's additional arguments had he known them. Valverde shows a specific knowledge of Servetus ... he takes an intermediate position between Servetus and Colombo; he modifies certain assumptions of Servetus in the light of the observations he made (together with Colombo); he cannot be dependent on Colombo for his whole doctrine. Colombo ... shows a specific knowledge of Servetus, whose ideas he develops and elaborates."

101 Bainton, 1931; 1951; 1953, loc. cit. in note [2] concerning the Paris manuscript Bibl. Nat. Latin 18, 212. It is not in the hand of Servetus and differs in some points from the printed edition. It is not merely a loose copy of the printed work but a transcript of the draft which is known to have been sent by Servetus to Calvin in 1546. For the manuscript lacks the three quotations from Clement of Alexandria which are extant in the printed book. Servetus had been trying to obtain the works of Clement since 1530 (*De Trinit. Error.* 52b), but they did not appear in Greek until 1550 and in Latin in the following year. The Paris manuscript would therefore date from before 1550 (Bainton, 1931, p. 373). This is borne out by the Philo-quotations given in Latin in the Paris manuscript, whereas two such citations appear in Greek in the printed work—the first printed Greek Philo dating from 1552, by contrast with earlier Latin editions.

102 Tollin, 1876, loc. cit. in note [2], p. 33–38, with reference to manuscript copies of the *Restitutio* possibly communicated to Italian Servetians such as Jean de la Vau, Jerome Bolsec, Giorgio Biandrata, Caelius Horatius Curio and others. Bayon's critical remarks to this (*William Harvey*, IV, *Ann. Sci.* 1939, IV, p. 95 seq.) do not seem convincing.

103 Valverde de Hamusco, *Historia de la composicion del cuerpo humano*, Roma 1556 (preface dated 1554); 2nd edition here also cited: 1560.

Valverde tells us that, under the guidance of Realdus Columbus, he had observed that the pulmonary vein contains nothing but blood which cannot have entered it from the heart. He also says quite unequivocally at one place that nothing passes from one ventricle to the other directly, but that blood from the right ventricle is so "disposed" as to generate vital spirit whilst the left ventricle receives the blood so "disposed", converts some of it into vital spirit and discharges the remainder together with the spirits into the artery. He refers to a further discussion of the matter later on. In the latter place he says that certainly blood from the pulmonary artery "sweats" into the substance of the lung; here it is attenuated and so "disposed" as to be easily converted into spirit, mixing with air and then carried to the left ventricle. Here it is mixed with the thicker blood which passes from the right ventricle into the left—if any of it does pass. For so far I have never succeeded to see where it can pass. But if it does pass there emerges from both bloods some matter disposed to conversion into vital spirits. In my opinion—and everybody can convince himself by inspection that it is true and need not only believed—the pulmonary vein contains blood (and, as he adds later: much of it). Hence it is necessary to say that blood comes to the left ventricle from the pulmonary vein and this is much more likely than to think that it is from the blood in the right ventricle—the latter being little different in quality from the blood in the big vein and obviously not able to be converted suddenly into vital spirit without having undergone a major change[105].

It is reasonable to assume that Valverde here gives the opinion of Columbus whom he quotes in the present context and praises as his guide and teacher. It is the cardinal point in which Columbus supersedes Vesalius whose *Fabrica* otherwise formed the model for Valverde's smaller and less sumptuously produced compendium of anatomy. From the evidence presented by Valverde within a year after the publication of the second edition of the *Fabrica* it must be assumed that Columbus was independent of it.

Nor was he necessarily indebted for his new knowledge to Servetus (see above 166), or for that matter to Ibn an-Nafis. Yet this does not exclude Vesalius as the first source for doubts into the permeability of the ventricular septum. For both Servetus and Columbus first guidance and inspiration may well have been provided by the strange discrepancy between observation and belief which Vesalius expressed in the first edition of the *Fabrica* in 1543 (see above p. 157).

104 Schacht, loc. cit. p. 330, in a closely reasoned argument, suggests that "a possible influence of the theory of Ibn al-Nafis on the three sixteenth century authors in the light of what we now know of Andrea Alpago, cannot be ruled out any longer" and with this in mind concludes that "Servetus shows a specific knowledge of the theory of Ibn al-Nafis on whom he is dependent more than his two contemporaries; he made additions of his own, partly anatomical, partly theoretical, which recur, elaborated and partly modified, in Colombo ... Colombo probably had direct knowledge of the theory of Ibn al-Nafis."

105 I quote from the Italian version of the *Composition: Anatomia del corpo humano composta per Giouan Valuerde di Hamusco et da luy con molte figure di rame, et eruditi discorsi in luce mandata.* In Roma per Ant. Salamanca et Antonio Lafreri. 1560, fol. 105 verso in Lib. IV, cap. 9: ma niuno passa da l'un ventricolo all'altro, come dicono, quanti che insino ad hora ne hanno scritto. – Fol. 131 verso ... dell'arteria portar l'aere da gli polmoni al ventricolo manco del cuore; parendo loro che in questa arteria non potesse in modo alcuno essere sangue. Ma, se havessero di cio fatto esperienza (come ho fatto io molte volte insiemo col Realdo, cosi in animali vivi, come in morti) haverebbero ritrovato, che non meno è piena questa arteria di sangue, che qual si voglia dell'altre vene ... in questa arteria è sangue, e che dal ventricolo manco non vi può entrare ...
... credo certo che dalla vena arteriale risudi il sangue alla sustanza del pulmone doue si assotiglia, et dispone a poter piu facilmente conuertirsi in spiriti; et di poi si mescola coll'aere, che entrando per gli rami della canna del polmone, va insieme con esso al l'arteria venale, et indi al ventricolo manco del cuore; mescolandosi col sangue alquanto piu grosso, che dal diritto ventricolo del cuore passa al sinistro (se puto ve ne passa); perche io insino a adesso non ho potuto vedere, per doue possa passare; ma se passa, d'amendue questi sangui si fa una materia, disposta a convertirsi ne gli spiriti, che danno la vita. *The passages are literal translations from the 1556 ed., fol. 76 r and 97 v.*

Neither this nor even the possibility of a loan from Servetus (or indirectly from Ibn an-Nafis) detract from the merit of Columbus. He was ahead of Servetus in the completeness and distinctness by which he denied any interventricular communication and which he built up in a pure atmosphere of observational empiricism, insisting on the pulmonary vein as a carrier of blood which cannot derive from the heart, but must come from the lung. This is one of the points in which he disagreed with Vesalius, and it is these points through which his achievement is further brought into focus.

Vesalius and Servetus accepted Galen's idea of a smoky excrement formed in the left heart and drained away through the lungs. Columbus flatly rejected it. He did this well in advance of Cesalpinus and thus provides an important stepping stone for Harvey. According to Vesalius, here closely following the Galenic tradition, the air goes partly through holes in the skull to the brain, partly to the lungs and thence by the pulmonary vein to the left ventricle of the heart where it serves to nourish the substance that maintains heat (*substantia caloris*). This in turn consists of air and an exhalation of the blood. There is need for ventilation, as in this process soot is formed and removed to the lungs, again by the pulmonary vein[106].

Though still believing in air ascending through the ethmoid plate into the cerebral cavities[107], Columbus would have nothing of the nebulous *fumi capinosi* as they are called by those ignorant not only in Anatomy but also in elementary Latin[108]. The heart is not an oven that burns green wood. Vesalius still assumed that the pulmonary artery serves to nourish the lung and nothing else[109]. Columbus insists that it is far too big if designed for this purpose alone[110]—an argument that had been brought forward before by Servetus[111].

On the other hand Columbus denies the heart any muscular nature[112], whereas Vesalius had been careful in pointing out the essential features which the flesh of the heart has in common with muscle and those by which it differs from it[113]. Finally Columbus errs with Vesalius in the matter that is most important in our context: the direction of the venous blood flow. As the artery propels the blood *impetu* into the organs to which it thus carries the vital spirit that regenerates and tempers their heat, in the same way the substance of the parts is restored by the blood brought to them by the veins. This statement of Vesalius[114] well accords with the verdict of Columbus that the branches of the vena cava carry the blood that is prepared in the liver to the individual parts: for it is by blood that each part of our body is fed[115].

106 *Fabrica*, lib.VI, cap.1 and cap.15, in the first ed. 1543, p.569 seq. and 598. See above p. 164 and note [89].

107 COLUMBUS, lib.VIII, cap.1 (de cerebro), ed.cit. p.351.

108 See above note [54], alluding to *capinosus* instead of *capniosus* (as derived from Greek: *kapnos*) with reference to Mundinus, *Anathomia*, Strassburg 1513, sig. G 1 recto: ex arteria venali quae oritur ex sinistro ventriculo portans *vapores capinosos* ad pulmonem.

109 Arterialem venam organum soli nutritioni opportunissime subserviens *Fabrica*, 1543, p.596.

110 See note [55].

111 See above p. 138.

112 Nullo autem pacto potest cor inter musculos connumerari: quamvis divinus Hippocrates in libro de corde ipsum musculum esse non erubuerit. Columbus, *de re anatomica* (1559), lib.VII, ed. cit. Francof. 1593, p.324.

113 Praecipua cordis substantia carne constat, musculorum carne paulo minus rubra, verum duritie, spissitudine et fibrarum quo intertexitur genere plurimum ab illa variante... Vesalius, *Fabrica* lib.VI, cap.10. First ed. 1543, p.586 *De cordis substantia.*

Ibid. p.587: carnis itaque cordis non postremus usus cum musculorum carnis usu in fibrarum firmatione correspondet... cordis fibrae alteri functioni subserviunt, qua cor ... et dilatatur et contrahitur, et aliquandiu inter contractionem dilatationemque quiescit. Dein quemadmodum cordis fibrae cum musculorum fibris nonnulla consequuntur communia, sic etiam ut et illae motui famulantur, sed prorsus diversorum musculorum enim motus arbitrarius est, cordis vero naturalis, absque lassitudine inscrutabili rerum Opificis industria indefessus ... neque ex cerebri nervis, ut musculorum motus, nulla ex parte dependens.

114 *Fabrica*, ed. 1543, p.570.

115 See above p. 154 and note [50].

In conclusion, then, we suggest that Vesalius, Servetus and Columbus were original and independent of each other in advancing those new observations and arguments which form landmarks in the pre-history of Harvey's discovery. At the same time we visualise the doubts in the permeability of the heart septum first expressed by Vesalius as a source of inspiration for Servetus as well as Columbus—indeed this may well explain the simultaneity and overlapping of some of their statements.

The point, however, that matters in our discussion more than the question of originality in the pronouncements of pre-Harveian anatomists is the direction of the venous blood flow. Here we must repeat that neither Servetus nor Columbus can be accepted as discoverers of the "lesser circulation"—for both believed in a centrifugal direction of the venous blood flow, with the exception of that portion of the blood which was sent from the liver up to the heart for the purpose of conversion into arterial blood. But this does not detract from their merit in establishing the pulmonary transit of this part of the blood. For by this the Galenic doctrine of inter-septal communication was not only doubted (as in the case of Vesalius), but definitely replaced—in the case of Servetus less distinctly and scientifically as by Columbus.

V. Cesalpinus as a Forerunner of Harvey (pl. 33)

In assessing Cesalpinus' (1525–1603) position with regard to Harvey's discovery of the circulation of the blood two points stand out as focal:

1. Cesalpinus' statement that there is a perpetual movement of blood into the heart from the veins and from the heart into the arteries, and

2. the linking of this statement with a corollary to the effect that the venous flow to the heart applies not only to the blood conveyed by the inferior vena cava, but to peripheral veins as well.

Cesalpinus' basic propositions and their linkage (pl. 34)

It is these two propositions which we have to discuss and to compare with other passages from Cesalpinus which seem to be contradictory.

1. For more than thirty years Cesalpinus consistently and at prominent places in his books reiterated that there is "a perpetual motion of blood from the veins into the heart and from the heart into the arteries".

This statement appeared for the first time in 1571, in the first edition of his *Peripatetic Questions*[1]. We have evidence that it was actually written earlier, namely before the middle of 1566: in a letter dated August 7th of that year Cesalpinus says that he has communicated the manuscript of his book to P. Vettori prior to submitting it for publication to the Junta Press[2].

The statement was then repeated in his great work *On plants* of 1583[3], and again in the second edition of the *Peripatetic Questions* in 1593—a work that was issued together with a new work: the *Medical Questions*, and in the latter we see the statement re-appear as well[4].

We finally meet with it in Cesalpinus' last work—that on the *Medical Art*, first published, one year before his death, in 1602, and reprinted on several occasions thereafter[5].

Although basically identical in all versions from its first appearance in 1571 up to 1602 the wording of the statement varied somewhat in detail. The wording in the *Medical Questions* of 1593: *sic enim perpetuus quidam motus est ex vena cava per cor et pulmones in arteriam Aortam* seems less generalised than the wording in the *Peripatetic Questions* (in both editions) and in the late *Ars medica* of 1602: *ut continuus quidam motus fieret* ex venis *in Cor et ex Corde in Arterias*. Here the movement of the blood is asserted not only with reference to that portion which is conveyed by the vena cava and the aorta, but to blood carried by veins and arteries in general.

In most versions the statement is closely associated with the anatomical properties of the valves which either admit or educe, but prevent any backflow of the blood. By contrast it is the attraction by the heart of nutritious blood from the veins that is emphasised in the work *On plants*, as it serves here as one of the features that distinguish plants from animals.

Cesalpinus, then, remained acutely aware of the singular import of his statement throughout the many years of his literary activity and with advancing years he appears to have become more and more convinced of its truth.

2. Yet the statement, at least in its narrow formulation, as given in the *Medical Questions*, was no advance on Galen. The latter had correctly described the pathway of blood from the liver through the vena cava into the right heart and followed up one portion of it through the lungs into the left heart and the aorta. He also realised that the tricuspid valve prevented by its arrangement any backflow of blood into the vena cava. As is well known he erred in letting a large portion of the blood in the right ventricle reach the left chamber through his imaginary interventricular pores[6]. But

1 Lib. V, quaestio 4.

2 MORTARA, A., *Alcune lettere di celebri scrittore italiani raccolti e publicate*. Prato. Alberghetti. 1852.

3 *De Plantis libri XVI*. Lib. I, cap. 2. Florent. 1583, p. 3.

4 *Quaest. Peripatet.* Venet. 1593 fol. 123 r. *Quoest. Medicar.* 1593, fol. 234r.

5 Quoted from: *Catoptron s. speculum artis medicae Hippocraticum* lib. VI, cap. 19. Francof. 1605, p. 473 and: *Praxis universae artis medicae*. Tarvisii 1606, p. 503 (wrongly numbered: 465).

6 See above in: Galen's Ideas on the Heart p. 130 note [18].

then Cesalpinus, too, mentions though only once and in passing, that blood is heated in the heart and transmitted from the right ventricle to the left, partly "*per medium septum*", partly "*per medios pulmones*[7]. Cesalpinus, by contrast with Galen, is clearly more interested in the pulmonary transit of the venous blood and states shortly afterwards—opposing Galen—that of the large amount of blood that passes into the lung only a portion is used for the nourishment of the lung substance which does not need much, as it is "rare"[8]. Instead, the real purpose of the transmission of blood through the lungs is its cooling—as Aristotle had taught. For the blood is heated in the heart in order to achieve "perfection".

One of the advances due to Harvey's work was the rectification, once and for all, of Galen's description of the pathways of the blood. The essential point of his discovery, however, was the demonstration that—*not some*—but *all* venous blood flows in a centripetal direction. This stands in sharp contrast with Galen's idea that—apart from the blood that reaches the right heart through the inferior vena cava—the veins carry their blood from its origin, the liver, directly to the periphery in order to nourish the organs and limbs.

This keynote in Harvey's discovery—the "closed" and exclusive flow of venous blood from the periphery to the heart—is indeed the yardstick by which we must judge all of Harvey's predecessors, and Cesalpinus in particular. The latter's statement of the "continuous motion of the blood through the veins into and through the arteries away from the heart" marks a breakaway from Galen and a stepping stone for Harvey if it was meant to appertain to peripheral veins as well.

Cesalpinus and the centripetal flow of venous blood as revealed by venous ligature (pl. 35)

Cesalpinus did not assert this *expressis verbis;* moreover he remains lamentably short of Harvey's demonstration of the "closed" circle and ambiguous remarks can be found in his writings which have been interpreted as an indication of his ignorance of the centripetal flow of all the venous blood. We do not believe this to be justified and shall return to this question presently.

What appears to us to be of principal importance is the evidence which seems to show that Cesalpinus indeed entertained the correct view of the centripetal flow of blood not only in the vena cava, but also in peripheral veins.

It is in his *Medical Questions* of 1593 that we find his basic state-

7 *Quaest. Peripat.* V, 4; ed. cit. 1593, fol. 126r.

8 *Quaest. P ripat.* ibid. fol. 126r.

ment of the continuous flow of blood into and from the heart consciously and expressly linked with the further statement that the flow of venous blood from the periphery to the heart applies not only to the vena cava, but to peripheral veins as well[9].

The argument in which the two statements appear in intimate association is complicated and will have to be given in full.

Its subject is the suffocation occurring in quinsy (*angina*) and its immediate causes. Cesalpinus raises the question whether it might be due to the overfilling and stasis of the blood in the jugular veins rather than to simple constriction of larynx and trachea. Indeed in ancient medicine overfilling and immobility of venous blood had been envisaged as inhibiting the flow of air (*spirit*) through the windpipes (*arteries*), i. e. as a cause of suffocation. Perhaps, Cesalpinus goes on, it is not easy to see how suffocation can follow from the closure of veins in that form of angina which is due to mucinous dyscrasia. Nor can angina (and suffocation attending it) pass as a form of apoplexy in which respiration, on Galen's showing, is affected through a lesion of motor activity communicated by the brain. For sensation and motion can be abolished without affecting respiration. Hence in swellings of the neck either the mouth of the larynx is closed, followed by obvious suffocation, or the closure of the veins involves incapacity of the lungs to expand and subside. Aristotle in his book on *Sleep and wakefulness*, cap. 3, says that in epilepsy the veins swell from spirit whereby the duct by means of which we breathe is constricted[10]. The same should apply when interception and occlusion of veins is followed by sudden muteness. For when the veins in the neck are occluded, blood and spirit being unable to go upwards must of necessity regurgitate to the heart and lung whereby the latter is overfilled and can no longer expand or subside—and this means that the duct through which we breathe, namely the bronchial tree (the "arteries of the lung"), is constricted. This is also the more likely cause of suffocation in apoplexy—more likely than an inhibition of motor activity. Indeed it would be strange if sometimes, in lesions of the principal organ, the brain, motor power should be abolished in the whole body and only be preserved in the thoracic muscles because of the "necessity of breathing", as Galen says. The reason, then, why seizure of the veins in the neck causes sometimes only deep sleep and sometimes also suffocation is that the "virtue of the heart" is not communicated to the brain and hence sensation and motion are abolished in the whole of the body—without any overfilling of the lung which could account for suffocation.

9 *Quaest. medicar.*, lib. II, quaest. 17, fol. 234.

10 *De Somno et vig.* cap. 3, 457a: "sleep is like epilepsy, and, in a sense, actually is a seizure of this sort. Accordingly, the beginning of the malady takes place with many during sleep, and their subsequent habitual seizures occur in sleep, not in waking hours. For when the spirit (evaporation) moves upwards in a volume, on its return downwards it distends the veins, and forcibly compresses the passage through which respiration is effected" tr. J. I. Beare, Aristot. *The Parva Naturalia* Oxford 1908. "hotan gar poly pheretai to pneuma ano, katabainon palin tas phlebas onkoi, kai synthlibei ton poron di hou he anapnoe ginetai" ex rec. I. Bekker Oxon. 1837, p. 295.

However, Cesalpinus continues, it is worth considering what causes the veins to swell peripherally to the site of a ligature and not centrally (*sed illud speculatione dignum videtur, propter quid ex vinculo intumescunt venae ultra locum apprehensum, non citra*), as those who practise venaesection know by experience (*experimento*). These apply the ligature centrally to the site of incision, not peripherally (*vinculum enim adhibent citra locum sectionis, non ultra*), because the veins swell peripherally, not centrally (*quia tument venae ultra vinculum non citra*). If, then, blood and spirit were to move from the viscera into the periphery of the whole body (*si motus sanguinis et spiritus a visceribus fit in totum corpus*) and its contents cannot move on as in a closed duct, the opposite (of what in fact is seen) should occur and therefore the swelling of the veins should take place centrally to the site of ligature (*debuisset autem opposito modo contingere ... tumor igitur venarum citra vinculum debuisset fieri*).

Perhaps the difficulty can be solved through what Aristotle says *On sleep*, cap. 3: "For what evaporates is of necessity driven somewhere and changed like (the tidal wave of) the Euripus; for what is warm in every animal is destined to be carried upwards, but when it has dwelled in the upper parts much of it returns and is taken downwards." Thus far Aristotle[11]. For the explanation of this passage the following must be known: the pathways of the heart are so arranged by Nature that from the vena cava blood is allowed to flow into the right ventricle of the heart from which its exit is open to the lungs. Besides this, there is another entry from the lungs into the left ventricle of the heart, from which finally the exit is open into the aortic artery—certain membranes being so attached to the ostia of the vessels that they impede backflow: for thus a perpetual movement takes place from the vena cava through the heart and the lungs into the aortic artery, as we have explained in the *Peripatetic Questions*. As in the state of wakefulness innate heat moves towards the periphery to the sense organs, but in sleep centrally, namely to the heart, we have to assume that in wakefulness much spirit and blood are taken to the arteries, since from there is the way into the nerves[12]. In sleep, however, the same heat returns through the veins to the heart, not through the arteries: for its natural entry is through the vena cava into the heart, not through the artery. This is indicated by the pulse which in those awake is large, strong, quick and frequent with some vibration, but in sleep small, feeble, slow and scanty. For the native heat tends less to the arteries in sleep, but breaks into them more strongly in those waking up. The veins, however, behave in a con-

11 Aristotle *De Somno* ibid. 456b: "sleep arises from the evaporation attendant upon the process of nutrition. The matter evaporated must be driven onwards to a certain point, then turn back, and change its current to and fro, like a tide-race in a narrow strait. Now, in every animal the hot naturally tends to move upwards, but when it has reached the parts above (sc. becoming cold) it turns back again and moves downwards in a mass. Tr. J.I. Beare loc. cit. 1908. "hypnos... ek tes peri ten trophen anathymiaseos ginetai ... anankaion gar to anathymiomenon mechri tou otheisthai, eit' antistrephein kai metaballein kathaper euripon. To de thermon hekaston ton zoon pros to ano pephyke pheresthai. hotan d'en tois ano topois genetai, athroon palin antistrephei kai katapheretai." *Parva Natur.* loc. cit. in note [10] p. 294.

12 Cesalpinus endorsed the ancient belief that the nerves are organically connected with terminal processes of the arteries. It was thus that he tried to implement Aristotelianism in which the heart was made the source not only of all vessels but also of the nerves. *Quaest. Peripat.* fol. 120 verso:

"Vena aorta appellata nervosa est; meatus igitur quos scribit Aristoteles ad oculos pervenire ex venulis quae sunt circa cerebrum quid aliud sunt quam nervi appellati visorii"—with ref. to Aristotle, *Hist. Anim.* III, 3–5; 513b 10 and 515a 30: "he d'aorte stenotera men tautes (sc. than the vein) sphodra de neurodes kai apoteinomene porro pros te ten kephalen kai pros ta kato moria stene te ginetai kai neurodes pampan" ed. I. Bekker cap. 3, p. 68 Oxon. 1837, and with ref. to tendons: "kai he kaloumene aorte neurodes esti phleps, ta men teleutaia kai pantelos autes. akoila gar esti kai tasin echei toiauten hoian per ta neura" ed. Bekker loc. cit. p. 73, in cap. 5. On Praxagoras as the main exponent of the idea: Galen., *De placitis*, I,6; ed. Kühn, V, 188.

trary way: for in sleep they are more swollen, but they are smaller in those awake, as is obvious when the veins in the hand are inspected. For in sleep the native heat transfers from the arteries to the veins through ostia common to each other and called anastomoses and from there (i.e. the veins) to the heart. But as the Euripus-like overflow of blood towards the superior parts and its backflow to the lower parts are manifest in sleep and wakefulness, so a motion of this kind is clearly observed wherever in the body a ligature is applied to veins or where these are occluded for any other reason. *When the passage is impeded the rivulets swell* where *they normally flow* (*cum enim tollitur permeatio, intumescunt rivuli qua parte fluere solent*). Then perhaps blood returns to its source lest it be cut off and annihilated. Not every interception of veins causes suffocation, but only interception of those which are taken to the head because of their importance and size.

Thus far Cesalpinus. The whole chapter and its argument has to be considered carefully in order to assess the real significance of the statements that seem to amount to a fundamental break-away from the traditional doctrine about the venous blood flow.

There are two such correct statements; they concern

(a) the centripetal direction of the venous flow, as demonstrable by the experience (*experimento*) of the blood-letters, and

(b) the perpetual movement of blood from the vena cava through the heart and the lungs into the aortic artery.

Moreover these two propositions are here linked together and clearly meant to supplement each other. Indeed they seem to provide good evidence for Cesalpinus' full knowledge of the venous flow—the first requisite for the discovery of "closed" blood circulation.

Contradictions, doubts and their resolution

This *favourable* impression is *strengthened* when the correct statements are *read in context*. In the chapter in which they occur Cesalpinus had given expression to his idea that the brain receives the "virtue of the heart" or "something of the heart" not only through the arteries, but also through the veins. Their interception in the neck may, he argues, prevent the virtue of the heart from reaching the brain and thereby cause paralysis. This may be combined with suffocation, if the back-pressure of the regurgitating blood is great enough. This idea can also be found in the *Peripatetic Questions*, issued in first edition some twenty years earlier.

The idea as such would seem to convey the frank confession of

Cesalpinus' traditional ignorance of the truth in the matter of the venous blood flow.

However, the correct statements are found at the end of the chapter. Their very position and tenor leave no doubt that they were meant as *critical points against the idea of a venous transmission to the brain.* This would be in harmony with the whole purport of Cesalpinus' book: it is to raise *questions* and to discuss them in the light of Aristotelian natural philosophy—rather than to give dogmatic answers. In this lies at the same time the weakness of his book and the cause of ambiguities, at least for its peruser to-day. The correct statements on the venous blood flow are brought forward as counter-argument against his own idea, but are left standing as such. They and their consequence, namely the refutation of the traditional belief in the centrifugal venous blood flow, would, then, seem to have occurred to Cesalpinus in a late phase of his life, i.e. when writing his *Medical Questions.* Insight into the truth of the matter, however, would not have been strong enough to cause him to eradicate the wrong proposition altogether, either in the second edition of the *Peripatetic Questions* or in the *Medical Questions* that were issued with the former. Perhaps he hoped to hit upon something that would reconcile traditional belief with contradictory factual evidence, at some later date.

In other words Cesalpinus stopped short of following up a line that should have led him to anticipate Harvey's discovery. He saw the contradiction of evidence versus theory, but, though endorsing the former, failed to withdraw the latter. This seems to be the source of the twilight in which the figure of Cesalpinus appears in the history of the discovery of blood circulation and of the doubts in his knowledge of the venous blood flow.

To see the matter in the right perspective we should also remember that in Cesalpinus' work the blood supply of the brain forms the subject of a special theory fitting a special case. In fact it was less traditional than usually believed.

To understand it we must turn back to the *Peripatetic Questions.* Here Cesalpinus recalls that Galen had produced unconsciousness by ligaturing the nerve in the neck, but had failed when he had blocked the artery. Cesalpinus has no intention of denying this, but assumes that after closure of the artery the brain is still supplied with blood through the veins, because of the extensive anastomoses that exist between veins and arteries, not only via the heart, but throughout their whole course in the body. He thus confirms the saying of the Master, that "those whose veins are interrupted in the neck become unconscious". Seizure of the artery, then, will not be followed by unconsciousness, unless all the neck veins have been seized as well[13].

In this passage at least the transmission of blood to the brain by the neck-veins need not mean a normal physiological mechanism. Cesalpinus here seems to resort to an auxiliary "shunt" as a welcome tool to solve a difficulty which has arisen owing to contradictory statements by Aristotle and Galen, and moreover to solve it in favour of the former. Had he really assumed that the brain normally receives blood through the veins, he would not have felt urged to emphasise arterio-venous anastomoses which take charge when the main artery is blocked.

It must also be borne in mind that Cesalpinus goes out of his way to defend another Aristotelian teaching, namely that the aorta finally, near the brain, assumes nervous structure, in other words that the nerves are terminal continuations of the artery[14]. It is thus that Cesalpinus finds confirmation of the Aristotelian doctrine that not only the vessels but also the nerves derive their origin from the heart. The blood supply to the brain is therefore primarily through the arteries. Cesalpinus may well have believed that nutritive (venous) blood is also brought through the arteries to the brain by arterio-venous anastomoses. These he certainly assumed to take over when the artery is closed.

At all events it is for the reason of these obscure theories found in strange juxtaposition with the correct statements that it has been said[15] and repeated[16] that Cesalpinus "knew of the so called greater circulation, but knew of it only as an exception obtaining in the three cases of sleep, impending suffocation and in venaesection. In these three instances the blood, lest it be entirely impeded, takes the only still patent *unnatural* way and does not run in a forward direction. like any other stream, but *backwards*"[17].

Centripetal venous flow not exceptional

We cannot endorse this statement which deprives Cesalpinus of *any* knowledge of the venous blood flow and interprets what appears to the modern observer as correct in Cesalpinus' discourse as a description of what are to the author exceptional and pathological phenomena.

Cesalpinus says that in wakefulness much spirit and blood are taken by the arteries to the sense organs (hence the wakefulness) and that in sleep the same (i.e. arterial) heat returns to the heart through the veins, not through the arteries, since its *natural entry* is into the heart through the vena cava, and not through the artery.

13 *Quaest. Peripatet.*, fol. 121 D: si venae omnes ad cerebrum tendentes in collo interciperentur, non amplius ex corde virtus influeret in nervos.

14 See above note [12].

15 TOLLIN, H., *Andreas Cesalpin* Bonn 1884 (reprinted from *Arch. ges. Physiol.* XXXV, 295–390), pp. 382–390.

16 PELLER, S., *Harvey's and Cesalpino's role in the History of Medicine, Bullet. Hist. Med.* 1949, XXIII, 218–219.

17 TOLLIN loc. cit. in note [15], p. 382.

The differences between sleep and wakefulness as due to the blood-factor are in Cesalpinus' own words of a *quantitative*, not a qualitative nature: it is a quantitative modification of the blood flow which Cesalpinus seems to intend. For he says: In waking *much* spirit and blood, in sleep *less* "heat" are taken to the arteries, which is reflected in the pulse. For the arteries are distended *more* vehemently in waking, whereas the opposite is true of the veins. From this wording Cesalpinus would appear to have implied that *some* arterial outflow towards the sense organs would still obtain in sleep and *some* venous backflow in waking, though it is palpably less in waking and sleep respectively[18].

Moreover Cesalpinus regards sleep and waking as events which make *manifest* the application by Aristotle of a *general* principle to the movement of the blood: evaporating matter is driven up to a point and then reversed like a tide race in a narrow strait. For what is hot is driven upwards in every animal; when it has sojourned there, much returns and is carried downwards. Aristotle himself in no way limited the application of this principle to the special conditions of sleep and waking. He says: since the veins are the place of the blood, while the origin of these is the heart—an assertion that is proved by anatomy—it is manifest that, when the external nutriment enters the part fitted for its reception, the evaporation arising from it enters into the veins, and there, undergoing a change, is converted into blood and makes its way to their source (sc. the heart). And later on: in every animal the hot naturally tends to move upwards, but when it has reached the parts above, it turns back again and moves downwards in a mass. And again: when the spirit moves upwards in a volume, on its return downwards it distends the veins, and forcibly compresses the passage through which respiration is effected[19].

In the basic Aristotelian text on which Cesalpinus comments the upward and downward movement of the blood, away from and back to its source, namely the heart, therefore appears as the manifestation of a general physical principle and not as an exceptional instance, although it serves to explain such phenomena as sleep, wakefulness, drowsiness and suffocation. Venous backflow is here seen as part of a tidal flow—comparable to the Euripus—that leads the blood back to its source, the heart, in rhythmical repetition. This movement is one of *antiperistasis*—a "circular thrust" or reciprocal replacement of hot evaporating matter and the product of its condensation in the periphery. The general application of these principles as intended by Aristotle is unlikely to have escaped Cesalpinus' attention. For, as Aristotle says,

18 *Quaest.medicar.*, lib.II, quaest. 17, fol. 234B.

19 *De somno et vigilia*, 457a and ibidem, 456b. See also above note [10 and 11]; tr. J.I. BEARE, Oxford 1908, loc.cit.

antiperistasis is everything. It is the mechanism that underlies and makes possible all movement in space[20].

Finally Cesalpinus speaks of *that part of the vein which swells when a ligature is applied as the part along which the contents are accustomed to flow*. In other words the venous flow is *normally*—and not in the exceptional case of venaesection—from the periphery to the centre. This is corroborated by Cesalpinus' statement that it should be just the other way round, if blood and spirit were to move from the viscera to the periphery. Against this the cryptic sentence—"that when the passage is impeded perhaps blood returns to its source lest it be cut off and annihilated"—weighs little. This again may have been meant as a quantitative consideration: the *rapid* collection of a *mass* of blood where the normal flow is hardly perceptible may perhaps be due to anxiety on the part of the blood not to be cut off from its source (towards which it normally tends) and thus to perish. The sentence in no way warrants the interpretation that venous blood normally running from the heart to the periphery turns round when a ligature is applied in order to force its way back to its source out of anxiety lest it be annihilated[21].

We would therefore *conclude* that Cesalpinus was aware of the centripetal flow of blood through the peripheral veins, but stopped short of the essential synthesis, i.e. the integration of this fact with the movement of the blood as a whole. In this he was encumbered by his failure to drop his earlier scheme of arterio-venous blood supply to the organs and notably the brain.

Pseudo-contradictions

3. It remains to examine some further passages from Cesalpinus which at first sight provide evidence against his knowledge of the centripetal flow of venous blood.

(a) On several occasions Cesalpinus pronounced that the heart is the source of all vessels and that arteries as well as veins emerge from it like the four rivers that spring from Paradise.

The comparison of blood vessels with water conduits goes back to Greek antiquity. Plato speaks in the *Timaeus* of the water-carrying in the body (*hydreia*, *hydragogia*), and how the gods made provision for it[22]. The analogy was taken up by Aristotle who said that the channels for the conveyance of the blood are like the numerous dividing and subdividing water courses in gardens. As the garden plants grow at the expense of the water, blood is the material out of which the whole fabric of the body is made[23].

Aristotle also said that the venous system is not so easy to

20 *Antiperistasis*—the circular thrust—underlies and explains all movement in space: *antiperistasis panta*, *Analyt. post.* lib. II, cap. 15; 98a 25; *Meteor.* lib. I, cap. 12; 348b 2; *De somno*, 3; 457b 2 (as cited in notes [10] and [19]). The concept stands for the change of objects, their place and situation in space. As there is no vacuum the antiperistaltic movement is *circular*—one body occupying the place of the other body which it has expelled from it "while that which has been thrust out pushes the adjoining body from its place until the last moved in this series finds itself in the place of the first which extruded something else"—Simplicius, as quoted by J.I. BEARE loc. cit. to 457b with further loci. On the Platonic source of the concept see CORNFORD, F.M., *Plato's Cosmology* London (1937) 4th ed. 1956, p. 319 to Plato's *Timaeus* 79 et seq., referring to Plutarch, *Quaest. Platon.* VII, 1004 D seq.

21 CESALPINUS, *Quaest. Medicar.* lib. II, 17, fol. 234B.

22 PLATO, *Timaeus* 70c; 77a; 78b; tr. CORNFORD, F.M., *Plato's Cosmology*, London 1937, 4th impress. 1956, p. 284; 307; 308.

23 ARISTOTLE, *De partibus animal.* lib. III, cap. 5; 668a 13; tr. OGLE, W., *Aristotle on the parts of animals*, London 1882, p. 73.

demonstrate in little animals, because in them the passages get clogged like water channels with slush[24]. Galen finally refers to the need for a fine subdivision of water channels in gardens (*en tois kepois ocheton*) in order to reach the areas remote from the main stream. The same was necessary in the body. It is for this reason that we find the origin of the vessels where the main conduit is largest[25]. According to Galen the vena cava has its maximum size near the liver and the latter is therefore the source of the veins. By contrast, to Cesalpinus it is the heart *qua* source of all blood, that irrigates the body through these vessels[26]. Found in the *Prooemium* to Cesalpinus' last comprehensive work on Medicine, it is a rhetorical, poetical and ornamental pronouncement and to all intents and purposes a way of expressing and amplifying the Aristotelian doctrine of the supremacy of the heart. It is in the same work[27] that we find Cesalpinus' basic statement that blood moves continually from the veins into the heart and from the arteries out of it. Indeed it is given here in its most generalised form. No contradiction can be seen in these two statements if each passage is read in its proper context. Nor does the pronouncement in the *Prooemium* provide evidence against any awareness which Cesalpinus may have had of the centripetal flow of blood in the veins.

It is of no little interest that the same pronouncement was made —by Harvey. In his *Lectures on the Whole of Anatomy* (1616–1618) he says: "Hence I do not see why the artery originates from the heart rather than the vein ... regarding the origin of the veins, I believe from the heart, the larger of them from the smaller, and all from the centre from which they grow and diminish in size (*hinc cur potius arteria oriri a corde quam vena non vidio ... Quaere de principio venarum puto a corde quarum maiores a minoribus omnes a centro a quo crescunt et extenuantur*)[28]. Again this is no more than a defence of Aristotle against Galen, who propounded the origin of the veins in the liver, and not a contradiction to any knowledge which Harvey may have had of the venous blood flow at the time of writing his lecture notes. It is one of the points in which Harvey, the Aristotelian, endorses the view of the Aristotelian Cesalpinus.

Indeed at a later time when the circulation of the blood had become commonplace knowledge the rhetorical phrase of the main vessels from the heart resembling the four rivers of Paradise was used in close connexion with a short account of blood circulation; in this the merits of its discoverer, Harvey, are specifically singled out for praise. It is found in Tobias Cohen (1653–1729), *Maasseh Toviyah*, an encyclopedia of natural philosophy and medi-

24 ARISTOTLE, *Historia animalium* lib. III, cap. 4, 15; 515a 24, tr. D'ARCY W. THOMPSON, Oxford 1910.

25 GALEN, *De naturalib. facultat.* lib. III, cap. 15 ed. Kühn vol. II, p. 210.

26 *Catoptron s. speculum artis medicae Hippocraticum* Francof. 1605, p. 1–2 Praxis universae artis medicae. Tarvisii 1606, p. 2.
The comparison with the rivers of Paradise occurs in Harvey's time in Riolanus, *Anthropographia*, loc. cit. p. 212 in note [11], p. 367.

27 CESALPINUS, *Praxis*, 1606, lib. VI, cap. 19, p. 503 (wrongly numbered: 465); *Katoptron*, 1605, p. 473.

28 HARVEY, *Praelectiones anatomiae universalis*, London 1886, fol. 74 recto. See also ibid. fol 75 recto and PAGEL, W., *A Harveian prelude to Harvey*, *Hist. Sci.* 1963, II, 114–125.

cine, first published in 1707, at Venice, and forms one of the "Harveian items in Hebrew medicine"[29]. Here it says: "numerous have been the attempts of the older physicians to conceive of the right way in which the blood is propelled to and fro. They dipped into deep waters, but raised only fragments until ... there was among the Christians one physician of great sagacity in the land of England named Harveus practising the wisdom of anatomy who found the right way to the consent of all physicians of our time. And he taught us that the heart does receive blood not from the liver alone but from all parts of the body ... and further said the wise Harveus that the rest of the blood, after having imparted nourishment to the organs, returns through the veins to its place. *So the Lord creator prepared four wells to moisten the body ... and they are almost like the four streams which went out of Eden to water the garden*[30]."

Cesalpinus' analogy, then, had lost nothing of its value as an epitome of the principate of the heart and proved fully compatible with the truth about the movement of the blood to and from the heart. Its use by Cesalpinus in itself is therefore no indication of his ignorance of the venous blood flow.

(b) In his work *On Plants* Cesalpinus compares the veins to the roots—the former drawing nutriment from the abdomen, the latter from the earth, "in order to distribute it to the whole of the body" (*venarum, quae alimentum ex ventre hauriunt, ut illud in universum corpus distribuant*)[31]. This is followed—not long afterwards—by the statement: "we see that in animals nutriment is carried by veins to the heart as the producer of innate heat, and, after acquiring ultimate perfection there, is distributed through the arteries over the whole body by action of the spirit which is generated from the same nutritive material in the heart" (*nam in animalibus videmus alimentum per venas duci ad cor tanquam ad officinam caloris insiti et adepta in ibi ultima perfectione per arterias in universum corpus distribui agente spiritu, qui ex eodem alimento in corde gignitur*)[32].

When these two passages are considered in juxtaposition, the former appears to present a general statement which is substantiated by the latter. The former therefore seems comparable to the general pronouncement which we discussed above under (a). Indeed it is the veins which in the last resort distribute nutriment to the whole body—but as the second passage explains, they do not do so directly, but through the mediation of the heart, the spirit which is formed therein and the arteries. As it was expressed in *De plantis* and later by Caspar Hofmann only that blood which has acquired spirituous quality in the left heart and in the arteries really qualifies to nourish the organs[33].

29 Leibowitz, J.O., *Harveian items in Hebrew Medicine. Hebrew Med. J.* 1957, II, 1–4.

30 *Maasseh Toviyah*, 1707, fol. 114 (quoted after Leibowitz).

31 *De plantis*, 1583, p. 1.

32 Ibidem, p. 3.

33 Hofmann, Caspar, *De Thorace ejusque partibus commentarius tripartitus* Francof. 1627 lib. III, cap. 12, p. 96 with ref. to Cesalapinus *Quaest. Peripatet.* V,4: "conficit quidem hepar omnem sanguinem, sed is nutrire non potest, nisi formam sanguinis adipiscatur. Adipiscitur autem admistione sanguinis arteriosi, qui in arteria magna it." See to this in the present book, below, note [117] concerning the convincing interpretation of the relevant Aristotelian passages by Caspar Hofmann.

If this interpretation is found unconvincing, one would have to assume that Cesalpinus had in mind two venous systems: one carrying nutriment from the abdomen directly to the periphery and another represented by the inferior vena cava which takes nutriment from the liver to the heart to be perfected and converted into spirit.

Any such double venous system, however, is difficult to reconcile with the wording of the second statement[34]. For here it is said advisedly and unmistakably that nutriment is taken to the heart through vein*s* (or perhaps: *the* vein*s*)—and not through one vein (i.e. the inferior vena cava). Moreover in the same passage in *De plantis* the *arteries* are stated to *distribute the nutriment* all over the body after its perfection and that this distribution is brought about by the activity of the spirit which is the product of the very same nutriment.

The meaning intended by Cesalpinus would then be as follows: Nutritive blood is brought to the heart by the veins. It is here partly converted into spirit and by the action of the latter driven from the heart into the organ by the arteries. This—partly nutritious and partly spirituous—blood (*sanguis et spiritus*) enables the body as a whole and its parts to exist and to live—it is the *nutriens quod esse praebet toti et partibus*. In addition there is venous blood which looks after growth—the *sanguis auctivus—quod accessionem ad magnitudinem facit*[35]. This blood is also conveyed to the organs by the arteries, but it is received by them from the veins directly through *oscula*—the arterio-venous anastomoses[36]. With a distinction between primigenial blood and blood for growth Cesalpinus took up again the Aristotelian heritage[37].

The close linking of arteries to veins through ubiquitous anastomoses—though part of the Galenic doctrine[38]—is a matter of importance for Cesalpinus: it is thus that the transference of the virtue of the central organ—the heat of the heart—over the widest possible distance is ensured. He sees the heart itself as the largest and most central place through which veins and arteries communicate with each other. In the periphery arterio-venous plexuses fulfil the function of the heart. The chief purpose of the cardiovascular system is nutrition of the parts, the supply of blood and spiritus, both of which are carriers of the heat of the heart. It is the latter which is the source of all blood and which by virtue of its heat attracts all nutriment that enters the body and converts it into blood.

When all this is considered we can understand such sentences as: nutrition is not accomplished, by the action of the individual

34 *Quaest. Peripatet.* V, 4 fol. 123r C: "motus enim fit ex venis in cor caliditate alimentum trahente, simul autem ex corde in arterias, quia hac solum patet iter propter membranarum positionem: idem enim motus utraque oscula aperit venae scilicet in cor, cordis autem in arterias. Posita autem sunt hoc modo membranae, ne unquam contingeret contrarium motum fieri, quod accidere posset in vehementis animi perturbationibus aut aliis causis, a quibus sanguinis retractio fit ad cor: obsistunt enim huic motui membranae."

35 *Quaest. Peripatet.* fol. 117 verso E, lib. V, cap. 3.

36 *Quaest. Peripatet.* fol. 123r B, lib. V, cap. 4: "auctivum ex venis elicit (sc. arteria) per osculorum communionem".

37 Aristotle, *De gen. anim.* II, 4; 740b: "to haima men trophe estin—he men oun auxesis to kyemati ginetai dia tou omphalou ton auton tropon honper dia ton rhizon tois phytois". The translation of auctive blood as *Mehrblut*—surplus blood—(Tollin, loc. cit. 1884 in note [15], p. 328) does not seem to be adequate.

38 Galen on ubiquitous arterio-venous anastomoses: *De usu partium* VI, 10 ed. Kühn vol. III, p. 455.

parts (as physicians believe), but by the heat which flows in from the heart through arteries and veins (*nutritionem fieri non a temperamento proprio singularum partium sed a caliditate per arterias et venas influente a corde*)[39]. This "influx" of heat through the veins does not necessarily mean a flow of venous blood directly to the periphery, in other words a contradiction to Cesalpinus' basic and often repeated statement of the venous flow to the heart. Nor can we assume a double direction of the venous blood: one into and one from the heart, as on Cesalpinus' own showing an emission of blood from the right heart into the veins is excluded by the anatomical arrangement of the tricuspid valve. The only interpretation which seems possible is that, as all blood is from the heart, that venous blood which reaches the peripheral parts is also from the heart—and it reaches them through the arteries which communicate with the veins by anastomoses. It is by virtue of the latter that "the heart is everywhere, for everywhere the vein is joined up with the artery—the heart being the biggest conjunction of veins and arteries" (*ut quasi ubique cor sit, quia ubique vena cum arteria coniuncta est ... cor enim coniunctio est venarum et arteriarum*)[40].

Moreover, why should Cesalpinus have felt the need of emphasising and repeatedly asserting the accession of venous blood to the organs by arterio-venous communications, i.e. by the arteries, if he believed in a venous blood flow from the heart to the periphery? The ambiguous passages which have been interpreted in this way find in fact their explanation in the idea of arterio-venous communication which he must have thought compatible with a basic venous blood flow from the periphery to the heart.

Moreover, belief in a *double venous system* would imply belief in *two kinds of blood:* one which is merely nutritious and carried by the veins direct to the organs and the other which is converted into spirit in the heart and conveyed by the arteries. No such belief can be substantiated from the works of Cesalpinus—on the contrary, he was criticised by his main adversary Nicolaus Taurellus for having emphasised the oneness of blood—like his master Aristotle[41], and, we may add, like Harvey, the Aristotelian.

(c) "As rivulets draw water from a source, veins and arteries do so from the heart ... but it is evident from dissection that all veins are continuous with the heart alone" and: "from the right chamber the vena cava, from the other the aorta springs[42].

This is a corollary to what we said under (a) and has nothing to do with the direction of the blood flow in these vessels. Nor has the passage following not far from the above: "the vein must be

39 *Quaest. Peripatet.* V, 6 fol. 133r.

40 *Quaest. Paripatet.* lib. V., quest. 6, fol. 131 recto.

41 TAURELLUS, NICOLAUS, *Alpes caesae hoc est Andreae Caesalpini Itali monstrosa et superba dogmata discussa et excussa.* S.l. (Francof.) 1597 ap. M. Zach. Palthenium, lib.V, quaest. 4, p. 893: "qui discrimen inter venarum et arteriarum sanguinem noverunt, facile intelligunt, quam absurda haec sit venosi sanguinis cum arterioso confusio. Non venosum, sed arteriosum in corde factum sanguinem in arterias transmitti oportet." See below note [111].

42 *Quaest. Peripatet.* V, 3, fol. 116: "ut igitur rivuli ex fonte aquam hauriunt, sic venae et arteriae ex corde ... Patet autem ex dissectione omnes venas soli cordi continuas esse. – Fol. 118B: "ex dextro ventriculo vena cava ... ex altero egreditur aorta."

continuous down to the ventricles of the heart in order that *from here all virtue may descend:* nor is it anywhere disconnected, for the *blood deprived of the heat of the heart* coagulates and finally putrifies"[43]. For in other passages from Cesalpinus a backflow of blood from the heart through the vena cava is ruled out—the "descent" of the virtue of the heart would therefore have to be through the artery[44].

The Capillamenta of Cesalpinus

Much attention has been given to the use of this term by Cesalpinus, by those who accorded as well as those who denied him the laurels of priority. Harvey too used the term[45]. However, neither the latter nor Cesalpinus were original in doing so. Galen had spoken of synanastomoses[46]. He had distinguished between small spider-like vessels (*mikrai arachnoeides*) and hair-like (*trichoeides*) vessels[47]. Not long before Cesalpinus, Peter Brissot (1478–1522) speaks in his famous treatise on blood letting of the smallest veins which are disseminated through the body like hair (*quae capillamentorum modo per corpora disseminantur*)[47a].

Cesalpinus followed this usage. He made it quite clear that they stand for the finest branches into which the vena cava and the aorta "dissolve" after having penetrated to the organs[48]. It is thus that the continuity of the vessels with the heart is maintained. There is no free effusion of blood into the organs. It is only in the heart that blood is found free, but then the heart is but a large arterio-venous anastomosis. It is true that Cesalpinus believed that nerves were the terminations of arteries (see above p. 176). Where he propounds this Aristotelian idea, however, the term *capillamenta* does not occur[49].

The reason why the latter have been thought to mean arterio-nervous filaments[50] is probably Cesalpinus' view that nerves are possessed of a small lumen just as is hair. It is stupid, Cesalpinus says, to deny nerves central canals, simply because such are not visible to the naked eye, as we know hair to be centrally perforated (*ut enim capillum perforatum esse scimus, non tamen visui ob parvitatem meatus apparet*)[51]. Nor is the identity of the *capillamenta* with arterio-nervous terminals proven by Cesalpinus' description of the brain receiving venules from the choroid plexus into its substance in which they seem to disappear—*capillamenti modo*. For, Cesalpinus continues, they can still be recognised through the droplets of blood which emerge when the brain substance is cut[52]. Even where Cesalpinus speaks of the vasculo-nervous canals in the

43 *Quaest. Peripatet.* fol. 118E: "venam igitur continuam esse oportet usque ad cordis ventriculos ut inde omnis virtus descendat. nec ullibi contingit disiunctam esse, sanguis enim calore cordis destitutus concrescit et tandem putrescit."

44 *Quaest. Peripatet.* V, 4, fol. 123r C—as cited in note [34].

45 HARVEY, *De motu* cap. XV, ed. 1628, p. 58; tr. WILLIS p. 68–71. Ibidem, cap. XVII, ed. 1628, p. 72; tr. WILLIS p. 85. See above p. 57 in the present work. Shortly before HARVEY we find *vasa capillaria* (of the skin) in CASPAR HOFMANN, *De thorace*, II, 10, loc. cit. 1627 in note [33], p. 34.

46 See WILSON, L.G., *The transformation of ancient concepts of respiration in the seventeenth century. Isis* 1960, LI, 161–172, p. 166. See above note [38].

47 With reference to GALEN, *De venarum arteriarumque dissectione* ed. Kühn vol. II, p. 799: Steudel, J., *Beitrag der Schule von Salerno zur anatomischen Nomenklatur. Atti del XIV Congr. Internaz. di Storia della Medic.* 1954, II. – The Galenic term recurs in the Salernitan *Anatomia porci ex Cophonis libro*. The present author refers to DRYANDER, JOH., *Anatomiae hoc est, corporis humani dissectionis pars prior, item Anatomia porci, ex traditione Cophonis*. Marpurgi 1537, sig. h 2 (fol. 30): vena ibi magna fit de arteriis capitis condensans quae venit usque ad renes, et bifurcatur, et ibi fit vena chilis, in qua infiguntur *capillares venae*, quae prae nimia parvitate sui videri non possunt, per quas urina cum quattuor humoribus, mittitur ad renes. See also above p. 57 and note [20].

47a PETRI BRISSOT *Apologetica disceptatio, qua docetur per quae loca sanguis mitti debeat in viscerum inflammationibus, praesertim in pleuritide*. Paris 1525, sig. e 4 verso.

48 Vena cava et arteria aorta reliqua viscera excepto corde, postquam adierint ... in capillamenta resolvuntur, non in ventrem aliquem transfundunt sanguinem, nullibi enim continetur sanguis in ventre extra venas praeterquam in corde: CESALPINUS, *Quaest. Peripatet.*, lib. V, qu. 3, fol. 116 recto. With ref. to Aristotle, *Hist. animal.* lib. III, cap. 3 and *De part. animal.* lib. III, cap. 4.

49 Fol. 120 verso and 131 recto.

50 JOHNSON, GEORGE, *The Harveian Oration*, del. June 24th 1882, 2nd ed. London 1883, p. 26; 32; 35. One of the points advanced by Johnson against Cesalpinus and his modern Italian admirers, is that the *capillamenta* were not used by Cesalpinus in

brain which cannot be seen, but must be there in the same way as the continuous but not visible canals between the two venous systems of the liver, the term *capillamenta* is not used[53].

These, then, stand for the finest branches of veins and arteries at large. As such they could have been also used to indicate the vasculo-nervous terminals. There is no evidence, however, that they were used in this meaning, let alone that they were so used exclusively.

Capillamenta and Continuity of Arterio-venous blood Flow

In *conclusion*, then, the *capillamenta* of Cesalpinus do constitute an important and original component of his doctrine of the blood flow. In the first place it is noteworthy for the correctness of the anatomical idea. What is perhaps more important in the present context is the continuity of the arterio-venous blood flow which Cesalpinus expressly associated with the *capillamenta*. For he insisted that there is no free blood anywhere in the organs and tissues outside the vessels, with the exception of the cavities of the heart, visualised by him as a large and indeed the principal arterio-venous anastomosis. As we shall see presently (p. 185) he established the same principle for the liver, demonstrating the continuity of the portal and hepatic venous branches.

Cesalpinus thus feels he has proved a fundamental Aristotelian point. For Aristotle had predicated of the heart that it is "hollow to serve for the reception of the blood while its wall is thick, that it may serve to protect the source of heat. For here, and here alone in all the viscera and in fact in all the body, there is blood without blood-vessels, the blood elsewhere being always contained within vessels (*ton d'allon morion hekaston en tais phlepsin echei to haima*)[54]."

The blood, then, according to Cesalpinus, never leaves its vascular containers—it is sent out from the heart through the arteries and returns through the veins, without any interruption in the periphery, other than a mutual give and take via ubiquitous arterio-venous anastomoses. Apart from this it would follow that Cesalpinus regarded the blood as a single stream which is continuous and permanently connected with its source, the heart. However, Cesalpinus does not seem to have stated that where the arteries dissolve into *capillamenta* the veins begin and vice versa, but it may be argued that his view of the continuity of the blood flow implied such an idea.

the modern sense of capillaries, but meant the arterial filaments which become nerves. According to Johnson, Cesalpinus nowhere says that blood passes from arteries to veins through *capillamenta*. Junctions between arteries and veins were in Johnson's opinion called by Cesalpinus inosculations and anastomoses. From our above analysis there seems to be little doubt that the *capillamenta* served to ensure the continuity of intravascular bloodflow and for this reason alone are comparable to our capillaries (to this see SCALZI, FR., *In difesa di Andrea Cesalpino scopritore della grande circolazione del sangue. Riposta all Doctor Johnson di Londra*, Roma 1883, p. 19 (reprinted from Bollet. R. Acad. med. di Roma, 1883, vol. IX).

Other points adduced by Johnson against Cesalpinus' knowledge of the bloodflow included his description of neck-veins as ascending to the brain (p. 39), his failure in recognising the propulsive power of the heart (p. 37) and the use of the analogy with Euripus implying flux and reflux through the same channels (p. 44). Even this, however, does not seem to have settled the Cesalpinian question once and for all.

51 *Quaest. Peripatet.* lib.V, 3; fol. 120 verso.

52 Ibidem.

53 Ibidem, fol. 121 recto.

54 ARISTOTLE, *De partibus animal.* Lib. III, cap. 4; 666a; ed. Bekker Oxonii 1837, p. 69. Tr. W. OGLE, London 1882, p. 67. – See also *Hist. animal.* lib. III, cap. 3; 513b.

The Venous Supply of the Liver

(d) Some other passages have been used[55] as evidence against Cesalpinus' knowledge of the correct venous flow; these do not belong to Cesalpinus, but have been taken from his report of the opinions of Galen which he proposes to refute.

One such piece is the description of the venous supply to the liver and of the distribution of blood to all parts of the body by the vena cava.

It is Galen, not Cesalpinus who said that the liver does not prepare blood for the heart, but for the whole body, as only a part of the blood is sent to the heart through the inferior vena cava and another part from the liver directly to the periphery. It is Galen's argument that in the liver the branches of the portal and hepatic veins do not join and that therefore blood must openly traverse the organ where it is prepared in a special way. It is Cesalpinus who opposed this very argument, trying to demonstrate communications between the two venous systems in the liver. Galen failed to see them. Hence, Cesalpinus says, he asserted that they did not exist and from this Galen concluded that the liver is the origin of the veins. When the organ parenchyma is washed away, however, a network remains that consists of the anastomosing plexuses of the two venous systems (*si hepatis particulam diutius lavemus ut sanguis concretus contabescat: relinquitur enim veluti retis cuiusdam tenuissimae contextus*)[56]. This incidentally confirms Cesalpinus' own statement that he set great store by anatomical investigation and often attended dissections (*cum saepe anatomicis administrationibus interfuissemus*)[57], a feat that has occasionally been denied[58].

Cesalpinus further argued that there must be such a direct communication of the two veins in the liver as otherwise the blood being extravasated could not remain unclotted.

It is well known how much the question of the anastomoses between the portal and the hepatic veins agitated the minds of anatomists at Harvey's time and after when Glisson had denied their existence and argued that the blood must flow through the parenchyma of the liver before reaching the finer branches of the hepatic veins (*eundem—sc. sanguinem—non quidem per fictas illas anastomoses elabi, sed ipsum hepatis parenchyma percurrere*)[59].

Glisson thus confirms the view taken by Harvey. Already in the *Praelectiones* Harvey had denied the existence of venous anastomoses in the liver—differing from Bauhinus. *Non est anastomosis*—he had declared. It followed that the liver contained blood—against Aristotle: *sanguinem contineri in iecore contra Aristotelem*[60]. This ob-

55 WILLIS, ROBERT, *William Harvey. A History of the Discovery of the Circulation of the Blood*, London 1878, p. 120, note 1 with ref. to *Quaest. Peripatet.* lib.V, 3 fol. 116F to 117B.

56 *Quaest. Peripat.* lib. V, quaest. 3, fol. 118 verso.

57 Ibidem, fol. 119B.

58 WILLIS, ROBERT., loc. cit. 1878, in note [55], p. 119.

59 GLISSONII, FRANC., *Anatomia hepatis*, cap. XXXIII: de venae portae et cavae in hepate connexionibus, ed. used: Amstelod. 1665, p. 266.

The situation is well described in Henry Power's manuscript on the circulation of the blood of 1652 (Brit. Mus. Sloane MS. 1343): "Again take that excellent experiment of our noble Professour Dr Glisson, which at once both proves the circulation of the blood and its transcribration through the parts of the Body ... thrust the glyster pipe into the vena porta ... you shall see the water to run into all the branches of the Cava and from thence to passe into the right auricel and ventricle of the heart ... In which experiment if you Cutt into the liver you shall see all the blood and ruddinesse of it to be washed cleere away not only out of the veines and arteryes thereof, *but also out of the very parenchyma of the Liver itselfe* which then will look of a duskish yellow colour which does not only confute all anastomoses in that organ of the vessels but also excellently shows the naturall streame and channel of the blood itself runing in ..." Cole, F.J., *Henry Power on the circulation of the blood. J. Hist. Med.* 1957, XII, 291–324, p. 323–324. Italics are of the present author. – See also ibidem p. 318: "In excarnated livers.... I have seene a Cohesion and union of the veines and arteryes and especially of the Portall Branches with those of the Cava ... yet I could never discover the least sensible miscalcution open'd whereby the one by any sensible orifice disgorged the blood into the other, which our famous Professour (sc. Glisson) hath since Confirmed as is observable in the Synanastomosis of the Embryo ... Therefore ... the transvasation ... of the blood is performed by percolation or transcribration through the Spongious Substance and porosityes of the flesh." – Cole draws attention to Power's manuscript antedating Glisson's book on the liver by 2 years.

Of the *protagonists of anastomoses* between the branches of the portal and hepatic veins *before and after Harvey*, Bauhin and Bartholinus should be mentioned in the first place.

viously refers to the passage from *Parts of the Animals* which had been cited by Cesalpinus when defending the presence of anastomoses (see above p. 184 note 54), to the effect that blood can nowhere be found in the body outside vessels, with the exception of the heart. Later, in the first *Exercise to Riolan*, Harvey boldly affirms (*audacter igitur affirmare ausus sum*) that no anastomoses exist between the veins in the liver. This result is embedded in an argument against the ruling—Galenic—opinion favouring arterio-venous anastomoses throughout the body. Harvey has used up "not a little oil and labour" (*non parum olei et operae*) in exploring the question of anastomoses, but nowhere succeeded in tracing them (*nusquam autem invenire potui vasa invicem, arterias scilicet cum venis, per orificia copulari*)[61]. This was finally confirmed by an experiment which at the same time proves the truth of blood circulation: when the vena cava is tied near the heart and then the carotid arteries are opened and emptied of blood, the veins remained filled. Hence blood does not anywhere pass from the veins into the arteries except through the ventricles of the heart[62]. Harvey noted, however, that the hepatic veins running through the convex part of the liver have their tunics pierced by infinitely many small holes—a feature missing in the branches of the portal vein[63].

To *conclude*
the points from Galen which are sometimes mistakenly attributed to, but were in fact criticised by Cesalpinus, it was Galen's contention that the liver possesses the virtue of a foster-mother (*vim altricem*) whereby the blood prepared in the liver acquires its nutritive quality (*vim alendi*). This was directly opposed to the Aristotelian view advocated by Cesalpinus that the origin of all vessels (arteries as well as veins), and of nutriment (blood as well as spirit) is the heart.

Another such point is Galen's argument derived from the size of the vena cava near the root of the liver in comparison with its smaller size at the heart. It was expressly rejected by Cesalpinus[64].

All this, then, appears in Cesalpinus' discourse as a review of Galen's opinions preceding their refutation in the light of old Aristotelian doctrines which, according to Cesalpinus, came nearer to the truth than those of Galen. This is in keeping with the whole purpose of Cesalpinus' work and its title: *Peripatetic Questions*. He therefore concludes this section: "This and similar things are the means whereby he (i.e. Galen) combats Aristotle's views on the origin of veins and blood" (*haec igitur et huiusmodi sunt, quibus Aristotelis placita impugnat circa venarum et sanguinis principium*)[65].

Bauhin illustrated such anastomoses in: *Anatomes Caspari Bauhini Basil. Liber Secundus partium similarium spermaticarum tractationem ... continens*. Basileae. Seb. Henricpetri. 1592, p. 525 (to cap. LIII). This may be compared with: *Thomae Bartholini Casp. fil. Anatomia*, Hagae Comitis 1655 libellus I (de venis), p. 407 and idem, Lugd. Batav. 1673, p. 591.

60 Fol. 37 recto (near the end): branches of the portal vein do not normally penetrate towards the convex part of the liver, whilst hepatic venous branches are absent from the central parts of the organ. Like Harvey himself many others have failed to find anastomoses. Bauhinus who claims to have seen them, found only one such anastomosis.

61 *Exercit. duae de circulatione sanguinis ad J. Riolanum*, I, Roterod. 1649, p. 40–41; tr. Willis, p. 103.

62 Ibidem, p. 44–45 (1649); tr. Willis, p. 104.

63 Ibidem, p. 41 (1649); tr. Willis p. 103: propagines venae cavae, per gibbam hepatis perreptantes, tunicas habere infinitis puncticulis cribrosas, tanquam in sentina, ad decumbentem sanguinem recipiendum fabrefactas (comparison with the sieve-like bottom of a ship letting through bilge water).

64 *Quaest. Peripatet.* lib. V, qu. 3, fol. 119B.

65 Ibidem, fol. 117B.

Without any doubt Cesalpinus meant to and did oppose Galen and it is reasonable to assume that this opposition embraced Galen's doctrine of a direct venous blood flow to the organs. He replaced it by the more sophisticated idea of arterio-venous plexuses in which the blood is conveyed to the organs by the arteries, although part of it comes from the veins. With this Cesalpinus seems to have taken a progressive step in the direction of the truth—however far this is still removed from Harvey's idea of the closed arterio-venous circle. But Cesalpinus supplemented this step by still more advanced views concerning the flow of peripheral venous blood, as we have seen (p. 173). We shall soon return to these.

The Transit of Blood from the Arteries into Veins

(e) It is true that Cesalpinus tells us more about the reception of venous blood by the arteries through anastomoses than about a transit of blood from the arteries into veins. He does mention, however, his experience that in prolonged venaesection the blood undergoes a colour change from that of venous to that of arterial blood[66]. He also adduces the Aristotelian principle that "evaporating matter is driven up to a point and then reversed like a tide race in a narrow strait. For what is hot is driven upwards in every animal; when it has sojourned there, much returns and is carried downwards[67]."

Cesalpinus characteristically sandwiched this quotation from Aristotle between the statement of the centripetal venous blood flow as seen in venaesection and the basic pronouncement of continual motion through veins into the heart and through arteries away from it.

From the arrangement of his statements in itself Cesalpinus is likely to have referred the upward movement of hot evaporating matter to the arterial blood flow and the downward movement after cooling (in the "cold" brain) to blood returning via the veins to its origin—the heart. He had described the same mechanism of hot blood being driven upwards through the artery and returning through the vein after cooling for the pulmonary blood-flow and had called it "*circulatio*" (see below p. 188). In other words, the idea of arterial blood returning to the heart via the veins was not foreign to Cesalpinus.

66 *Quaest. Medicar.* II, 5 fol. 212 C: "venas cum arteriis adeo copulari osculis, ut vena secta primum exeat sanguis venalis nigrior, deinde succedat arterialis flavior, ut plerumque contingit."

67 See above note [11].

Final Assessment of Cesalpinus in the History of the Discovery of Blood Circulation

Without any doubt Cesalpinus has *no claim* on the possession of any clear conception of the closed circulation of the blood, in other words on having been its "Discoverer". His discourses contain ambiguous statements which have led to an unequal and sentimental distribution of light and shadow in this matter. He had no idea of the *exclusive* centripetal movement of the blood in *all* veins, but instead allowed some part of it to be drawn into the arteries while on its course towards the heart. Though once mentioning in passing interventricular pores, he certainly reduced the importance of such communications and the quantity of blood supposed to pass through them to a minimum by emphasising the transfer of the blood through the lungs for the purpose of refrigeration. He had, however, no knowledge of the sequence of the movements of the heart, but assumed that its dilatation led simultaneously to the entry of venous blood and the emission of arterial blood[68].

On the other hand Cesalpinus cannot be denied awareness of the correct venous blood flow at large—although this knowledge was bound to remain lamentably short of fruition, because it was encumbered with the important position which Cesalpinus attached to arterio-venous anastomoses. These concerned the larger vascular branches, whereas his *capillamenta* implied the idea of arterio-venous continuity and transfer in the periphery and thus constitute a sound element in his doctrine. Moreover we have good reason to believe that what he did know and state about the correct flow of blood in the veins from the periphery to the centre was not meant as an exceptional instance, but as the basic mechanism whereby blood that was sent out from the heart returned to its source and foster-mother.

Cesalpinus' idea of "Circulatio" (distillatio)

It is also in the work of Cesalpinus that we find the motion of blood visualised as a rhythmic to and fro movement in accordance with the Aristotelian principle of hot evaporating matter being driven upwards and returning to its source after cooling. The two cooling organs in Aristotelian physiology were the brain and the lung—the former because it was connected with the production of—cold—phlegm and the latter because of its close contact with air. Cesalpinus enlarged on this idea developing it along the pattern of *chemical distillation.*

68 *Quaest. Peripatet.* lib.V, qu.4, fol.123r: idem enim motus utraque oscula aperit venae scilicet in cor, cordis autem in arterias.

Distillation was also called *circulation*—to denote the rhythmical repetition of the process. Indeed Cesalpinus said of the transit of blood from the right ventricle of the heart through the lungs and back to the heart, i.e. the left ventricle: "this circulation of the blood from the right ventricle of the heart through the lungs into the left ventricle is well borne out by dissection[69]".

Obviously the term *circulatio* has here a largely chemical connotation in the sense of distillation—but it also conveys a rhythmically repeated process. It was Cesalpinus who insisted on *continuity* with regard to the cardio-vascular system as such and to the movement of blood therein. This may well be seen in the light of the Aristotelian doctrine that *continuity is circularity*. For, according to this doctrine, it is circular movement alone that is continuous and explains the continuity of coming into being[70]. Finally it is this rhythmically repeated and continuous process of "circulatory" distillation which provides in Cesalpinus' physiology the link by which venous and arterial blood are joined. It is therefore pertinent to look closer at his concept of *Circulatio*.

As we have just mentioned, Cesalpinus speaks of a circulation of blood from the right ventricle of the heart through the lungs into its left ventricle. In the same setting Cesalpinus insists on the cooling function of the lungs and the particularly hot quality of the blood in the right ventricle. In the preceding chapter the brain is compared to the alembic of the chemists who want to distill brandy (*aquam ardentem*) from wine. It is thus through the brain and its cooling action that loss of spirits from the arterial blood is prevented. The term *circulatio* is not used for this process, however. Perhaps Cesalpinus did not intend to connote here the rhythmical repetition and continuity which he envisaged for the movement of blood from the heart into the lungs and back into it. Nevertheless there is little doubt that it largely conveys the meaning of chemical distillation. This is evident from certain lecture notes from Pisa dated November 3rd 1590 taken by a pupil of Cesalpinus[71]. Here it is said that "the blood that is hot in the heart is refrigerated during its transit through the lung owing to inspiration and expiration of air. It runs from the right ventricle through the artery and into the left ventricle through the vein. As in the instruments for the distillation of hot liquor a certain *circulation* takes place by virtue of contact with the cold. Thus the vessels that lead away from the heart are true arteries. Those which intromit veins. The lung is very much filled with blood, not merely to be thereby nourished, but for the blood to become perfected through a certain *circulation*." (*Aeris inspiratione ac expiratione re-*

69 *Quaest. Peripatet.* lib.V, 4, fol. 125 verso: huic sanguinis circulationi ex dextro cordis ventriculo per pulmones in sinistrum eiusdem ventriculum optime respondent ea, quae ex dissectione apparent.

70 Aristotle, *Physicor.* lib.VIII, 8; 262a seq., ed. C. Prantl, Leipzig 1854, p. 439. Continuity is circularity—mian ousian kai syneche, kai haute estin he kyklo. Also: *De generat. et corrupt.* lib.II, 10; 336b–337a.

71 Bayon, H.P., *Allusions to a "Circulation" of the Blood in MSS. anterior to De Motu Cordis 1628. Proc. Royal Soc. Med.* 1939, *32*, 707.

frigeratur sanguis in corde fervens dum per pulmonem ex dextro ventriculo per arteriam in sinistrum per venam permeat. Ut in organis distillationis aquae ardentis frigido contactu circulatio quaedam fit. Sic vasa educentia ex corde uere arteriae. Introducentia venae. Pulmo sanguine refertissimus non ut eo tantum nutriretur, sed ut circulatione quadam ipse (sc. sanguis) perficeretur)[72].

Caspar Hofmann, Fludd and Quercetanus on Circulatio-Distillatio

Perhaps even better proof of this meaning of *circulatio* in our context is afforded by the work of Caspar Hofmann—an important figure in the history of Harvey's discovery and one of the few contemporaries quoted in Harvey's book. Hofmann follows Cesalpinus closely, and we shall have to say more about him anon. Here it will suffice to quote from his work *On the chest* which preceded Harvey's *De motu* by one year.

Hofmann rejects with great emphasis and finality the interventricular pores of Galen. They do not exist, either in cattle or in man. If they did exist and were used for a simple percolation of blood from the right ventricle to the left, where should the blood be refrigerated? The difficulties raised by Galen's doctrine can in Hofmann's opinion only be removed by recognising a dual function of the pulmonary artery: (a) its primary purpose, the transference of blood from ventricle to ventricle, a *circuit* (*ambitus*) which also accomplishes its refrigeration and (b) the alimentation of the lung.

Proof of the transference of the blood through such a process of *circulation—to use the language of Chymists*—lies in the great size of the vessel which speaks in itself against its purpose for the mere nutrition of the lungs. Another proof is its substance. As its function is the driving out of blood, this could not work without pulsation particularly as it operates against a gradient—hence it could not be less strong than the aorta (*transferri sanguinem per circulationem talem, ut cum Chymistis loquar, probat magnitudo utriusque vasis...*)[73].

In the same decade in which Hofmann's and Harvey's great work was published the *Amphitheatrum anatomiae* by Robert Fludd, the mystic, Rosicrucian and personal friend of Harvey, had appeared (Francof. 1623).We have discussed the man and his work before (p. 113). Fludd in his mystical anatomy of the heart likens the motion of the blood to a series of chemical distillations. The liver, right ventricle of the heart and brain are compared to three chemical *athanors*, two of them joined by a neck with a fur-

72 Ibid. as note [71].

73 Hofmann, Caspar, *De Thorace* III, 11 Francof. 1627, p. 95.

ther receptacle: the liver with the right heart by the vena cava, and the right ventricle with the lungs by the pulmonary artery. The right ventricle of the heart—the second *athanor*—*circulates* the blood which has already been subjected to one distillation, redistilling it into the lungs after it has been thinned and purified. From the arterial system the vital spirit rises to the brain where it is further distilled and made suitable for the function of the intellect by still greater rarefication[74].

Fludd thus elaborated on the original Cesalpinian concept and gave it his own alchemical twist. "How hateful and worthy of contempt", he says, "those men are who are accustomed to hold in derision the Alchemists, since a chemist undertakes to do nothing that nature has not already delineated in the human body[75]".

As Debus points out, Fludd is preceded and evidently influenced in this by the great Paracelsian Du Chesne (Quercetanus 1544–1609). Already in 1604 the latter had called the heart a *pelican of nature*, i.e. a *vas circulatorium*, a still. In this the blood that comes from the abdomen is sublimated and acquires like a *quinta essentia* the virtue of an ardent sulphureous liquor (*aquavitae*), the origin of the innate and cognate heat. The same *aqua vitae* is transferred through the arteries into the *Balneum Mariae* of the brain where it is again sublimated in the *rete mirabile* by *circulations*. Hence is born the animal spirit, the main instrument of the soul... and thus in blood (which by right we compare with wine) those three principles are contained which by their very nature fulfil the offices of a true Alchemist and are wisely and exactly distributed and diffused to all parts of the body—each member receiving its due[76].

Circulatio-Distillatio: Harvey and after

The original Cesalpinian meaning of the "circular" movement of the blood from ventricle to ventricle had been somewhat diluted by the more generalised and less distinct version given by the Chemists and Fludd. Nevertheless the connotation of a rhythmically repeated and automatic process remained and was even accentuated later on.

Whatever claims may have been raised on Cesalpinus' behalf on the strength of his use of the term *circulatio* appeared to be shattered when its chemical connotation was realised. It should be borne in mind, however, that this very connotation remained prominently alive in the work of Harvey himself and in that of his followers. Moreover it was Harvey who, like Cesalpinus, linked

74 Debus, A.G., *Robert Fludd and the Circulation of the Blood. J. Hist. Med.* 1961, XVI, 374–393.

75 Fludd, *Anatomiae Amphitheatrum* Francof. 1623, p. 226: "quam sint illi homines odio et contemptu digni, qui Alchimistas in derisione habere solent, cum verus chimicus nihil aggredi conetur quod natura non in corpore humano delinearit." Cited from Debus loc. cit., in note [74], p. 377. – On other aspects of Fludd's ideas on "*Circulatio*" see above p. 113.

76 Quercetanus (Du Chesne), Jos., *Ad veritatem Hermeticae Medicinae ex Hippocratis veterumque decretis ac therapeusi* Paris 1604, p. 226–227.

it with the Aristotelian idea of a cyclical—"circular"—moving up of water in the form of vapour and its descent in the form of rain.

Harvey used the analogy to introduce and illustrate his idea of blood circulation: *Coepi egomet mecum cogitare, an motionem quandam quasi in circulo haberet*—I began to think whether it (sc. the blood) might not have motion, as it were in a circle. Which motion, he continued, may be allowed to be called circular, after the same manner that Aristotle says that the air and rain imitate the circular motion of the superior bodies. For the moist earth warmed up by the sun evaporates, the vapours lifted upwards are condensed, descend again as rain, make the earth moist, and so on. In the same way through the motion of the blood all parts are nourished, cherished and quickened by the warmer, perfect, vaporous, spirituous and so to speak alimentative blood: by contrast, in the parts the blood is cooled down, coagulated and as it were effete, whence it returns to its beginnings (*principium*), namely the heart, in order to restore its perfection: here, through the natural, potent and fervid heat, it is liquefied again, impregnated with spirits and so to speak a balsam, and hence it is distributed again[77].

Harvey here describes under the heading of *circulation* not only the cyclic circuit of the blood around the body, but also a cyclic heating and evaporation with subsequent cooling down and condensation of the blood fluid—what is known in chemistry and alchemy as *distillation*. It is the same rhythmically repeated and continuous process of cooling down, condensation and respiritualisation which Cesalpinus had envisaged for the venous blood passing from the right ventricle through the lungs into the left ventricle of the heart.

In the above passage from the eighth chapter of *De motu* the Cesalpinian principle of blood distillation is applied by Harvey to the venous blood, cooled down in the periphery and heated up and respiritualised at the centre—as against the Cesalpinian idea of the heating up of venous blood in the right heart and its cooling down on passing through and returning from the lung. However, Harvey was acqainted with this original Cesalpinian meaning and application of the principle of distillation and indeed elaborated on the chemical change which the blood undergoes owing to its cooling down in the lungs. In the Lumleian lectures on anatomy he gives it as his own contribution that the lung retains the fatty and oily exhalation, just as oil or balsam or alimentary fat *cools down in an alembic*[78]. This use of the chemical analogy by Harvey is all the more remarkable in view of his lack of sympathy for the chemists—of which we are apprised by Aubrey[79].

77 *De motu*, cap.VIII, ed. Roterod. 1648, p. 102. – For full text see above p. 82–83.

78 *Praelectiones* fol. 86 recto.

79 "He did not care for chymistrey, and was wont to speak against them with undervalue", *Lives of eminent men*, London 1813, vol. II, p. 385.

The chemical pattern of distillation was linked with the circulation of the blood by such followers of Harvey as Descartes, Walaeus, Power, Thruston, Swammerdam, de le Boe and Mayow.

According to Descartes (1596–1650) the heart contains a "fire" whereby it swells and dilates as soon as blood enters. The flesh of the lung is so scarce and by virtue of the air so cold that the blood coming in a vaporous condition from the right ventricle is condensed and reconverted into fluid blood whereby it is enabled to maintain and nourish the "fire" of the left heart. Hence the necessity of respiration: for the condensation of blood vapour, the maintenance of the heart fire and the preservation of life. Arterial blood differs from venous blood because the former becomes "rarefied and as it were distilled" (*rarefactus et veluti distillatus*) during its transit through the heart. This "subtle, vivid and hot" blood is capable of opening the arterial outlets in the heart, and it is the difference between arterial and venous blood in heat and density which maintains circulation at large[80].

Blood circulates for the sake of perfection, says Joh. de Wale (Walaeus, 1604–1649). By virtue of continuous movement it is attenuated. It warms up and becomes rarefied in the heart and subsequently condensed and as it were concentrated in the periphery of the body. For none of its parts is warmer than the heart and none cooler than the body surface. Hence a kind of "*circulation*" operates, not unlike that by means of which *chemists* utterly refine and perfect their "spirits"[81].

Henry Power (1623–1668), an early Fellow of the Royal Society (1662–1663), microscopist and possibly a personal acquaintance of Harvey, wrote in his Manuscript entitled *Circulatio sanguinis Inventio Harveiana*, 1652: "Nature like an excellent chymist continually channells (or as they phrase it) Pellicanizes the Blood that the crude and inconcocted parts thereof might acquire a perfect elaboration the noxious and excrementitious parts avoidance and Separation, as we shall shortly show in an excellent parallel twixt chymicall and naturall operations, and all the parts of the Body their respective nutriment heat and refocillation for by these repeated Circulations, every part receives its appropriate and specificall nutriment for what one part refuses, another embraces, and by this perpetuall motion all particles in the Blood, are at some time or other offered to all parts indifferently, and the whole fabrick thereby kept up by Continuall reparations.[82]" It should be noted that this was written in Harvey's life time by an eminent though nowadays somewhat neglected naturalist, a friend and

80 DES CARTES, R., *Specimen philosophiae s. dissertatio de methodo recte regendae rationis et veritatis in scientiis investigandae*. Amstelod. 1672, p. 32 seq. – idem, *De homine* ed. Lud. de la Forge, Amstelod. 1677, p. 8.

81 WALAEUS, JOH., *De motu chyli et sanguinis ad Th. Bartholinum in*: Th. Bartholinus, *Anatomia ... ad sanguinis circulationem reformata*, Hagae-Comitis 1655, p. 561 and Lugd. Bat. 1673, p. 790: unde quaedam quasi circulatio contingit, non absimilis qua Chymici suos spiritus tenuissimos reddunt et perfectissimos.

82 COLE, F.J., *Henry Power on the circulation of the blood. J. Hist. Med.* 1957, XII, 291–324, p. 320.

"disciple" of Sir Thomas Browne, who, moreover, may have been personally known to Harvey.

Thruston (ab. 1644) ascribed to venous blood a tendency to become ebullient and overheated owing to its richness in particles and its brisk mixture with lymph when entering the lungs. The same mechanism is used by *chemists* who mix fluids and let them effervesce, often causing the vessel to break. Hence the necessity of feeding at regular intervals whereby chyle is produced, the blood regenerated, kept in motion and prevented from coagulating and cooling down excessively when achieving contact with air in the lungs[83].

Respiration is the means by which blood attains perfection, said Swammerdam (1637–1680). It effervesces when emerging from the right ventricle, is kept moving, ventilated, then condensed, cooled down by the air, and purified from hot vapours whereby it is rendered more "spirituous" and apt for preserving life[84].

De le Boe (Sylvius, 1614–1672) still speaks of the setting alight of blood by the innate fire of the heart which causes its rarefaction and expansion. Hence it dilates the blood and finally breaks through into the arteries. True to his "iatro-chemical" philosophy he compares the effervescence of blood with the reaction between acid and alcali. Inspiration serves to temper this process by giving access to a salt in the air into the blood[85].

Similarly Mayow (1641–1679) saw in particles of the air—his famous nitro-aerial bodies—the cause of an ebullition of arterial blood owing to fermentation[86].

Opposition to effervescence and indeed to the concept of innate heat in blood and the heart had been voiced earlier on by Van Helmont (1579–1644). At the same time he envisaged a "ferment" from the air combining with blood passing through the lungs, whereby a "certain residue" was eliminated from the venous blood through its conversion into "volatile salts" and subsequent escape—a remarkable anticipation of more modern theories of respiration[87].

It may be said that the great Richard Lower (1632–1691) followed this Helmontian lead in deprecating any ebullition of blood and its supposed role in the movements of the heart and in denying the existence of a "focus" of fire and heat in the heart[88]. Similarly Walter Needham (1631?–1691) emphasised the purely muscular structure of the heart which alone is responsible for the pumping of the blood and incompatible with its ebullition or vaporisation or the presence of a fiery "focus" of life—*biolychnos*—in the heart[89].

Returning to Cesalpinus and his *circulatio*, we can *conclude:* any

83 THRUSTON, MAL., *De respirationis usu primario* Lond. 1670 Cited from: *Bibliotheca Anatomica* ed. le Clerk and Manget, Genev. 1685, vol. II, p. 166 seq. (p. 176 in sect. XIII). Ed Lugd. Bat 1708, p. 49.

84 SWAMMERDAM, JOH., *Tractatus physico-anatomico-medicus de respiratione usuque pulmonum. Bibl. Anat.* loc. cit. II, 151 seq.

85 SYLVIUS, FR. (de le Boe), *Disputat. medicar.* VII, 52 seq. *Opp. med.* Amstelod. 1679, p. 32.

86 MAYOW, JOH., *Tractatus quinque ... secundus de respiratione* Oxonii 1674, p. 301: "probabile est tamen spiritum nitro-aereum particulis sanguinis salino-sulphureis admixtum, fermentationem debitam in eodem excitare ... neque tamen putandum est, effervescentiam istam sanguinis in corde solo fieri, sed statim in vasis pulmonalibus, et postea in arteriis non minus quam in corde...

87 VAN HELMONT, *Blas humanum* 37 seq. in *Ortus medicinae* Amstelod. 1648, p. 187. – PAGEL, W., *Van Helmont. The 300th anniversary of his death. Brit. med. J.* 1945, I, 59. – Idem, *J.B. Van Helmont (1579–1644)* Nature 1944, CLIII, 675.

88 LOWER, R., *Tract. de corde* Amstelod. 1669, p. 18: "cordis substantia omnino muscularis est"; p. 79: cordis eadem est ac reliquorum musculorum actio; pp. 65–66: "nullum in corde fermentum aut ebullitio sanguinis"—for the heart and even small particles of its substance removed from the chest pulsate; pp. 69–73: "cordis motum non dependere a sanguinis ebullitione; p. 75: "tantum etiam abest ut credam sanguinis motum a sua in corde accensione ulla dependere..."

89 NEEDHAM, GUALT., *Disquisitio anatomica de formato foetu.* London 1667 cap. VI —digressio de biolychno et ingressu aeris in sanguinem item de sanguificatione—pp. 129 seq.

diminution which his standing in the pre-history of Harvey's discovery may have suffered through the realisation of the largely chemical meaning of the term in his usage, is amply compensated by the strong undercurrent which the same chemical connotation of the term formed in the usage of Harvey himself and his followers until its final rejection by Lower and Needham. Indeed the mere fact that the term had this connotation in the work of Cesalpinus in itself is of no particular significance. What *is* worthy of attention, however, is that it was eminently compatible with the "modern" meaning of the term as conceived by the discoverer himself and elaborated upon by his supporters. It was the same Robert Fludd who in 1623 had propounded a system of subsequent distillations—circulations—of the venous blood as the mechanism responsible for its motion who came forward some eight years later as one of the earliest (if not the earliest of the) supporters of Harvey's discovery[90].

Harvey and Cesalpinus—The Role of Caspar Hofmann

Cesalpinus not Mentioned by Harvey

The works of Cesalpinus contain observations and speculations which later assumed importance in the process and presentation of Harvey's discovery. Cesalpinus may or may not have influenced the latter in this way—we have no means of deciding this. It is quite a different question, however, whether Harvey was acquainted with Cesalpinus' work. Even here we have no direct evidence. For some long time it was generally accepted as a fact that Harvey mentioned Cesalpinus by name in his Lumleian lectures on anatomy which date back to 1616–1618[91]. The passage in the *Praelectiones* reads as follows: "*J. Caes. Aratii| v. Arter. qut. ij d.|Art. venalis 4 dig.|admitt: unde Aditus|major Aspera Art.|*. This was transcribed by the editor of the *Praelectiones* in 1886: *J. Caesalpinus Aretinus vena Arterialis quantiate ij digitos Arteria venalis 4 digitos admittit unde Aditus major Aspera Arteria*. F.N.L. Poynter has not only shown that the correct reading is: *Julius Caesar Arantius* (instead of J. Caesalpinus Aretinus), but also discovered the locus to which the passage refers: it comes from the *third edition* (1587) of Arantius *De humano foetu*[92].

In other words *Harvey has not mentioned Cesalpinus*, and the latter's name does not occur in the Harvey-literature prior to Conring, Nardi and Power (1642–1655)[93]. It was Nardi who probably mentioned Cesalpinus to Harvey some thirty years after the publication of *De motu*.

90 PAGEL, W., *Religious motives in the medical biology of the XVIIth century. Bullet. Hist. Med.* 1935, III, 277–278. See also Debus loc. cit. in note [74], p. 375 and 388; see also our account above, p. 115.

91 HARVEY, *Praelect. Anatomiae universalis* London 1886, fol. 75v.

92 POYNTER, F.N.L. in *Addendum* to PAGEL, W., *The philosophy of circles—Cesalpinus—Harvey. J. Hist. Med.* 1957, XII, 152–153.

Doubts in the reading of the passage had already been voiced in passing by Bayon, but not substantiated or verified by the demonstration of the locus referred to in Arantius. This is due to the work of Poynter. See: BAYON, H.P., *The life work of William Harvey and modern medical progress Proc. R. Soc. Med.* 1951, 213–218, p. 214.

93 GIOVANNI NARDI (d. 1655), *Noctes geniales* Bonon. 1655, p. 274. See also: BAYON, H.P., *William Harvey. Physician and Biologist. His precursors, opponents and successors*, part V. Ann. Sci. 1939, IV, 353.

At the very same time and in the same connexion Cesalpinus was mentioned by Henry Power (see above p. 193, note [82]) in a letter to Ralph Widdrington (d. 1688), one of Power's older contemporaries (M. A. 1639) who corresponded with him on scientific matters, notably physiology and chemistry. The letter of the 2nd of January 1655/(56) is found in BM *Sloane* MS 1326, ff 9–11. It is also of interest that here Cesalpinus is bracketed with Sennert as forerunners to Harvey. The author is indebted for this to Dr. Charles Webster who reviewed Power's work as a whole and Dr. P. Rattansi who checked the passage for him in the manuscript.

CONRING, HERMANN, *De sanguinis generatione et motu naturali* (1642). Lugd. Bat. et Amsterod. 1646, p. 263: etiam Caesalpino observata fuisse illa de sanguinis circulari motu, quae triginta quinque post annis luculente docuit Harvejus (with reference to the venous blood flow after ligature). Visa autem isti...non nisi per umbram. Nor was he consistent about it or self-confident in this matter. Longe exactius patuit haec veritas Harvejo.

It is, however, hardly conceivable that Harvey remained unacquainted with Cesalpinus until this late date. He possessed an encyclopaedic knowledge of ancient as well as contemporary literature which shows up well in the *Praelectiones*. Like Cesalpinus himself Harvey was steeped in Aristotle and intent on defending the views of an "author so diligent and faithful"[94] as far as possible. He could not have failed to notice Cesalpinus' *Peripatetic Questions* which had been written for the very purpose of vindicating Aristotle through the whole realm of natural philosophy. Nor could a work of this nature have escaped someone who had studied at Padua—the stronghold of Aristotelianism—and had done so only a few years after the publication of its second edition. In fact Cesalpinus' work had a tremendous influence on the academic youth, not only in Italy, but also in Germany. It was there that Taurellus compiled a point by point refutation of the book in order to counteract this very influence which he regarded as harmful[95].

Caspar Hofmann (1572–1648; pl. 36–38)

The extent of the influence of Cesalpinus is reflected in a more positive way in the works of Caspar Hofmann, notably his authoritative commentary on Galen's *Use of the parts* and his work *On the chest*[96]. The former of these was well known to Harvey, as it is one of the literary sources that are expressly quoted in *De motu*[97] and there is no reason why Hofmann's book *On the chest* should have remained unknown to him.

Hofmann forms an important figure in the life of Harvey whose visit and demonstration to him of the circulation at Nuremberg in 1636 is one of the landmarks in the history of the reception of Harvey's discovery[98]. It is further illustrated by Harvey's correspondence[99].

There is a tragic streak in the personal relations between Harvey and Hofmann. It is well known how the latter could not persuade himself to acknowledge the truth of Harvey's discovery—inspite of Harvey's personal demonstration and the enthusiastic support of Hofmann's pupil Marquard Slegel. There may even be some truth in the story that it was Hofmann who, prior to the publication of *De motu*, first talked about a "circulator"—an itinerant quack believing in blood circulation[100].

The objections which Hofmann raised against the circulation clearly reveal the difficulties which Harvey's contemporaries must have felt when confronted with his challenge. It was the absence of purpose why the blood should run the new course prescribed

94 *Praelect. anat. univers.* fol. 74v.

95 TAURELLUS, *Alpes caesae* loc. cit. in note [41]. *Epist. dedicat.* p. 4: "ex Italia superatis alpibus aliam philosophandi rationem (i.e. other than the philosophy of the "moderate" Aristotelian Jac. Scheck of Schorndorf), nescio, quibus excogitatis, et assumtis principiorum loco hypothesibus, a vera et Aristotelica philosophia alienissimis, in omnes Germaniae angulos irrepsisse. Et eo quidem id mihi magis grave molestumque fuit: quod Caesalpinianis hisce paradoxis, et falsis opinionibus, plurimis in locis, Germana iuventus magna verae philosophiae jactura imbueretur..."

Of modern authors compare PAYNE, JOS. FR., *Harvey and Galen* London 1897, p. 12: "Harvey had evidently studied the works of the contemporary Peripatetic school in Italy, especially Cesalpino, the great Aristotelian, and Cesar Cremonini and was probably somewhat influenced by him (sc. Aristotle)."

96 HOFMANN, CASP., *Commentarii in Galeni de usu partium corporis humani libri XVII cum variis lectionibus*. Francof. 1625 and idem, *De thorace* 1627 loc. cit. in note [33].

97 HARVEY, *De motu cordis* cap. VII ed. pr. Francof. 1628, p. 40. Tr. WILLIS p. 44.

98 See: FERRARIO, E.V., POYNTER, F.N. L. and FRANKLIN, K.J., *William Harvey's debate with Caspar Hofmann on the circulation of the blood. New documentary evidence. J. Hist. Med.* 1960, XV, 7–21.

99 Extracts published in *Opp. omn.* London 1766, p. 635. Tr. WILLIS p. 595–596.

100 The well known story of Helvicus Dietericus (1601–1655), *Vindiciae adversus Othonem Tachenium*. Hamburg 1655, p. 194 —as retold by BAIER, J.J., *Biographiae professorum medicinae qui in Academia Altdorfina umquam vixerunt* Nürnberg 1728, p. 48–49; R. LANDAU, *Ein deutscher Vorläufer Harveys. Janus* 1902, VII, 60–63; POYNTER loc. cit. in note [98], p. 11 and others.

by Harvey. This is the very point with which Hofmann sets out and to which he finally returns.

According to traditional doctrine blood was perfected in the heart and then distributed by it—an office which the heart should accomplish at a single attempt. On Harvey's showing, however, the same blood was subject to a continual repetition ("recrudescence") of the process—as if Nature were redundant in her works and did things in vain.

What worried Hofmann was thus the same question which agitated the mind of Harvey, the "life-long thinker about the purpose of circulation". Indeed, in Hofmann's opinion, Harvey was trying to scrutinize the inscrutable—the same Harvey who more than once had pointed out how difficult it was to reach certainty concerning the motion of the heart and arteries and the nature of systole and diastole[101]. One may be allowed to argue indefinitely, but to reason is one thing, to prove one's arguments by the judgment of the senses another. The former is easy enough, the latter not so easy and yet the only thing that matters. In fact, Hofmann says, Harvey's reasoning is at fault, because owing to ebullition the actual quantities of blood that pass through in the unit of time are rendered unquantifiable. This had already been observed by Primrose, the first critic of Harvey. It is not a matter of ounces and drachms, as Harvey assumed, but of grains. Nor is there any question of a flooding with blood which would threaten the organs were there no circulation. For this would be controlled by the attractive and retentive virtue of the organs. Harvey thus neglected what is obvious to the anatomist's eye in favour of computing and reasoning. The anatomist is unable to say by which channels the blood should find its way from the arteries into the veins, as nobody ever dreamed of anastomoses between the finest vessels through which the peripheral organs receive their aliment. Should alleys that have been blind for so many centuries in the past thus have been opened up by the Englishman (*viae quaedam caecae, et a tot retro seculis ignoratae, quas primus aperuerit hic Anglus*)?

Hofmann concludes: Once the heart has expelled the blood into the arteries it has no means to call it back through the veins. In fact it sends out blood through arteries as well as veins. Nor could there be any "re-cooking" of blood in the heart, for its result would not be blood, but bile. And yet on Harvey's showing the blood would have to be "re-cooked" not twice, three or four times, but *ad infinitum*. Finally, reverting to his point of departure, Hofmann asks again: why all this? Indeed the question of the cause of causes is that without which all that is being said is said in vain.

101 Re vera, Harvee, persequeris *pragma anexereuneton*, rem inexputabilem, inexplicabilem, imperscrutabilem. HOFMANN, C., *Digressio in circulationem sanguinis, nuper in Anglia natam. Cap. 48 Manuscripti physiologici.* In: JO. RIOLANI, *Responsio ad duas exercit. anatom. postremas G. Harvei de circulatione sanguinis.* Paris, 1652, p. 360.

It is here given as a "chapter from a manuscript on Physiology" which Guy Patin had acquired and made accessible to Riolan. The chapter is incorporated in Hofmann's posthumously published *Apologiae pro Galeno, sive chrestomatheion libri III*, Lugduni 1668, in lib. II, sectio 4, cap. 48, p. 104–107, a book which, according to the dating of the preface had been written in 1635 (see JOH. JAC. BAIERI *Biographiae professorum medicinae qui in Academia Altorfina unquam vixerunt*, Norimbergae et Altorfii 1728, p. 56–57).

Hofmann's criticism of Harvey would thus appear to have taken shape not long before the meeting at Nuremberg which fits in well with the tenor of Hofmann's letter of May 19th 1636 to Harvey and the reply of the latter, dated the following day, both as published by FERRARIO, POYNTER and FRANKLIN, loc. cit. 1960, in note [98].

Hofmann's argument, then, in its main point resembles that advanced by Riolan (p. 75): Harvey tried to quantify the unquantifiable. Indeed Riolan must have felt satisfaction at the discovery of Hofmann's manuscript and its publication as an appendix to one of the former's own works against Harvey was most fitting.

And yet Hofmann should have been the first to see the light—for he finally and decidedly rejected the Galenic pores in the interventricular septum[102]. Moreover he unmistakably stated that arterial blood is driven into veins through anastomoses[103] and that in the embryo the heart forms two vessels—the artery and the vein—through which the blood "goes and returns"[104].

What is of particular interest in this context is Harvey's letter written on May 20th 1636—the day after the demonstration—to Caspar Hofmann. For a long time only a fragment was known, but it has recently been re-published in full and commented upon by F.N.L. Poynter[105]. Here Harvey himself seems to express his surprise at Hofmann's unwillingness to see the truth of his discovery. For, he says, there were not a few people in England who denied me priority as the "inventor" of the circuit; they did so in public lectures on Anatomy, and, quoting your (sc. Hofmann's) writings, argued that it was instruction and teaching learnt from you which brought me to my opinion. Thus I had to produce a face to face comparison of our writings and the times when they were written to clear and defend my name[106].

At all events Hofmann's work as quoted in Harvey's *De motu* contains many important references to Cesalpinus, and in many respects Hofmann follows the Cesalpinian and Aristotelian lead. We mentioned Hofmann's acceptance of Cesalpinus' *circulatio* for the transference of blood from the right ventricle to the left through, and its refrigeration in, the lungs. Like Cesalpinus Hofmann used it in the chemical sense of distillation and said so *expressis verbis*[107]. Hofmann largely follows the Aristotelian tradition as revived and presented by Cesalpinus in the following points of detail: he supports Cesalpinus' view that blood formed in the liver has no nutritional virtue and is not immediately taken to the organs, but acquires such quality by arterialisation in the heart[108]. Hofmann agrees with Cesalpinus that there is no need for Galen's "natural faculty" in explaining respiration. Its cause is simply the expansion of the lung subsequent to the in-flow of ebullient blood[109]. He endorses the view of the heart as the source of all blood, arterial and venous, and of all vessels, arteries as well as veins[110]. He also insists on the virtual unity of all blood which

102 Hofmann, C., *De thorace* lib. III, cap. 9, p. 94 and *Commentarii*, pp. 110–111.

103 *De thorace* lib. II, cap. 10, p. 34.

104 *Commentarii*, lib. XV, cap. 4, p. 337: cor non potest id (sc. fabricationem reliquarum partium) autem sine vasis, quae sunt illi instar aquae ductuum, per quos sanguis *it reditque*, statim facit sibi ... venam et arteriam, quae sunt duo illa gemina, quae Coiter vidit primo die (italics are of the present author).

105 Poynter, loc. cit. in note [98], p. 14 (transl. p. 17–21).

106 Poynter ibidem p. 15.

107 *De thorace* III, 11 loc. cit. p. 95. See above note [73].

108 *De thorace* III, 12, p. 96 with ref. to Cesalp. *Quaest. Peripat.* V, 4; see above note 33. Also *de thorace* II, 23, p. 56: "aliud esse docere, ubi sanguis omnis conficiatur; et aliud ubi sanguis ille conficiatur, qui vere nutrit. Verum est, omnis sanguis in hepate fit: at falsum est, sanguis in hepate factus nutrit solus."

109 *De thorace* II, 16, pp. 43–44: "tu autem, si placet, vise ante omnia ad Cesalpinum 5 Quaest. perip. 4 qua de facultate vitali. p. 96: "et hoc est quod pulcerrime deduxit Cesalpinus 5 quaest. perip. 4.

110 *De thorace* II, 23, p. 56.

is proven by a limitless number of anastomoses between arteries and veins[111].

All these points had been made by Cesalpinus and none of them could have been lost on Harvey—perhaps least of all the unitarian view of the blood, venous and arterial, as against Galen's dualistic conviction in this matter. A further point is the analogy drawn by Cesalpinus between veins and the roots of plants[112].

Hofmann pays tribute to Cesalpinus' demonstration of the continuity of the branches of the portal vein and the inferior vena cava—a point mentioned in Harvey's letter to Hofmann[113]. There are further quotations from Cesalpinus in Hofmann's work which are relevant—for example Hofmann supports Cesalpinus' contention that the vena cava is not only not smaller close to the heart than near the liver, but—as anatomical studies had taught the latter—bigger[114].

Wherever Hofmann refers to Cesalpinus he has a word of praise—"what Cesalpinus most beautifully deduced"; "on this point Cesalpinus should be consulted before all"; "on this compare the praiseworthy Cesalpinus[115]". There is no need to enumerate in detail further passages from Hofmann in which Cesalpinus is quoted or praised[116], but it may be mentioned that Hofmann's interpretation of Aristotle is closely reminiscent of Cesalpinus: Not without indignation, says Hofmann, do I hear those who prattle about a passage in Aristotle as if it were to show that he had taught that blood leaves the heart through the veins when he obviously speaks about arteries alone[117].

All this,we believe, provides ample indirect evidence for Harvey's acquaintance with the work of Cesalpinus. We also believe that this did not come to him through the writings of Hofmann, but through perusal at first hand.

As we have mentioned *acquaintance* as such tells us nothing about *influence:* it could be argued without much difficulty that there was no such influence whatever and even that Harvey might have run the risk of being misled rather than assisted in his research by following Cesalpinus' lead.

The *argumentum ex silentio* is hardly productive of information either way. On the other hand one cannot help feeling that the parallels which we noted between Cesalpinus and Harvey were not accidental and that at least some of Cesalpinus' observations and speculations had not been lost on Harvey. These seem to lie in the strengthening of the Aristotelian background of Harvey's discovery which was due to Cesalpinus and is best epitomised in the latter's denial of the role of the liver in forming venous blood,

111 *De thorace* II, 23, p.56: "idem sensus convincit, Venas cum arteriis *synanastomousthai*, fierique communicationem seu potius confusionem utriusque sanguinis..."

112 *De thorace* II, 26, p.63: "de quibus videre est laudatum Caesalpinum".

113 See Poynter loc.cit. in note [98], p.16 and 20.

114 De thorace II, 26, p.63: "at vena cava circa hepar est latior (i.e. as stated by GALEN). Hoc ego simpliciter inverti, et nunc probo autoritate trium insignium virorum. Venae cavae orificium, inquit Vesalius 1.3 cap.6 ad dextrum cordis sinum amplius est etc. Cum saepe interfuerimus Anatomicis administrationibus, Caesalpinus ait, 5 Perip. quaest. 3 non vidimus venae partem juxta cor magnitudine superari ab ea, quae juxta hepar est: imo etiam superare, a multis animadversum est... docet Acorambonus ... venam cavam triplo latiorem meatum habere circa cor, quam in jecore..."

115 *De thorace* l.c.p. 96; 44; 63.

116 For example: *De thorace* II, 19, p.46: "modulamur ab anima sentiente". – I, 8, p.11: Aristotle—according to Hofmann—observed but two ventricles; this is in no way negatived by Cesalpinus' observation (*Quaest. peripat.* V, 3) of three ventricles in fishes. – III, 16, p.98: the firm substance of the heart is suitable to protect the "aetherea facula", as it is called by Cesalpinus. – p.91: role of the heart in initiating respiration.

117 *De thorace* II, 26, p.59: "non sine indignatione audio illos, qui illa ... crepant ek tes kardias epocheteuetai eis tas phlebas. Eis de ten kardian ouk allothen, sanguis ex corde in venas it: in cor autem aliunde non venit (with reference to ARISTOTLE, *De partibus animal.* lib.III, cap.4; 666a). Intelligit enim heic arterias solas, in quibus it sanguis arteriosus."

At the same locus Hofmann convincingly argues that by "the parts fitted for the reception of nutriment" (*dektikous topous*) Aristotle in *De somno et vigilia* (cap.III, 456b) understands stomach and gut, and that "veins" in this connexion embrace liver and spleen, in addition to the mesenteric vessels, as a system for the preparation of blood from the nutriment taken in (*mediatae sanguinis officinae*). For, according to Aristotle, the liver is made for the sake of concoction (*pepseos charin*) of the food (*De partibus animal.* lib.III, cap.7; 670a). As far as the production of blood is concerned the liver is second in dignity only to the heart (ibid. cap.12; 673b), the spleen forming a kind of "bastard-liver" (*nothon hepar*). From these organs the blood passes to its immediate source, its *arche*, the heart.

and of its distribution by the latter directly to the periphery and also his insistence that the heart is the origin of all the blood and all the vessels—the organ from which the blood goes to the periphery and to which it returns. It was thus that Cesalpinus paved the way for an understanding of the venous blood flow and the basic identity of venous and arterial blood. It is indeed in Cesalpinus' work that the first steps in this direction and thereby towards Harvey can be recognised.

Cesalpinus' role as a precursor of Harvey thus largely coincides with the revival and defence of Aristotle that was professed by both. However much Galen's observations and reasoning remained fundamental to Cesalpinus as well as Harvey (p. 132), vindication of Aristotle by the latter implied anatagonism to the former. This was in the best tradition of Padua which owed its preeminence to the forging and maintaining of the link between the study of Aristotle and nature (p. 19). Nor is there any doubt that the progressive elements in Cesalpinus as well as in Harvey are closely bound up with their rejection of Galenic views—a rejection that went with the vindication of Aristotle who in turn had been opposed by Galen.

Parallels and Contacts between Cesalpinus and Harvey in Detail

1. There is first the whole shift of emphasis from the liver to the heart as the origin of *all* vessels, not only of the arteries, as recognised by Galen, but notably of the veins which Galen had located in the liver—in opposition to Aristotle.

With the dethronement of the liver as the site of blood formation and the origin of the veins this organ lost its role as the central distributor of venous blood not only to the heart, but particularly to the whole periphery of the body and to the organs.

Concentration on the heart thus immediately made the liver subservient to it and brought the correct direction of the flow of venous blood to the heart into focus. Indeed the view that not only part of the venous blood, but all of it turns to the heart may be regarded as the logical conclusion of the genuinely Aristotelian belief in the supremacy of the heart as the metropolis of blood and blood vessels. It is this vista of the centripetal flow of all venous blood which forms the backbone of Harvey's discovery. Its traces can be found in Cesalpinus, as we have seen, and it is in the work of the latter that they are connected with venous ligature—the very "experimental" proof in the hands of Harvey and his followers.

2. Admittedly opposition to Galen made Cesalpinus as well as Harvey neglect points in which the former was in advance, for example the fundamental difference between arterial and venous blood. Harvey believed in the basic unity of the blood which was driven around as such and only strained in transit through the lungs. Similarly Cesalpinus regarded blood as essentially uniform.

3. Cesalpinus as well as Harvey[118] deny the entrance of air or any airy product into the left heart and herewith profess to follow the Aristotelian lead against Galen. As we have seen (p. 188) Aristotle rejected any communication of the tracheal system with the vessels in the lung. His idea that breath was transmitted to them "by contact" in Cesalpinus' interpretation merely meant a cooling action and this would indeed appear to have been Aristotle's intention. For, as Cesalpinus adds, the Philosopher had referred to fishes which take in water and not air. The latter, according to Aristotle, cannot create heat; nor does it engender spirit which is rather the result of the warming up of fluid. Hence, Cesalpinus concludes, heat and animal spirit are not the product of air, but of the nutriment which is taken to the heart by the veins[119]. Nor could Cesalpinus agree with Galen's doctrine of the discharge of soot through the left auricle and lung—here following Columbus and again foreshadowing Harvey. How, Cesalpinus asks, would a separation be conceivable of the air which has entered the left ventricle and the soot which is about to leave it? And what would prevent spirit and air to leave together with the soot, since on Galen's own showing the mitral—unlike the tricuspid-valve is not tight? Instead Cesalpinus emphasises the blood flow from the lung to the left heart, the oneness of its direction and its continuity—undisturbed by a complicated mechanism concerned with the inflow and outflow of air and vaporous products.

4. In intimate connexion with this Cesalpinus presents a closely reasoned argument against the way in which Galen had made respiration subservient to the heart—again anticipating, however remotely, Harvey and doing so in following up the Peripatetic tradition. For already Aristotle had refuted any dependence of the motion of the heart upon the lungs, in quite general terms. If it were so dependent, Aristotle had argued, the motion of the heart should be identical and uniform in all animals endowed with lungs; but it is in man alone that palpitation can be observed, since hope and expectation—the causes of such palpitation—are emotions that occur in man alone[120].

118 Already in the Lumleian lectures Harvey said that spirits are not from air—*spiritus non ex aere*, fol. 85 verso. This is associated with the rejection of the "vulgar" idea that spirits are distinct and separate substances in the humours and parts, as if they were formed in different places or contained in others. By contrast, spirit and blood to Harvey are one thing (*spiritus et sanguis una res*) comparable to whey and cream in milk—following Aristotle according to whom the spirit in blood assumes the same position as light in a candle, representing function and actuality of the latter (with reference to Aristotle, *De part. animal.* 649b 19–27; see Curtis loc. cit. on p. 135, 1951, p. 28). Harvey returned to the subject in *De motu*, Introduction, tr. Willis, p. 12, almost literally, and again in the *Second disquisit. to Riolan*, tr. Willis, p. 116 and *On generation*, Exerc. LXXI (of the innate heat), tr. Willis, p. 504. – The experimental proof against the entry of air into the heart is also found in the Introduction to *De motu*, tr. Willis, p. 16: when air is forced into the lungs of a dog by means of a pair of bellows and then the trachea is tied securely, abundance of air is found in the lungs down to the investing membrane, but none in either the pulmonary veins or the left ventricle of the heart. – Cooling action of the air thus remained its most likely function in the lung—an interpretation apparently abandoned by Harvey at a late date in his life. Curtis (p. 28) in this connexion cites *On parturition*, tr. Willis, p. 530: air is neither given for the "cooling" nor the nutrition of animals, for once the fetus has breathed it may be more quickly suffocated than if it had been entirely excluded from air; it is as if heat were rather enkindled within the fetus than repressed by the influence of the air (Willis' translation). See: Sir Henry Dale, *Some epochs in medical research. Harveian Oration*, London 1935, p. 12 (The meaning of respiration).

119 *Quaest. Peripat.* V, 4 fol. 121 verso with ref. to Aristotle 2 *de Respir.* and III *de Gener. Animal.* 10.

120 Aristotle, *De partibus animal.* lib. III, cap. 6; 669b; tr. Ogle, p. 75. See to this Ogle's note [7] on p. 205 with reference to *De respir.*, 20 where the distinction between jumping palpitation (*pedesis*) and ordinary heart action (*alsis* and *sphygmos*) is elaborated.

The Galenic subordination of cardio-vascular function to respiration—Cesalpinus' opposition and Harvey's criticism of Galen

Cesalpinus argues against this Galenic view in the fourth *Quaestio* of the fifth book of his *Peripatetic Questions* under the heading that there is *no access of external "spirit" (air) to the heart*[121].

Galen, he says, assumed a dual purpose for respiration: (a) the preservation of heat inside the heart which is accomplished by moderate refrigeration through air during inspiration and removal of smoke during expiration, and (b) the nutritional maintenance of animal spirit by air admitted in inspiration.

Aristotle, on the other hand, had denied the nutritional role of respiration, as fishes draw water and not air[122].

Nor, according to Aristotle, can heat be generated by spirit—it is rather the product of heated humours. Cesalpinus concludes that neither heat nor animal spirit are from the air, but that they derive from the nutritional fluid which flows from the stomach through the veins to the heart and is comparable to fuel. Air reaching the heart in any appreciable quantity should have to find ways and means of escaping from it again. If it did, what would prevent spirit and soul from escaping as well? For it is easier for spirit to escape into the open from a narrow and enclosed space than to go the opposite way, i. e. from the open into a narrow space that is already filled, namely with blood. Nor would the valves hinder its egress—for, on Galen's own showing, the two leaves of the mitral valve afford easy escape to smoky excrement from the heart with the breath in expiration. But what could possibly insure separation of spirits and air designed to remain in the heart from the smoke that has to leave it (*at quae separatio spirituum, et quae commixtio remanentis in corde aeris excogitari potest*)?[123]

Moreover a chain of absurdities would follow from the contrariety of movements which Galen's theory implies (*accedit motuum repugnantia*)[124]. The assumption is that in inspiration when the lung and thorax are dilated air is admitted to the heart which is dilated at the same time and that smoke escapes from it in expiration, i. e. when the lung, chest and heart are contracting. Hence the heart and lung must dilate and contract simultaneously. This, however, is at variance with the fact that the rate of respiration can be modified at will, whereas that of the heart beat cannot. In fact the former is normally less frequent than the latter.

If, on the other hand, it were assumed that air reaches the heart in expiration, in other words that the heart dilates when the lung is constricted, smoke would have to escape from the heart when

121 Quaest. Peripat., fol. 121 verso.

122 Aristotle, *De respirat.*, cap. VI; 473 a: It is certain that we must not entertain that it is for nutrition that respiration is designed. There is no generation of heat from the breath. Observation shows rather that it is a product of food. – cap. V, 472 b: It is non-sense that respiration should consist in the entrance of heat, for what is breathed out is hot and what is breathed in is cold. When it is hot we pant in breathing, for, because, what enters does not adequately perform its cooling function, we have as a consequence to draw the breath frequently.

Cap. VII, 473 b–474 a: Against Empedocles' theory that inspiration takes place through arterial pores that communicate with the outside world and alternates with a moving down of the blood and forcing out of air through the same pores—comparable to what happens in a water clock (*clepshydra*).

Cap. I, 470 b: It is untrue that all animals breathe. Ibidem: In animals with a bloodless and spongy lung there is less need for respiration. – Animals which have the lung charged with blood have greater need of respiration on account of their amount of heat.

Cap. II, 471 a: It is impossible for fishes to draw air and water, for these must meet and obstruct each other.

Cap. IV, 472 a: in hot weather we grow warmer, and having more need of respiration, we always breathe faster. But when the air around us is cold and contracts and solidifies the body, retardation of the breathing results.

Cap. XVI, 478 a: Respiration is the means of affecting refrigeration of which those animals make use that possess a lung as well as a heart. But when they, as for example the fishes, possess the latter organ without the former the cooling is effected through the gills by means of water. Tr. J. I. Beare. Oxford 1908.

123 *Quaest. Peripat.*, fol. 121 verso.

124 Ibidem.

the lung is inflated in inspiration—which is again plainly impossible.

Further absurdities result from a consideration of the pulmonary vein which is supposed to admit air (or spirit) from the lung into the heart. If, as Galen assumed[125], this vessel is endowed with pulsation (as it derives from the left heart and contains spirit), it should have a double pulse: one which it shares with the rest of the arteries—the pulse *ad motum cordis*—and another that corresponds to the movement of the lungs—*ad motum pulmonis*—from which it receives spirit through the bronchial tree. Dilating in inspiration and contracting in expiration, it would be subject to contrary motion engendered by the pulse of the heart which differs in time and rate from the respiratory motion of the lungs.

Still more absurdities are encountered in *Galen's doctrine of the pulse*. This he supposed to achieve for the whole body what respiration was to do for the heart, namely to receive air (spirit) from outside and to expel its product (smoke). It was to take place through the terminal parts of the arteries—air entering through the skin when these are dilated and smoke leaving when they are constricted. If that were true, Cesalpinus says, the arteries destined to distribute spirit from the heart would be unable to receive anything from the latter, as the multitude of terminal arterial openings (however small) would already fill them to overflowing.

If, however, that portion which is received from the heart exceeds in quantity the rest of the air (spirit) received through the terminal arteries the former must be so hot that it cannot serve for refrigeration of the innate heat. Indeed the heat inside the heart and that attracted by the dilating arteries would be greater than any refrigeration obtainable by reception of outside air.

What would be the purpose of the pulse after all? It would not be the preservation of the heat, for this, in Galen's opinion, is accomplished by respiration. The pulse would therefore be superfluous.

In the last resort, Cesalpinus *concludes*, all these absurdities are due to Galen's insistence that it is a *special faculty* that makes the heart dilate and thus draw blood from the vena cava and spirit from the pulmonary vein and contract for the expulsion of smoke into the lungs and of spirit into the aorta.

Galen's Pulse-making Force

It is the same faculty which was assumed to be transmitted from the heart to the arteries through their coats (*tunicae*), and to account for the arterial pulse[126]. There is no need for such a pulse-

125 GALEN, *De Anatomicis Administr.* lib. VII, cap. 4; ed. Kühn vol. II, p. 596: It is impossible to perceive the pulsation of the arteries inside the lungs, but one may assume (suspect) their arterial nature from their continuity with the left ventricle (tas d'en to pneumoni diagnonai me pany ti saphos aisthesei dynaton esti sphyzousas. ek de tes pros ten aristeran koilian synecheias auton hyponoeseien an tis).

126 GALEN, *De anatomic. administrat.* lib. VII, cap. 16, ed. Kühn, vol. II, p. 646–647 —the experiment supposed to demonstrate the *vis pulsifica*. Galen's experiment was repeated and finally disproved by FORRESTER, J. M., *Proc. R. Soc. Med.* 1954, XLVII, 241 and AMACHER, M. P., *Arch. f. Gesch. d. Med.* 1964, XLVIII, 177–180. See also p. 212 and note [10d].

making force (*vis pulsifica*). Distension of the heart and arteries is brought about by the heat of the blood and its conversion into spirituous blood. If the heart were dilated by dint of a special faculty at the time when the ebullition of the spirit subsides, then contraction would have preceded it at a time when the spirit was rising and expanding. If it were dilated, however, when the spirit, rises, the latter would be enough reason for the cavity to enlarge.

Indeed Aristotle was nearer the truth: if pulsation of heart and arteries is a secondary phenomenon (*accidens quoddam*) to the effervescence of the fluid in the heart, then all arteries should dilate simultaneously and at the same time as the heart[127]. This dilatation is due to the ebullition of the blood—through the latter blood is perfected, the arteries are filled and spirit is distributed throughout the body[128].

When this is accomplished the empty artery subsides. The continuous repetition of this cyclical movement—inflation and subsidence—of the heart and arteries is the pulse, and through it the continuous and most rapid distribution of spirituous blood into all parts is insured. It carries with it aliment which remains in a condensed and coagulated form in the organs after its spirituous component has evaporated into the ambient air. It is thus that the heart and arteries pulsate at the same time—to deny this is to deny sense and to doubt reason (*est negare sensum et quaerere rationem*)[129]. For the pulse is the means of sending out the contents of the arteries and it is for this reason that the veins which do not do so, but merely serve for the intromission of the vascular contents do not pulsate. Hence the vessel coming from the right heart pulsates in the lung, for it receives blood from the heart just as does the aorta, and is similar to the latter in structure. The vessel to the left ventricle, however, does not pulsate, as it merely admits blood and has its structure in common with the other veins[130].

Cesalpinus' main points and Harvey's Prooemium

The main points of Cesalpinus' argument are therefore directed against:

1. Galen's assumption of a simultaneous motion and function of the heart and lung

2. Galen's inference that air (or a product of air) enters the left heart and provides spirit, and that its smoky excrement leaves the heart

3. Galen's interpretation of the pulse as the means of maintaining innate heat and spirit by cooling

127 ARISTOTLE, *De vita et morte*, cap. II (*De respirat.* XX), 480a: all the veins pulse and do so simultaneously with each other owing to their connexion with the heart... palpitation, then, is the recoil of the heart against the compression of the cold and pulsation is the volatilization of the heated fluid (kai sphyzousin hai phlebes pasai, kai hama allelais, dia to ertesthai ek tes kardias ... anapedesis men oun estin he ginomene antosis pros ten tou psychrou synosin, sphyxis d'he tou hygrou thermainomenou pneumatosis). ED. BEKKER, Oxon. 1837, tom. III, p. 353; tr. J. I. BEARE, Oxford 1908.

The passage was referred to by Harvey as well: *De motu*, cap. III, 1628, p. 25; tr. WILLIS, p. 25. In addition Harvey refers to *Hist. animal.* "III, 9" which is actually found in III, 19 (old III, 14): blood palpitates in all animals within their arteries ("veins") *everywhere simultaneously* (sphyzei de to haima en tais phlepsin en hapasi pante hama tois zoois; tr. D'ARCY W. THOMPSON, Oxford 1910: "alike all over their bodies"; tr. R. CRESWELL, London (Bohn), 1862: "alike in all animals").

128 ARISTOTLE, *De Vita et Morte* loc. cit. (in note [127]) 479b: there is a similarity between the beating of the heart and boiling, for boiling is due to the volatilization of fluid by heat and the expansion consequent on increase of bulk (esti d'homoion zesei ... he gar zesis ginetai pneumatoumenou tou hygrou hypo tou thermou. airetai gar dia to pleio ginesthai ton onkon).

129 *Quaest. Peripatet.* fol. 122 recto.

130 Pulsat igitur in pulmone vas dextri ventriculi, hoc enim e corde recipit ut arteria magna, et similiter fabricatum est eius corpus. Vas autem sinistri ventriculi non pulsat, quia introducit tantum, et eius corpus simile est reliquis venis. *Quaest. Peripatet.* fol. 125 verso F.

4. Galen's idea of a special faculty controlling cardiovascular contraction and dilatation.

By contrast, Cesalpinus stipulates that the heart and arteries expand simultaneously and that this dilatation occurs when the main driving force in the cardio-vascular system is at work—namely the ebullition of blood that is heated up in the heart, as soon as it reaches the latter through the veins. Effervescence of blood and its consequence—the dilatation of the heart and arteries—is followed by subsidence or contraction. This "cyclic" sequence is the pulse—a continuous movement that serves the rapid distribution of aliment and spirit to the periphery.

Because of its continual repetition this cyclic effervescence and subsidence of the blood which forms the main driving force behind it is seen as a "circulation", i.e. a process of distillation (p. 188). It is the pulse which maintains this circulation which is in fact a dual one. It is true that Cesalpinus uses the term *circulatio* only with reference to the blood that reaches the lung from the heart through the pulmonary artery. He does, however, hint at the same mechanism for the blood that is driven from the left heart into the aorta and provides spirit and nutrition for the peripheral organs (p. 189; 204).

It is immediately evident how far Cesalpinus is led astray by his loyalty to Aristotle and hostility to Galen. Indeed he seems to deprive the heart of any physical and mechanical function of its own and to reduce it to a nidus for the formation of truly nutritious and spiritual blood. It is the latter which initiates and maintains its movement by its own power and impetus.

And yet it is through this anti-Galenic argument—retrogressive in many ways—that Cesalpinus anticipated some of the critical points which were later raised by Harvey and led to the vista of a dual "circulation".

These points are among those with which Harvey opened *De motu cordis et sanguinis*, in the introductory *Prooemium* in which he professes to show "that what so far has been written on the motion and use of the heart and arteries stands on insecure grounds[131]".

1. Most anatomists, physicians and natural philosophers agree with Galen that pulse and respiration have an identical purpose. Thus Fabricius of Aquapendente regarded the lungs as the instrument for the ventilation and refrigeration of the blood, for which the heart and arteries by themselves would not be sufficient. The motion of the heart and the arteries, their systole and diastole, have consequently been looked upon in correlation with the movement of the lungs.

131 *Prooemium* quo demonstratur quod quae hactenus scripta sunt de motu et usu cordis et arteriarum minus firma esse. HARVEY, *de Motu Cordis* ed. princ. Francof. 1628, p. 10.

But the structure as well as the movements of the heart differ fundamentally from those of the lungs and the motions of the arteries from those of the chest[132].

2. The arteries are commonly supposed to draw air into their cavities in diastole and to emit smoky excrement in systole by the pores of flesh and skin.

But, then, Galen himself wrote a treatise to the effect that the arteries contain nothing but blood. Moreover if it were true that the arteries draw air, submersion of the body in a bath should immediately change the pulse, as no further air could enter and no smoke could leave[133].

3. If the arteries emit smoke in systole, why not also the spirit which they are supposed to contain as well, as spirits are much finer than smoky vapours?[134]

4. From the cooling and paralysing effect of arterial ligature, it would appear that the arteries carry heat to the parts rather than serve for fanning and refrigeration[135].

5. How can the arteries draw spirit from the heart in order to convey heat to the body, and at the same time air from without with the result of cooling and tempering it?[136]

6. If the arteries are said to be filled not only with blood (sc. from the heart), but also with air from the ambient atmosphere, how and when can they receive blood from the heart? If in (arterial) systole, this will be quite impossible, for the arteries would have to fill up while contracted—they would have to fill up and yet not dilate. If in diastole, they would receive blood and air, heat and cold, for contrary purposes at the same time—which is unlikely[137].

7. The artery is distended by the impulse of the blood, and it is not so by Galen's *vis pulsifica* which he supposed to emanate from the heart and to extend through the coats of the arteries. This is shown by arteriotomy and in wounds: for the blood is poured out from the arteries with a spurt (*saliendo*) under an impulse (*cum impetu*), now farther, now not so far, "leaping by fits", and the leaping always takes place in (arterial) diastole, never in systole. The artery, by its own force, could not throw the blood with such strength. Indeed they are filled like bladders or leather bottles—they are not filled because they expand like bellows (*arterias distendi, quia replentur, ut sacculi et utres, atque non repleri, quia distenduntur ut folles*)[138].

8. Acceleration of pulse and respiration during exercise does not prove an identity of purpose for the two functions—for against this there is the experience that by immoderate repletion the pulses grow greater and breathing lesser, and in young persons

132 Cum vero aliter se habeat motus, et constitutio cordis, quam pulmonum, aliter arteriarum quam pectoris, alios exinde usus et utilitates, exoriri verisimile est, differreque plurimum cordis, et similiter arteriarum pulsus, et usus, a pectoris et pulmonum. Ibid. p. 10–11. Tr. WILLIS p. 9.

133 Ibid. p. 11; tr. WILLIS p. 10.

134 Et si in systole arteriae per poros carnis et cutis, fuligines e cavitatibus illorum expellunt, cur non item spiritus, quos dicunt etiam in illis contineri, cum spiritus multo tenuiores fuliginibus sint ibid. p. 11; tr. WILLIS p. 10.

135 Magis arterias calorem partibus deferre, quam refrigerium, et eventationem. Ibid. p. 12; tr. WILLIS p. 11.

136 Quomodo Diastole simul spiritus a corde attrahat, ad caleficiendas partes, simulque ab externo refrigerium? Ibid. p. 12 tr. WILLIS p. 11.

137 Nam si etiam aere ab ambiente repleri dicant, quomodo et quando recipient e corde sanguinem? Si in systole id fiat, continget impossibile repleri arterias, cum attrahantur, vel repleri et non distendi; sin autem in Diastole, in duos usus contrarios, et sanguinem, et aerem, et calorem, et frigus simul recipient; quod est improbabile. Ibid. p. 13; tr. WILLIS p. 12.

138 Ibid. p. 13; tr. WILLIS p. 12. – Ibid. p. 14; tr. WILLIS p. 13: Impulsu sanguinis arteriam distendi.

Willis' translation in this passage is rather free: for the blood spurting from the arteries escapes with force, now farther, now not so far alternately or in jets. The early English translation (London 1673, p. 6): "the blood is poured out of the arteries with a forcible leaping, sometimes farther, sometimes nigher, leaping by fits" seems preferable (in arteriotomia ... sanguis enim saliendo ab arteriis profunditur cum impetu, modo longius, modo propius, vicissim prosiliendo, et saltus semper est in arteriae Diastole, et non in Systole).

the pulse is quick whilst respiration is slow. So it is also in fear, care and anxiety of the mind; sometimes in fevers the pulses are frequent and respirations slower[139].

9. The heart is commonly regarded as the fountain and workshop of the vital spirit—yet the right ventricle is denied this function and merely supposed to provide nutriment for the lungs. But how can this be reconciled with the structure, identical in both ventricles? In other words, how can one possibly serve the "private" office of nourishing the lungs, and the other the "public" office of providing for the whole body? As Realdus Columbus already stated, the size of the pulmonary artery and the quantity of blood passing through it far exceed anything that the lungs could claim for their keeping. Moreover, what is the use of the pulse of the right ventricle if this were its only function?[140]

10. The left ventricle is supposed to receive air and blood from the lungs and to return smoky vapour to the latter. If that were so, how and by what means is the separation of spirit (to be propelled into the aorta) and smoke (to be ejected into the lungs) effected, in other words, how can spirit and smoke pass hither and thither without mixing and confusion (*quid est quod separationem facit, et quo modo huc illuc spiritus et fuligines citra permistionem aut confusionem commeant*)?[141]

Moreover if the mitral valve is not made to prevent the egress of smoke to the lungs, how should it oppose the escape of air?

If they will have it that smoke runs from the heart and air to the heart through the same canal, surely Nature is not wont to design (*fabricare*) one and the same vessel and pathway for such contrary motions and uses, nor is this seen anywhere[142].

In addition to these ten points from Harvey's *Prooemium* we may refer to the third chapter of *De motu* where Harvey inculcates the simultaneous filling of the arteries by the pulse—comparing them to the fingers of a glove being blown up. Like Cesalpinus Harvey refers in this connexion to Aristotle's opinion expressed in a passage of *De vita et morte* (as appended to his treatise *On respiration*) and adds a concurrent passage from the *Historia animalium* (see above, footnote 127).

If we compare these points from Harvey's *Prooemium* with the four points in which we summarised Cesalpinus' argument against Galen and in favour of Aristotle (p. 204), the similarity is obvious and hardly accidental.

This parallel is no proof nor even forms a piece of circumstantial evidence that Harvey used Cesalpinus' points or was influenced by them. For we must not forget that Harvey's argument con-

139 Ibid. p. 15, tr. WILLIS p. 14.

140 Ibidem, p. 16; tr. WILLIS, p. 15.

141 Ibidem.

142 Ibidem, p. 17; tr. WILLIS, p. 15–16.

tains one essential point in which he fundamentally differs from Cesalpinus: diastole and systole of the heart and arteries cannot be simultaneous. For how, asks Harvey, can two bodies that are connected with each other attract or draw anything from one another when they are simultaneously distended, or, contracting simultaneously receive anything from each other?[143] By contrast, Cesalpinus believed as we have seen, in the simultaneous dilatation of the heart and arteries—the result of an ebullition of the blood which also provided its driving force.

It should be borne in mind, however, that according to Harvey the whole movement of the heart is initiated by the ebullition, the "seething" of the blood as a part that is possessed of sensibility and intrinsic motion.[143a]

In making the ebullience of the blood the main driving force that controls the movement of the heart and arteries Cesalpinus closely followed the Aristotelian lead.

This idea, however, was by no means alien to Harvey. On the contrary, it was intimately associated with his categorical denial that any suction or attraction might be operative in diastole. Instead, according to Harvey, diastole was indeed brought about by the ebullition of the blood, and systole followed it as a reactive contraction. Thus, as Curtis said, "the Harveian heart beat is caused and initiated by an Aristotelian swelling up of the hot blood", although Harvey shifted the Aristotelian emphasis on the heart as the prime source of innate heat to the blood. It was Harvey, however, who "established anew the Aristotelian seething, making this the result of what we to-day may style a localised automatism of the conjoined heart and blood. He has localised this automatism of the hot blood in the vena cava, close to the base of the heart and to the right auricle, i. e. close to that region ... where the physiology of to-day places, not within the blood but in the texture of the walls which contain it, the seat of what is prepotent in determining the rhythm of the mammalian heart beat[144]".

In arriving at this modern view, however, Harvey was clearly foreshadowed by Cesalpinus. It is true that the latter had no clear conception of systole and diastole and remains far behind Harvey and for that matter even Columbus[145]. Harvey distinctly limited the action of the seething blood to the causation of diastole, while deriving systole and the consequent motion of the blood from the muscular force of contraction inherent in auricles and ventricles. In doing so, however, he referred to Aristotle whose opinion of the heart's pulsation—namely that it is produced after the manner of ebullition—he thought to be in some measure true.

143 Amplius cum affirmant, simul Diastolen cordis et arteriarum esse, et simul systolen, alterum est inconveniens. Quomodo nam cum simul distenduntur duo corpora a se invicem connata, alterum ab altero attrahat, vel cum simul contrahuntur, alterum ab altero recipiat aliquid? Ibid. p. 13; tr. WILLIS p. 12.

143a *Sec. Exerc. to Riolan*, ed. Roterod. 1649, p. 114; tr. Willis p. 132.

144 CURTIS, *Harvey's views*, loc. cit. 1915, p. 89–90. See Harvey's letter to R. MORISON, 1652, (tr. WILLIS, p. 604; *Opp.* Lond. 1766, p. 620–626) expressing much hesitation towards a recognition of Pecquet's discovery of the receptacle of chyle and the thoracic duct.

145 See the discussion above, p. 155 and 205.

Diastole, then, in Harvey's own words, is produced by the blood that swells up as if with interior spirits or the internal heat—a movement that is also regulated by the soul in conformity to nature, and is kept up for the health of living things. Pulsation in so far as it involves expansion and dilatation is thus accomplished by the blood, whereas systole is produced by the membrane of the vesicle in the *ovum* and later by the auricles and ventricles. These two alternating movements propel the blood through the whole body, and thus the life of animals is perpetuated[146].

In conclusion it must be admitted that Cesalpinus' critical argument against Galen does include essential points that were taken up and utilised on a higher level by Harvey.

In spite of some fundamental differences from Harvey and although lacking any certainty and synthesis, Cesalpinus remains an important forerunner of Harvey—if not the most important. He owes his kinship to the world of Harvey to his adherence to Aristotle and the Peripatetic tradition.

146 *Second Exercit. to Riolan*, ed. Roterod. 1649, p. 128; tr. WILLIS, p. 137: neque eandem esse causam diastoles et distentionis, quae systoles et contractionis, sive in arteriis, sive in auriculis, sive ventriculis cordis, arbitror: sed pulsus pars quae dyastole dicitur aliam habet causam a systole diversam ... distentionis primam causam, calorem innatum esse, primamque distentionem esse in sanguine ipso (fermentantium in modum) sensim attenuato et turgente, in eoque ultimo extinctam puto. Aristotelis, pultis vel lactis in modum, exemplo assentior ... – *On generation* Exerc. LI, ed. 1662, p. 191; tr. WILLIS, p. 375: distentio ... sanguini competere: constrictionem vero, a vesicula pulsante in ovo (ut a corde in pullo) propriis fibris institui ... certumque est, vesiculam dictam et cordis auriculam postea (unde pulsatio primum incipit) a distendente sanguine, ad constrictionis motum incitari. Fit, inquam diastole, a sanguine ab interno quasi spiritu intumescente: adeoque Aristotelis sententia, de pulsatione cordis (fieri enim scilicet ad motum ebullitionis) aliquatenus vera est with ref. to Aristotle, *De respirat.* XXVI (XX); 479b–480a: similarity between the beating of the heart and boiling; the beating is produced by expansion through the action of heat constantly supplied by food. It occurs when the fluid rises to the outer wall of the heart, and it goes on continuously ... all the "veins" pulse, and do so simultaneously with each other, owing to their connexion with the heart. The heart always beats, and hence they also beat continuously and simultaneously with each other and with the heart (see for this also: *Historia animal.* lib. III, cap. 19; 521a).

VI. Harvey – the Predecessor of Harvey

Introduction: The Spark that lit up Harvey's Way to Discovery

What made a genius of the past arrive at his discovery? Was it a chance observation which, like a spark, touched off a chain of thoughts leading to it? Or was it the whole scenery of the time set ready for the discovery to be accomplished? Was it the treasure of contemporary knowledge, experience and ideas out of which it emerged as from "the air", the climate of a time that was ripe for it?

In Harvey's case the answer seems to be easy, at all events at first sight.

As Robert Boyle was told by Harvey himself, it had been a meditation on the venous valves which had stimulated his new view and vision[1]. Here, then, we have a well defined single and leading observation, interpretation and trend of thought.

However, the present day observer may find it difficult to separate this point from several other facts and ideas with which Harvey's correct view of the purpose of the venous valves and thereby of the direction of the venous blood flow seems to be bound up.

1 "That so provident a cause as nature not so plac'd many valves without design" BOYLE, ROB., *A disquisition about the final causes of natural things wherein it is inquired whether and (if at all) with what cautions a Naturalist should admit them*, London 1688, p. 157. – "Boyleius physicus ille celeberrimus, in libro, quem de finibus rerum naturae conscripsit, narrat Harveium illi dixisse primam lucem sibi sanguinis itinera perlustranti a valvulis venarum Fabricio ab Aquapendente primum observatis effulsisse. Cum enim ex forma atque nexu valvularum pateret sanguinem a corde venarum ductu in singulas corporis partes deduci non posse; nec naturam labore irrito et inani artificio valvulas illas construxisse certum esset; nihil verisimilius excogitari posse sibi visum esse, quam sanguinem a corde arteriarum ramulis quaquaversum deferri, venarumque finibus exceptum in cor rursus reportari; siquidem a venis in cor via pateat, sanguini vero nitenti contra

First: the uniform "look" of the venous valves towards the major trunks and the heart, suggesting a directional arrangement identical with the semilunar valves at the aortic and pulmonary arterial conus[2]. From this the uni-directional course and in turn the oneness of the blood[3] seem inescapable conclusions. This, in a broader setting, would amount to a recognition of the singleness not only of the blood, but also of its source: the heart. Blood came from it and went back to it. This, however, was the old Aristotelian view[4]. Against it there was the Galenic doctrine which had made provision for two separate kinds of blood: the nutritional blood of the veins and the spirituous blood of the arteries. Accordingly two different sources had been stipulated: the liver for the former and the heart for the latter. Harvey took the Aristotelian view and in doing so was fully conscious of the historical connexion. He was even dogmatic about it and tried to argue against the obvious differences between arterial and venous blood and their significance[5]. As we have seen Galen had already talked about a "yellowish" tinge of the arterial blood—*xanthos*, *flavus*, he had called it, a term that had later been revived by Vesalius and Servetus[6].

No doubt, Harvey knew best what had ignited the spark of his discovery, and there seems to be no place for speculation as to what else might have. Nevertheless we cannot separate the single "spark", in his case the venous valves, from the tangle of ideas which seem indissolubly bound up with it and form the complex background of his discovery. Nor would it be easy to say which came first: idea or observation, or even philosophy or observation. As we have endeavoured to show (p. 54) there is support for the view that indeed the idea came first. Harvey had been a staunch Aristotelian all the time—by upbringing as well as by inclination. Perhaps this and all that it had taught him about the heart and blood influenced the way in which he looked upon the venous valves. So possibly did his firm conviction of the oneness of the blood—a point that has been rightly emphasised as a leading idea in Harvey's mind[7].

There is, then, a marked contrast between the scarce hints which illuminate the development of the discovery in Harvey's, the discoverer's, own mind and the bulk of information which we possess about his predecessors. Nothing had been published by Harvey before his masterpiece made its somewhat diffident appearance in Germany, a country stricken by the Thirty Years' War at its height and setting its stamp on the production of one of the greatest and at the same time least sumptuously produced books of scientific literature.

valvulae opponantur. Hac felici conjectura usus rem omnem experimentorum indicio patefecit." T. LAWRENCE, *Harvei vita* in: *Guilelmi Harveii Opera omnia: a collegio medicorum Londonensi edita.* 1766, p. XXIII. – On the place of this matter in Boyle's qualified teleology and—deistic—natural theology: PAGEL, W., *Religious motives in the medical biology of the XVIIth century. Bullet. Hist. Med.* 1935, III, 97–312 (p. 309).

The Boyle-passage fittingly appears as motto preceding the *Bibliographical Preface* in KEYNES, SIR G., *Bibliography of the Writings of Dr. William Harvey.* Cambridge 1953, p. 1.

2 *De motu* cap. XIII, 1628, p. 54–58; p. 57: "hoc, cum pluribus in locis experiri quis potest, apparet valvularum officium in venis idem esse cum sigmoidarum illarum trium, quae in orificio aortae et venae arteriosae fabrefactae sunt, videlicet: ut ad amussim claudantur, ne retro sanguinem transeuntem remeare sinant." WILLIS p. 66.

3 See for example: *Second disquisition to Riolan* ed. Roterod. 1649, p. 60 seq.: "contra eos, qui aliam speciem sanguinis in arteriis fingunt, quam in venis" p. 62: tria potissimum apta sunt ad hanc opinionem inducendam de diversitate sanguinis—followed by detailed rejection. Tr. WILLIS p. 113–116. Leading to the discussion of the *spiritus*.

4 "... since the veins are the place of the blood, while the origin of these is the heart —an assertion which is proved by anatomy —it is manifest that, when the external nutriment enters the parts fitted for its reception, the evaporation arising from it enters into the veins, and there, undergoing a change, is converted into blood, and makes its way to their source (the heart)"—tes thyrathen trophes eisiouses eis tous dektikous topous, ginetai he anathymiasis eis tas phlebas ekei de metaballousa exaimatoutai, kai poreuetai epi ten archen—ARISTOTLE, *De somno et vigilia* cap. III, 456b tr. J. I. BEARE, Oxford 1908; ed. Imman. Bekker, Oxford 1837 (*Opp.* vol. III), p. 294. See Caspar Hofmann's interpretation in *De thorace* lib. II, cap. 26, Francof. 1627, p. 58 et seq. and above, p. 199.

5 See above in note [3].

6 See in the present book, p. 137; 149; 164.

7 LORD COHEN OF BIRKENHEAD, *The germ of an idea or what put Harvey on the scent.* J. Hist. Med. 1957, XII, 102–105.

However, Harvey had made no secret of his opinions for some time before the publication of his discovery. The *Dedicatio* of his work bears witness to this: "I have already and on not infrequent occasions disclosed my new opinion regarding the motion and the use of the heart and the circuit of the blood in my lectures on Anatomy. Having now for nine years and more (*per novem et amplius annos*) confirmed it with the help of many ocular demonstrations in your presence ... I have acceded to so many requests by all and entreaties by some and made it public[8]".

With these words Harvey calls upon those who have listened to his *Lectures on the Whole of Anatomy* to support his case as being borne out by what they have been shown in dissections and ocular demonstrations. For, Harvey continues, as his book goes so much against the traditionally ruling opinion he would have felt himself open to a charge of presumption, had he not repeatedly and for some considerable time proposed its subject to his auditors, answered their doubts and objections and achieved the assent of the President of the College of Physicians.

Harvey's Lecture Notes on Anatomy and the Circulation of the Blood

What, then, could form a better source of Harvey's thought than his own notes for the *Praelectiones Anatomiae Universalis*, the Lumleian Lectures for 1616 and the following years that are extant in a manuscript in the Sloane Collection at the British Museum?[9]

However, these notes jotted down in a kind of colloquial Latin interlarded with short sentences or catchwords in the vernacular, do not seem to provide the clue.

It is true that they contain what looks like the first account of the circulation of the blood and what is more, in Harvey's own hand: "From the structure of the heart it is clear that the blood is constantly carried through the lungs into the aorta (*sanguinem per pulmones in Aortam perpetue transferri*) as by two clacks of a water bellows to rayse water. By means of a bandage it has become established that there is a transit of the blood from arteries into veins, wherefore the beat of the heart produces a perpetual circular motion of the blood (*constat per ligaturam transitus sanguinis ab arteriis ad venas. Unde perpetuum sanguinis motum in circulo fieri pulsu cordis*)[10]".

This indeed is the crucial statement, and also of great interest is the fact that it is immediately followed by the reflections of the true Aristotelian, the "lifelong thinker about the *purpose* of the circulation": "Is this for the purpose of the nourishment, or more for the conservation of the blood and members by the infusion of

8 "Meam de motu et usu cordis, et circuitu sanguinis sententiam E.D.D. antea saepius in praelectionibus meis Anatomicis aperui novam: sed iam per novem et amplius annos multis ocularibus demonstrationibus in conspectu vestro confirmatam, rationibus et argumentis illustratam et ab objectionibus doctissimorum et peritissimorum Anatomicorum liberatam, toties ab omnibus desideratam, a quibusdam efflagitatam, in lucem et conspectum omnium hoc libello produximus." *De motu* 1628, *Dedicatio* sig. A 3 recto. Tr. WILLIS p. 5 (with the unfortunate omission of: *et circuitu sanguinis*).

9 *Sloane 230.* First published in facsimile with transcript prepared by EDWARD SCOTT in: *Praelectiones anatomiae universalis by William Harvey.* London 1886. – O'MALLEY, C.D., POYNTER, F.N.L. and RUSSELL, K.F., *William Harvey Lectures on the whole of Anatomy. An annotated translation of Praelectiones anatomiae universalis.* Berkeley and Los Angeles 1961—to this see PAGEL, W., *An Harveyan prelude to Harvey Hist. of Science* 1963, II, 114–125. – WHITTERIDGE, G., *The anatomical lectures of William Harvey. Praelectiones anatomie universalis. De musculis. Edited with an introduction, translation and notes.* Edinburgh and London, 1964—an extensive work, containing a new transcript with improved reading throughout facing a new translation and equipped with critical apparatus and notes. It also provides a substantial Introduction and the first edition of Harvey's work on the muscles (Sloane 486). See W. PAGEL's review in *Medical Hist.* 1965, vol. IX, p. 187–190 and WILKIE, J.S., 1965, loc. cit. on p. 55, note [13a].

10 Fol. 80 verso.

heat; and in turn, is the blood that warms the members cooled down and does it carry heat again from the heart?" This statement implies the idea of a constant regeneration of the blood, its perpetual preservation by virtue of the circular movement that leads it from the heart and back to it—a special biological instance bearing out the Aristotelian idea of the preservative function of circular motion.

The Heart as a Pump

Harvey's summary of his discovery in the *Praelectiones* is also remarkable for introducing the comparison of the heart with a pump. This, however, was not as new as it is often presented. Galen had employed the comparison with the blacksmith's bellows (*hai ton chalkeon physai*, *fabrorum folles*) to illustrate the attractive action of the heart in diastole. The cavities of the heart, according to Galen fill up rapidly owing to its attractive faculties. These may be compared with the blacksmith's bellows that attract air when dilated (*diastellomenai sposin eiso ton aera*), the wick of a burning lamp that attracts the oil or else the magnet that attracts iron[10a]. Galen based this on a critical appraisal of the views of Erasistratus.

The latter had made a distinction between the heart which is filled because of the vacuum created therein—it is filled because it is distended—and the arteries that are distended while and because they are filled—the former acting like the bellows of the blacksmith, the latter like bladders. From this Erasistratus had concluded that distension and contraction of the heart and arteries alternate, a point that was supported by Riolan and Harvey against Galen who believed that the movements of the heart and arteries coincide[10b]. The idea that the arteries were filled like bladders was rejected by Galen outright; that they might move like bellows he admits for the sake of argument[10c], but does not really subscribe to any arterial motion by distension and contraction as assumed by Erasistratus. Instead he favoured an active pulse-making faculty that inheres in the heart and is propagated along the arterial walls[10d]. In Harvey's account the rejection of Galen's pulse-faculty and the experiment adduced to prove it follows accordingly the rejection of the simultaneous movement of the heart and arteries as maintained by Galen against Erasistratus.

At Harvey's time the comparison with a pair of bellows (*follis*) was employed by Riolan who was to become Harvey's most serious and persistent adversary[11]. I have observed, he says, that the heart is distended like a pair of bellows and compressed (*ego vero saepius observavi Cor instar follis distendi, et comprimi*).

10a GALEN, *De usu partium*, lib. VI, cap. 15; ed. Kühn vol. III, p. 481; tr. DAREMBERG, vol. I, p. 434.

10b GALEN, *De pulsuum differentiis*, lib. IV, cap. 2; ed. Kühn vol. VIII, p. 703; *De pulsuum usu*, cap. 4, ed. Kühn, vol. V, p. 164. HARVEY, *De motu*, ed. 1628, p. 13–14 (*Prooemium*); tr. WILLIS, p. 12–13.

10c GALEN, *De usu partium*, lib. VI, cap. 21; ed. Kühn, vol. III, p. 512; tr. DAREMBERG, vol. I, p. 455.

10d GALEN, *De pulsuum differentiis*, lib. IV, cap. 2; ed. Kühn, vol. VIII, p. 714. See above, p. 203.

11 RIOLANUS, JOH. (the younger), *Anthropographia et Osteologia* (1618), Ed. used, Paris 1626, lib. III, cap. 12, p. 371–372 and lib. VII, cap. 1, p. 658 (where the sentence quoted is found).

No such comparison, however, occurs in De motu of 1628; it is only found in the *Second Anatomical Exercitation on the Circulation of the Blood to Riolan*, of 1649. Here it says that the arteries have no inherent pulsative power, neither do they derive any from the heart, but that they undergo their diastole solely from the impulse of the blood ... precisely as in the water that is forced upwards, through leaden pipes, through the force and impulse of a bellow pump (*sipho*—fire engine), we can observe and distinguish individual compressions of the instrument (though they may be many stades distant) in the flux of the outcoming water, the order of the single strokes, a beginning, increase, end and vehemence, as from the opening of a cut artery[12].

The "clacks" mentioned in the *Praelectiones* are likely to refer to bellows as the use of the term *follis* by Riolan suggests, or more precisely correspond to the valves in "water-bellows" which ensure a uni-directional flow of the water—just as the atrioventricular and semilunar valves in the heart do for the blood. Like the latter the clacks were flexible, being made of leather, as Basalla has shown[13]. Early known examples of such "*Balg—or Sackpumpen*" go back to about 1460–1474 when they were used for emptying moats or filling wine vats. *Sipho*, the term used by Harvey in 1649, means fire-engine and evidence has been adduced by C. Webster that Harvey indeed meant the pumping device of a fire engine. One such engine which made use of the bellow pump was well known in London between 1625 and 1680[14].

Harvey's statement and the dating of his discovery

Harvey's short statement of his discovery in the *Praelectiones* thus remains of acute interest.

Unfortunately, however, there is nothing in the notes leading to it. It stands by itself on an otherwise empty space on the back of a sheet without internal connexion either with the foregoing or the following page of the manuscript. Indeed it breaks off with four dots after the last word—a dramatic tailing off which is clearly visible in the original[15]. Moreover it is written in a ductus that is different from the rest.

All this goes to suggest that it is an addition, inserted later than 1616–1618, when the bulk of the manuscript was written, and perhaps even much later[16]. This is also supported by the use of the comparison with the pump which is missing in *De motu* and cannot therefore have been of major significance for the discovery as such. It is another question whether its use in 1649 brings of ne-

12 Harvey, *Exercit. anat. secunda*, ed. Roterodami 1649, p. 121: quemadmodum cum aqua vi et impulsu syphonis, per fistulas plumbeas in altum cogitur, singulas compressiones instrumenti (per multa licet stadia distent) in ipso aquae exeuntis fluxu, singulorum ictuum ordinem, principium, incrementum, finem, vehementiam observare et distinguere possumus, ita ex abscissae arteriae orificio. Tr. rather "freely" by Willis, p. 135.

13 Basalla, G., *William Harvey and the heart as a pump. Bullet. Hist. Med.* 1962, XXXVI, 467–470, referring (for the definition of "clack") to John Bate, *The mysteries of nature and art* (1634), third ed. London 1654, p. 13 and for an early example of water bellows to the German translation of Vegetius of 1511. – See also: Whitteridge, 1964, loc. cit. in note [9], p. L–LI.

14 For early examples of "*Balg-Pumpen*": Feldhaus, F. M., *Die Technik der Vorzeit, der geschichtlichen Zeit und der Naturvölker*, Leipzig und Berlin 1914, p. 838, with ref. to Valturio (1472), the *Atlas* to the German Vegetius of 1476 (fol. 9 verso) and Mendel's *Portrait-Book* (fol. 194; Feldhaus' fig. 549 showing wine receptacles filled by means of a *Balg-Pumpe* in 1474).

On *Sipho*-fire-engine and its use in London, ab. 1625: Webster, C., *Harvey's conception of the heart as a pump, Bullet. Hist. Med.* 1965, XXXIX, 508. In this paper it is convincingly suggested that walter Warner [1550–1640]) was instrumental in Harvey's use of the concept, some time between 1628 and 1935 when the bellows pump fire engines were introduced into London. Warner was particularly interested in the heart as a hydraulic mechanism. – On Warner and his manuscript see Rolleston, G., *The Harveian Oration 1873*, London 1873; on p. 50: on the claims raised on Warner's behalf concerning Harvey's discovery. See also Bayon, H. P., *William Harvey, Annals of Sci.* 1938, III, 111–112 and ibidem, 1939, IV, 371–372.

On the term *sipho*, meaning fire-engine since antiquity and early examples see Feldhaus, loc. cit. in note [14], p. 308–316.

15 Pagel, W., *A Harveian prelude to Harvey, Hist. Sci.* 1963, II, 115.

16 This was mooted by Malloch, A., *William Harvey*, New York and Oxford 1929, p. 17 et seq. with reference to an earlier suggestion by Underhill, C. E., *Harvey as a teacher, Scot. Med. and Surg. J.* 1905, XVII, 109–129. It was further substantiated by O'Malley, Poynter and

cessity the date of the statement as far forward as this or not. As we mentioned, the comparison was used before the publication of *De motu*, i.e. some twenty years before it appeared in a printed work by Harvey.

The Lecture Notes on the Heart

What can we conclude from the rest of the *Praelectiones* concerning the development of the idea in Harvey's mind?

The main information should be expected from the chapter on the heart which starts on fol. 72 recto. The conclusion that has been drawn, however, is not unanimous. On the one hand it has been said that "it is from the fabric of these short notes on the heart that *De motu cordis* was built[17]". On the other hand it has merely been admitted that the lecture notes anticipate much of Harvey's knowledge of the movement of the heart as later incorporated in the first seven chapters of *De motu*, but that "from chapter VIII onwards all parallels with the *Praelectiones* cease[18]". What was anticipated in the Lecture-notes, however, was said to be nothing essentially new and "more or less in accordance with the findings of Galen and Columbus[19]". The latter is presented as "leading the way"—particularly in his demonstration that what was commonly called diastole was in fact systole and vice versa. At all events the circulatory idea does not seem to be even touched upon in the Lecture-notes—indeed from several passages Harvey appears to have been unaware of the centripetal direction of the venous blood[20]. Thus it has been pointed out that the venous valves and their setting—the crucial point that on his own showing led him to the idea—are barely mentioned in the notes[21]. We shall return to this below.

Evidently, the bulk of the notes does not contain any clear hint, let alone an exposition of the circulatory idea. But then, these notes do not constitute an original work, but were meant to aid the memory of a lecturer concerned with the wealth of the extant literature. Harvey here follows such textbooks as those of Bauhinus[22], Laurentius and others. Yet he saw the data which he found in the literature with the eyes of a critical and original observer with a sound sense for the correct way through a tangle of contradictory and confusing theories. Partly he achieved this through his own selective appraisal of the somewhat more correct idea of Columbus which at the time was still subject to controversy.

RUSSELL, 1961, loc. cit. in note [9] and in particular by WHITTERIDGE, 1964, loc. cit. in note [9]. – There is further evidence for the composition of the notes at various times after 1618, for example the note on the post mortem findings in Harvey's father (fol. 26 v) who only died in 1623 (see KEELE, as quoted in note [20] below).

17 O'MALLEY, POYNTER and RUSSELL, 1961, loc. cit. in note [9], p. 17.

18 WHITTERIDGE, G., 1964, loc. cit. in note [9], p. XLV.

19 WHITTERIDGE ibidem.

20 KEELE, K. D., *William Harvey as morbid anatomist*, *Proc. Roy. Soc. Med.* 1962, LV, 677–684: "in the 'Praelectiones' a branch of the azygos vein conveys the pleural fluid to the renal vein and so to the kidney along a fairly orthodox Galenic pathway. In '*De Motu Cordis*' Harvey suggests that such fluid is absorbed into the pulmonary vein, and passes through the left ventricle of the heart to reach the kidneys". For further examples see WHITTERIDGE, G., 1964, loc. cit. in note [9], p. XLVII–XLVIII.

21 WHITTERIDGE, 1964, ibidem.

22 Bauhinus as source to Harvey's anatomical lectures was emphasised by WHITTERIDGE, 1964, loc. cit. in note [9], p. XXXII et seq.

The Lectures and De motu cordis

However, though not explicit about the circulation of the blood, the chapter on the heart in the *Lectures* did in fact form the substructure of *De motu.* For the latter was meant to deal not only with Harvey's discovery, but also with its essential basis: the motion of the heart. Hence its title: *De motu* cordis *et sanguinis.*

Systole and Diastole. The Lead of Columbus.

Moreover even where Harvey follows the lead of Columbus in his lecture notes he is distinct and definite where Columbus remains ambiguous. Let us take for example the statement of Columbus repeated in its entirety, though with modifications, in the lecture notes and compare it with Harvey's own statement following it[23]. The former is admirable in itself and should not be reduced to a "wisp of wool"—*neque hoc floccifacias,* in Columbus' own words. Yet Columbus somewhat loosely states: the heart is pulled upwards and appears to swell when it is constricted. When it thrusts itself out (*exerit*), however, as if relaxed, it tends downwards and at that time the heart is said to be at rest: and this then is the systole of the heart, because it assumes it more easily and with less effort, whilst when it transmits (sc. the blood) it requires more force. Columbus follows this up with the warning that the matter should not be underrated in importance, for you may find not a few who are convinced that the heart is dilated at that time when it is really contracted[24].

In the *Lectures* as well as in *De motu,* Harvey tells us how difficult he found it to say what is systole and what diastole. In the *Lectures:* Though observing for whole hours I have not easily been able to discern them either by sight or by touch:... see how arduous and difficult it is to judge either by sight or by touch concerning dilatation or constriction and what in quality is of systole and what of diastole[25]. In *De motu:* I could not correctly distinguish how systole and how diastole occurred, nor when or where, or where dilatation and constriction occurred, because of the swiftness of the motion which in many animals offered itself to sight and then withdrew again in the twinkling of an eye or the flash of lightning; so that I thought to perceive now systole here and diastole there and then again everything was the opposite, the motions being varied and confused. Hence my mind wavered and I was ignorant as to what I should state myself and what to believe from others[26].

In spite of all this lingering doubt and the ambiguities besetting the subject, Harvey already in the *Lectures* had arrived at a clear-

23 *Praelect.,* fol. 77 recto et verso.

24 *Realdi Columbi Cremonensis De re anatomica libri XV* (1559). Francof. Martin. Lechler, 1593—the fourth edition and that used by Harvey—, Lib. XIV, *de viva sectione,* p. 474. The main *modification introduced* into the passage by Harvey is as follows: Columbus has "atque eo tempore dicitur cor quiescere: *estque* tunc cordis systol*e*", as against Harvey "*esseque* tunc cordis systo*len*" (italics are of the present author).

25 *Praelect.,* fol. 77 recto.

26 *De motu,* cap. I, ed. 1628, p. 20; tr. WILLIS, p. 19.

cut conclusion: Erection is the proper motion of the heart, for it is first strengthened and then relaxed and void of strength. Erection is systole: 1. it strikes the chest in the act of erection 2. from soft it becomes hard and can only be felt when erected ... 3. the auricles are visibly contracted, become whiter and the blood is thrust forth ... the pulse begins from the auricles and progresses towards the tip of the heart ...[27].

Harvey thus introduces distinctly termed physiological facts instead of the somewhat loose and vague terminology of Columbus: erection, a distinctly active movement, whereas Columbus had spoken of the heart as being pulled upwards. Harvey clearly identified this active motion as the proper movement of the heart and its systole.

Columbus—Riolan—Harvey on Systole and Diastole (pl. 39, 40)

By contrast Columbus inspite of his better and forwardlooking insight into the movements of the heart, had called systole what had been and is now termed diastole.

This is quite clear from the account given of the matter by Riolan and his rejection of Columbus' terminology. It occurs in his *Anthropographia* at two places[28]. Riolan says that according to Erasistratus diastole was due to a distracting and elevating movement of the heart and systole to the falling back and pressing together of its walls as in a pair of bellows (see above p. 212). Galen envisaged diastole as an attraction of the apex towards the base of the heart by the action of the straight fibres—the heart thereby becoming bigger and assuming a spherical shape, its "length being commuted into width" (*longitudine in latitudinem mutata*). In systole, he thought, the straight fibres relax and the apex is removed from the base by virtue of the transverse fibres. Riolan himself does not subscribe to this. He feels that the apex does not move by itself—it is the *immobile principium* around which the fibres pivot, as against the base which is soft and easy to move. Hence it is the latter that approaches the apex in diastole and recedes in systole. Riolan here adduces the observations of Volcherus Coiter[29]. The latter had found that in diastole the corrugated base is constricted and pulled down towards the apex, thereby gaining in roundness what it loses in breadth. The sides of the heart are thus distended and the conus drawn upwards. The motion of the heart, Riolanus continues, is similar to that of the auricles, but occurs at a different time. For when the heart is dilated the auricles are contracted and vice versa. In Galen's view the heart is filled because

27 *Praelect.*, fol. 77 verso.

28 RIOLAN, *Anthropographia* (1618), ed. used Paris. 1626 at the loci quoted in note [11].

29 COITER says that he would have agreed with the opinion of Columbus—*expulsion* of blood and spirit in "*diastole*" and *reception* (without attraction) in "*systole*"—but for the fact that the movements of the auricles are opposed to those of the heart. COITER, VOLCHER, *Externarum et internarum principalium humani corporis partium tabulae*, Noribergae 1573, p. 124–125.—For a general appreciation of Coiter as an original observer: HERRLINGER, R., Volcher Coiter (1534–76), Nürnberg 1952, p. 88–89.

it is distended, but the auricles are distended because they are filled, acting as they do as diverticula to be filled with blood and air during systole of the heart.

Riolan concludes: from the way in which the auricles are filled and emptied, Columbus' view is manifestly wrong. For he believes that in diastole blood and spirit were expelled whilst they were freely (though without attraction) received in systole. Riolan objects that active power (*robur*) is needed for expulsion.

Riolan returns to the subject later in his work. Many believe with Galen, he says, that the heart was dilated when by virtue of the straight fibres the apex was drawn towards the base and that the heart is contracted when by relaxation of the straight fibres and constriction of the circular ones the apex receded from the base. Again, Riolan refers to the divergent observations of Coiter which have shown that in diastole the corrugated base was constricted and drawn towards the apex and that in systole the apex was drawn towards the base. The latter was carried downwards when the apex was erected, ascended and lightly beats the chest wall. What the heart lost in breadth in the diastolic motion it recovered in roundness, whilst in systole the heart was thinner, broader, longer, more flaccid and pale. As against all this Riolan records his own observation according to which *the heart was distended and compressed like a pair of bellows* (*ego vero saepius observavi Cor instar follis distendi, et comprimi*)[30]. It was distended and dilated when, in diastole, it admitted venous blood and air, and constricted when, in systole, it expelled smoke and arterial blood. It should be noted, however, that the apex cannot be rolled back towards the base because of its hardness, nor can the base be brought back (*reduci*) towards the apex as it is firmly anchored to the great vessels. Riolan expresses doubts as to whether it was the apex which accounted for the heart beat, although it was obvious in the heart of a salmon removed from the chest (*exemptum*) that it was lifted up in a straight direction with a declination sideways (*Cor Salmonis piscis exemptum, quod manifeste recta sursum in motu elevari, atque ad latus declinare vidimus*)[31]. But, says Riolan, owing to the connexion of the pericardium with the diaphragm the heart apex was directed downwards—how could it then beat against the chest?

Meanwhile, Riolan concludes, you can *put aside the opinion of Columbus* about the movement of the heart—that when it is pulled upwards and seems to swell it is then constricted; but *when it is relaxed and tends downwards, that there is systole. For it receives with greater ease and less effort, but when it transmits it needs greater strength.*

This excerpt from Riolan which first appeared at the time of

30 RIOLANUS, Anthropographia, loc. cit. in note [11], p. 658.

31 RIOLANUS, ibidem, p. 659. – At the same place Riolan *opposes further Galenic ideas:* (a) in stating that the *artery is dilated when the heart is contracted and* (*b*) in *rejecting the pulse-making force of the arterial wall,* maintaining that the *pulse* is *due to the blood infused into the arteries by the heart*—for it persists when the arterial wall is damaged in aneurysm. This latter point was mentioned by HARVEY (*De motu,* Introd. tr. WILLIS, p. 14).

Harvey's Lumleian lectures (1618), is interesting in several respects. First of all it contains the comparison of the heart with a pump, or more precisely a pair of bellows. This is usually associated with Harvey; but, as we have seen (p. 212) the connexion is not as significant, prominent and early as is commonly believed.

Moreover, Riolan entertains views about the movement of the heart which formed an advance over the Galenic tradition (see note 31 above). In this he followed Coiter.

Finally, though remaining behind Columbus in certain points, he correctly insisted on calling the expelling motion of the heart systole and its receiving state diastole—against Columbus. So did Harvey, already in the *Praelectiones*: "*erectio est Motus proprius, vigoratur enim relaxatur enim et innervatur. Erectio systolen esse*". (Erection is the proper movement of the heart, it is made full of strength first, then relaxed and devoid of strength. Erection is systole.)[32]

Harvey had thus achieved a substantial step forward which led him to a position well ahead of Columbus and became instrumental in building up *De motu* some ten years later. This is well seen against the background of Riolan and the latter's rejection of the terminology of Columbus.

Original Observations in the Praelectiones

The *Praelectiones*, then, are *productive* of *original observations* and *interpretations*. Further examples are: the spurting out of blood at the heart's erection and the recognition that this causes the pulse; the implied assessment of the heart's movement as muscular action which had been denied by Columbus and above all the rejection of Galen's "pulse-making" force of the arteries in favour of his clear insight into the nature of the arterial pulse as the result of the thrusting forth of the blood by the heart (*hinc pulsus arterialis non ex innata facultate sed protrudente corde; ex autopsia vivo, mortuo, ex ratione, ex experimento ligaturae*)[33].

It is true that the *Praelectiones* are reticent about the movement of the blood in the veins or even contain hints that Harvey at the time of jotting down his notes still believed in its centrifugal direction. However, we find there the strange pronouncement that the "viscera are rather for the sake of the veins than the veins for the viscera" (*potius venarum gratia quam venae viscerum*)[34]. And all, Harvey continues, are for the sake of the innate heat and the blood.

With this we are reminded of a passage in the fifty second chapter of his work *On generation:* if the venous blood is considered as

32 *Praelectiones*, fol. 77 verso.

33 *Praelectiones*, fol. 77 verso and 78 verso. See on this point Riolanus, loc. cit. in note [31].

34 *Praelectiones*, fol. 38 recto and 35 verso.

a whole, there is nothing against the belief that it contains nourishment in itself, concocts it and serves it up to all parts of the body—thus nourishing and being nourished, forming both the matter and the efficient cause of the body[35].

In the light of this, written in a late period in Harvey's life and at all events after his discovery of circulation, the former passage from the *Praelectiones* may well indicate a tendency to connect the veins with the preparation of the material offered them by the viscera for the concoction of the blood, implying its direction away from the viscera.

This interpretation is not negatived, but rather strengthened by the Aristotelian reminiscences which it evokes and which may well have prompted Harvey in making his statement about the veins and their relationship with the organs. For it had been Aristotle who had located the first coction of the blood in the veins. The evaporation arising from the external nutriment, he had said, enters the veins, and there, undergoing a change, is converted into blood and makes its way to their source, namely the heart[35a]. Galen had retained this doctrine to some extent, leaving a subsidiary role in haematosis to the veins in order to allow additional time to the principal and primary blood formation which he allotted to the liver[35b].

Later on, in the *Praelectiones*, while dealing with the differences in wall texture between arteries and veins, Harvey speaks of an *attraction* to which the veins are subject, in contrast with the pulsating arteries, and gives as his original observation that the veins do not pulsate because of the valves which would break the pulse[36]. There is, then, a drawing action upon the veins and no pulse therein because of the adverse position of the venous valves. This may have been conceived in the traditional pre-circulatory trend of thought; on the other hand it may not.

In Conclusion:

The *Praelectiones* thus retain their historical value as a prime source for our knowledge of the development of Harvey's ideas. First and foremost in a positive sense: the ideas and observations which form the substructure of *De motu* and concern the movement of the heart are indeed essentially found in the *Lecture-notes* and thus go back to an early period in Harvey's life. Of his discovery itself, the circular movement of the blood, as based on the correct appraisal of the venous blood flow, we have no such evidence. Harvey himself intimated in 1628 that he had demonstrated and confirmed his personal view not only of the motion and use of

35 HARVEY, *De generatione*, Exercit. LII, ed. Amstelod. 1662, p. 202; tr. WILLIS, p. 386.

35a ARISTOTLE, *De somno*, cap. III, 456b 4–5. – In *De partibus animal.* lib. II cap. 3; 650a 27 seq. and III, 5; 667b 17, the role of the veins as a receptacle of aliment for the organs (*hai de phlebes hoion angeion haimatos eisi*) seems to be emphasised rather than their part in forming it.

35b GALEN, *De usu partium* lib. IV, cap. 13, ed. Kühn, vol. III, p. 306 et seq.; tr. DAREMBERG, CH. *Œuvres de Galien*, Paris 1854, vol. I, p. 310–311. Ibid. I, 16; IV, 12 and 17.

36 *Praelectiones*, fol. 80 recto.

the heart, but also of the circuit of the blood (*meam de motu et usu cordis*, et circuitu sanguinis *sententiam*) for nine years and more, taking us back to 1618, the very time of his Lumleian *Lectures on the whole of anatomy*. We have no reason to doubt his word—even if it is not fully borne out by fugitive lecture notes which are likely to have accumulated at various times. It would be unwise to attach over-optimistic expectations to them, but their historical importance for the history of Harvey is difficult to overrate.

Some controversial minor points

A look at the detail contained in the heart chapter of the *Praelectiones* is therefore likely to be rewarding.

1. The *central position of the heart:* The heart lies "in the centre" (*in medio*). It does so in three respects (*trifariam*): from it all measurements are taken, above-below, front-back, right-left. Hence it is not only the principal, but the most principal part (*principalissima pars*) because it occupies the most principal site (*locum principalissimum*) like the centre in a circle (*ut centrum in circulo*)[37].

This is essentially the Aristotelian doctrine as propounded in *Parts of the animals*[38]. However, Harvey gives it an interesting personal twist: he compares the heart to the centre of a circle. Aristotle had used no such comparison—he simply spoke of the *meson*, the middle of the chest, not the *kentron* or *kyklos* in this respect. Nor did Cesalpinus, the most prominent of the Aristotelians in Harvey's early days[39].

Harvey supplied the microcosmic analogy of which he made use in the *Dedicatio* and the famous eighth chapter of *De motu*. In Harvey's own time the heart had been compared with the centre of a circle by Giordano Bruno and before him by Charles Bouelles —both under the influence of the philosophy of Nicolaus Cusanus. We discussed this "circular symbolism" with reference to the heart and the motion of the blood and its significance for Harvey in another chapter of this book[40]. Here it may suffice to say that it is unlikely that Harvey based his analogy of the heart with the centre of a circle, and for that matter with the macrocosmic centre, the sun, on the works of Bruno. We have, however, every reason to believe that such ideas were popular in academic circles at Harvey's time, especially at Padua. Moreover Harvey's friendship with Robert Fludd, Rosicrucian symbolist and mystical naturalist, must be considered important in this respect—a point which was also discussed above[41].

37 *Praelect.* fol. 72 recto.

38 ARISTOTLE, *Parts of animals* lib. III, cap. 4; 666a: "en meso keisthai tou anankeiou somatos". Ed. Bekker, Oxon. 1837, p. 68. "There is a tendency in the heart to assume a similar position (i.e. in animals similar to man) in the centre of the necessary part of the body which terminates in the vent for excrement", tr. OGLE, W., *Aristotle on the parts of animals*, London 1882, p. 67.

39 "In medio est, qui locus est commodissimus, ut omnibus partibus vitam impartiatur." CAESALPINUS, AND., *Quaest. peripateticarum*. lib. V, quaest. 3 (1571), ed. used: Venet. 1593, fol. 115 verso.

40 See the chapter on *Circular Symbolism* in this book p. 112.

41 See ibidem, p. 117.

2. *Pericardium and Adamas:* Before and at the time when Harvey was preparing the Lumleian Lectures, much discussion was devoted amongst anatomists to such strange questions as to whether the pericardium was normally endowed with fat and the ante- and postmortal formation of pericardial fluid. Vesalius' famous observation of a post-mortal increase in pericardial fluid and its significance in the theological discussion of the blood and water exuding from the spear wound in Christ's body is a leading example[42], referred to by Harvey[43]. The latter incidentally recalls the concretion of the pericardial sac in a consumptive—an important morbid-anatomical observation—and finally cites a case report by Jasolinus, one of his lecturers at Padua, in which hydropericardium was connected with the suspicion of poisoning[44].

This is followed by a problem-passage: "Cachexia vel prava qualitate. W H remediis (? radiis)[45] veneni: ex pulvere: Adamas. comprensi (?, compensari?)[46] hic humorem et cor Aqua acrimoniae et salsedinis expers tam W H Nitrosum slippery scowring as in Butchers hands."

Only a conjectural interpretation can be offered: "Cachexia also comes from its (i.e. the pericardial fluid's) bad quality. WH (i.e. a personal note added to the literature) for remedies against poisoning; from powdered diamond fluid as well as heart are affected. Thus the fluid (is rendered) free of sharpness and salt and yet WH (containing) salt of nitre slippery scowring as in butchers hands."

This interpretation is based on the translation of *Adamas* by *diamond.* This makes good sense if it is remembered that the diamond formed a generally recognised item in the traditional list of mineral poisons—and antidotes.

Fernel, for example, placed it in the same class with sulphur, lapis caeruleus (a preparation from *nitre*, alum and vitriol used as *caustic* in the treatment of ulcers), mercury and cinnabar[47]. He also mentions *pulvis adamantis* among the corrosive remedies (*exedentia medicamenta*) which, like colocynth, can cause dysentery[48].

According to Cesalpinus the powdered diamond (*adamantem comminutum*) is regarded as an eroding poison against which there is no remedy. However, in Cesalpinus' personal opinion its effects are not due to the diamond, but to *argyrodamas*, a kind of talc[49].

What is perhaps more important in the Harveian context is the use of the *diamond as an antidote in poisoning: Adamas madendo venena irrita reddit*—the diamond renders poison ineffective by moistening[50]. This is probably the rationalisation of a very old and popu-

42 Vesalius, *De corporis humani fabrica*, Basil. 1543, lib. VI, cap. 8, p. 585; Pagel, W., *Vesalius and the pulmonary transit of blood. J. Hist. Med.* 1964, XIX, 327–341 (p. 332). – See above p. 159.

43 *Praelectiones* fol. 72 verso.

44 Jasolini, Julii Hipponiatae, *De aqua in pericardio*, cap. 2 at the end. In: *Collegium anatomicum Cl. trium virorum Jul. Jasolini Locri, Marci Aurelii Severini Thurii, Bartol. Cabrolii Aquitani.* Francof. 1668, p. 37. – In a case of sudden death with suspected poisoning hydropericardium was referred by Jasolinus to palpitation of the heart.

45 "WH radii venenosi" is the reading of Whitteridge, loc. cit. p. 248.

46 "Ex pulvere Adamas compensari hic humorem et cor" is the reading of Whitteridge ibidem—"Adamas compensari" marked as "doubtful" in the apparatus.

47 Fernel, Joh., *De abditis rerum causis*, lib. II, cap. 15 (*de venenatis morbis*). In: *Universa medicina* ed. J. and O. Heurnius. Traj. ad Rhen. 1656, vol. II, p. 513.

48 Fernel, Joh., *Pathologia* lib. VI, cap. 10 (*De morbis intestinorum*). Ibidem, vol. II, p. 167.

49 Caesalpinus, And., *Praxis universalis artis medicinae* lib. III (*de venenis*, cap. 32), Tarvisii 1606, p. 197. – Ibidem, *Katoptrum s. speculum artis medicae Hippocraticum*, Francof. 1605, p. 190.

50 This is one of the many miraculous effects of the diamond listed by Martin Ruland, *Lexicon Alchimiae s. Dictionarium Alchemisticum*, Francof. 1612, p. 5: in summa adamas ligat magnetem, et viribus privat. O Deus admirabilis in operibus suis! Ceterum adamas venena irrita facit, abigit lymphationes, lemures, incubos, succubos: reddit animatos fortes, propterea anachitis dicitur.

From the alchemical lit. see also: *Aureum vellus* lib. II, cap. 1 in *Theatrum Chemicum*, vol. V, 1622, p. 434: Adamanti vires divinas ... contra venena ac incantamenta amuletum esse praesentaneum testantur, qui adamantem praesente toxico madere confirmant. – See also: Rattray, Sylv., *Causae sympathiae et antipathiae* in *Theatrum sympatheticum* Norimbergae 1662, p. 24: Adamas madendo venena irrita reddit.

lar belief in the protective properties of the diamond against evil demons, the evil eye, possession, poison and mental disturbances of all kinds—properties that were attributed to the fiery sparkling and the sharp edges of the stone[50a].

Harvey's notes are jotted down in a Latin far removed from Ciceronian correctness and elegance; they bear evidence of haste in many places[51]. That he should have written the grammatically correct: *Ex pulvere Adamantis* instead of: *Ex pulvere: Adamas* cannot therefore be accepted as a legitimate objection.

The alternative interpretation of *Adamas* as *Adam* meets with insuperable difficulties. Apart from Gnostic writings[52] Adam is nowhere called Adam*as*, although Adam*us* occasionally occurs[53].

What is most important, however, is that *Adamas—diamond* makes sense in the present context.

3. *Cor a currendo:* Harvey makes that etymology of "cor" his own which is found in contemporary text-books of anatomy, notably that of Laurentius[54]. The heart is called *cor*, as it perpetually "runs" (*currere*). The word thus conveys its constant motion. Laurentius' definition sounds quite correct: "The Greeks call the heart *Kardia* and *Kradia* from *kradainesthai* which is to vibrate, *aei kinetos gar*, for in perennial motion the heart is moved." A possible connexion with the Arabic *kalb* from *kalaba*, to turn or to jump or skip, and the Hebrew *leb* may also be mentioned[55]. By contrast mediaeval writers such as Isidorus and other encyclopaedists, notably Bartholomew the Englishman, derived *cor* from *cura*, care[56].

4. *Principalissima pars non propria ratione... sed copia sanguinis.* The heart is the most principal part of the body, not because of its own structure which is hard, cool and fibrous, but because of the abundance of blood and spirits in its ventricles whence (a) it is the source of all heat (b) the right auricle in the recently dead looks like an inflammatory swelling[57], and (c) fishes have as it were a pool of blood.

With this, we believe, Harvey somewhat modifies his adherence to the Aristotelian primacy of the heart in favour of the blood—a point which is developed more fully shortly below this passage. Here it is also made quite clear that it is a personal and original view which Harvey wishes to express.

The heart, then, is indeed fortress and homestead of the heat, the household deity (hearth) of this building, fountain and conduit-head, as it imparts heat to all the parts without receiving it

50a The best *literary source* is KONRAD VON MEGENBERG's *Buch der Natur* (first half of the fourteenth century). It is based on Thomas of Cantimpré's Encyclopaedia from the thirteenth century. In Book VI, on precious stones, we find in chapter 3: "*Von dem adamas*... man sprichet auch, daz der stein guot sei in der zaubraer kunst: wer in tregt den sterkt er gegen seinem veint und vertreibt uppig traem und *schäuht und melt die vergift.* man spricht auch daz er switz, wenn vergift pei im sei... (adamas is useful in the magic art; he who carries it is strengthened against his enemy; it drives away bad dream and drives out and announces poison. It is also said to sweat when poison is near it). Ed. F. Pfeiffer, Stuttgart 1861, p. 434.

In certain cases the true meaning of *adamas* is steel and has often been confused with diamond in the history of magnetism, chemistry and metallurgy. To this the fundamental papers by E. O. VON LIPPMANN should be consulted: *Beiträge zur Geschichte der Naturwissenschaften und Technik*, Berlin 1923, p. 213 and vol. II, Weinheim, 1953, p. 158.

On the *popular beliefs* connected with the virtues of the diamond as prophylactic against evil demons and diseases caused by them some material can be found in *Bächtold-Stäubli*, *Handwörterbuch des Deutschen Aberglaubens*, vol. II, p. 194. The diamond was worn as an amulet, but also used internally as a "salt" or liquor, especially in epilepsy, although a warning was attached to the internal use, as it was thought to tear up the viscera.

51 For examples of grammatical mistakes: fol. 80 recto—unde venis plurimae valvulas. – Fol. 73 recto—puto enim ventriculi fieri. – Fol. 72 recto—medium corpori necessarii, and passim.

52 ADAMAS denotes the archetype of man in the writings of such Gnostic sects as the Ophites and Naassenes and frequently occurs in Irenaeus whose work was well known in Harvey's time, also in others, notably Hippolytus (whose book was not then known). With ref. to the Mandaeans see: LADY DROWER, *Adamas* in *Theolog. Litzeitg.* 1961, col. 173–180, as quoted by G. SCHOLEM, *Ursprung und Anfänge der Kabbala*, Berlin 1962, p. 136, n. 149, and eadem, *The secret Adam*, Oxford 1960.

53 PAGEL, W., *An Harveyan prelude to Harvey* loc. cit. 1963, in note [9], p. 122–123.

54 *Historia anatomica corporis humani* (1600) Francof. 1602, p. 746.

55 KRAUS, LUDW. AUG., *Kritisch-etymologisches medicinisches Lexikon*, 3rd ed. Göttingen 1844, p. 267.

from any of them. However, the heart assumes this principality, *qua* domicile of blood and heat, and not by virtue of specific structural merits of its own.

5. *The principality of the blood. Nec principalis origine ... ventriculi ... fieri ex gutta sanguinis:* Harvey's view is further strengthened by *embryological* observation. This is an important point to which Harvey returns in *De motu* as well as in his last great work *On generation*, and it is from the *Praelectiones* that we learn that he must have formed this view early in life.

In Harvey's opinion it is not the heart itself, as taught by Aristotle, but a drop of blood that is the first thing to develop in the fetus—*ventriculi fieri ex gutta sanguinis, quae in ovo.* Aristotle had emphatically propounded the first appearance and primacy of the heart in the embryo, as the *arche physeos* and *arche zoes*[58]. Harvey was consistent in this deviation from the Master, for in his last work, that *On generation* of 1651 we read: "So far as my observations enable me to conclude, the blood has seemed to go before the pulse[59]." We shall return to this later on in this book (p. 252).

Seen *ex post facto* and by way of a digression, one may even speculate whether this Harveian idea could have had a bearing on the vision that led to the discovery of blood circulation. The high priority and dignity of the blood—so Harvey may have felt—was incompatible with its consumption in the peripheral organs. Blood and heart were seen as a unit in which one is unthinkable without the other. The heart acted as the fountainhead of the blood for the body, but the blood in turn was the source of the heart. Hence it was not to be consumed in the periphery, but to return to it—moving in a circle.

Further support for the principality of the blood is derived from the observation that it is the abundance of blood that keeps isolated parts of the heart going. This seems to be the meaning of a passage which has caused some difficulty in interpretation. In the opinion of the present author it is connected with the ancient observation that

6. *the auricle is the last to die.* The passage may be read as follows: "in so far as it (sc. the heart) is distended and not contracted life is possible wherefore the auricle pulsates after the heart has been separated (? ceased to function), through the large quantity of blood[60]."

This would imply an explanation of the persistent movement of the auricles after death or for that matter after removal of the rest of the heart in terms of a persistent blood supply.

56 Isidorus Hispalensis *Liber etymologiarum* Venet. 1483, lib. IX, cap. 1 *de homine et partibus ejus*, fol. 56 recto; Bartholomaei Anglici *De proprietatibus rerum*, Argentinae 1491, lib. V, cap. 36, sig. f recto.

57 An allusion to Aristotle, *De respiratione* cap. XXVI (XX)—*de vita et morte* II—, 479b 27: the beating of the heart, which, as can be seen, goes on continuously, is similar to the throbbing of an abscess ... there is a similarity between this phenomenon and that of boiling; for boiling is due to the volatilization of fluid by heat and the expansion consequent on the increase of bulk ...

Aristotle, *Parva Naturalia* tr. J.I. Beare and G.R.T. Ross. Oxford 1908.

58 Aristotle, *De generatione animalium* lib. II, cap. 4; 740a. – Ibid. cap. 6; 741b–743b and elsewhere.

59 Quantum mihi observare licuit, videtur sanguis esse ante pulsum ... Exerc. XVII, ed. Amstelaed. 1662, p. 64; tr. Willis p. 237.

60 *Praelectiones*, fol. 73 recto.

The auricle as the "last to die" (*ultimum moriens*) is Galenic. Galen speaks of a weak and short motion which appears in the auricles after death—*amydra kai bracheia kinesis ... en tois osi tes kardias phainetai*[61]. Harvey refers to this in *De motu:* "and finally, all the other parts being at rest and dead, as Galen long since observed, the right auricle still continues to beat; life, therefore, appears to linger longest in the right auricle[62]." Between Galen and Harvey this observation had not been forgotten. It is not without antiquarian interest that it should have occurred in the "First English Anatomy" of 1532, a short, crude and rather philological recital of traditional anatomical lore[63].

Vesalius on the Auricles and the Passage under Discussion

What is even more important in our present Harveian context and palpably helps in its interpretation is what Vesalius has to say about the function of the auricles.

Following tradition he points out that the auricles act as a storeroom for the blood preventing its rush to the ventricles and a rupture of the thin-walled vena cava at the "impetuous" (*valido impetu*) attraction of the blood by the heart. They also help in the preparation of the blood that takes place in the ventricle. Vesalius emphasises the abundance of blood in the auricle (*sanguinis plena*). These functions, however, do not even seem to be the principal ones, which is apparent from their movement when the heart is completely collapsed *or in the living animal bisected in a transverse direction*—just as the auricles are observed to palpitate, to be distended and contracted when in the living animal the movement of the heart has already ceased and the ventricles are not dilated (*quod vel ex illarum—sc. auricularum—motu corde penitus concidente, et in vivis sectionibus transversim dissecto queas animadvertere, quoties in vivo animante cordis motu iam cessante, neque dilatatis cordis ventriculis, auriculas tamen adhuc palpitare, distendique ac contrahi observas*)[64].

Our passage from Harvey sounds almost like a scholion to the text of Vesalius just quoted. Emphasis is laid in both on the abundance of blood in the auricles (a traditional doctrine) and their continued motion after cessation of the movement of the heart as a whole and even then when the latter is transversely bisected in an experimental animal. This corresponds well to Harvey's: *unde auriculae pulsant post emotum cor sanguinis multitudine*[65]. In explaining the survival of the auricles, then, Harvey would seem to have begun by using the traditional item of knowledge of the abundance of blood flow through the auricles from the veins.

This interpretation is further strengthened by Harvey's reversion to the point later when discussing the ventricles[66]. Here he

61 GALEN, *De anatomicis administrat.* lib. VIII, cap. 15; ed. Kühn, vol. II, p. 641.

62 HARVEY, *De motu*, cap. IV, ed. 1628, p. 26; tr. WILLIS, p. 27.

63 EDWARDES, DAVID, *Introduction to Anatomy*, 1532, facs. reprod. with English translation by C. D. O'MALLEY and K. F. RUSSELL. Oxford 1961, p. 61–62.

64 VESALIUS, *De corp. humani fabrica*, Basil. 1543, lib. VI, cap. 15, p. 597.

65 *Praelectiones*, fol. 73 recto.

66 *Praelectiones*, fol. 74 verso.

speaks of the greater heat on the right side, "*and* the right auricle being the last to pulsate"—implying that it is the greater quantity of blood traversing the right heart which makes it hotter and maintains pulsation longest, as seen in the right auricle.

It should also be borne in mind that Harvey saw in the blood and its inherent pulsating movement the first stimulus for the motion of the heart. As we have discussed elsewhere (p. 208) it was the ebullience of the blood that in Harvey's opinion accounted for the distension in diastole which was to touch off the reactive contraction of systole.

Admittedly the reading of our passage from the *Praelectiones* is beset with difficulties. It baffled John G. Curtis some fifty years ago when he commented: "In his lecture notes Harvey says ... that the auricles pulsate after removal of the heart because of the multitudinous blood. But this jotting, written only as a brief reminder for himself, is obscure to others. By the word "heart" Harvey means sometimes the ventricular mass without the auricles and sometimes the ventricular mass and the auricles taken together. Hence it is uncertain whether the above reference be to auricles left attached to the body or removed with the ventricular mass. In neither case is it easy to imagine effective distension produced by the seething even of the "multitudinous blood". However in the same lecture notes a few pages further on (77v, l.15) Harvey says: "Nevertheless, the heart pulsates, cut away from the auricles[67]".

Nor are things made easier by the fact that Harvey wrote on top of "auricles": "ventr"—meaning ventricles. If the latter reading is chosen[68], the meaning would simply be: the ventricles continue to beat after the heart is removed from the body. This would correspond to the statement in *De motu* that the hearts of an eel and several fishes, taken out of the body, beat without auricles[69]. That the word used for "taken out" in *De motu* is *exemptum* and not as in the passage under discussion *emotum* seems of little consequence. But how are we to explain Harvey's main point that the continued beat is due to the abundance of blood, if we adopt the reading *ventricles*?

With the evidence at hand we would therefore *conclude* that our Harveian passage refers to the long survival of the auricle as due to the continued and abundant blood flow through it from the veins—a survival that can be seen when the function of the heart as a whole has ceased or else the rest of the heart has been removed (*emotum*). At all events it serves to show the principality of the blood which antedates the formation of the heart in generation,

67 CURTIS, J. G., *Harvey's views on the circulation of the blood.* New York 1915, p. 92.

68 As by G. WHITTERIDGE, 1964, loc. cit. in note [9], p. 250.

69 HARVEY, *De motu* cap. IV, ed. 1628, p. 27—cor anguillae, et quorundam piscium, et animalium etiam exemptum sine auriculis pulsat. Tr. WILLIS p. 28.

when a small pool of blood is seen at the site of the heart or possibly *only in the auricles* (*an est gutta tantum sanguinis in Auriculis*)[70].

7. *Heart disease as incompatible with life and the rarity of morbid changes in the heart*—the former being traditional knowledge, the latter given as an original Harveian observation. Harvey objects to Galen's assumption that the heart suffers from drying out in consumptives[71]. In the latter Harvey found the heart sound by contrast with the lungs which he always found consumed. He sides with Aristotle who referred the failure of the heart in old age to drying up of the lung: the source of life, Aristotle said, is lost to its possessors when the heat with which it is bound up is no longer tempered by cooling ... the lung in the one class and the gills in the other get dried up, these organs become hard and earthy and incapable of movement, and cannot be expanded or contracted. Finally things come to a climax, and the fire goes out by exhaustion[72]. And in a more general context: When bodies age they must become dry, and therefore the fluid in them requires to be not easily dried up. The reason why certain things such as fat do not easily decay is that they contain air; now air relatively to the other elements is fire and fire never becomes corrupted[73].

8. *The heart is the origin of all vessels*[74]—arteries as well as veins. This is the Aristotelian viewpoint, hotly contested at Harvey's time by the Galenists who regarded the liver as the origin of the veins and only granted the heart to be the source of the arteries. In Harvey's case this is merely a way of expressing and amplifying the primacy of the heart in the body. It has nothing to do with the blood flow in these vessels—derived as it is from the anatomical analogy between the ramification of the veins with that of the arteries and from the similarity in texture between the veins and the auricles. At the time of his decision in favour of the Aristotelian point of view Harvey may not have been in possession of the circulatory idea (see above p. 213)—yet Harvey's statement concerning the heart as the source of all vessels in itself cannot imply belief in a centrifugal venous blood flow.

This is well shown by the way in which Harvey describes in *De motu* the distribution of the veins that eventually form the portal vein. Here he speaks of a dissemination of the veins *in ventriculum*—*towards* or *upon* the stomach—and *in intestina*—just as the mesenteric vessels are *towards* or *upon* the gut. Similarly the vena haemorrhoidalis *deo sum in colon et longanonem usque deducitur*—the haemorrhoidal vein is aken downwards *towards* or *upon* the

70 *Praelectiones* fol. 73 recto.

71 *Praelectiones*, fol. 73 verso.

72 Aristotle, *De respiratione*, cap. XXIII (XVII)—De vita et morte I—479a 10.

73 Aristotle, *De longitudine et brevitate vitae*, cap. V, 466a 21. *Parva naturalia* tr. J. I. Beare and G. R. T. Ross, Oxford 1908.

74 W H hinc cur potius arterias oriri a corde quam venas non vidio. Quattuor digitis W H. *Praelect.* fol. 74 recto.

colon and rectum. The following text makes it quite clear that Harvey is fully conscious of the "returning" of the blood in these veins and its conveyance to the porta of the liver[75].

As we have seen (p. 178) the same applies to a similar pronouncement of Cesalpinus[76].

9. *The three ventricles of Aristotle.* Harvey expresses his surprise that Aristotle should have described three ventricles instead of two. But, he continues, Aristotle could have meant the left auricle —*nisi auriculam sinistram pro ventriculo salvare posse*[77]. In other words Aristotle's view is possible if we can *claim* (literally: *salvage*) the left auricle as a ventricle. It was T.H. Huxley who made precisely this interpretation of the Aristotelian doctrine his own in one of his classical essays[78]. Huxley demonstrated that for Aristotle the right auricle did not form a special compartment, but was merely the entrance lobby of the venae cavae. This seems to conform with Harvey's findings as given in the *Praelectiones:* the vena cava can be probed down to the groin when a rod is inserted into it—*vena cava Immisso Bacculo ad Inguina*[79]—, experimental evidence for the straightness of the vertical line along which the venae cavae and the right auricle are joined with each other. Consequently the three chambers remained, in Aristotle's view, the two ventricles proper and the left auricle, i.e. the third ventricle. The same view was taken by Ogle[80].

However, Harvey suspects that with the passing of time anatomical changes may have taken place in certain animals. For at all events he cannot believe that Aristotle—so diligent and faithful an observer (*author tam diligens fidelis*) could have fallen into an observational error[81]. The argument is strangely reminiscent of that brought forward by Jacobus Sylvius in favour of Galen against Vesalius[82].

10. Harvey briefly returns to the *primacy of the blood* which he also upholds for the liver. Aristotle had decided for the heart as the source of all blood and against the liver, because it is only in the heart that blood is found free in its cavities whereas it is enclosed in vessels throughout the liver[83]. As we have seen before[84] Cesalpinus had made this the basis of an anatomical demonstration: the continuous network of the branches of the portal vein and the vena cava which he thought to emerge when the liver parenchyma is washed out[85]. According to Harvey, however, blood is the origin not only of the liver but also of the heart. He rejects the venous anastomoses in the liver[86], and subscribes to

75 HARVEY, *De motu* cap.XVI ad finem, ed. 1628, p.63; ed. Roterod. 1648, p.182–183. Tr. WILLIS, p.75. – See also COLE, F.J., *William Harvey (1578–1657) Nature* 1957, CLXXIX, p.1103–1105.

76 CAESALPINUS, *Praxis universae artis medicae*, 1606 loc.cit. p.179 in note [26], p.2; *Katoptron*, 1605, p.1–2.

77 *Praelectiones* fol.74 verso.

78 HUXLEY, T.H., *On certain errors respecting the structure of the heart attributed to Aristotle*, *Nature* 1879, XXI, 1–5; *Scientific Memoirs* vol.IV, p.380.

79 *Praelectiones* fol.76 verso.

80 OGLE, W., *Aristotle on the parts of animals*, London 1882, p.198 ad: lib.III, cap. 4, note 23.

81 *Praelectiones* fol.74 verso.

82 SYLVIUS, JAC., *Vaesani cuiusdam calumniarum in Hippocratis Galenique rem anatomicam depulsio*, Paris 1551, fol.8 verso. See: O'MALLEY, C.D., *Andreas Vesalius of Brussels 1514–1564*, Berkely and Los Angeles 1964, p.249. – H.W. JANSEN, *Apes and ape lore in the Middle Ages and the Renaissance* (*Studies of the Warburg Institute* vol.XX), London 1952, Appendix on *Titian's Laocoon caricature and the Vesalian-Galenist controversy*, p.355–368, has suggested that the famous Laocoon parody, with three apes, of about 1550, was a "pictorial rebuke to the Galenists in general and to Sylvius in particular" (p.361). See PAGEL, W., and RATTANSI, P., *Vesalius and Paracelsus. Medical History* 1964, vol.VIII p.320.

83 *Praelectiones*, fol.37 recto and fol.75 recto.

84 The present work, p. 185.

85 CESALPINUS, *Quaest. Peripatet.*, lib.V, quaest.3; ed. 1593, fol.118 verso.

86 *Praelectiones*, fol.37 recto. See above p.185 seq.

the belief that the organ parenchyma (notably that of the liver) consists of extravasated and solidified venous blood—an *affusio quasi sanguis effusus extravenatus concretus*[87].

11. *Interventricular septum and pores*. Recognition of the fictitiousness of the interventricular pores—one of the buttresses of the discovery of blood circulation—has a long pre-Harveian history, going back to Massa and Vesalius, as has been discussed in the present book elsewhere[88]. It was Harvey, however, who finally established it. For at his time the matter had by no means been settled. It is true that shortly before *De motu* Caspar Hofmann—one of the few contemporaries quoted by Harvey—had rejected them in definite terms[89]. That he had to do so in itself shows that the pores were still on record, as the wording of the anatomical textbook by Laurentius reveals: "the middle septum is permeable by means of many little holes (foramina) so that there is easy access from the right cavity to the left—*whatever the younger ones may clamour against Galen*[90]." In view of all this the cautious wording in the *Praelectiones* is of great interest. Harvey says: "some (*alii*) believe that blood passes through the interstitial septum (*per septum interstitium*)—the wall being gibbous on the right and convex (should read: concave) on the left side and hence—so they say—porous[91]". By *alii*—some—Harvey presumably meant *others*, thereby implying his own opposition to the pores. If his is so, the *tamen*—"however"—a few lines below falls into its proper place, the meaning of the whole passage being: although I object, others believe in the pores; however (*tamen*) Bauhin found it (sc. the porous septum) conspicuous in the cooked heart of the ox.

In Conclusion

Our analysis of Harvey's Lumleian Lectures—the *Praelectiones anatomiae universalis*—was short and of necessity selective. Even this, however, seems to us to reflect Harvey as the predecessor of Harvey, i.e. the critical and original observer of nature against the background of contemporary doctrines and traditional beliefs. Harvey here appears to us as if groping his way towards the great illumination which must have come to him some time between the period of the Lecture-notes and the publication of his great work some ten years later.

Although the short and clear exposition of the discovery which is found in Harvey's own hand in the *Praelectiones* bears marks of a later addition, the notes contain much of the material on which

87 *Praelectiones*, fol. 38 recto.

88 See the present work p. 157 seq. and PAGEL, W., *Vesalius and the pulmonary transit of blood. J. Hist. Med.* 1964, vol. XIX, p. 327–341.

89 HOFMANN, CASPAR, *De thorac· ejusque partibus commentarius tripartitus*, Frankfurt 1627, lib. III, cap. 9, p. 94. – *Comment. in Galeni de usu partium*, Frankfurt 1625, p. 110–111.

90 LAURENTIUS, *Historia anatomica* Francof. 1602, p. 750.

91 *Praelectiones* fol. 76 recto.

92 COLE, F. J., *William Harvey*, 1957, loc. cit. in note [75] and idem, *Harvey's animals. J. Hist. Med.* 1957, XII, 106–113.

93 KEELE, K. D., *William Harvey as morbid anatomist*, 1962, loc. cit. in note [20].

the first part of his great work, namely the treatise on the movement of the heart—*De motu cordis*—is based. It includes original statements and observations which led to the clarification of a matter that had been left in a state of controversy and doubt. There are also occasional remarks which may be interpreted as pointing in the direction of the discovery, although this is open to contradiction.

With these forward looking aspects, to *Lectures* lead us into the presence of a youthful and energetic Harvey with all the facets which a truthful and patient historical appraisal of the "savant" reveals: Harvey the cool and rational man of science, the comparative anatomist[92], the keen explorer of form and function in health and disease[93], the shrewd physician and experienced pathologist. On the other hand there is Harvey, the staunch Aristotelian, the life-long thinker about the purpose of the movements of the heart and blood, the believer in the analogies between macrocosm and microcosm, accessible to him through the symbol of the circle. There is finally Harvey following up blind alleys[94], and, in spite of all his admiration and piety towards Aristotle, the author so "diligent and faithful[95]", Harvey, the critic of Aristotle. In short here is Harvey, as "he really was".

94 For example in the question of *lung pores* and the *function of the lungs*. These—according to *Praelectiones* fol. 71 verso—provided a cooling system for the heart—an old Aristotelian doctrine, expounded by Cesalpinus (p. 201). Later in the *Praelectiones*—fol. 83 verso—Harvey describes the small holes by which he believed the lung to communicate with the chest cavity. They are, Harvey says, closed in inspiration when the lung is stretched. To this Harvey persistently adhered. For in the third chapter of his late work *On generation* (1651) Harvey claims these pores as a discovery of his own in the lung of birds. "The perforations", he says, "of the lung discovered by me ... are neither obscure nor doubtful, but, in birds especially, sufficiently conspicuous ... you will find that a probe passed downwards by the trachea makes its way out of the lungs and is discovered lying naked and exposed in ... the abdominal cavities... We may even be permitted to ask whether in man whilst he lives there is not a passage from openings of the same kind (sc. as those seen in birds) into the cavity of the thorax. For how else should the pus poured out in empyema and the blood extravasated in pleurisy make its escape? In penetrating wounds of the chest, the lungs themselves being uninjured, air often escapes from the wound; or liquids injected into the cavity of the thorax are discharged with the spit." Exercit. III, ed. 1662, p. 6; tr. WILLIS, p. 174.

The sound principle of comparative anatomy would thus seem to have carried away Harvey and with him many contemporaries who would welcome just another divergence from Galenic tradition, regardless of the accuracy of Galen's view of the lungs as a pair of bellows suspended in the airless pleural cavity and following the suction and compression exerted by the chest wall. For we find the idea of the lung pores developed at length by VAN HELMONT *Catarrhi deliramenta*, cap. 43 et seq. in *Ortus Medicinae*, Amstelod. 1648, p. 439–440. To this: PAGEL, W., *J.B. Van Helmont Einführung i. d. philos. Medizin d. Barock*, Berlin 1930, p. 81 et seq.; id., *Prognosis and Diagnosis. A comparison of ancient and modern medicine*, *J. Warburg Institute*, 1939, II, 382–398 (p. 397). Van Helmont seems to be independent of Harvey in this matter. Indeed the doctrine of the lung pores forms a standing piece of contemporary text-book information, as shown for example in Th. Bartholinus' *Anatomia reformata*, The Hague 1655, p. 280, and it was not before Haller that it was ultimately rejected.

95 *Praelectiones*, fol. 74 verso.

Harvey on Generation—Epigenesis

Harvey and the Pre-Harveian History of the Concept Aristotle—Severinus—Harvey

The term *Epigenesis* in its modern-embryological sense was created by Harvey. It stood originally for something supervening to something else, notably a symptom as an epiphenomenon of disease (*Epigennema*)[1], but was also used for a morbid cause spreading by propagation (*kat'epigenesin*)[2]. Its Latin form was introduced ("usurped")[3] by Harvey to denote the formation of the fetus and of animals by addition of one part after another.

Harvey on Epigenesis and Metamorphosis

Epigenesis was stipulated by Harvey in all its aspects:

1. its main element, the successive formation of parts
2. the first development of the principal part
3. the formation of each individual part *de novo* which implies
4. the rejection of preformation of parts supposed to be all there from the first but too small to be discernible and
5. the simplicity and uniformity of the seed substance.

In all these points Harvey followed the Aristotelian lead and opposed contemporary medical teaching (p. 235 seq.).

In the forty-fifth Exercise on *The Generation of Animals* Harvey distinguishes the process called *Metamorphosis* from *Epigenesis*. In the former "all parts are fashioned simultaneously, each with its distinctive characteristic ... and in this way a perfect animal is at once born; on the other hand, there are some in which one part is made before another, and then from the same material, afterwards receive at once nutrition, bulk and form: that is to say they have some parts made before, some after others ... The structure of these animals commences from some one part as its nucleus and origin, by the instrumentality of which the rest of the limbs are joined on, and this we say takes place by the method of epigenesis, namely, by degrees, part after part; and this is, in preference to the other mode, generation properly so called[4]."

Metamorphosis is synonymous with *spontaneous generation*, as seen when a worm is born from an egg or from putrescent material by the drying up of a moist substance or by the moistening of a dry one. It works as though through the impression of a seal or through the shaping of material in a mould, i. e. by transformation of the whole material. In this all is left to chance—an accidental factor such as heat or moisture will uncover preformed structures that are ready for life, but as it were waiting for a stimulus that will awaken them. Thus "bees, wasps, butterflies, and whatever is

1 *Epigennema:* "Symptoma nosematos hoper enioi ton iatron epigennema kalousin". GALEN, *de Diff. Symptomat.* cap. 1. Ed. Kühn vol. VII, p. 42–43.

2 CASTELLI, *Lexicon Medicum* Lips. 1713, p. 308 sub: *Epigennema.*

3 "Epigenesis etiam latinitati donatum usurpatur de modo formationis foetus et animalium, qui fit per additionem partis post partem quemadmodum patet ex Harveji *de generatione animalium* Exerc. 45." Castelli *loc. cit.*

4 HARVEY, *de gener. animal.* Exerc. 45. *Opp.* London 1766, p. 351; ed. 1662, p. 154; tr. WILLIS London 1847, p. 335.

generated from caterpillars by metamorphosis, are said to have sprung from chance and therefore not to be preservative of their own race."

"An animal, however, which is created by epigenesis attracts, prepares, elaborates, and makes use of the material, all at the same time." In other words formation and growth coincide. There is no cutting up and distribution of material as in metamorphosis, but parts are created in succession out of material that is varied in disposition in accordance with the varied disposition of the parts. The power by which the chick is formed acquires and prepares its own material instead of finding it already prepared and there is no other agency to form the chick and cause it to grow but the chick itself.

In short, then, in generation by metamorphosis the whole is divided *into* parts and thus differentiated; in epigenesis, however, the whole is composed and constituted *from* parts in a certain order (*denique in generatione per metamorphosin totum in partes distribuitur et discernitur; per epigenesin vero, totum ex partibus certo ordine componitur ac constituitur*)[5].

Harvey had prepared this conclusion carefully in the foregoing chapters. In these he refuted the *common mistake of seeking for the cause of diversity of parts in diversity of matter*, as if soft parts came from soft and hard parts from hard matter (*communis error ... quaerere varietatis partium caussas, ex diversa materia, unde oriantur*)[6].

The same *anti-materialist* line is taken by Harvey—as before him by Aristotle—against the followers of Democritos according to whom all things are composed of atoms and against those of Empedocles who see everything as built up from elements, as if generation were nothing but separation, aggregation or composition of things. Admittedly these are necessary when one thing is to be produced from another; but generation is different from them all (*quasi generatio nil aliud foret, quam separatio aut congregatio, aut dispositio rerum ... generatio tamen ipsa ab iis omnino diversa est*)[7]. In this Harvey finds the true Aristotle.

Indeed it is Harvey's intention to show that all the parts of the organism are formed from a material in which nothing is preformed, or in Harvey's own words: "It is my intention to teach that out of the *same albumen* (which all allow to be uniform, not composed of diverse parts) all the parts of the chick, bones, nails, feathers, flesh etc are produced and nourished[8]." Those who assume preformation invoke a *material cause* for generation and at last resort to the concurrence of elements—spontaneous or accidental—or to atoms—variously disposed—as the causes of na-

5 HARVEY, *On generation*, Exerc. XLV, Opp. loc. cit., p. 352; ed. 1662, p. 155; tr. WILLIS, p. 335.

6 Ibidem, Exerc. XI, Opp. p. 219 seq; ed. 1662, p. 36; tr. WILLIS, p. 206 seq.

7 Ibidem, Opp. p. 220, ed. 1662, p. 36; tr. WILLIS, p. 207.

8 "docebo ex eodem albumine (quod omnes fatentur similare esse, non autem ex diversis partibus compositum) singulas pulli partes, ossa, ungues, plumas, carnem ceterasque omnes procreari et nutriri". Ibid. *Opp.* p. 220; ed. 1662, p. 36; tr. WILLIS p. 207. Based on Aristotle, *De gen. anim.* I, 18; 724b25 (simplicity and homogeneity of semen).

tural objects. They thus miss what is first and foremost in the works of nature and in generation and nutrition of animals; nor do they recognise that divine *efficiens* and *numen* of nature which operates with the highest art, providence and wisdom, leading everything to a certain end and good. Indeed they derogate from the honour due to the divine Architect "who has not contrived the shell for the defence of the egg with less of skill and foresight than he has composed all the other parts of the egg of the same matter, and produced it under the influence of the same formative faculty[9]".

Already in an earlier chapter Harvey had opposed those who assume any prepared material such as the semen or the menstrual blood to be the source of the embryo: "Some will have it that the semen or the blood is the matter whence the chick is engendered; others that the semen is the agent or efficient cause of its formation. Yet to him who dispassionately views the question is it quite certain that there is no prepared matter present, nor any menstruous blood to be coagulated at the time of intercourse, as Aristotle will have it; neither does the chick originate in the egg from the seed of the male, nor from that of the female, nor from the two commingled[10]".

As in all other fields Harvey's opinion concerning Epigenesis is based on empirical observation—the ocular inspection of the successive stages in the generation of the chick. It also has a strong metaphysical background, however. Again this is in keeping with Harvey's method of scientific invention and discovery. The idea behind epigenesis is the *vitalist* point of view. It is the view that had been advocated by Aristotle.

Aristotle on Epigenesis

Aristotle first of all examined the theory of *pangenesis* according to which the semen is a derivative of all parts of the body. This theory was propounded by the Atomists (Democritos), was modified in the Hippocratic Corpus and refuted by Aristotle[11]. Naturally this theory implicitly favoured preformation. Aristotle asks: how will those parts that came from all the body of the parent be increased or grow? If what is added (the *prosgignomenon* or *proselthon*) can be changed, as the pangenesists say it can, then why not say that the semen from the very first is of such a kind that blood and flesh can be made out of it, instead of saying that it itself *is* blood and flesh? Nor is there any other alternative, for "surely we cannot say that it is increased later by a process of mixing, as wine when water is poured into it. For in that case each element of the mix-

9 Ibid. *Opp.* p. 220; ed. 1662, p. 36, 37; tr WILLIS p. 207.

10 Ibid. for example Exerc. 14. Opp. p. 241–242; ed. 1662, p. 56; tr. WILLIS p. 228: "alii nimirum sanguinem aut semen *materiam* esse censent, unde pullus constituatur: aliis semen videtur opifex, seu causa efficiens, quae eundem fabricet. Cum tamen accuratius rem omnem perpendenti certum sit, nullam ibidem paratam esse materiam; nec sanguinem menstruum adesse, quem semen maris coitus tempore coagulat, ut voluit Aristoteles; nec pullum ex semine maris, aut foeminae, aut utrisque commistis, in ovo oriundum esse."

11 LESKY, E., *Die Zeugungs- und Vererbungslehren der Antike und ihr Nachwirken.* Wiesbaden 1950, p. 70 seq.; p. 128 seq; p. 166.

ARISTOTELES, *De generatione animal.* I, 18; 722a; I, 20; 729 a ed. H. Aubert and Fr. Wimmer, Leipzig 1860 (*Aristoteles' Fünf Bücher von der Zeugung und Entwicklung der Thiere übersetzt und erläutert*), p. 109.

ture would be itself at first while still unmixed, but the fact rather is that flesh and bone and each of the other parts is such later[12]".

Neither the semen nor the female part can contain any of the future tissues and organs in a pre-formed state. For the semen does not contribute any material, but solely acts by its initiating and formative power, not by its body (*soma*), but by some inherent faculty and efficient cause (*hexis kai arche geneseos gennetike*)[13]. Indeed, the male does not lend anything to the quantity (*poson*), but only to the quality (*poion*)[14]. This is empirically suggested by the fact that some males, for example insects which unite with the female, do not insert any part of themselves into the female, but on the contrary the female inserts a part of herself into the male[15]. It is therefore not necessary that anything at all should come away from the male, and if anything does come away it does not follow that what develops comes from it as something present in the developing. It is not present in the embryo as such, but merely provides motion and form, comparably to the carpenter who brings a bed into being or the form that makes a ball out of a lump of wax or the medical art which cures the patient[16]. This also emerges from the pneumatic nature of semen, its intrinsic vital heat—a heat that has nothing to do with fire[17].

Nor are any parts preformed in the female germ, just as little as the piece of furniture is preformed in the wood that is fashioned by the carpenter. They are only preformed in the material (*hyle*) potentially (*dynamei*)[18]. As ocular observation shows, the parts develop in succession (*ephexes*), or as we would say to-day by *epigenesis*, rather than simultaneously, nor is it true that this is simulated by smaller parts which escape attention though present. For the lung in spite of its size, clearly follows the—smaller—heart in development[19]. Hence it is only one part—the heart—that comes into being first and it is this that provides the origin (*arche*) of the parts. "And what comes into being first is the first principle; this is the heart in the sanguinea and its analogue in the rest... This is plain not only to the senses (that it is first to come into being), but also in view of its end; for life fails in the heart last of all, and it happens in all cases that what comes into being last fails first, and the first last, Nature running a double course, so to say, and turning back to the point from whence she started. For the process of becoming is from the non-existent to the existent, and that of perishing is back again from the existent to the non-existent[20]."

Epigenesis thus forms the keynote of the Aristotelian Theory of Generation and Embryology. The same may be said of Harvey's

12 Aristot. *de gener. animal.* I, 18; 723a tr. A. PLATT. Oxford 1910. Aubert and Wimmer p. 78–79.

13 Aristoteles *de gener. animal.* I,19; 726b tr. PLATT. Aubert-Wimmer p. 98–99.

14 Aristoteles *de gener. anima*. I,21; 730a tr. PLATT. Aubert-Wimmer, p. 114–115.

15 Aristoteles *de gener. animal.* I,21; 729b tr. PLATT. Aubert-Wimmer p. 112–113.

16 Aristoteles *de gener. animal.* I,21; 729b tr. PLATT; Aubert-Wimmer p. 112–113.

17 Aristoteles *de gener. animal.* II,3; 737a tr. PLATT; Aubert-Wimmer p. 150–151.

18 Aristoteles *de gener. animal.* I,21; 729b tr. PLATT; Aubert-Wimmer p. 113; "the parts of the embryo exist potentially in the material" (enhyparchonton en hyle dynamei ... ton morion): II,5; 741b tr. PLATT. Aubert-Wimmer p. 175.

19 Aristoteles *de gener. animal.* II,1; 734a, tr. PLATT; Aubert-Wimmer p. 137. – Only one part comes into being first and not all of them together (*ouch hama panta*) ibid. II,1; 735a; Aubert-Wimmer p. 141–142. – Ibid. II,6; 742b tr. PLATT; Aubert-Wimmer p. 179. – Ibid. II,6; 741b; Aubert-Wimmer p. 175.

20 Aristoteles, *de gener. animal.* II,1; 735a Aubert-Wimmer p. 140–143. – II,4; 740a Aubert-Wimmer p. 166–169. – II,6; 741b; Aubert Wimmer p. 175. See above p. 84.

ideas on the subject. In this as in so many other fields, Harvey seems to be a direct follower of Aristotle. How he gave a definite lead towards the Aristotelian theory of Epigenesis can be seen from a comparison with the ruling opinion of his time.

Theories of Generation current at Harvey's Time
Galen—Fernel—Laurentius

At Harvey's time the theory of generation was largely based on Galen as modified by Jean Fernel (1485–1558).

Galen as well as Fernel opposed Aristotle's epigenetic point of view in general and on several counts in detail:

1. Neither of Aristotle's opponents would admit of succession in the development of parts. The formative faculty separates the hard particles from the soft ones and assembles the former in the periphery already at the very first (*en arche*). Nothing of this is seen, however, because of the extreme smallness of these parts, until much later, when from the hard and dry peripheral layer the bones emerge[21].

In other words everything is there from the first and there is no epigenesis. As Fernel expresses it: the part is formed or rather steps out into visibility (*gignitur, id est genita apparet*)[22]. There is no order or time schedule which the formative agent in the semen follows in modelling first this and then that organ—if the ancients had suggested such a schedule, it was not of the nature of the agent (*non agentis est naturae*), but it would mean the order in which the further perfection of parts takes place as required by the work as a whole—this schedule is in the nature of the finished work (*effícti operis*)[23].

Fernel refers to Hippocrates who had said that all members are formed simultaneously, none earlier or later than the other, but those that are larger by nature appear earlier[24].

2. Galen would not unequivocally recognise a principal part that is formed first. He nevertheless emphasised, against the claim raised by Aristotle for the heart as the principal organ, the very early and expeditious formation of the liver. Its substance is closely akin to blood from which it is therefore readily formed. At all events it is the liver and not the heart which the fetus needs in its early stages—for then it leads the vegetative life of the plant. In the latter there is nothing analogous to the heart, nor any need for pulsation and the animal spirit which is maintained and diffused by it[25].

21 Galen, *de semine* Lib. I, cap. 8 ed. Kühn vol. IV, p. 540–541: a "firm house" is formed—"steganon heauto ton oikon ergazetai tes perieilephyias auto tou spermatos hygras ousias, hoson en pachyteron te kai skleroteron apothoumenon eis ten ektos perigraphen hoper emellen en to chrono thermainomenon te kai xerainomenon ostoun esesthai." This is achieved by the formative faculty in the very beginning: "touto *en arche* he diaplattousa to zoon dynamis ergazetai", but the result is invisible because of the smallness of the parts—"phainetai de oudepo kata ten archen hypo smikrotetos".

22 Fernel, *Physiologia* lib. VII de hominis procreatione et de semine cap. 10. *Universa Medicina* ed. Heurnius. Traj. ad Rh. 1656, p. 186.

23 Fernel ibidem.

24 Hippocrates *Regimen I*, cap. 26: "and all the limbs are separated and grow simultaneously, none before or after another; although those by nature larger become visible before the smaller, yet they are formed none the earlier..." (kai diakrinetai ta melea panta hama kai auxetai, kai proteron ouden heteron heterou oud'hysteron. ta de mezo physei protera phainetai ton elassonon, ouden protera ginomena). ed. and tr. W.H.S. Jones, *Hippocrates* vol. IV, p. 262–265 London Loeb Class. Lib. 1931. – German tr. by Rob. Fuchs, *Hippocrates Sämtl. Werke* München 1895, vol. I, p. 301 with cross references.

25 Galen, *de Foetuum Formatione* cap. 2 ed Kühn, vol. IV, p. 658 seq; cap. 3, p. 665: "to kyoumenon out' arterion echon anankaian chreian en arche tes geneseos, oute sphygmon, oute kardias, hosper oude ta phyta".

3. Galen concludes that at an early date the three principal parts—liver, heart and brain—appear separated into three and are therefore formed simultaneously[26]. Again he is followed by Fernel who insists that this conclusion was arrived at not by theory, but by observation after the first two weeks of conception (*observatione constat omnes partes simul conformari*)[27]. Hence there is no formation *de novo*, there is only perfection of parts already outlined and formed.

4. Aristotle had visualised the semen entering the female matter, but here merely acting as the igniter which touches off a series of developmental motions in the germ. The semen initiates motion, it acts as the *arche kineseos*, but its material substance is of no import. It is simple and homogeneous, and discharged when it has issued the developmental stimulus. It forms no part of the fetus.

Galen takes Aristotle to task for all this. The latter, he says, did not really believe in the discharge of the male semen, although elsewhere he compared it to the whey that emanates from curdled milk[28]. Nor is there any idea of a pneumatisation of the semen as envisaged by Aristotle—for it is just impossible in view of the firm embracement of the germ by the uterus which is found when the female is opened at an early stage after cohabitation[29]. At all events we would be left with the ridiculous alternative between a discharge of the male semen or its annihilation after conception[30].

Moreover at an early stage there is much in the embryo that is identical in quality with semen[31]. Indeed, the material substance of the semen is the structure in which such parts as the veins, arteries and nerves are preformed. These are white, bloodless and tensile and therefore not derived from blood. If they were, i.e. if the blood were capable of secreting such semen-like substances, nature would have made something in vain—the semen.

Nor is the semen of a simple and even texture, as Aristotle believed. On the contrary, as Fernel points out, it consists of soft parts that are pure and possessed of active spirit (*purior et vegetior portio*) and solid parts which are not. The semen is therefore not simple, although it thus appears (*hoc enim simplex non est et uniusmodi, quanquam tale apparet*)[32].

In the semen the formative spirit arises as it were from a state of numbness to break out into activity, diffusing itself and pervading all the semen's parts. It thus separates what is thick and cold from what is warm and of fine texture. All these various structures are materially there, but they attain to perfection at various stages—those in the centre that form the three principal parts, liver, heart

26 Galen ibid. cap. 3 ed Kühn, vol. IV, p. 662–663: after the 30th day liver, heart and brain have clearly emerged—"saphos phainetai ta tria tauta tou zoou moria ... mona d'allelois engys horatai tria tauta kathaper artios eipon, he te kardia kai ho enkephalos kai to hepar".

27 Fernel *loc. cit.* p. 185.

28 Galen, *de Semine* Lib. I, cap. 3 ed Kühn vol. IV, p. 517.

29 Galen ibidem Lib. I, cap. 4, Kühn p. 521.

30 Galen ibid. Lib. I, cap. 3, Kühn p. 517 —"hoste tis auton sphodra hemon kategelasen, ei nomizoimen palin antekkrinesthai to sperma para tou theleos eis touktos, e menon endon eis to meden analyesthai".

31 Galen ibid. Lib. I, cap. 5, p. 528 seq. Kühn.

32 Fernel, *loc. cit.* p. 185.

and brain, earlier than those at the periphery which are condensed into bone, muscle and tendon[33].

In Harvey's own time anatomical textbooks reflect the Galenic doctrine as modified and summarised by Fernel. Among such books the Anatomy of Laurentius may be briefly examined.

Laurentius decides against both components of Epigenesis: (a) the successive formation of parts following the development of a principal and central organ and (b) the homogeneity of the germ. The heart, he says, is not the first to live, as Aristotle believed. In eels and serpents the principle of life is found in the caudal parts. Nor is the heart the first to be nourished and informed by soul. For all nutrition is through the blood, all blood comes through the veins and all veins are from the liver. Laurentius visualises Galen as a believer in successive formation of parts, who failed to reach a decision as to which part was formed first. He thought, however, that the fetus leads a vegetative plant-life for which the liver was best adapted, whereas no organ analogous to the heart was present in plants[34]. By contrast Laurentius approves of the old Hippocratic verdict that all parts are formed simultaneously[35] and that the body should be likened to a circle in which no beginning or end can be found[36]. His conclusion is: the rudiments of all germinal parts and first "warps" are outlined at the same time (*spermaticarum omnium partium rudimenta et prima stamina simul et semel delineari*)[37]. An exception from this is claimed for the "membranes", i.e. amnios, chorion and allantois. These Laurentius holds to be formed first from the thicker peripheral material of the germ.

Concerning the preformation of parts, his view is in keeping with the rejection of their successive formation. The germ, he says, appears to be uniform, but is in reality not homogeneous in structure. It is endowed with dissimilar parts from the very beginning, i.e. before the spirit, the instrument of the soul starts to act upon it. This is primarily a process of *separation* of these dissimilar parts, placing the finer, nobler and more spiritual components in the centre and the thicker, colder and more viscid ones towards the periphery. It is from the latter which stem from the semen that the "membranes" are formed[38].

Epigenesis between Aristotle and Harvey – Severinus on Epigenesis (pl. 41)

Opposition to Epigenesis, though overriding at Harvey's time, was not unanimous, however. Indeed, *between Aristotle and Harvey*, the epigenetic point of view had found an able advocate in the

33 FERNEL, ibidem.

34 LAURENTII, ANDREAE *Historia Anatomica Humani Corporis* Lib. VIII, cap. 2 *de principiis generationis, semine et sanguine*. Francof. 1602, p. 576 seq. In particular quaest. 15; p. 631 seq.: An omnes partes simul conformentur. "Cor non est primum vivens. – Anguillis et serpentibus vitae principium erit in cauda. – Cor nec primum alitur nec primum animatur".

35 HIPPOCRATES, *Regimen I cap. 26, loc. cit.* in note [24].

36 HIPPOCRATES, *De locis in homine* cap. 1 ed Kühn, Lips. 1826, vol. II, p. 101; Fuchs, München 1897, vol. II, p. 566.

37 LAURENTIUS *loc. cit.* cap. 5, p. 635.

38 LAURENTIUS ibid. p. 627.

Paracelsist Peter Severinus (1542–1602). He was born as Peder S. Soerenssen at Ribe in Jutland, studied and lectured at Copenhagen University, travelled and practised medicine in Italy and Germany, became physician to King Frederic II. of Danmark in 1571 and died of the plague[39].

His main work is the *Idea medicinae philosophicae fundamenta continens totius doctrinae Paracelsicae, Hippocraticae et Galenicae*. It first appeared in 1571[40]—at the time when the bulk of the Paracelsean treatises was being discovered and eagerly printed, translated and reprinted. In fact it was the year after the *Archidoxen-Sturm* which saw a series of editions of the *Archidoxis*—reflecting the widespread desire to recover and preserve the main chemical work of Paracelsus. Severinus' *Idea* was praised by Sir Francis Bacon as the eloquent presentation and philosophically harmonious system of Paracelsus of whom he thought little otherwise[41]. Severinus was attacked *qua* Paracelsist by Herman Conring and in turn defended by Olaus Borrichius[42]. In Sprengel's excellent account the attacks on Severinus were repeated, chiefly for his traffic with panaceas, his claim to be able to cure gout, epilepsy and leprosy, his use of Galenic remedies alongside those of Paracelsus and his overlooking of important tenets of the latter in favour of unimportant detail[43]. He was again defended in turn by Haeser for the clarity of his exposition, his piety and his erudition—in spite of his adherence to the belief in the analogies between macrocosm and microcosm, in the causation of diseases by germs as well as by sin, in signatures and in antimony as a universal medicine[44].

Severinus' position is anti-materialist and vitalist. He thus rejects the humoral theories of the ancients which are the "source of defeat and have contaminated all of philosophy". For they are content with external appearances such as the fallacious qualities and complexions and have confused "elements" with "principles". Ancient naturalists would have been more successful had they based their doctrine of elements on the diversity and specific properties of creatures, the vital principle that is active in every one of them and accounts for their specific individual and generic differences. They would then have learnt that each of the elements releases its specific "fruit", i. e. objects that are related to each other by virtue of their origin in one of the four "mother"-elements, and of the "seal" which it impresses on them. Thus minerals and metals are kindred by virtue of their common origin in water, plants and animals by virtue of their common "mother" earth. Manna, dew and meteoric phenomena wrongly ascribed to inane, "empty" vapours and exhalations are specific "fruit" of the firma-

39 Petersen in: Hirsch-Gurlt, *Biographisches Lexikon der hervorragenden Ärzte* vol.V, Wien und Leipzig 1887, p.456. – Thorndike, L., *History of Magic and Experimental Science* vol.V, New York 1941, p.630. – Pagel, W., *Will. Harvey and the Purpose of Circulation. Isis* 1951, XLII, 34. – The most comprehensive account is by Sprengel, Kurt, *Versuch einer pragmatischen Geschichte der Arzneykunde* 3rd ed. vol.III, Halle 1827, p.503–508.

40 Basileae, Henr. Petri. Reedited: Erfurt 1616 and Hagae Comitis 1660 (preceded by Will. Davisson's Commentary—on this see W. Pagel, *Das Medizinische Weltbild des Paracelsus. Seine Zusammenhänge mit Neuplatonismus und Gnosis*. Wiesbaden. Steiner. 1962, p.131–133). A reprint of the 1660 edition in 1668 is mentioned by Sudhoff, K., *Ein Beitrag zur Bibliographie der Paracelsisten im 16. Jahrhundert, Centralbl. f. Bibliothekswesen* 1893, vol.X, p.403.

41 "Quaevis enim *Philosophia* integra se ipsam sustentat: atque dogmata ejus sibi mutuo et lumen et robur adjiciunt: quod si distrahantur, peregrinum quiddam et durum sonant ... sicut illam Theophrasti Paracelsi, eloquenter in Corpus quoddam, et Harmoniam Philosophiae redactam a Severino Dano..." Fr. Baconis de Verulam *De Augmentis Scientiarum* lib.III, cap. 4. Amstelod. Henr. Wetsten. 1694, p.192.

42 Borrichius, O., *Hermet. Aegypt. et Chemicor. Sapientia*. Hafniae 1674, p.290.

43 Sprengel *loc. cit.* in footnote [39].

44 Haeser, Heinr., *Lehrbuch d. Geschichte d. Medicin* vol.II, 3rd ed. Jena 1881, p.109.

mental element. "Elements" thus understood convey life, support and preservation to their offspring—a function that could never be achieved by such qualities as hot, cold, moist or dry or their combination[45].

In all this Severinus follows the teaching of Paracelsus, but also refers to Hippocrates who in his work *On ancient medicine* had rejected the humoral hypotheses based on humoral mixture and quality, in favour of the "forces" called by him the adstringent, the acid, the bitter and the sweet[46]. It is these that cause and have power to cure disease. In other words the overriding principle is what is "alive in nature" (*to embion tes physeos*) and through which all is alive and active. Paracelsus called it variously: *balsam*, *mummy*, *mercury*, *quinta essentia*, *arcanum*, *elixir*, *materia perlata*, *manna* or *chaerionian power*. These are the *logoi* (*rationes*) which the Platonists derived from the *soul of the world*. Through the ministry of these powers and *logoi* nature was enabled to unfold all that is in it: nature became *seminal*—propagating and preserving its *semina*.

This is the vitalistic idea on which Severinus' doctrine of *seed* and *semen* is based. The latter is primarily something spiritual—potentially present in all parts of the body, but brought to perfection in the generative organs. It is "astral" in that it harbours the superior and magisterial power of life. Hence it is invisible, but easily converted into a body—in fact spirit and body overlap, the coarser spirits being body and subtle bodies being spirit, and the invisible kernel of an object may be made visible by removing its coarse vestments[47].

The seed committed to earth putrefies and perishes by dissolution; its radical power persists, however. For in it there is its total "anatomy and power" which enable it to step out again into the mundane scene and to start a new circle by fashioning a new body for itself, adapted to its destined function[48]. A study of the semina thus promises the most illuminating information as to the nature of the elemental world.

From such a study we learn:

1. The semina are connected with certain places—the "mother-*elements*" which in themselves are "empty and hidden".

2. The semina are bound to a *time* schedule which includes praedestination, the laws of motion and the office of generation. They thereby watch over the continuity and preservation of things which without them would sink into infinity that is into nothing.

3. The semina maintain the consensus and communication of things by virtue of *sympathy*.

45 SEVERINUS, *Idea*, 1571, cap.V, p.42.

46 SEVERINUS, *Idea*, 1571, cap.II, p.20; cap.VII, p.65. – See above p.98.

47 SEVERINUS ibid. p.26: "ex spiritibus corpora produci, et rursus corpora in spiritus resolvi." The basic statement of the reciprocal nature of spirit and body is found in Ficinus, Mars., *De Vita coelitus comparanda* lib.III, cap.3 ed. Aldina Venet. 1516, fol.153r: the spirit as it were not body but already soul, or not soul but already body ("ipse vero est corpus tenuissimum, quasi non corpus et quasi iam anima. Item quasi non anima, et quasi jam corpus"). This was verbally repeated by Agrippa of Nettesheym, *de Occulta Philosophia* lib.I, cap.14 ed. Lugd. 1550, p.33. On its significance in the philosophy of Paracelsus and his speculation on the power of Imagination see PAGEL, W., *Paracelsus. An Introduction to Philosophical Medicine in the Era of the Renaissance* Basle and New York 1958, p.121 seq, p.181 (with ref. to the causation of plague), p.221 (Ficinus), p. 297 (Agrippa) and on the underlying Neoplatonic tradition: PAGEL, W., *Das Medizinische Weltbild des Paracelsus* 1962, *loc.cit.* in footnote [40], p.39–40. See also below footnote [52] for the application of the principle to the *semina*, and below in the present book, p. 264.

48 SEVERINUS Idea cap.II, p.29.

4. The semina are *independent* of the physical *laws* by which *masses* are directed and limited in motion, space and dimension. They penetrate the abyss of the elements obeying the laws laid into them by the Creator. They are thus also independent of *astral* inclination and impression, of the action of rays, atoms and mixture (e.g. of humours and qualities).

5. The semina are bound to a periodic *circuit* of generations and act through *rays* which are of great penetrative power and can arise suddenly.

Semina are usually defined as particles of matter that can preserve the fertility of their own kind. This definition is too narrow, for it only applies to animals and plants, but not to minerals, although there are semina in the mineral kingdom too[49]. A more comprehensive definition should be based on the coming and going of semina and their products, their periodicity of motion, their *circular property* (*circularis seminum proprietas*), and their action by virtue of *rays*—features that enable them to work as links (*vincula*) connecting the visible and invisible, the nether and upper worlds. These semina are indestructible, and generation as well as corruption merely indicate the flux and reflux—the periodicity—of semina. It is for this reason that Orpheus called Night—the abyss from which the semina emerge—and Nature "cyclically returning" (*enkyklia*) and "round" (*kykloteres*)[50]. Hence *semen is the intrinsic vital principle of an object*, the bearer of its "mechanical spirits" and the *Quinta Essentia* of the whole anatomy proper to its species. It provides the means by which a body is built up with colours, flavour, qualities, size, figure and other features (*signatures*) appropriate to its function and predestination[51]. It is a spirit, possessed of an internal "*knowledge*" (*scientia innata*) which at the same time means a mechanical art and infallible notion of the properties of the object to be formed. The semina are at the same time bodies, but spiritual ones[52]. This explains why even a *minimal part of the semen* (*minima gutta seminis*) contains the whole anatomy of the species (*universam anatomiam totius speciei continet*)[53].

It is from this vitalistic and spiritualistic—Augustinian—view of the Semina that Severinus arrives at *Epigenesis*.

We do not believe, he says, in dissimilar parts being preformed in the semen, although they are represented in it by tendency (*specie*). The multitude of the organs emerges from one and the same semen by virtue not of its matter and a material diversity of parts, but of the variety of its inherent endowments, rational plan and awareness of what has to be done (*neque existimare debemus in semine partes esse dissimilares, quamvis similari specie representententur, ita*

49 SEVERINUS ibid. cap.VI, p.55. – See below Marci's criticism of the idea of "mineral semina", p. 297.

50 SEVERINUS ibid. cap.VIII, p.90.

51 SEVERINUS ibid. cap.VIII, p.96.

52 SEVERINUS ibidem cap.VIII, p.101: "corpora tamen sunt, sed spiritualia et spiritus rursus sed corporei"—hence their name: *prima materia* see above footnote [47] concerning the reciprocity of spirit and body.

53 SEVERINUS ibid. cap.VIII, p.106: "minima gutta seminis universam anatomiam totius speciei continet: quia spiritus mechanici et principia generationum a dimensionibus et corporum angustiis excipiuntur."

quod aliud sit corpus cerebri, aliud cordis, aliud hepatis ... sed hanc multitudinem temporis progressu ex uno semine exituram, non mole, non corporum multitudine, aestimari oportet: sed Donorum, Rationum, Scientiarumque varietate, qua pollent spiritus mechanici)[54]. Such is the power of spirits that if they have the idea (*scientia*) of the heart they will form it from the nutriment which they attract ... and this in appropriate order and at predestined times (*tanta est spirituum potestas, ut si scientiam habuerint cordis, ex alimento attracto cor formabunt ... idque debito ordine definitisque temporibus*)[55]. In this lies the divinity in each individual being. It is divine through the *Light of Nature*—a nature that in the words of Hippocrates is untaught (*apaideute*)[56].

The semen is alive—as manifested by its perceptible movement. First it is contracted and thereby forced to assume *globular shape*. At the same time it is agitated by a *pulsation*, however small and starts attracting most refined nutriment (*alimentum spirituosum*). This is followed by contraction of the matrix—a friendly embrace of the seed which it contains. By virtue of the awareness (*scientiae*) and endowments inherent to the semen the elemental body is then *unfolded* (*explicatio*) in methodical fashion[57].

The first stages of development are thus: (a) motion as the first sign of life, (b) contraction into globular shape, (c) pulsation and (d) unfolding of a—rational—schedule underlying the formation of the elemental body. Again this is *not* accomplished by the *evolution of parts that are preformed* in the seed-matter, but by *free building up* of organs and tissues from the *same—homogeneous—* elemental *material* (*elementa constituuntur ... non quia in elementis tales jam contineantur partes vel partium proportiones: non quod ex ossibus, venis, arteriis, nervis, ex corde, cerebro, hepate elementorum exordia profecta sint: neque quod in semine contineantur totidem spiritus ex similibus parentum partibus derivati: sed quia tot talesque scientiae, in generationum principiis et mechanicis spiritibus latent. Ii enim ex iisdem elementis cor, cerebrum, hepar, nervos, venas, arterias, ossa conformare noverunt*)[58].

In fact it is the same process by which from the same bread a dog produces canine and man human flesh (*quemadmodum ex eodem pane canis canina membra producit, homo humana et coetera animalia similiter*). In the light of this epigenetic view the ancient theory that the constituents of the semen derive from the corresponding parts of the parents (pangenesis) refutes itself[59].

Severinus leaves no doubt that it is his anti-materialist conviction which leads him to epigenesis. He admonishes us that it is *not matter* from which number, substance, site, form and seals derive, but from what is really efficient—the spirit (*hoc tueri consilium est numerum, substantiam, situm, conformationem et signaturas*

54 SEVERINUS ibid. cap. VIII, p. 107.

55 SEVERINUS ibidem.

56 SEVERINUS ibidem: "ita quaelibet herba refert presentem Deum ... hoc est Lumen Naturae..."

57 SEVERINUS ibid. p. 110: (a) semen vivit in utero ... motu quoque manifesto vitae inditia ostendit (b) globular shape and pulsation of germ: contrahitur enim et in globum cogitur vitalique pulsu quamvis exiguo ac tantulo semini proportionato movetur alimentumque spirituosum attrahere incipit (c) contraction of matrix: et amico favore arctissime semen complectuntur (d) unfolding of the Scientiae et Dona spirituum.

58 SEVERINUS ibid. p. 110.

59 SEVERINUS ibid. p. 110.

omnes non ex materia, sed ex efficiente proficisci)[60]. Even the smallest and most paltry animals reveal the greatest miracles in nature—emulating the creation of the whole universe. For as in the latter, first from invisible principles, then through a methodical arrangement of elemental matter by virtue of an innate awareness of a time schedule and plan of construction, the highest differentiations are achieved and adapted to predestined functions. To those who attribute the development of the parts to the matter of the semen and their nutrition and growth to the maternal blood, Severinus answers that he denies the bodily and largely material nature of the semen (*negantes corpoream et nimis materiatam seminis naturam*)[61].

And finally: from his epigenetic point of view Severinus concludes that the ancient controversy as to which part develops first is futile."They quarrel about goat's wool", he says: Aristotle thus regarded the heart as the root of the life-principle which provides motion, sense and nutriment. Against him the medical schools denied the heart its foremost position among the organs, notably as the suppositious source of vessels and nerves. Instead they held that the three principal organs: heart, brain and liver, are formed first simultaneously to act as the root of the others and that then the arteries are produced by the heart, the nerves by the brain and the veins by the liver. They all erred, Severinus believes, because of their neglect of the power of the internal "knowledge" of the seed from which everything derives by "mechanical sculpturing" ("stone-masonry"—*lithurgia*) and the undue attention paid to its material part. For in the latter they *imagine to be corporeal rudiments of the parts* (*corporea partium rudimenta in semine fingunt*). Here they suffer from an illusion: When the principal viscera are separated and contract by virtue of heat, the members finally emerge—so they believe (*maximeque principalium viscerum, quibus separatis et a calore coactis, membra tandem ostendant, quorum exordia obtinuerant*)[62]. In other words their adherence to a theory of preformation, their preoccupation with the building materials, in short their materialism led them into blind alleys and error. Already in Hippocrates *de Diaeta* they could have found that the members are separated simultaneously, no part before or after the other, although parts that are by nature bigger than others appear, though they are not formed, earlier. Indeed Hippocrates compared the body to a circle in which there is neither beginning nor end, but everything is beginning as well as end—for when a circle is drawn no beginning can be found[63]. It is its simplicity and uniformity which makes the circle illustrative of the nature of seed. By con-

60 SEVERINUS ibid. p. 111.

61 SEVERINUS ibid. p. 111.

62 SEVERINUS cap. X, *de generatione humana et transplantationibus generationi supervenientibus*, p. 162 et seq. The controversy between the followers of Aristotle and the "Medici" as to which part develops first: "de lana caprina rixantur quaestionibusque otiosis fatigantur".

63 See above in footnotes [24, [35], [36].

trast the preformationists must resort to angular figures such as the triangle, quadrangle and pentagon. It is by virtue of its spirituality and its attraction of spiritual nutriment that unity and circularity are preserved. Only at a later stage, however, when more copious nourishment is attracted, do angular patterns and with them solid bodily structures emerge[64].

Aristotle granted superior rank to the heart—and rightly so, if this is understood to appertain not to the heart as the bodily organ, but to its function which is the "office" of the vital spirit. This refutes those who argue against Aristotle that the fetus leads a plant-like vegetative life and that there is no analogous part to the heart in plants[65]. In fact the difference between animal and plant life does not lie in the absence of comparable organs or tissues, but in the superior quality of vital spirit which enables the seed to display the "offices" of the heart and to form it. Equally absurd is the opinion of those who attribute the origin of the veins to the liver, of the arteries to the heart and of the nerves to the brain. Again this is a *nimis materialis partium origo*—a materialistic view which was already repudiated by such diligent anatomists as Falloppia. It is true, however, that veins, arteries and nerves carry out the functions (*officia*) proper to liver, heart and brain respectively. Indeed veins, arteries and nerves just like muscle, bone, membranes, blood and humours act as the "links" (*vincula*) that are responsible for the harmonious continuity of the life of the organism, the "consensus" and "conspiratio" of its parts[66]. Nor should one underrate the value of the bodily organs which serve as focal points for the concentration and unification of the virtues of the spirits that are dispersed throughout the body (*partes corporis sunt quasi matrices, radices, penuaria, Astra, in quibus concentrantur et uniuntur virtutes spirituum, per orbem, id est, per totam Anatomiam, dispersae*)[67]. It would be wrong, however, to make such differences as between motion and sensation dependent upon differences in the structure of nervous fibres. The primary cause of such differences is conditioned by the spirit responsible for them, but it is the latter which needs properly organised fibres in order to translate an impulse into reality. At all events this applies to visible motion, whereas more "obscure" motion is administered by the "benefit of the spirits" alone, as most frequently occurs in natural actions and "in the vital poise of the whole body". From all this there follows the even greater—"puerile"—absurdity of those who attribute motion to the posterior, i. e. the spinal, and sensation to the anterior, i. e. the cerebral nerves[68].

Thus the first origin of everything remains the spirit—it is the

64 SEVERINUS cap.X, *loc. cit.* pp. 163–164.

65 "Qui Aristotelem reprehendunt, quod cor primum conformari dixerit in Animalibus, iecori primas attribuunt, quod primo plantae vitam vivat in utero foetus, neque in plantis reperiri quippiam proportione cordi respondens. Quibus antea satisfecimus. Diximus enim copiosum spiritum vitalem semini conjunctum esse, et pulsu ac respiratione, quamvis occulta, cordis officium absolvere: et quid dico cordis officium, cum non cordis, sed spirituum proprium sit." SEVERINUS ibidem, p. 164.

66 SEVERINUS ibidem, p. 164.

67 SEVERINUS cap. XI: *de usu partium actionumque omnium administratione et de fructibus Astrorum in Revolutione humanae Astronomiae*, p. 176.

68 SEVERINUS, ibidem, p. 177—obviously meant as an allusion to Galen. According to the latter the "softer"—sensory—nerves are from the brain and the "harder"—motor—nerves from the cerebellum and spinal cord (*de usu partium* lib. IX, cap. 14 ed. Kühn vol. III, p. 740 et seq.; *de anatomicis administrat.* lib. VIII, cap. 8 ed. Kühn vol. II, p. 613; *de placitis Hippocratis et Platonis* cap. 5 ed. Kühn vol. V, p. 621). The emphasis here lies on the soft and hard structure of the nerves, the soft ones being more akin to that of the brain, the others being "hardened" in proportion to their distance from the brain and thereby enabled to serve as motor nerves. The theory was well summarised and widely opposed by sixteenth century anatomists, notably Columbus: "Animadvertendum praeterea est Galenum velle nervos sensum deferentes ab anteriori cerebri parte exoriri, motivos vero dictos a posteriore". However, with due deference to Galen, it is obvious that hard and motor nerves also originate in the brain. Moreover all nerves apart from the optic and purely sensory nerves, conduct not only sensory but also motor impulses. (*De re Anatomica* lib. VIII, cap. 3. Francof. 1593, p. 366.) LAURENTIUS (*Historia Anatomica* loc. cit. Francof. 1602, p. 292 et seq., lib. IV, quaest. 10: An nervi motorii a sensificis distinguantur) writes in the same vein: Galen's doctrine is false if taken to be applicable in general "non enim sensorii omnes a cerebro, sed plurimi a spinali medulla, nec motorii omnes a cerebello, sed quidam a cerebro ortum ducunt...").

latter that watches over the maintenance of unity, but by attracting nourishment and continually mixing with it, spirits are "thickened" (*spiritibus mixtione continua crascescentibus*)—whereby "distances, separations and divisions of endowments" and with them impurities are introduced. The *formation of parts* is thus seen as the *result of a degeneration of spirits into body components* (*in corpoream familiam degenerant*)[69]. There is one component, however, which has a claim to a place above the rank of the other parts: the *blood*, by virtue of its eminent necessity for the keeping together (*societas*) and direction (*gubernatio*) of the human republic[70].

69 SEVERINUS ibidem, p. 172–173.

70 SEVERINUS, ibidem, p. 181.

Assessment of Severinus as Epigenesist

Severinus would thus appear to be the most eloquent exponent of Epigenesis between Aristotle and Harvey. However there is hardly any embryological observation on which his contentions are based. His main task is an exposition and defence of the ideas of Paracelsus and consequently the demonstration of the superiority and priority of the spirit, the spirit of life and its creative role with regard to matter and the body[71].

71 On the physical effects of spirits and the power of imagination (Ficinus, Agrippa, Paracelsus) see note [47] above.

Moreover it is true that Severinus emphasised the unity of the spirit that develops the germ and paid little attention to the development of the material parts. But although he referred to the Hippocratic adage of the circle, implying simultaneous separation of parts "without beginning and end", it would not be true to say that he denied the successive formation of each member at its appointed time. On the contrary he underlined this as an indication of the intrinsic "knowledge" and power of the seed. It is in the latter that all faculties are "at once and once only", i. e. without succession. In other words there is multiplicity and succession of solid parts, but not of faculties and intra-seminal tendencies.

Indeed Severinus' view amounts to a defence of epigenesis. For he ridicules those who believe in the simultaneous formation of the three central organs: liver, heart and brain. Moreover his motive in doing so is his characteristic vitalist attitude. Through this he finds fault with the preformationist view which forms a necessary corollary to the opinion of those who deny successive development of organs *de novo*.

Severinus thus insisted with Aristotle that the seed substance is simple and homogeneous—a view that was later taken up by Harvey with decisive emphasis (p. 261). He also strongly upheld the primacy and superiority of the heart as stipulated by Aristotle and later supported by Harvey (p. 84; 236). Here again, Severinus is actuated by his spiritualist conviction—he will not grant supremacy to the heart *qua* material part of the body, but only *qua* bearer of the vital spirit. For this, Severinus says, is concentrated in its fulness at the point where the heart afterwards develops. For the same reason he goes further than Aristotle and thereby *even more closely approaches Harvey in according to the blood a position of dignity and priority superior to the heart*. For he, like Harvey, saw in the blood the first shrine of the vital spirit. Consequently it is only natural that he should again side with Aristotle in rejecting material quality and complexion as causative agents in generation—in favour of spirit and Logos[72].

We have dealt with Severinus at some length because his ideas largely overlap with those of Harvey and their Aristotelian source. Severinus in fact clearly illustrates the *vitalistic background* of the theory *of Epigenesis* as propounded by Harvey.

His book was well known at Harvey's time, when it went through three editions[73]. Bacon should have been well acquainted with it, as he had accorded to it words of praise[74]. It is reasonable to assume that it was not unknown to Harvey, however little its affiliation to Paracelsean ideas and Lord Bacon's praise may have impressed him as commendable features.

72 Aristotle *de generatione animal.* 734b ed. Aubert-Wimmer *loc. cit.* p. 140.

73 See footnote [40] above.

74 See footnote [41] above.

Harvey's Vitalistic Criticism of Ancient Materialism

The Elements, Qualities and Humours
The Position of Semen and Ovum

Harvey advocated vitalism. Of this we found ample evidence in the discussion of *Epigenesis* (p. 233). Here he showed himself a staunch follower of Aristotle—just as much as in the comparative-anatomical approach which he practised.

However, in a number of questions, not always of mere detail, he had much to say against "The Philosopher". Such points in which he differed concerned the function and fate of the male semen, the activity of the female part (denied by Aristotle) and the independence of the *ovum* as a structure in its own right endowed with a "psychic" impulse and direction of its own (p. 272). Harvey also opposed Aristotle in granting the blood primacy, even over the heart. The blood, according to Harvey, is the first to develop and the true "seat of the soul".

Contagion from a Distance—the Operative Force in Fertilisation

In some of these points Harvey was actuated by vitalistic leanings which exceeded those of the master. The latter had regarded the female part in generation as a menstrual product, as residual matter that provides the "stuff" for the—active—male seed to unite with and work upon.

Harvey denied any real unification of the male and the female parts in favour of action at a distance, comparable to *contagion*. This Harvey visualised as a specific mechanism, a divine artifice, an act that is "momentary ... a transitory thing which is neither found to be remaining, nor touching, nor contained, as far as the senses inform us, and yet works with the highest intelligence and foresight, beyond all art[1], and which even after it has vanished, renders the egg prolific, not because it now touches, but because it formerly did so" (*non quia jam tangit, sed quia olim tetigit*)[2]. It is the same event as when "epidemic, contagious, and pestilential diseases scatter their seeds and are propagated to a distance through the air, or by some tinder (*fomes*) producing diseases like themselves, in bodies of a different nature and in a hidden fashion silently multiplying themselves by a kind of generation[3]".

The male semen, then, does not act upon the female part as matter acts on matter, i.e. by unification, but by virtue of *sympathy*. This action is *spiritual* and is prompted by a mere touch that has taken place in the past.

1 *On Generation of Animals* Exerc. XLI. Amstelod. 1662, p. 143., tr. WILLIS London 1847, p. 321.

2 Ibidem, similarly in: Ex. XLIX ed. 1662, p. 175. WILLIS p. 358. – See also Ex. XLI as quoted in note [1]: "So noble a work ... the contagion of intercourse, an act ... so momentary". – Also *On Conception* ed. 1662, p. 378. WILLIS p. 575.

On the other hand Harvey admits that no touch may have ever taken place: "For in the egg there is no semen, neither does any touch it, nor has ever done so (nam in ovo nullum semen inest, aut tangens ovum, aut quod illud umquam tetigerit)" Ex. XLVII, ed. 1662, p. 167. WILLIS p. 349; Ex. XLIX, ed. 1662 p. 175. WILLIS p. 358: "nay contact is not necessary; a mere halitus or miasm suffices and that at a distance and by an inanimate medium and with nothing sensibly altered". Based on Aristotle, *De gener. anim.* 734b, 10–15, lib. II, cap. 1

3 "Seminaria sua eminus per aerem aut fomitem aliquem spargant aut propagent morbosque sui similes in alienis corporibus producant atque abscondito modo per generationem quendam ... se tacite multiplicant". Ex. XLI, 1662, p. 143. Willis p. 322. – See also Letter of November 30 th 1653 to Joh. Nardi of Florence; letter V in WILLIS p. 610–611.

The Influence of Fracastor

Here Harvey followed closely Fracastor (1483–1553). By *contagium* the latter understood a manifestation, on earth and in man, of a *sympathy* that was operative in the cosmos at large. Already Fracastor connected it with *generation*. He distinguished it from *putrefaction:* contagion is a *generatio*, putrefaction is not. For the former implies a chain of consecutive digestive processes which is not found in simple putrid corruption. Thus, for example, vinegar develops from wine by generation and not by putrefaction. In contagion we recognise an orderly sequence of events directed by an *idea* and manifested in a digestive process that is associated with a specific taste and smell[4].

Humours, Blood and Spirits

Aristotle, in Harvey's view, could not entirely emancipate himself from interpreting biological phenomena in terms of ancient elemental and humoralist doctrine, in other words from ancient materialism. This doctrine is criticised by Harvey in the two concluding chapters of his work *On Generation*, which are devoted to *Innate Heat* and *Primigenial Moisture* respectively[5].

Against Aristotle Harvey entered a plea in favour of the priority and supremacy of the Blood. He also opposed the Fernelian "spirits" which had been given a leading role as offspring of the stars and source of animal heat[6].

At first sight it is therefore Harvey and not Aristotle who appears to have been actuated by materialist leanings. However, this is not so. For Harvey does not deny the spirit and its power—the spiritual "heat" or power that is *inherent* in the blood. What he does deny is that blood is inert matter with spirits *superadded*—a separate spiritual authority that gives the blood its functional impulse and direction.

In other words Harvey would only recognise blood that is alive owing to its own—inherent—spirit. Its vitality is maintained as long as blood runs in the vessels. As soon as it ceases to circulate it becomes *cruor* or gore and no longer deserves the name of blood deprived as it is of *spirit* and *heat* (*sine spiritu aut calore, non sanguis, sed cruor appellandus*)[7].

Blood had been denied its eminently spiritual quality, chiefly because—since antiquity—it had been regarded as a *material* constituent of the body and as composed of the four elements. Hence the quest for a spirit endowed with power of action beyond the

4 Utrum contagio omnis putrefactio quaedam sit. The answer is: no. "circa putrefactiones est intelligendum, quod interdum sola misti dissolutio fit, et sola evaporatio humidi atque innati caloris, *generatio* autem nova nulla consequitur". Hence putrefaction is attended by abominable odour and taste. Not so generation with its "digestio ordoque partium pro certa forma". For example: "vinum quandoque simpliciter putrefit ... interdum non simpliciter putrescit sed et simul *generatio* aliqua sequitur ut aceti". Hieron. Fracastorius, *De Contagione* lib.I, cap.9. Venet. 1546, fol.34 recto. *Opp. omnia* Venet. 1555, fol.110 verso; ibid. cap.12, fol.112 recto (1555): "eam seminariis inesse vim ut sibi simile propagare et gignere possint, sicuti et spiritus faciunt". and fol.112 verso: "differt autem seminarium contagionis a vapore simplici". (1546, fol.36 recto et verso.)

5 Ex.LXXI and LXXII ed. 1662, p.314–330. Willis p.501–518. With reference to Aristotle on semen and blood as composed of water, earth and air, e.g. in *Meteora* IV, 10; 389a 19 and *De part. animal.* III, 5; 669a and ibid. IV, 10; 686a 6 (*haimatos krasis*).

6 For example: Ex.LXXI, ed. 1662, p. 315 and 322. Willis p.502 and 507.

7 Ex.LXXI, ed.1662, p.314–315, Willis p.502.

This refers to Aristotle, *De Partibus Animal.* II,3; 650a. To this see Averroes, *Commentary* in: *Aristotelis Libri Omnes cum Averrois Cordubensis variis in eosdem commentariis.* Venet. apud Juntas 1562, vol.VI, fol.134 recto: "Verum nomine sanguinis eum intelligi volo, qui intus lateat in animali vivente. nam extra corpus, aut obeunte animali per accidens frigescit atque siccescit".

elements, "a body of perfect simplicity, most subtle, attenuated, mobile, rapid, lucid, ethereal[8]".

Such ethereal spirits, Harvey says, had been looked upon as the paramount authority, coming from outside, which gives the body orders that are conveyed by the blood.

Of the authors who followed this tradition Harvey singles out Scaliger and Fernel for criticism. They have, he says, never demonstrated such a spirit or shown its superiority over the elements and indeed the power of the blood itself. Fernel had referred to the empty spaces of the heart, the arteries and the brain as the receptacles suitable for an extremely subtle aura or vapour that is cherished by the air which we breathe[9].

Harvey can see no truth in this, as the cavities of the heart and the arteries are filled with blood as long as life persists. Nor are the ventricles of the brain empty, but they contain a product of secretion.

Further arguments against the spirits are the absence of cerebral ventricles in some animals and nature's abhorrence of a vacuum. Moreover, a mere element such as the air cannot act as the main aliment of a spiritual, i.e. super-elemental power, all the more so as the spirits are believed to be extremely vulnerable and short-lived and thus to require continual regeneration. This, by general consensus, is achieved by the blood and the spirits are said to be unable to survive, when separated from it even by a nail's breadth. Why then, asks Harvey, introduce a spiritual power coming from outside and acting *on* the blood, instead of one that resides and acts *in* the blood—a power that is comparable to the flame of a lamp or candle and inseparably bound up with the oil or tallow that feeds it?[10]

Pneumatic Theories and Harvey's Ideas

Blood thus qualifies as the immediate instrument of the soul, as it is present and moving everywhere[11]. Indeed it is blood itself that shares the nature of a substance that is more divine than are the elements. For the heat innate in the blood is derived neither from fire nor from air—mere elements and for that reason severely restricted in activity and power. The blood "acts above the forces of the elements" and what Aristotle said about the soul is true of the blood, namely that it "seems to have a connection with a matter different from and more divine than the so-called elements... All have in their semen that which causes it to be productive; I mean what is called vital heat. This is not fire nor any such force,

8 Ex.LXXI ed. 1662, p.315. Willis p. 503.

9 Fernel refers to Aristotle *De Gener. Animal.* II, 3; 736b: "recte prodidit Aristoteles, in semine spumosoque corpore spiritum, in spiritu naturam contineri, quae proportione respondet elemento stellarum.". Obviously, Fernel continues, this spirit is intermediate (interponi) between body and divine nature as some common link. It is an "ethereal body", the seat and link of the animal heat and the faculties, the first instrument making function possible. To know more about its substance and status, one should look upon the structure of the body, notably the arteries, the cavity of the heart and the ventricles of the brain which will show up empty and void of any fluid (quos dum inanes ac nullius prope humoris participes videbit). Yet such big spaces cannot be without their proper purpose. If follows that as long as life persists, they are filled with a very fine *aura* (praetenuem auram eos tum implevisse). This derives its nutriment (pabulum) from the air which we breathe—the main purpose of respiration being not so much refrigeration (which could be obtained in other ways), but to cherish and foster (fovendae gratia) this thin and spirituous substance (si nulla in nobis esset tenuis et spirituosa substantia, vix ulla profecto nos ad inspirandum necessitas impelleret). Fernel, *Physiologiae* lib.IV, cap.2. *Universa Medicina* ed. J. et O.Heurnius. Trajecto ad Rh. 1656, p.81–82. – See below p. 264 and note [67].

10 Ex.LXXI, 1662, p.317; Willis p.504.

11 "Est igitur sanguis sufficiens et idoneus, qui sit immediatum animae instrumentum; quoniam et ubique praesens est et huc illuc ocyssime permeet". – Ibid. (l.c. note [10]). Here Harvey also refers to Cremoninus (1552–1631), the successor to Zabarella as Professor of Philosophy in the University of Padua since 1590, i.e. at Harvey's time, the last of the Paduan "Averroists", the defender of observational experience (albeit hampered in practical life by loyalty to Aristotelian doctrine). Harvey calls him: "Aristotelicae philosophiae eximie peritus" who rejected additional non-corporeal spiritual qualities and more divine forms of heat such as light, opposing Albertus Magnus. See: Cremoninus, Caesar, *De Calido Innato et Semine. Pro Aristotele adversus Galenum*, Lugd. Batav. 1634, Dictatio VII, p.71: movetur (sc. spiritus) quocumque et quacumque prout sibi paratae sunt viae, et instrumenta, per quae a facultate animae huc, et illuc transferatur. Sic a corde et ad cor...

but it is the spiritus included in the semen and the foam-like (*emperilambanomenon en to spermati kai to aphrodei pneuma*), and the natural principle in the spiritus (*he en to pneumati physis*), being analogous to the element of the stars. Hence whereas fire generates no animal and we do not find any living thing forming in either solids or liquids under the influence of fire, the heat of the sun and that of animals does generate them. Not only is this true of the heat that works through the semen, but whatever other residuum of the animal nature there may be, this also still has a vital principle in it (*zotiken archen*). From such considerations it is clear that the heat in animals neither is fire nor derives its origin from fire[12]".

Harvey thus attributes to blood what Aristotle had called the *Connate pneuma*[13]. The latter had insisted that this *Pneuma* is neither from without nor identical with air nor for that matter with any other of the elements. It assumes a higher position in dignity and power than that of the elements. With this Aristotle finds himself at variance with his predecessors, notably Diogenes of Apollonia and the Hippocratic writer *On the sacred disease*[14]. It was these who had made life, sense perception, thought and also movement dependent upon the air that we breathe and that runs in the vessels, whilst blood had been reduced to a minor and restricted role. By contrast Aristotle saw the connexion between *Pneuma* and organism as much more intimate: it is born with *Pneuma*—a physical substance of finest corporality (*aither*) that hails from the stars and is endowed with generative power, unlike the elements which are not. It has its "seat" in the central organ, the heart, which sends it out to the periphery with the blood, enabling the latter to ensure nutrition, growth and the production of semen[15].

Harvey used the term *connate genius* (*connato ingenio*) to denote *natural* action as against action that emanates from "forecast, instruction or reason" (*providentia, disciplina aut consilio*). Natural action is untaught (*autodidaktos*) in contrast to knowledge and action that are acquired by virtue of art, intellect or foresight (*ars, intellectus, providentia*). Thus the spider weaves her web, birds build nests, incubate their eggs and cherish their young, bees and ants construct dwellings and lay up stores for their future wants—all this is done naturally and from a *connate genius*. In the same way the vegetative faculty of the parents and the semen arrive at the form of the foetus. Hence it is from such *natural* processes that the pattern of *artful* operations should be derived and judged rather than that one should refer to art and artifice as judges of Nature[16].

The semen as well as the blood are, according to Harvey, endowed with the superelemental power of *Pneuma* and it is to the

12 *De Gener. Animal.* II,3; 736b–737a; tr. A. PLATT. Oxford 1910.

13 See: PECK, A.L., *The Connate Pneuma. An essential factor in Aristotle's solutions of the problems of reproduction and sensation. Science, Medicine and History. Essays*, ed. E.A. Underwood, Oxford 1953, vol. I, p. 111–121.

14 SOLMSEN, F., *Greek Philosophy and the Discovery of the Nerves. Museum Helveticum* 1961, XVIII, p. 150–167; 169–197 (notably p. 174 seq.).

15 PECK loc. cit. (note [13]) 1953, p. 119; Solmsen loc. cit. (note [14]) 1961, p. 177.

16 Ex. L, ed. 1662, p. 185; WILLIS p. 369.

latter that blood owes its emergence in the embryo as the first part of the new organism[17]. It is equally due to the *Pneuma* that from the primigenial drop of blood all the other parts are formed in succession—the blood that is "proceeding at all times with such foresight and understanding, and with definite ends in view, as if it employed reasoning in its acts[18]".

The blood therefore, "*is spirit* by reason of its admirable properties and powers" (*sanguis itaque est spiritus, ob eximias ejus virtutes et vires*)[19]. Harvey continues: "It is also celestial, for nature (that is the Soul) that which answers to the essence of the stars, is the inmate of the spirit, in other words it is something analogous to heaven, the instrument of heaven, vicarious to heaven[20]".

This is not negatived by the material and elemental composition of the blood. For blood does not stand alone in displaying superior power to that of the elements. Indeed there is hardly any body composed of elements that does not exceed their power, when in action. Thus the winds and the ocean "waft navies to either India or round this globe, when they grind, stamp, sift, dig wells, cut timber, kindle fire, bear up some things, overwhelm others and perform many other innumerable and wonderful offices—do they not seem to act above the powers of the elements?[21]" This is also true of the many varied effects brought about by fire, the magnetic power of iron and the precise work of clocks. Bodies do not accomplish such effects as such, i.e. as "primary agents" or "prime efficients", but as "instrumental agents". In other words they do not act by their own virtue, but by the virtue of a superior agent[22].

There is no need, then, to fetch down from heaven all sorts of—astral—"spirits" to explain generation—a process that surpasses in divinity and power any spirit, nay the soul itself, the vegetative as well as the sensitive and even understanding by the rational soul. This also applies to nutrition—itself a kind of generation[23]. For "the nature of generation and the order that prevails in it are truly admirable and divine, beyond all that thought can conceive or understanding comprehend[24]".

Blood not a Humour, but an Integral Part of the Body

Outside its functional sphere—the all-pervading blood vessels—blood loses its power. It becomes an inert conglomerate of elemental matter—a "cruor" that exhibits but a few hardly perceptible effects and virtues.

By contrast: "contained within the veins it forms a *part* of the body and at that one that is animated and engendering (*genitalis*)[25]".

17 "quemadmodum in semine inest aliquid, quod ipsum foecundum reddat, et in fabricando animali vires elementorum excellat; spiritus nempe, et natura in eo spiritu respondens elemento stellarum: ita pariter in sanguine, inest spiritus sive vis aliqua, agens supra vires elementorum (in singulis animalis partibus nutriendis et conservandis valde conspicua) et natura, imo anima in eo spiritu et sanguine, respondens elemento stellarum" Ex. LXXI, ed. 1662, p. 318. WILLIS p. 506.

18 "cum jam pars primogenita et calor innatus existens (ut fit in semine et spiritu) reliquas totius corporis partes ordine fabricat, idque summa cum providentia et intellectu, in finem certum agens, quasi ratiocinio quodam uteretur." Ex LXXI, ed. 1662, p. 319; WILLIS p. 507.

19 Ex. LXXI, ed. 1662, p. 320; WILLIS p. 507.

20 Ex. LXXI, ed. 1662, p. 320; WILLIS p. 507.

21 Ex. LXXI, ed. 1662, p. 321; WILLIS p. 509. – The first English translation London 1653, p. 456 is more literal than Willis, notably in the following sentence concerning the power of fire.

22 Ex. LXXI, ed. 1662, p. 321; WILLIS p. 509.

23 See p. 310 and Ex. LXXII, ed. 1662, p. 326; WILLIS p. 514.

24 "Natura enim generationis ejusque ordo, admirabilis plane est et divinus, supra quam quispiam cogitatione capere aut mente complecti possit". Ex. LXXI, ed. 1662, p. 322; WILLIS p. 510.

25 "Quatenus pars corporis eademque animata et genitalis" Ex. LXXI ed. 1662, p. 322. "An *Animate* and *Genital* part"—tr. London 1653, p. 458. – "is animated and regenerate"—tr. WILLIS p. 510. Sensibility of blood denied by Aristotle: *De part. anim.* II, 3; 650b; II, 5; 651b5; II, 10; 656b19 and elsewhere.

Harvey attached much importance to the blood forming a *part*—a member just like any other member or organ.

Blood, Sensation and Irritability

In accordance with this he was emphatic in attributing sense and motion to the blood, as Temkin rightly pointed out[26]. Indeed the blood perceives things that tend to injure by irritating or to benefit by cherishing it[27]. This is associated with Harvey's views on the priority of blood, even over the heart. The latter is thus not identical with the *salient point* in the embryo, but develops from it. For, as Harvey says, the *salient point* as the animated generative part must derive from the soul of the ovum which is transferred into the *salient point* and hence into the heart[28]. *Qua* blood and thus endowed with sensibility and motion the *salient point* is liable to irritation, reacting as it does to touch with a needle, a probe or a finger or to differences in temperature or any other molesting circumstance or thing. Its reaction is expressed in alteration of its pulse[29]—the outward sign of an "irritability" that is independent of the central nervous system, and, as Temkin has shown, an important example foreshadowing the ideas of Glisson[30].

In thus attributing sensation to the blood Harvey is conscious of his divergence from Aristotle[31]. This divergence is part and parcel of the whole argument concerning the priority and supremacy of the blood which thus assumed the position of a member or part and the one with the highest responsibility and dignity in the body at that—a position expressly denied by Aristotle in favour of the heart.

Harvey continues: Even if it were devoid of sensation this would not disqualify the blood from forming a part and even a very principal part of a body endowed with sensibility. For neither does the brain nor the spinal marrow nor the crystalline or the vitreous humour of the eye, feel anything, though by common consent, these are parts of the body. Nay even the heart itself, the most distinguished part of the body, appears to be insensible. Here Harvey reports the case of young Viscount Montgomery whose heart had been laid bare in consequence of a severe fall in early childhood and tolerated palpation without any discomfort. Harvey was thus enabled to confirm in the live human body that in diastole the heart is drawn in and retracted, that in systole it comes forth and is thrust out, that systole of heart is simultaneous with diastole of the artery at the wrist, and that systole, the proper motion of the heart, makes the latter prominent, causing it to beat the breast, lifting it upwards and contracting it into itself[32].

26 TEMKIN, O., *The classical roots of Glisson's doctrine of irritation Bullet. Hist. Med.* 1964, XXXVIII, 297–328 (p. 321) with ref. to Harvey, *On generation* Exercit. LII, ed. 1662, p. 197; tr. WILLIS p. 381: utrumque autem, *sensum* scilicet et *motum*, sanguini inesse ... etiamsi Aristoteles id negaverit.

27 HARVEY ibidem, 1662, p. 195; WILLIS p. 380: eum et irritantis injuriam, et foventis commodum persentiscere.

28 MEYER, ARTHUR WILLIAM, *An analysis of the De generatione animalium of William Harvey.* Stanford Univ. Press and London 1936, p. 96 with ref. to Harvey, *On generatioh* Exerc. XLVII, ed. 1662, p. 166; tr. WILLIS p. 347–348: punctum saliens partemve genitalem animatam, ab ovi anima proficisci (nihil enim sui ipsius autor est) animamque ab ovo, in punctum saliens; mox in cor, et deinde in pullum traductum.

29 HARVEY, *On generation* Exerc. XVII, ed. 1662, p. 66; tr. WILLIS p. 239: ego vero pluribus experimentis certus sum non motum solummodo puncto salienti inesse (quod nemo negaverit) sed sensum etiam. Nam ad quemlibet vel minimum tactum, videbis hoc punctum varie commoveri et quasi irritari (perinde omnino ac sensitiva corpora, sensus sui indicia propriis motibus exhibere solent), et ad iteratam saepe injuriam extimulari, atque in pulsuum rhythmo et ordine conturbari. See below note [98a] and p. 330.

30 TEMKIN, loc. cit. in note [26], especially on parallels and differences between the views of Glisson, Harvey and Galen.

Temkin has also shown that Vesalius recognised a principle of motion as a general property of living tissue. The motions, he said, that are particular to all parts and do not aid other parts are effected completely without the help by fibres, by a force simply implanted in the parts (*De humani corporis fabrica*, Basil. 1543, lib. III, cap. 1, p. 257–258). Vesalius is in this more definite than Galen who merely spoke of an "innate tension" present in all parts of the body whereby surplus material could be passed from a stronger to a weaker part. By contrast Galen attributed attraction, retention and discharge to the operation of fibres. TEMKIN, O., *Vesalius on an immanent biological motor force. Bullet. Hist. Med.* 1965, XXXIX, 277–280.

31 See the passages quoted in note [25] and [26].

32 HARVEY, *On generation* Exerc. LII, Opera Londini 1766, p. 399, ed. 1662, p. 198; Tr. WILLIS p. 382 seq. Tr. Lond. 1653, p. 285–287. – See also VIETS, H. R., *Young Montgomery and his beating heart. New Eng-*

Harvey himself tells us that the blood was not unanimously regarded as a part or member of the body, but that Aristotle counted it among the "similar parts" and so by implication did Hippocrates, since according to him the body consists of containing, contained and impelling parts, blood thus coming under the second category, i.e. the parts that are contained[33].

It is not without interest that Harvey's view had been expressed in alchemical sources when it had been put forward in conscious opposition to Galen. Thus the commentator to the *Golden treatise on the secret of the natural stone*, a Dominicus Gnosius (Belga, writing in about 1600) speaks about the "rubicund spirit" which is like blood, emerging from the *pelican*, i.e. a still formed like the large water fowl, fabled to feed its young with its own blood. Also in the human body the blood is not only rubicund, but also that *part* in which the spirits are most abundant—although it is unjustly excluded from the number of parts by the crowd of Galenic physicians, whilst some regard it as the foremost seat of life[34].

The blood, then, *qua part* of the body acts as the immediate instrument of the soul and its first ranking seat (*sedes primaria*). It thus partakes of another more divine body—perfused as it is by divine animal heat. For all this it obtains extraordinary force and emulates the element of the stars[35]. It is the Sun of the Microcosm, a *Platonic Fire*, for unlike ordinary fire it preserves, nourishes and makes things grow by virtue of a vagrant (*vago*) and perpetual motion[36].

Blood, Semen and Primigenial Dew

In short, then, blood incorporates in itself the two vital principles of the ancients: *Innate Heat* and *Radical Moisture*. It derives from the crystalline colliquament which forms the immediate germ of the embryo and all its parts. This germinative liquid, though "simple" and formless in itself, is capable of assuming all forms—potentially[37]. It is Protean, it is *Prime Matter*. Being generative implies that it is also nutritive—for all generation is a form of nutrition and vice versa. The body "is what it eats"—no physician nor any philosopher ever denied this.

The primordial fluid, then, is a nutritious *dew*, a *ros primigenius*[38].

The Ancient Sources for the Primigenial Dew

Harvey though referring for this term to the Arabs[39], here develops an Aristotelian theme that was taken up by Galen, transmitted

land J. Med. 1957, CCLVI. 702, with special reference to H. MILNE EDWARDS, *Leçons sur la physiologie et l'anatomie comparée de l'homme et des animaux.* vol. IV, Paris 1857–1881 (in 14 vols), p. 15.

33 Ibidem, Opp. 1766, p. 398; tr. WILLIS p. 382; tr. 1653, p. 285. Arist., *de part. anim.* II, 2, 648a and PECK, A.L. ed. Loebs Lib. 1937, p. 28.

34 *Hermetis Trismegisti tractatus aureus de lapidis physici secreto in capitula septem divisus: nunc vero a quodam Anonymo scholiis illustratus* in *Theatrum Chemicum* vol. IV, Argentor. 1613, p. 722: "in corpore etiam humano nullam invenies partem (quamvis is ex partium numero immerito excludatur a medicorum Galenicorum turba) quae plus abundet spiritibus, quam ille ipse (sc. sanguis), ita ut a medicis quibusdam praecipua vitae sedes dicatur". See for detail about the treatise which is probably of mediaeval-arabic origin and the commentator from the first decade of the XVIIth century: W. PAGEL, *Hermetic alchemy at Bruno's time.* Appendix to review of YATES, F.A., *Giordano Bruno and the Hermetic tradition.* London 1964 in *Ambix* 1964, XII, p. 72–76.

The Hermetic *Tractatus Aureus* first appeared under the title *Septem tractatus s. capitula Trismegisti aurei* in the *Ars Chemica*, Argentorati 1566, pp. 7–31. – See also below, p. 276, note [114].

35 Ex. LXXI, ed. 1662, p. 322. WILLIS p. 510.

36 Tr. London 1653; p. 458: "Free perpetuall motion". WILLIS p. 510: "vague and incessant motion".

37 Ex. LXXII, ed. 1662, p. 325. WILLIS p. 513.

38 Ex. LXXII ed. 1662, p. 326. WILLIS p. 514.

39 HARVEY here undoubtedly alludes to Avicenna, as quoted in note [43].

by such mediaeval writers as Avicenna and Arnaldus of Villanova and elaborated upon and summarised in the era of the Renaissance by Fernel.

Blood, according to Aristotle, in a more advanced stage becomes semen in the male who can thus concoct the *nourishment in its ultimate phase* (*peptikon tes hystates trophes*). He owes this capacity to the first principle and the part which contains the principle of natural heat. Indeed the semen is the ultimate secretion of nutriment (*perittoma trophes on to eschaton*) and as such carried *to* all parts of the body—rather than coming *from* them (as assumed by the Pangenesists; see above p. 235). Though it is the last extract of nutriment spread to all parts of the body (*prosion eschaton; peritton genomenon*) it is by no means a waste product and it is small in quantity—as Aristotle says: the final secretion is smallest in proportion to quantity of nutriment (*to teleutaion ek pleistes trophes oligiston*)[40]. In Averroes' commentary to this passage we read: blood is the ultimate nutriment of the first member which is the heart (*sanguis est alimentum ultimum primi membri quod est cor*) and semen is the ultimate secretion of the nutriment of the members which is the blood (*semen—excrementum ultimum nutrimenti membrorum quod est sanguis*), and finally it is gathered in small quantity from much nutriment (*parum aggregatur ex nutrimento multo*)[41].

Galen speaks of a substance that is dispersed and continually absorbed through all animal parts *like dew* (*drosoeidos*) by a process of nutrition[42].

Mediaeval and Renaissance Sources

Following Avicenna[43], Arnald of Villanova (1235–1311) enumerates the three kinds of fluid that are contained in the substance of the parts: first the moisture that exudes into the porous substance of the members from the cavities that naturally contain blood. This liquid is called *dew*, because it sweats through in very small dew drops. It becomes *cambium* when it is more assimilated to the substance of the part in colour and complexion and finally *glue* (*gluten*), the moisture that keeps the parts together, and has given up the functions of a mere fluid[44].

Fernel distinguishes between an oily—primigenial—fluid that maintains the vital spirit and "secondary" humours. He names four such humours: 1. fleshy substance understood as a product of condensation of fluid 2. the immediate nutriment that becomes attached and incorporated ("agglutinated") into a part, its "glue" (*gluten*) 3. fluid that is not yet tissue-bound, but poured forth into

40 Ability of the male to concoct blood into semen which carries the principle of the *form* and the first moving cause: Aristotle, *De Gener. Animal.* Lib.IV,1; 765b.– Concoction of nutriment in its last stage ibid. 766a 35. – Semen as the ultimate secretion of nutriment 766b 8. – Semen as a secretion or excretion (*perittoma*) ibid. I, 18; 724b 28. – Semen as residue of nutriment bid. 724b 34–35. – Semen not a part as it is simple and homogeneous ibid. 724b 29. – Semen not *from*, but going *to* all parts ibid. 725a 23. – Small quantity of final secretion ibid. 725a 18. – Semen not a waste product 725a 25. – Semen as secretion of useful nutriment in its last stage of digestion 726a 26.

41 Averroes to Aristotle *De Gener. Animal.* IV, 1–2 loc. cit. 1562 (note [7]), vol. VI, fol. 114 recto and ad I,18 fol. 57 verso.

42 Galen, *De Methodo Medendi* lib. VII, cap. 6 ed. Kühn vol. X, p. 471.

its substance and covering it *like dew* ("roris vice") and 4. humour exuded from the terminals of the finest vessels into empty tissue spaces. These four represent the prime and principal fluids and juices of the body. Though themselves in the last resort derived from blood, they are quite separate from that blood which runs in the large vessels. They are closely related to the *semen*, however, for this is a product of the immediate—"last"—nutriment of the parts, i.e. the thin, pure and spiritual part of the blood. This spermatic humour is continually "sprinkled" into the blood—like *dew* (*semperque sanguini spermaticus humor roris modo inspergitur*)[45].

44 Arnaldus de Villanova, *Speculum Introduct. Medicinal.*, cap.IV. *Opp. omnia* ed. Nicol. Taurellus, Basil. 1585, p. 13E.

45 Fernel, *Physiologia* IV,5. *Universa Medicina* loc. cit. (note [9]) 1656, p. 86—on *Humidum primigenium* and the four *Humores secundarii*. – Ibidem lib.VII, cap. 2, p. 170: spermatic fluid is "sprinkled" into the blood.

43 Avicenna, *Canon*, Lib.IV, Fen 1, tract. 3, cap. 2. *Libri in re medica omnes*, Venetiis, Valgrisius, 1564, vol.II, p. 61, l. 39–53.

Hebrew sources—Maimonides and Kabbala:

Dew, as J.O. Leibowitz informed the present author, is a symbol of resurrection in Jewish religious literature and through its association with life connected with blood; it is visualised as blood distillate. Thus Maimonides, closely following Galen, speaks of the contents of the arteries as being thin and of the nature of a vapourous dew. The term used is *ejd*. The Galenic equivalent is *atmos kai pneuma* (*vapor et spiritus*)—*De usu partium*, lib.VI, cap. 16; ed. Kühn, vol. III, p. 491; tr. Daremberg, vol. I, p. 440: *de vapeur et d'air*. – *Vapor et spiritus* is also used by Nicolaus Regius, Paris. 1528, p. 185. Maimonides, *Aphorismi*, partic. I, ed. Wilna 1888, fol. 1 verso. For the interpretation of *ejd* as dew: *Midrash b'reshith rabba*, ed. Theodor, Berlin 1912, p. 119.

Maimonides would seem to distinguish three contents of the arteries: blood, pneuma and *ejd* (i.e. vapour and dew). Not far from the passage quoted above, he says that the most subtle and hidden in the body is the pneuma, whereas the *ejd* (vapour) is less so and blood still less.

The Crystal-dew of the Kabbala

This is called *tala debedulcha* and indicates the fluid between the meninges and in the brain at large. For this Prof. G. Scholem referred the author to *Sohar* II, *Sifre de-Zeniutha* fol. 176b, *Sohar* I, 225b; II, 136b; III, 49a and in particular to the *Idra Rabba* elaborating on *Sohar* II, 176b.

See also: Scholem, G., *Vuillaud's Übersetzung des Sifra de-Zeniutha aus dem Sohar* in *Monatschr. Gesch. Wiss. d. Judent.* 1931, LXXV, 353 where it says: "Dabei (wie auch später) wird im mystischen Gleichnis die arabisch-galenische Anatomie des Mittelalters benutzt, der '*Kristalltau*' zwischen Dura Mater and Pia Mater".

The present author would like to add the corresponding *loci* from the *Kabbala Denudata: Siphra de Zeniutha sive Liber mysterii*, paragr. 48: "Ros copiosus super eo duorum colorum (sicut in Macroprosopo albus tantum, ita hic albus et ruber est, ob judicia vide in *Idra magna* paragr. 44)". – *Idra Rabba s. Synodus magna* sectio IV. *De Rore seu humiditate cerebri Senioris seu Macroprosopi* paragr. 44 et seq.: "Et ex illo cranio destillat ros versus illum, qui est extrinsecus; et replet caput ejus quotidie. – Et ex illo rore, quem excutit de capite suo, ille qui est extrinsecus, excitabuntur mortui ad mundum venturum". *Kabbalae Denudatae Tom. secundus id est Liber Sohar Restitutus.* Francof. 1684, p. 364 and 393.

These passages suggest a knowledge of the cerebral liquor by the mediaeval authors of the *Sohar* which is remarkable in view of the few and sketchy hints which we possess from ancient and mediaeval authors (see for example: Woollam, D.H.M., *The historical significance of the Cerebro-spinal Fluid. Med. Hist.* 1957, I, 91–114; pp. 105–108: the discovery of the cerebrospinal fluid).

However the cerebral liquor seems to have been generally known. According to Prof. Scholem (personal communication to the present author of June 25th 1963), Eleazar of Worms (about 1200) speaks of the *lechah saviv l'moach*—the liquor around the brain (*Chochmath ha-nephesh*, 1876, fol. 33a). Eleazar is known to report preferably facts that were general knowledge at his time. It has to be borne in mind, of course, that since antiquity (notably including Aristotle) the brain was thought to be muciparous.

Fernel's version of the matter was quoted and given qualified acceptance by Van Helmont who restricted humoral transmission of the essentials of the organ substance to the juvenile body. For wherever he could, Van Helmont laid emphasis on local production rather than humoral transmission, either through the blood in normal life or through "catarrh"-fluid in disease[46]. Nevertheless Van Helmont does speak of the *mucoid dew* and spirit which emanates from the blood on its *third journey* through the liver and the veins themselves, providing as it does for the growth of the parts. It thus operates in what he calls the *Third realm of the body*, and corresponds to the *secondary humour* of the Schoolmen, visualised as an intermediary between blood and tissues[47].

Harvey mentions the *ultimate aliment* of the parts—an Aristotelian concept, as we have seen. Moreover in his reference to the primigenial *dew* he enlarges on its condensation, adhesion and final incorporation into the tissues in the form of *gluten*—ideas and terms with which we are familiar from Galen, Avicenna, Arnald of Villanova and Fernel. Harvey here visualises a *cyclical* process: condensation of nutritive fluid into solid parts alternating with a re-conversion of the latter into *dew*. This is seen, for example, when the white of the egg is liquefied and, in the form of *colliquament*, provides the radical moisture and primigenial *dew* for the embryo[48].

The *dew* or *cambium*—the nutritive portion or *ultimate aliment* of the tissues emanating from the blood had been also discussed by Harvey in the *Second exercitation to Riolan*[49]. Here it is said to have more penetrative power than the blood at large, as it has to be added everywhere, even to the feathers, horns, nails and hair. Hence Harvey does not think that it must necessarily circulate with the rest of the blood. It is separated from the blood, but unlike the latter incorporated in the parts and without influence on the rate of circulation.

For Harvey the comparison with dew denotes the "simplicity" and "homogeneity" of the prime fluid and the semen. Aristotle had already emphasised the simplicity of the latter[50]. Harvey links the "most simple pure and sincere body definable"[51], i.e. the *primigenial dew* with *First matter*—the medium that is common to all things, as it contains all things—potentially. As an illustration Harvey refers to the crystalline humour of the eye: itself colourless it is susceptible to all colours. This follows the Aristotelian doctrine that "what is capable of taking on colour is what in itself is colourless, as what can take on sound is what is soundless[52]". Moreover, according to Aristotle, water as well as air can transmit

46 Van Helmont, *Imago fermenti impraegnat massam semine*, cap. 4; *Ortus medicinae*, Amstelod. 1648, p. 112: nutrimentum verum immediatum membrorum ... de quo dici solet: nutrimur iisdem, quibus constamus. Hoc autem alimentum volunt roris modo inspergi in singula membra (ego vero in singulis partium culinis minimis fabricari credo).

On Van Helmont's localist views and the significance of the organ-"kitchen": Pagel, W., *J.B. Van Helmont*. Berlin 1930, p. 44 and passim; idem, *Religious and Philosophical Aspects of Van Helmont's Science and Medicine*, Baltimore 1944, p. 38 et seq.

47 Van Helmont, *Triplex Scholarum digestio*, cap. 6 in *Ortus medicinae*, Francof. 1707, p. 198.

The expression: *Third journey* and *Third realm of the body*—reminiscent of the mystical parlance of the followers of Joachim of Fiore—is not found in the Latin text, but in the Flemish version as given in: *Auffgang der Artzney-Kunst* (the German translation of the *Ortus* by Knorr of Rosenroth), Sultzbach 1683, p. 260. The *Third realm* occurs again, also in the Flemish version, in *Tract. von der Pest*, cap. 19, Aufgang, p. 657: und wascht demnach das heiße Wasser durch einen schnellen Schweiß die Pest aus dem Dritten Reich des Leibes aus.

48 Exerc. LXXII, ed. 1662, p. 326; tr. Willis, p. 514. See note [38] above, p. 257.

49 "Pars nutritiva et ultimum alimentum, sive ros sive cambium magis penetrativa est... neque excrementa... neque ultimum alimentum (rorem et cambium) cum sanguine revolvi necesse puto, sed adhaerere quod nutrit, ut agglutinetur, oportere." *Exercit. duae anatomicae de circulat. sanguinis ad Joannem Riolanum filium*, Roterod. 1649, II, p. 89; tr. Willis, p. 124.

The denial of a conversion of blood into *dew* and *cambium* is one of the arguments advanced in favour of circulation and against Riolan by George Ent, *Demonstratio circulationis sanguinis* in *Opera omnia medico-physica nunc primum junctim edita*, Leyden 1687, p. 135. The blood should be more white than it is, in the capillary veins and in the peripheral parts at large, if it were converted into nutritious material and consumed by the parts. In Ent's opinion blood is not a nutrient.

50 Aristotle, *De Gener. Animal.* 724b 29 —homoiomeres.

51 "terminabilis"—"that can be defined" left untranslated by Willis. "imaginable" in the London 1653 transl. p. 463.

52 Aristotle, *De Anima* 418b 25–30; lib. II, cap. 7.

colour, both being transparent, and the eye proper is made of water[53]. Finally Harvey invokes the Thomistic-Averroistic *Intellectus Possibilis* which is capable of all forms. Hence it is called *potential* (*possibilis*) rather than merely *passive* (*passibilis*)[54].

If, then, Harvey concludes, the essential parts, namely blood and semen from which all the other parts of the body stem are "simple", the body is neither a product of *composition* (*congregatione*), nor of *mixture* (*mistu*), neither of the four elements nor of atoms of diverse figures. Indeed the primigenial fluid knows of no diversity or heterogeneity of parts. If it did, nothing would be "similar, one, the same, and continuous"; there would be no union other than in appearance, only a "congregation or colligation of very small bodies forming a congeries and a heap[55]". In other words there would be no organism. Nor would generation be distinguishable from aggregation and the due posture of parts[56].

Blood and Semen as Acting and Disposed Matter

What does all this amount to? At the very end of his great work on generation Harvey returns full circle to his main profession and philosophy which is summarised in *Epigenesis*. The basic vitalism by which this doctrine is inspired, is poignantly expressed: *Similar bodies exist before their material constituent* (*corpora similaria mista elementa sua tempore priora non habeant, sed illa potius elementis suis prius existant*)[57].

Harvey's allegiance to vitalism thus goes even farther than that of Aristotle. For the latter still believed in the Empedoclean elements—fire, air, earth and water—as the essential components of natural objects, and notably of blood (p. 252).

Nor would Harvey admit of the *Three Principles* (*Tria Prima*) of the Chemists—Salt, Sulphur and Mercury—as constituents of objects, or for that matter of the Democritean atoms. All these are residues; they are products of corruption rather than principles (*posteriora potius et reliquiae magis quam principia*). Nor are they the end-products of the dissolution of things, for nobody ever (Aristotle included) has demonstrated their separate existence or that they were the principles of "similar bodies[58]".

The question as to whether bodies consist of those substances into which they can be dissolved was one of the stock topics for contemporary discussion by naturalists. Its source is Aristotle (IV *meteoron* and II *metaphys.*). Thomas Erastus opposed Paracelsus on this score. The latter, Erastus said, had affirmed it, as he thought

53 Ibid. lib. III, 1; 425a 1–5. See also ARISTOTLE *De Sensu* cap. II; 438a 10–15—the visual organ is composed of water; water is easily confined, hence the pupil, i.e. the eye proper consists of water. – *De Partibus* Animal. II, 10; 656b—vision is of the character of water. See to this W. OGLE, *Aristotle on the Parts of Animals*. London 1882, p. 154 to II, 1 note [12] and note [16] to II, 10.

54 "Intellectum possibilem incorporeum", transl. London 1653: "potential understanding which is incorporeal"—this tr. more correct than WILLIS, p. 513: "possibility of an incorporeal intellect." With reference to: Aristotle, *De Anima* III, 5; 430a 10 seq. – AVERROES in: *Aristotelis De Anima libri tres cum Averrois commentariis et antiqua tralatione*. Ed. Mich. Sophianus Venet. apud Juntas 1562, fol. 136 recto ad Lib. III, cap. 1 in particular comment. fol. 138 verso and 161 recto. In the edition Papiae. Jacob Paucidrapus de Burgofranco 1521, fol. 121 recto: Summa prima: De potentia animae intellectiva. De Intellectus Possibilis essentia. Ipsius impassibilitatem non esse similem ei, quae sensus. On Averroes and the *potential intellect:* GEYER, B., *Patrist. u. Scholast. Philos.* (Überweg's Grundriß vol. II; 13th ed.), Darmstadt, 1956, p. 318–319. – On the *active* and *passive* intellect: WILKIE, J.S., *Body and Soul in Aristotelian Tradition*. In: POYNTER, F.N.L. (Ed.), *Hist. and Philos. of Knowledge of the Brain*. Oxford 1958, 19–29.

55 EX. LXXII, 1662, p. 328. WILLIS p. 516. "Colligatio" tr. by WILLIS with "collection".

56 Ibidem: "neque generatio ab aggregatione debitaque partium positura quicquam differret". Tr. London 1653; p. 467: "aggregation and convenient positure of several parts". WILLIS, p. 516: (mechanical) aggregation and arrangement of particles".

57 HARVEY, *On generation*, Exercit. LXXII, ed. 1662, p. 329; tr. WILLIS, p. 517.

58 Ibidem.

to have been able to isolate salt, sulfur and mercury from any given substance by chemical manipulation. Against this Erastus argued that bodies do not consist of those parts from which they were generated nor are the products of generation such as worms constituents of a putrefying body from which they develop. If they were we should regard pus as a component of lung, since the latter may degenerate into an abscess. By the action of heat bodies can be converted into many divers—heterogeneous—substances such as ashes, fluids, nitre—which cannot be possibly looked upon as constituents of the original bodies[59].

With all this Harvey reveals himself as a professed adversary of ancient humoralism, and even his loyalty to Aristotle stops short at this point.

It is not, however, the elements and humours of the ancients which he opposes as such, although he once clearly expressed his doubt as to the existence of elements in the strict sense[60]. He dismisses the *Tria Prima* of the Chemists just as distinctly as the atoms of Democritos. In other words what he rejects is *not this or that matter*, *but matter altogether*, i.e. matter that is made to serve as the feature distinguishing individual objects and in particular living individuals.

Nor is this all. Harvey would have nothing of any explanation in terms of mixture or composition. What composes or goes into a mixture is secondary to the object. This is not the product of a synthesis of the former. Indeed the object is prior to its material components.

Harvey's, then, is an idealistic view: If it is not matter that determines the object as an individual in its own right, it must be an idea or vital principle that directs it and is responsible for its formation and maintenance. In Harvey's opinion this idea is incorporated in the blood. It is not, however, found in the substance of the blood or in any of its constituents. Rather it is in the blood as an operative unit; it is in blood as long as it moves in the vessels; it is in the blood that is the first to be formed in the embryo and to become visible as a pulsating point—in short the blood that actively maintains life. Seen thus blood is the substratum and visible representative of the living individual and the idea that made it.

This idea and vital principle is truly divine. Harvey ascribed *numinous* inspiration to the fertilising principle (*spirit*) of the male semen—"it is spiritual and effervescent as if swelling with a fertilising spirit and a turgescence of numinous character (*numine turgescens*)". Here again it is not the semen or its emission as such

59 *Disp. de nova philos. Paracelsi medicina.* Pars altera. Basil. 1572, p. 72–73. In support of Paracelsus: VIOLET, FAB., *La parfaicte et entiere cognoissance de toutes les maladies du corps humain causées par obstruction.* Paris 1635, p. 77. – On Van Helmont's qualified opposition to these Paracelsian ideas and metaphors: *Imago ferm. impraegnat massam semine* cap. 7. *Ortus Med.* Amstelod. 1648, p. 112 and *Scholarum Humoristarum Pass. Deceptio* I, 65–66. *Ortus Med.* Amstelod. 1648, vol. II, p. 79–80 (in this connexion also referring to generation being the production of one single whole and not a sum of parts: "in generatione naturali oporteat partes constitutivas sic fieri unum quid, ut ab unica generati forma actuentur plenarie"). – On the Erastus-Paracelsus controversy: PAGEL, W., *Paracelsus* Basle and New York 1958, p. 320.

60 *On generation* Exerc. LXXI, ed. 1662, p. 329; tr. WILLIS p. 517.

that matters, but only in so far as "that fluid has a prolific quality and is imbued with a plastic power; that is to say is spiritual, operative and analogous to the essence of the stars ... imbued with the spirit and the virtue of a divine agent[61]".

In other places Harvey extols the order prevailing in generation as "divine"[62]. There is foresight and divine intelligence in the fertile semen as well as in the egg[63]. It is this divine power which is conferred upon the blood. For the latter is also "celestial"[64].

Harvey thus visualises *blood* as "*pneumatic matter*", i.e. something that is at the *same time matter and force*. It is *operative* or *acting matter*. It does not act because of a superadded spirit which calls it into action like an officer commanding a soldier, but because of its own spiritual nature. The latter in turn manifests itself by the effects which it brings about through its material side.

The Aristotelian, Stoic and Neoplatonic Background

What place are we to allocate to the Harveian view of operative matter in the history of European thought? In discussing this we shall have to refer back and to repeat some points which were made before in elucidating the background to Servetus (p. 146).

In Platonism a deep—dualist—gulf had been erected between —celestial—ideas and—sublunary—matter. The former really exist; they *are*, but never develop ,whereas matter *is not*, but continually develops. Matter was thus seen as non—(or pseudo-) existent, *qua* bare of any spirit, although it was allowed some share (*methexis*) in the world of ideas whereby the purposeful course of nature could be explained.

It was Aristotle who brought the lofty Platonic Ideas down to earth, from the transcendent world of Plato to the realm of visible and palpable objects. The *transcendent* idea became the active and formative power that is *immanent* to the individual object and through the latter open to investigation by the natural philosopher. It is thus "given" to the latter and his empirical experience. With this Aristotle anticipated much of the further development of the original Platonic ideas, notably the versions which they were given by the Stoics and Neoplatonists[65].

Nevertheless Aristotle as well as the Neoplatonists upheld the basic gulf between spirit and matter: spirit retained its superiority. It was the active, real and actualising force as against passive and formless matter.

It was only in Stoicism that a *monistic* solution emerged: one

61 "Maris genituram esse prolis opificem ... quia spiritosa est, et effervescens, tanquam foecundo spiritu, et *numine* turgescens" Ex. XL, ed. 1662, p. 136. WILLIS p. 315 translates: "because it is spiritual and effervescent as if swelling with a fertilising spirit, and a praeternatural influence". Somewhat better and more literal the London 1653 translation: "because it *is spirituous* and boyling as being inspired with a *fertile spirit*, and turgent like a thing possessed".

62 Ex. LXXI ed. 1662, p. 322. WILLIS p. 510.

63 Ex. XL ed. 1662, p. 137. WILLIS p. 315.

64 Ex. LXXI ed. 1662, p. 320. WILLIS p. 507.

65 HOFFMANN, ERNST, *Platonismus und Mystik im Altertum*. Heidelberg 1935, p. 106 seq.

spirit was made to pervade the whole world—the *World-Soul*. It entered the individual as his personal soul, a matter of highest subtlety: at all events something substantial—the *Pneuma*[66].

Related to this "pneumatic" version of the ideal world was the Neoplatonic concept of a *Cosmos in Steps*—the world forming a step-ladder with all gradations of increasing materiality of the Pneuma from the One and the Intelligences on High down to minerals and metals. However, the basic difference between spirit and matter—abandoned by Stoicism—was retained in Neoplatonism. The latter accorded to *Pneuma* a position intermediate between spirit and matter—that of a carrier of the soul (*Ochema*)—a carrier that was of finest corporality (*Astral Body*) and "ethereal" in nature (see above p. 146). It was through this tripartition that continuity was maintained in this vision of the world.

The super-element from the stars to which Harvey refers when criticising Fernel and Scaliger (p. 253) is in fact this *Astral Body* or *Quinta Essentia*—the Neoplatonic (Aristotelian) concept that had agitated the minds of the Renaissance philosophers not long before Harvey's own time.

Harvey himself was by no means averse to the idea of the *astral body* itself, as we shall soon see (p. 276). What he did criticise in Fernel's concept was the transcendence attributed to the *astral body* which had been made to be superadded to the body and in particular to the blood. Against this the blood, as Harvey saw it, displayed all the virtues of the *astral body* in itself, *qua* acting spiritual body. In other words it was immanent and not transcendent to the blood. It may well have been Fernel who formed Harvey's source for the knowledge and use of Neoplatonic parlance in this matter[67]. However Fernel was preceded and probably influenced by Marsilius Ficinus (1433–1499) and Agrippa of Nettesheym (1487–1535) who had given the concept of the astral body its classical formulation in the Renaissance—the former providing the source for the latter. The astral body, they had said, is no longer body and not quite soul, and no longer soul and not quite body. *Qua* vector of the soul, however, it makes liaison with the body possible[68].

By contrast with Platonism, ancient and new, Stoicism had arrived at a monistic system which was much simpler. Having removed the basic difference between spirit and matter, it paved the way to the concept of objects, each with a spiritual and material aspect—the concept of operative, of acting matter. In this, matter was graded up to the status of functional and active matter. Spirit on the other hand lost its elevated position to become the direct-

66 HOFFMANN loc. cit. (note [65]) p. 78 seq.

67 According to D.P. WALKER, *Spiritual and demonic magic from Ficino to Campanella*, London 1958, p. 39, Fernel adopted the idea of the *astral body* without any of that restraint which because of its heretical implications is noticeable in some of his contemporaries and even in Ficinus. That Harvey in fact embraced the idea was briefly mentioned by WALKER, D.P., *The astral body in Renaissance Medicin*. *J. Warburg and Courtauld Instit.*, 1958, XXI, 119–131 (p. 131).

68 "Ipse vero est corpus tenuissimum, quasi non corpus, et quasi jam anima. Item quasi non anima, et quasi jam corpus." MARS. FICINUS, *De Vita coelitus comparanda* lib. III, 3 ed. Aldina Venet. 1516, fol. 153 recto.

"Cum vero anima primum mobile sit, et, ut dicunt, sponte et per se mobile: corpus vero vel materia per se ad motum inefficax, et ab ipsa anima longe degenerans, iccirco ferunt opus esse excellentiori medio, scilicet quod sit quasi non corpus, sed quasi jam anima, sive quasi non anima, et quasi jam corpus, quo videlicet anima corpori connectatur. Medium autem talem fingunt spiritum mundi, scilicet, quem dicimus essentiam quintam." AGRIPPA AB Nettesheym, *De Occulta Philosophia*, lib. I, 14. Lugduni 1550, p. 32–33. See p. 147.

ing impulse, the *Seminal Logos* (*Logos spermatikos*), the vital principle inherent in things.

Harvey attributed the properties of operative bodies to the primigenial fluid of the *ovum* and its immediate product, the pulsating blood. With this he seems to stand in the Stoic tradition. He has no hesitation in finding his vital principle incorporated in such a substance as blood. Aristotle had expressly rejected this, for he had seen in blood nothing but the result of elemental composition and mixture.

At first sight Aristotle's position would seem to be more truly idealistic and vitalistic than Harvey's. However in disagreeing with Aristotle on the score of the blood, Harvey was actuated by opposition to humoralist materialism. As he saw it, the ancient view of semen and blood as elemental compositions and mixtures, the result of a process of adding according to certain quantities and ratios, implied a *preformationist* principle. Harvey opposed this in the same way as he opposed preformationism in Embryology (p. 234).

Harvey replaced preformationism by *Epigenesis*, because he could not accept generation—a creative process—as a mere addition of preformed parts. Instead he insists that something new emerges in generation from a homogeneous, "simple" albumen—*epigenesis*. Likewise blood in Harvey's opinion is not the product of an addition or mixture of elemental particles and humours. This it is when found "dead" outside the vessels, when as already Aristotle had said it has lost its heat and degenerated into *cruor*[69]. Blood as the principal operative *part* of the body, however, appears to Harvey as indivisible, as a *Logos*, i.e. a directing vital principle as well as matter specifically tuned to a single function and without parts.

Harvey thus favours the concept of *immanence:* an idea or vital principle is visualised in indissoluble union with matter, with which it forms a biological unit. There is no place for its interpretation in terms of addition and subtraction, of mixture and decomposition of material parts, nor of a psychic principle that supervenes and is added to matter.

Opposition to Aristotle, in Harvey's case, is therefore not directed against the vitalistic appraisal of the soul as the vital principle immanent to the object and directing it towards perfection (*Entelecheia*). Where Harvey differs is in the position of the blood which Aristotle had regarded as composite elemental matter. Consequently he had denied it supremacy, primogeniture and the privilege of being the "seat of the soul".

69 Exerc. LXXI, ed. 1662, p. 322; tr. WILLIS, p. 510.
Harvey does not here refer to Aristotle who has a related passage in *De partibus animal.* lib. II, cap. 3; 650a: blood is hot "in form", i.e. functioning blood, but it is not "in substance". See above note [25].

The Position of J.B. Van Helmont
Gas as the Embodiment of the Specific Principle of Individual Life

At Harvey's own time the main exponent of a monistic view in biology was J.B. Van Helmont (1579–1644). Van Helmont is chiefly remembered to-day for his discovery of *Gas*. This is in fact intimately bound up with the idea of operative units in nature that are spirit and body at the same time.

Van Helmont's concept embraces what is understood by *Gas* in modern Chemistry, i.e. well-defined chemical substances that appear as aeriform or completely elastic fluids. He had already realised their basic difference from air and water vapour. These were media common to many things in nature, whereas he saw in *Gas* a specific individual substance. However, in Van Helmont's world, *Gas* had a far more complex and wider significance than in modern Chemistry. It stood for the essential core that exists and must be looked for in any object of nature. It is, he believed, the divine seed that is responsible for the specific form and function of the individual. To isolate and visualise it one has to divest the object of its coarse material cover with the aid of heat or fire (*per ignem*). If, for example, coal is heated in a closed vessel, the body of the coal loses its normal appearance by conversion into a smoke. It thus loses however, nothing that is essential, and what is essential is volatile; it is its *Gas*. Coal roasted "even to its last day in a bright burning furnace, the vessel being shut..." loses nothing when prevented from escaping. For the coal as well as any other body which is not immediately converted into water or fixed in its solid state "do necessarily belch forth a wild spirit or breath" (*necessario eructant spiritum silvestrem*) [70]. How this observation was "quantified" by Van Helmont we discussed in a previous section of the present book (p. 79).

Gas is not a pure spirit, but is also matter. Van Helmont still believed in the existence of pure, inert matter. This he thought was water. Matter as such, however, takes no part in the formation of individual objects. It is only "disposed" or "organised" matter that does—matter that has received a "seal" through the agency of spirit or "form". Matter (water) so "disposed" or "sealed" is *Gas* and acts as the material vector of a specific schedule of form and function. Matter is transformed into an object, i.e. the bearer of individual specificity, when a "ferment" acts on it. In *Gas*, then, matter assumes spiritual qualities just as much as spirit acquires a material aspect. In other words *Gas* stands for an "acting body" which does not admit of a dualistic separation of spirit and body [71].

70 *Complexionum atque mistionum element. figment.*, 13–14; *Ortus Medicinae* Amstelod. 1648, p. 106; ed. 1652, p. 86; Hafniae 1707, p. 102; tr. CHANDLER, London 1662, p. 106.

71 For a detailed appraisal of Van Helmont's discovery of *Gas:* PAGEL, W., *The debt of science and medicine to a devout belief in God, as illustr. by the work of J.B. Van Helmont. Trans. Victoria Institute* 1942, LXXIV, 99–115 (p. 106). – Idem, loc. cit. 1944 (note [46]), p. 19 seq. Idem, *The position of Harvey and Van Helmont in the history of European thought. J. Hist. Med.* 1958, XIII, 186–199 (p. 194–195). – Idem, *The Wild Spirit* (*Gas*) *of J.B. Van Helmont and Paracelsus. Ambix.* 1962, X, 1–13.

The prototypes of *Gas* are *Archeus* and *Semen*. By *Archeus* Van Helmont understands a substance that contains the "image of the being". It is the product of an indissoluble union of spirit with matter and therefore occupies the key position in the world of individual objects. The *Archeus is* the object, and it is so *qua Gas*, the bearer not only of specificity, but of the *life* of this specific individual object[72]. Thus Van Helmont calls the life-spirit in the arterial blood *Gas*[73].

Van Helmont also ascribed *gaseous* nature to the *Semen*. For this is a substance endowed with *Archeus*, i.e. a spiritual *Gas* that is possessed of the transmuting power of a *Ferment* with the *image* of the thing to be performed and knowledge of how to achieve this[74]. The seminal image is the spiritual nucleus of the *Archeus*, and as such responsible for fertility. It directs the semen to embrace some impressions and to avoid others, in other words it operates by arousing sympathy and antipathy[75]. *Semen* being a special manifestation of *Archeus* is thus the master of destiny in the world—the semen that is which is the efficient principle in the visible semen, its coarse outer envelope, its "husk". "All necessity in Nature I have apportioned to the *Semina*", Van Helmont says[76].

In *defining generation* Van Helmont closely approaches Harvey's rejection of any explanation in terms of apposition of material and pre-formed components. Generation, in Van Helmont's opinion, is a creative act in which the semen brings about a transmutation of form by "disposing" its matter to produce a single whole and not an appositional collection of components[77]. In this act the generator contributes some of his own substance—as against a mere copulation of something active with something passive[78]. It is a unique process—"the flow towards perfection, the maturing of properties, the manifestation of hidden features and consummation of regular periods to the destined end[79]". Obviously a vital process such as this cannot be determined by matter, but requires forces that are capable of arranging, organising and disposing matter. Such a force is the *image* which forms the invisible kernel of the semen. It is therefore a *first principle* (*initium*) that is absolutely immaterial, yet eminently real and effective, that has precedence in the semen. It is the soul of the generator which "illuminates" (*lustrat*) the seminal body and sketches, in an *aura*, its own seal and figure and thereby renders the semen fruitful. The *anima* therefore is *figurata*, i.e. possessed of the outline of the body to be formed. Were it not and if the body developed its shape by itself, loss of limbs would cause limbless offspring[80].

Although mystical elements play a greater part in Van Hel-

72 *Complex. mistion. element. fig.* loc. cit. (note [70]) cap. 40–43. *Ortus Med.* 1648, p. 110.

73 Ibidem.

74 *Imago ferm. impraeg. mass. semine* cap. 12. *Ortus Med.* Amstelod. 1648 p. 113.

75 "Quae imago est essentia invisibilis seminum concitans ad complectendum vel abhorrendum". – The seminal image is also called the interior spiritual nucleus of the *Archeus* that makes the semen fertile. The visible semen is only the coarse envelope—husk (siliqua). *Archeus Faber* cap. 4. *Ortus* 1648, p. 40.

76 *Imago ferm. impr. mass. sem.* cap. 7 loc. cit. (note [59]), p. 112.

77 "At postquam optice scivi, quod nullum ens, existens in sui perfectione, attestetur partes dissimilares suae radicis seminalis, si quae superessent: sed quod semen disponat suam materiam, ut ex ea hoc unum quid fiat, et non per appositionem, sed per veram formalem transmutationem". *Scholar. Humoristar. Passiva Deceptio* I, 65. *Ortus Med.* Amstelod. 1648, p. 79 (vol. II).

78 *Ignotus Hospes Morbus* 87; *Ortus* 1648, p. 504. Ed. Hafniae 1707, p. 479.

79 Ibid. 38; *Ortus* 1648, p. 492; 1707, p. 468.

80 *Imago Mentis* 17; 1648, p. 270; 1707, p. 256.

mont's embryological speculation than in Harvey's ideas, these are akin to the former in principle. Van Helmont sees in generation the action of a spiritualised body—the *Archeus* in the semen which is materially transformed through direction by this *Archeus* and accomplishes the translation of a figure scheme that pre-existed in the *Archeus* into material reality.

Like Harvey, Van Helmont is basically inspired by opposition to ancient humoralist doctrine, like him he claims a level for generation that is above and utterly different from elemental mixture and composition—arrangements of matter that are secondary and subordinate to the vital force that does the arranging. In the same trend of thought Van Helmont's concept of *Gas* closely corresponds to Harvey's idea of the blood as spiritual matter, i.e. matter that is "disposed" and at the same time acting according to its specific "disposition".

The Liquor Vitae of Paracelsus

Harvey's opposition to any elemental constituents as *efficients* in generation was directed not only against the elements and humours of the ancients, but also against the *Three Principles* (*Tria Prima*) of the Chemists: Salt, Sulphur and Mercury[81].

This in itself should discourage any search for parallels and contacts between Harveian and Paracelsian ideas. Yet, as we have seen (p. 100), Harvey knew and appreciated Paracelsus. Moreover there is one Paracelsian concept which stands in close proximity to Harvey's appraisal of blood and semen as "spiritual" or "acting" bodies: the *Liquor Vitae* of Paracelsus.

Paracelsus believed this to be omnipresent as body-liquor in the organism. He thought it to be intimately bound up with body substance and related to, though not identical with, blood. As the earth has two water systems—one that runs in rivers and brooks and the other that is closer to the earth itself and filters through it—the body is possessed of two fluid supplies that carry salt. One is the blood and the other the *Liquor*. Eventually both are joined in a third "single river"—the urine into which they excrete their salt. If one of these fluids discharges its salt at a wrong place an ulcer develops[82].

So far the *Liquor* is merely presented as matter that carries other matter, namely salt. Raised to the status of *Vital Liquor*, however, it becomes semen, the seed of another living being. As such it is evenly distributed through the body and contains "all nature,

81 On the meaning and significance of the *Three Principles* of Paracelsus: PAGEL, W., *Paracelsus* 1958, p. 82 seq., 129 seq., 319 seq. Idem, *Das Medizinische Weltbild des Paracelsus* 1962, p. 8; 81; 105.

82 *Von Öffnung der Haut und irer natürlichen Verletzung. Ein Fragment* Lib. I, cap. 6 ed. Sudhoff vol. X, p. 550. – Also: II. *Buch der Großen Wundartzney* (1536) ed. Sudhoff, vol. X, p. 264; 292. – *Tractat von den offenen scheden* cap. 3; ed. Sudhoff vol. X, p. 295. – With reference to *sinovia*, the mucoid liquor in joints, bones and tendons: *Elf Traktat – von Farbsuchten* ed. Sudhoff, vol. I, p. 55.

property, essence and all kinds of members and spirits in itself. And as the body is essentially form, so is the *Liquor Vitae*, and the *Liquor Vitae* is but hidden man. For what is visible hides him. "The *Liquor Vitae* is thus comparable to a "shadow at the wall... so is the *liquor* which is microcosm, the internal shadow. It has in itself, however, a substance that is apprehensible and perceptible by the senses and imagination—that is the essence and nature of all the members of the body, and is the most noble in the whole body and in man[83]".

Paracelsus also calls "the sperma a product (*egestio*) of the *liquor vitae*" which confers upon the semen its own digestive and formative power. "For the *liquor vitae* is a form of the body. Hence the sperma contains such a form in itself and has the power of forming the body just as much as its *liquor*[84]".

And finally: "God has given man the phantasy induced by lust and desire—this he has given so that it becomes matter; this matter is the seed... this phantasy is a product of speculation[85]". And: "God endowed the body liquor with the power to become seed when ignited by the phantasy of man. It lies quiet all over the body. And as split fire wood, it is ignited, burns and becomes fire... phantasy is its fire[86]".

The *Liquor Vitae* of Paracelsus, then, foreshadows in many ways Van Helmont's *Archeus* in blood and semen. Like the latter it becomes active and fertile when "ignited" through human phantasy and speculation, i.e. a faculty that is productive of an *image*. The latter directs simple matter to be converted into "disposed" or "acting" matter. Disposition and action are consummated in the fertility of the seed—the formation of a new individual in the *image* of the parent.

Paracelsus made the semen to develop from all parts of the body—each of them contributing its own specific *vital liquor*. With this he revived the Democritean theory of *Pangenesis*[87] which had been refuted by Aristotle[88]. In its place the latter had regarded semen as a product of nutriment, and of secretion and excretion[89].

Harvey endorsed the Aristotelian argument against *Pangenesis* (p. 234). He was bound to find in it a materialistic ring consonant with the interpretation of generation in terms of elemental mixture and composition as against free creative action from "simple" matter. Paracelsus, however, gave the theory of *Pangenesis* a spiritualist twist. In his view it was not elemental matter that was contributed to the semen by each of the parts, but spiritualised, "acting" matter—the *Liquor Vitae*, i.e. matter "illuminated" and "ignited" by the spirit.

83 *Buch von der geberung der empfindlichen Dinge in der vernunft* Tr. II, cap. 2. ed. Sudhoff vol. I, p. 258.

84 Ibidem (l. c. note [83]) cap. IV, p. 260.

85 *De generatione hominis* ed. Sudhoff vol. I, p. 293 seq.

86 Ibidem (l. c. note [85]) p. 294–295.

87 Lesky, E., *Die Zeugungs- und Vererbungslehren der Antike und ihr Nachwirken.* Mainz 1950, p. 33 and 70. – Pagel, *Paracelsus* 1958, p. 124.

88 Aristotle *De Generatione Animal.* I, 18; 722a. See above p. 235, note [11].

89 Aristotle ibidem (note [88]) I, 18; 724b. – IV, 1; 766b. In the passage in Aristotle, *Metaph.* VII, 31; 1034 a 33, semen was interpreted to designate intellectus by mediaeval commentators (see Mitterer 1947, loc. cit. (on p. 46, note [104] p. 140.)

To mention Paracelsus in connexion with Harvey is therefore not as unnatural as it may appear at first sight. Though probably not directly influenced by Paracelsian speculation, Harvey's idea of the blood as "activated" or "spiritualised" matter is in fact affiliated to the Paracelsian *Liquor Vitae*.

Harvey was acquainted with Paracelsus' theory of *Tartaric disease* (p. 100)—there is no reason why he should not have had knowledge of the Paracelsian *Liquor vitae*. The congeniality of the Paracelsian world with some speculative aspects of Harvey's ideas had already impressed Henry Power, an eminent naturalist and microscopist, who was a contemporary and possible personal acquaintance of Harvey. His manuscript on the circulation of the blood, of 1652, ends: "Thus there is a Constant flux and reflux of this Red Sea of blood within us as well as in that without us. Had Paracelsus known this mystery, hee might farre better have made out his Analogicall philosophy and his Crocosmicall Conceits, then by those lank and farre fetch'd parallelisms which hee Sometimes uses[90]."

Imagination, Sensus Rerum and Generation

A final point: In the speculations of Paracelsus and Van Helmont the semen is closely connected with the imagination, phantasy and desire of the parents. It is this psychic factor which activates, "ignites" and endows the semen with fertility. There is also the resort to the magnetic attraction which the uterus and the female semen exert on the male generating agent (see p. 271).

All these speculations are based on the supremacy of spirit over body—and related ideas that were transmitted by the Neoplatonic Schools, ancient, mediaeval and contemporary[91]. The efficient principle in objects is spirit and for that reason not essentially different from perception, imagination and even thought. There is a *sensus rerum* which operates by sympathy and antipathy. This is evident in the magnet which "senses" the site of the pole by a kind of "imagination". In the same way Van Helmont says, the "principle" (*initium*) engendering beings that are alive "flows from the image either according to the idea fabricated by the conception of the generator or by cogitation—hence called imaginative force". Accordingly in the germ cells (*primis entibus*) of animate beings there are "seminal gifts" (*dona seminalia*) which correspond to imagination and instruct (*docent*) the object to follow the lines indicated by sympathy and antipathy[92].

90 Cole, F.J., *Henry Power on the circulation of the blood. J.Hist. Med.* 1957, XII, 291–324, p. 324.

91 Pagel, W., *Das Medizinische Weltbild des Paracelsus. Seine Beziehungen zu Neuplatonismus und Gnosis* Wiesbaden 1962, p. 46 seq. and passim.

92 In animantibus: "hoc autem initium ab imagine juxta ideam, a generantis conceptu, sive cogitatione fabricatam (quae proinde vis imaginativa vocatur) in vitalibus profluere facile mihi concedetur. Sed quod inanimata in suis primis entibus insita habeant dona seminalia, quae per modum recipientis, etiam analogice, quadantenus imaginationi respondeant, docent antipathia et inanimatarum sympathia—magnetem sentire quodammodo poli situm..." *De Lithiasi* cap. I,3 *Ortus Med.* ed 1648, vol. II, p. 11; 1707, II, p. 3.

However unexpected, these ideas are not alien to Harvey. On the contrary Harvey devoted a whole little treatise, that *On conception*[93] to the psychic or psychoid energies which in his view lay at the bottom of generation.

It would appear that Harvey turned to the realm of the spirit and its action at a distance because of his conviction that the "semen of the male does not so much as reach the cavity of the uterus, much less continue long there, and that it carries with it a fecundating power by a kind of contagious property[94]". Characteristically he immediately evokes the power of the magnet which by mere touch endows iron with its own powers of attracting other iron—in the same way it is through mere contact with the spermatic fluid without any sensible corporeal agent that the woman is made fertile. Though not without effect on the female organism as a whole, the main burden of conception devolves upon the uterus. Harvey finds the pregnant uterus in many ways similar to the brain and is inclined to regard conception as the "specific energy" of the womb which "conceives as we see by the eye and think by the brain[95]". Cohabitation then would excite in the uterus the same thing as or something analogous to "what is *phantasma* or *appetitus* in the brain[96]". Both are called *conceptions* and, both are *immaterial*, though one is of organic (*conceptus naturalis*) and the other of psychic (*conceptus animalis*) character. The latter leads us to fashion in our work something similar to the *idea* or *form* represented by the brain; the idea or form (*species*) of the generator induces the uterus to bring forth a fetus similar to him. Indeed it is an example of the identity of both structure and function which Harvey here sees realised in the uterus and brain.

It is the same imaginative faculty which makes a bird build a nest without ever having seen one, i.e. not from memory or habit—indeed the woman is made pregnant and becomes the "artificer of generation" by the "conception of a general idea without matter[97]".

Harvey is in no doubt that the big-nosed (*nasuti*) who believe nothing but what they think themselves will laugh at this. However it is a legitimate hypothesis that explains something that is not understood at the time as well as possible. It is a "fable" to which Harvey feels himself driven, since nothing is seen in the uterus after cohabitation. Hence the "something" responsible for fertility should be nothing material, but merely a "conceptus", i.e. the reception of "bodiless images"—a process that undoubtedly takes place in the brain. This, to Harvey, seems superior to the resort to subtle "atoms" believed to emanate from the male semen

93 *De Conceptione* occupies in the first edition of Harvey's *Exercitationes de Generatione Animalium* London, Pulleyn, 1651, pp. 293–301 sig. Rr3 recto to Ss3 recto. In the Amstelaedami, 1662, ed. pp. 378–388 transl. London 1653, p. 539–566. WILLIS p. 575–586.

94 *De Conceptione* WILLIS p. 575.

95 Quemadmodum oculis videmus et cerebro cogitamus, ita foemina utero suo concipiat, ed. 1662, p. 379; tr. WILLIS, p. 576.

96 Quod phantasma sive appetitus est in cerebro, istuc idem vel saltem eius analogum, a coitu in utero excitari; unde generatio s. procreatio ovi contingat? Functiones enim utriusque *conceptiones* dicuntur, suntque ambae immateriales" ibid. ed. 1662, p. 380; WILLIS p. 577. *Phantasma immaterial:* ARISTOTLE, *De anima*, III, 8. – See note [89] on: *virtus in semine* and *intellectus*.

97 "Nam quemadmodum nos, a conceptione formae, sive ideae, in cerebro similem ei in operibus nostris efficimus: ita pariter idea, aut species genitoris in utero existens, formatricis facultate ope, similem foetum generat; dum speciem nempe, quam habet immaterialem operi suo imponit. Non aliter sane, quam ars, quae in cerebro est eidos seu species operis futuri, similem in agendo profert, et in materia gignit. Ed. 1662, p. 381. WILLIS p. 578.

According to ancient doctrine the uterus forms a being by itself that is in many respects independent of the organism to which it belongs, actuated as it is by its own desires and appetites. Asthma and hysterical fits—the *pnix hysterike*, *suffocatio* or *strangulatio uteri*—was explained in terms of this theory. The uterus was believed to ascend into the hypochondria and thereby to narrow down the space of the viscera with the result of "strangulation". Sources of these pathogenetic ideas are Aretaios, Celsus and Galen. See: PAGEL, W., *Joh. Bapt. Van Helmont. Einführung in die philosophische Medizin des Barock*. Berlin 1930, p. 108. D.P. WALKER, *The Astral Body in Renaissance Medicine*, *J. Warburg and Courtauld Instit.* 1958, XXI, p. 119–133 (p. 133), refers to the possible Platonic origin of the theory.

like odour, incorporeal spirits, demiurges, demons or finally ferments which have been invoked as the efficient agents in generation. Harvey is confident that he could easily refute any of these on account of his personal observations, but it is easier to say what a process is not than what it is[98].

It is quite possible that with this Harvey has in mind Paracelsian and Helmontian ideas on generation. To the present observer, however, his own view would seem to be close to the identification of the seminal agent with imagination, sensus and idea as propounded by just such a Paracelsian thinker as Van Helmont. It is true that it was the latter who introduced and emphasised the action of *ferments*—but these were thought to be the transmitters of an idea resulting in a transformation of matter into something similar to itself, in other words of a generation "in its own image". As we have seen, the Paracelsians had—like Harvey—insisted on the identity of fermental and generative action with imagination and the representation of images.[98a]

The idea of a parallel between the formation of the embryo and cerebral function, congenial to Paracelsus, foreshadowed by the latter's followers and clearly expressed by Harvey, sounds unrealistic and fanciful to the present day student. However, as Lord Brain recently pointed out, the idea is not altogether foreign to modern molecular biology. In this structural modification of protein molecules in the brain tissue is held to be "equivalent to the prescribed storage of information in the chromosomes of the germ cell[99]".

98 Ed. 1662, p. 383. Willis p. 580.

98a It is of acute interest that "*ferment, vapour and odour*", i.e. typically Helmontian terms, occur in Harvey's marginal notes to the Pybus-copy of *De generat. animal.* (as transcribed and published by Jos. Needham, *Hist. of Embryology*, Cambridge, 1934, p. 127) under the heading: *What makes the seed fertile.* Elsewhere Harvey regards "odours" as "spirits" which are "excremental" by-products, for example of the blood, rather than active and creative forces (*Sec. Exerc. to Riolan*, ed. Roterod. 1649, p. 75; tr. Willis, p. 119).

Needham also pointed out that it had been from his *embryological* observations that Harvey formulated, *25 years before Glisson*, the view that *irritability* was an *intrinsic property of living tissues.* For Harvey observed sense and motion in the fetus before the first appearance of the brain (Exercit. LVII, tr. Willis, p. 430). – See Needham, p. 123, and above, p. 256, on *sense and motion attributed by Harvey to the blood*, and notes [26] to [30]. – Harvey's priority in this matter was recognised by Conr. Victor Schneider: "Ante Helmontium Harveus naturam naturalis Sensus exposuit", in *Liber de catarrhis specialissimus*, Wittebergae 1664, p. 230

99 Brain, Sir Russell, *William Harvey, Neurologist. Brit. Med. J.* 1959, II, 905, with reference to Elsasser, W.M., *The physical foundation of biology.* London. Pergamon Press. 1958.

Harvey's Views on the Ovum

Harvey's criticism of ancient humoralism was inspired by vitalism and yet was based on a divergence from his master Aristotle, the vitalist, in certain points. This notably concerned the position of the male "geniture", the semen. According to Aristotle it entered bodily the female matter, although not materially contributing to the future embryo. Harvey denied its entry into a union with the female "geniture"—assuming that it transmitted a "magnetic" impulse from a distance. He compared its action with contagion.

Even more decisive, though similarly motivated, was Harvey's deviation from Aristotle's ideas about the position of the female geniture and notably the *ovum*. Aristotle had regarded the female matter as of an excremental, menstrual nature (*katamenia*). He had assumed that it merely furnished the stuff out of which the male, like a workman, actively forms and fashions the embryo—actualising the female geniture and conferring *animal form* on it.

Harvey opposed this subordination of the female to the male. He believed in *primordia*—the independent precursors of all that is endowed with life. These *primordia* were *ova* and, with the exception of spontaneous generation by *metamorphosis*, were carried by the female body. *Ex ovo omnia*—the adage found on the frontispiece that adorns his work *On generation*— therefore well epitomises Harvey's idea. At the same time we should remember that Harvey was unaware of the Graafian follicles, let alone the mammalian *ovum*. Instead he transferred by analogy the properties of the egg of the oviparous animals to the mammalian *conceptus*, i. e. the developing embryo in its earliest stages, and saw in their common ovoid shape the symbolical expression of their productivity (p. 45).

Inevitably, then, the *ovum* assumes a position of high dignity. Harvey elaborated this for the *ovum* of the chick. There is little doubt, however, that it was meant to apply to all animals, including mammals and notably to man, even where it looks as if he presented the female geniture as a product of the uterus[100].

Harvey, no doubt, attributes much less significance to the ovary in mammals than to the analogous organ in oviparous animals. He speaks about the ovaries in deer as insignificant "glands" comparable to the prostate or mesenteric lymph-nodes, made for the secretion of a lubricant rather than the preparation of semen. For, in the rutting season, when in the male the testicles swell and are replete with seminal fluid, the "female testicles" neither swell nor change either before or after coition. Nor is there any other indication that they are involved in coition or generation[101]. By contrast Harvey points to the swelling of the uterine horns which is observable at the critical time, not only in deer, but also in the rest of the viviparous animals.

Moreover Harvey describes certain uterine "mucous filaments" which rise from the uterine horns like spider webbs, are joined together and form a membranous empty looking longitudinal "wallet". This is reminiscent of the chorioid plexuses in the brain. It contains a viscid fluid not unlike the thinner part of the white of an egg. This, Harvey says, is the *conceptus primus* of the hind and doe—obtaining as it does the nature and status of the *ovum*. Indeed it conforms to Aristotle's definition of the *ovum* as "that from part of which the young comes into being, the rest being nutriment for it[102]". It is the *primordium* of the future fetus and therefore called the *ovum* of these animals in accordance with the dictum of

100 This is accepted as one of the factual errors committed by Harvey in A.W. Meyer's *Analysis of the De generat. animal. of Harvey*, Stanford and London 1936, p. 140. – See also Marcus Marci's criticism of Harvey (1662) below, p. 321.

101 Harvey, *On generation*, Exerc. LXV ed. 1662, p. 286; tr. Willis p. 473. Also ibid. in Exerc. LXVII, ed. 1662, p. 290; tr. Willis p. 477. By contrast the description of the ovaries and their eminent position as the reservoir and supplier of the ova in chickens, fishes, frogs, crustacea and testacea, ibidem, Exerc. III, ed. 1662, p. 6–9; tr. Willis p. 175–177.

See also: Exercit. XL, ed. 1662, p. 138; tr. Willis p. 316: Ovorum primordia non fiunt in utero ... sed in ovario.

102 Aristotle, *De generat. animal.* lib. II, cap. 1 (not: 9, as given by Willis), 732a 30; tr. A. Platt, Oxford 1910. Also: Aristotle, *Historia animalium* lib. I, cap. 5; 489b 5: "what we term an egg is a certain completed result of conception out of which the animal that is to be develops, and in such a way that in respect to its primitive germ it comes from part only of the egg, while the rest serves for food as the germ develops". tr. d'Arcy Wentworth Thompson, Oxford 1910.

the Philosopher: "With animals internally viviparous the embryo becomes egg-like in a certain sense after its original formation, for the liquid is contained in a fine membrane, just as if we should take away the shell of the egg wherefore they call the abortion of an embryo at that stage an efflux[103]".

The difference, then, between the oviparous and viviparous animals concerns the position of the ovary rather than that of the *prime conceptus*, the *ovum*. The latter thus retains the exalted position attributed to it by Harvey throughout the animal kingdom. Hence the title of the sixty second exercise: *An Ovum is the Common Origin of All Animals* (*ovum esse primordium commune omnibus animalibus*). This also forms the key-note of the subsequent chapters. Whatever the generative process may be in detail, it always starts from *some principle* containing an *efficient cause* that is adequate for generation (*ut ex principio aliquo ad hoc idoneo, et ab efficiente interno in eodem principio vigente gignantur*)[104]. This *primordium* resides in all beings alive—indeed it is a resident rather than a product of the body, a material substance *per se existens*, apt to be converted into a "vegative form" by virtue of its indwelling principle. Such a *primordium* is the ovum and the seed of plants, such the *conception* of viviparous animals and such the *worm*—as Aristotle calls it—from which the insects emerge[105].

Harvey intends to go farther than Fabricius. The latter had assigned generation from an ovum to the majority of the animals. Harvey asserts that this applies to *all* animals (*nos vero*... cuncta animalia *quodammodo ex ovo nasci affirmavimus*)[106]. They have this in common with the chick, for in viviparous animals there is a pre-existing *conceptus* that is comparable to the egg produced by the former. And finally all this applies equally to man (*confessa enim res est et manifesta, foetus omnes*, etiam humanos, *a conceptu* [*seu primario quodam*] *procreari*)[107].

What is called *primordium* in *spontaneous generation* thus corresponds to the *seed* in *plants*, to the *egg* in the *oviparous* and to the *prime concept* in the *viviparous* animals.

To *conclude*, then, there resides in the uterus of all animals a *conceptus primus* which, on Aristotelian evidence, "looks like an egg enveloped in its membrane after removal of the egg shell"[108].

Indeed Harvey sees the *ovum* as a primordial element that is housed by and resident in, but not of, the mother. It is not a product of the uterus, but is stored in the repository of the ovary[109]. When fertilised by the "contagious" distance action of the male geniture it becomes the *conceptus*—a living being entirely in its own right[110]. In it is enshrined the *circular* pattern which ensures eternal

103 Aristotle, *De generat. animal.* lib. III, cap. 9 758b 1; tr. A. Platt, Oxford 1910.

104 Exercit. LXII, ed. 1662, p. 270; Willis p. 457.

105 Ibidem as in note [104], by contrast with Aristotle, *Hist. animal.* l.c. in note [102] who distinguishes between ovum and "grub" the latter, developing into the embryo, in its entirety. Harvey believes in the identity of ovum and grub: Exercit. LXII, ed. 1662, p. 271, tr. Willis p. 458: nec distinctio illa, quam Aristoteles affert inter ovum et vermem, admittenda est.

106 Exercit. LXIII, ed. 1662, p. 275; tr. Willis p. 462.

107 Ibidem, ed. 1662, p. 276; tr. Willis p. 463.

108 Aristotle, *Hist. animal.* lib. VII, cap. 7; 586a 20; tr. Thompson. Oxford 1910.

109 Harvey, *On generation*, Exerc. XL, ed. 1662, p. 138; tr. Willis p. 316. The ovum and its primogenital blood as independent of the mother was already emphasised in *Praelect. anat.* fol. 33r (sanguis nec a matre veniens in ovo, etenim non gutta).

110 *On generation*, Exerc. XXVI, ed. 1662, p. 97; tr. Willis p. 272.

duration for the species. For the ovum is both beginning and end (*quatenus principium et finis*)—it is the beginning as far as the offspring to be is concerned and it is the end by virtue of forming the *fruit* of both parents, the end which they propose for themselves to be achieved in generation[111].

Videtur etiam ovum medium quid esse[112]—the ovum also appears to be a certain mean, not only because it is a beginning as well as an end, but also for several other reasons. First of all it is the product of both sexes. Further it is endowed with matter as well as plastic force. Then it is the mean between the animate and inanimate worlds, for it neither is fully equipped with life nor entirely without vitality (*neque enim vita prorsus donatum est, neque eadem omnino privatur*). It thus stands midway between parent and child, between those who were and those who will be. It is the hinge and pivot around which the generation of the whole gallinaceous tribe revolves (*cardoque et centrum circa quod generatio totius gallinacei generis vertitur*). In short it is the terminus—*ex quo* as well as *ad quem*. *From it* male as well as female take their origin and *towards it* as the goal set for them by nature they tend throughout their lives. It is thus that the individual earns a claim to eternity for the service rendered to the species in engendering his own like.

The *ovum* thus is the ever returning circuit of this eternity (*est inquam ovum huius eternitatis periodus*), for it is not easy to say whether the *ovum* is the cause of the hen or the latter the cause of the *ovum*, nor which is earlier in time or by nature. In all this lies the analogy with the seeds of plants, whence the *ovum* is just as rightly called seed as the seed of the plant its *ovum*. For it provides the matter out of which the chick develops as well as the efficient cause through which it does so. It contains all parts of the individual to be, potentially, but none *actu*.

By definition, then, the ovum is a natural body endowed with a vital principle, the virtue of soul, i.e. the principle of motion, transmutation, rest and preservation. Moreover, when not in any way impeded, it is bound to assume animal form—just as naturally as heavy bodies when given freedom of motion tend downwards and light ones upwards. In this way again the ovum (or seed) is the fruit or end to that of which it is the beginning and efficient cause (*ovum itaque est corpus naturale, virtute animali praeditum; principio nempe motus, transmutationis, quietis, et conservationis: est denique ejusmodi, ut, ablato omni impedimento, in formam animalis abiturum sit nec magis naturaliter gravia omnia, remotis obstaculis, deorsum tendunt; aut levia sursum moventur; quam semen, et ovum, in plantam*

111 *On generation*, Exerc. XXVI, ed. 1662, p. 96; tr. WILLIS p. 271.

112 Ibidem. The term *medium quid* is also used by Harvey for the eggs of insects which present a mean between perfect and imperfect eggs (*On gener.*, Exerc. LXII, ed. 1662, p. 272; tr. WILLIS, p. 459).

aut animal, insita a natura propensione feruntur. Estque semen (atque ovum) ejusdem fructus et finis, cujus est principium, atque efficiens)[113].

The Neoplatonic Sources

Harvey's interpretation of the *ovum* as a *tertium quid* implies an allusion to Neoplatonic speculation. We discussed above (p. 264) the fine ethereal "carrier of the soul" which derives from the stars, the *Astral Body*. Indeed Harvey's formulation: the *ovum* is neither fully equipped with life nor entirely without vitality is immediately reminiscent of what Marsilius Ficinus said of the *Astral Body:* that it was not body and almost soul, and not soul and almost body. Repeated by Agrippa of Nettesheym the formula had been incorporated into the stock of ideas found in the works of Paracelsists and alchemists[114].

Harvey's use of this Neoplatonic idea and parlance with reference to the *ovum* was by no means accidental or an isolated instance of Neoplatonic influence. On the contrary it was deliberate. For he applied it to the *blood* and its immanent soul-like activity. In the seventy-first Exercise *On generation* he deals with innate heat and the properties of the blood that exceed those of the elements whereby it qualifies as seat of the soul. Indeed it is the instrument of the Creator (*summus opifex*) and no praise will be high enough to extol its admirable and divine faculties. It enshrines the soul primarily and principally—the soul that is not only vegetative, but also sensitive and motive. It permeates everywhere and is ubiquitous, and with it the soul soon perishes too. Hence there is not much difference between blood and soul; or at any rate blood should be regarded as the substance whose function (*actus*) is life (*anima*). I say, Harvey continues, such is the soul that it is *not all body and yet not entirely without body* (*talis, inquam, anima est: quae nec omnino corpus sit, nec plane sine corpore*)[115]. It partly hails from without and is partly engendered at home, forming part of the body in some way. On the other hand it acts as a principle and cause of everything contained in the body of the animal.

Harvey opposed Aristotle on two main counts and it would appear that it is these two positions in which he resorted to the Neoplatonic idea and formulation of the *tertium quid*, the middle and the mean.

These two counts were:

1. the position of the *ovum* for which Harvey claimed independence and the high dignity of a primordial shrine of life that ensures

113 Ibidem, Exercit. XXVI, ed. 1662, p. 97; tr. WILLIS p. 272.

114 See above the loci from Ficinus and Agrippa of Nettesheym, p. 264.

It is not without interest in our context that the Neoplatonic *tertium quid* formed a source for Paracelsus and can be followed up in the alchemical tradition from mediaeval to Harveian times. The "spirit" which combines occult power and matter and stands between heaven (*mercury*) and earth (*salt*) is called *sulphur*. It is the "third" that bridges and unites two contraries, namely spirit and body. So we are told in the *Hermetic Golden treatise on the secret of the Philosopher's stone*. This did not appear in print until 1566 (as *Septem tractatus s. capitula Trismegisti aurei* in *Ars Chemica*, Argentor. 1566, p. 7–31). It is much older, however, (not unlikely Arabic in origin) and was probably referred to by Paracelsus as "Hermes" indicating the intermediate position of Sulphur as the *tertium* between mercury and salt (*De natura rerum*, lib. I, ed. Sudhoff, vol. XI, p. 318). It is just this point that was taken up in the commentary to the Hermetic treatise published in 1600 (*opera Dominici Gnosii Belgae*), with special reference to Ficinus. See: PAGEL, W., *Hermetic alchemy at Giordano Bruno's time*, *Ambix* 1964, XII, 75. – Idem, *Paracelsus and the Neoplatonic and Gnostic tradition*, *Ambix* 1960, VIII, 125–166 (p. 128; 154). – Idem, *Das medizinische Weltbild des Paracelsus*, Wiesbaden 1962, p. 105–108. – See above note [34].

115 *On generation*, exerc. LXXI, ed. 1662, p. 323; tr. WILLIS, p. 511. In *De motu locali anim.* fol. 95 Harvey speaks of the *moving spiritus as a medium inter animam et corpus*. To this see Aristotle, *De motu animal.* IX–X, 702b15 to 703a15 (the seat of the moving body must be in the middle; see above p. 92).

the eternity of the species—as against the subordinate role assigned to it by Aristotle as residual—katamenial—matter, and

2. the similar exalted position granted by Harvey to the *blood* as the seat and embodiment of the soul—as against the view of Aristotle who expressly denied this in favour of the heart.

It should not be forgotten, however, that the idea of the mean as such does not originate with Neoplatonism, but is much older and indeed a concept much favoured by Aristotle (*mesotes*)[116].

Van Helmont's Middle Life

In 1648—three years before the publication of Harvey's *On generation*—the works of John Baptist Van Helmont (1579–1644) had been printed posthumously[117]. These included a treatise entitled *The great necessity* (*Magnum Oportet*)[118]. It is devoted to what Van Helmont called the *Middle Life* of things (*vita media*). Owing to this and its stubborn persistence it is impossible for one body to be entirely "digested" by another body. Thus anything taken in from outside leaves its characteristic seal by virtue of a mechanism comparable to contamination or contagion. It operates throughout the cosmos and nature at large, and not only in animated life. In fact through it order is maintained in nature so that "he who is the strongest remains master". The autonomy thus granted to each individual being is reminiscent of that ascribed to the *ovum* by Harvey.

In Van Helmont's concept *Middle Life* is also related to generation. There is, however, a slight difference. Van Helmont says, where there is *Middle Life*, there must be a first and an ultimate life. First life is that of the Semina—*in seminibus gliscit vita prima*[119]. When this is developed into the embryo, it has reached the stage of Middle Life, and ultimate life is attained with the full maturation and perfection of the individual. It is the last, the ultimate, life, however, which gives rise to new first life, to new seed. The first life of the fruit containing the new seed is therefore the last life of the previous seed, for this in itself dies in the process of giving life to the new offspring. However, the death of the mother-object is not complete: some of it remains, its Middle Life, the life that confers upon it autonomy and specificity as an individual, this *Middle Life* was termed by Van Helmont *Archeus*.

Van Helmont's speculation about the Middle Life is derived from Paracelsus or at all events from a Paracelsian tradition. The former said that all that matters in nature is activity, motion, operation and change, comparable to the work of a horse which

116 See for example: KLIBANSKY, R., PANOFSKY, E. and SAXL, F., *Saturn and Melancholy*, London 1964, p.33–34 where the use of the notion of the mean serves to support the genuine Aristotelian authorship of Problemata XXX, 1: "there is the notion of the "mean" (*mesotes*) which determines the ideal melancholic in the same way as it determines the ideal mental and physical performance in the genuine Aristotelian writings."

117 VAN HELMONT, JOH. BAPT. *Ortus medicinae id est initia physicae inauditae.* Amsterodami 1648.

118 *Ortus*, ed. 1648, p.149–163. Eng. translation by J. CHANDLER: *Oriatrike or Physick Refined*, London 1662, p.148–159 (*Magnum Oportet or a thing of great necessity or concernment*). – German translation by CHRISTIAN KNORR VON ROSENROTH: *Aufgang der Artzney-Kunst.* Sultzbach 1683, p. 193–210 (*Von dem großen Müssen*, niederländ. *der grosse Oportet, zu aller Verwandlung und Untergang der Dinge*).

119 *Magnum Oportet* cap. 27; Ortus, 1648, p.155.

pulls the cart. Hence a thing in its first matter is of just as little importance as an object in its ultimate form, i.e. the two stages at which it is at rest. "*Commotio* is not in prime matter, nor is it in ultimate matter, but it is in the middle between the two matters[120]." This concept of "*middle matter*" was taken up in a pseudo-Paracelsian treatise. Moreover it was here quite clearly associated with the life of the semina and seeds. "Everything grows through its *middle nature* which communicates its heat and humidity to it, whereby also all things are brought together. For *middle nature* is a *seed* and *sperma* in all things that grow and is the fire and the sixth essence in all things ... it is greenness that makes all things in the earth to become green[121]."

The Neoplatonic doctrine of the *tertium quid* which we mentioned above (p. 276) thus forms the basis of further interesting parallels between Harvey on the one hand and the ideas of Paracelsus and Van Helmont on the other[122].

120 Paracelsus, *Philosophia sagax* lib.I, cap.2; ed. Sudhoff vol.XII, p.257.

121 *De secretis creationis* (1575) quoted from Appendix to Huser's edition of Paracelsus, *Chirurgische Schriften*, Strasburg 1605, p.105. See: Pagel, *Das medizin. Weltbild d. Paracelsus* loc. cit. in note [114], 1962, p.56. – See on the interesting literary history of this pseudo-Paracelsian treatise: LIEB, FRITZ, *Valentin Weigels Kommentar zur Schöpfungsgeschichte und das Schrifttum seines Schülers Benedikt Biedermann. Eine literar-kritische Untersuchung zur mystischen Theologie des 16.Jahrhunderts.* Zürich 1962. Lieb discovered its ascription to WEIGEL, the Paracelsist (1533–1588), by his pupil Biedermann (ca. 1545–1621).

122 See above p. 270.

123 Edition used: Lugd. Batav. 1644. Issued with: PLAZZONUS, FR., *De partibus generationi inservientibus* libri duo.

Appendix

Gregory Nymman on the Life of the Fetus in utero

Gregory Nymman was the son of Hieronymus Nymman (1554–1594) and both were Professors of Medicine in the University of Wittenberg. He was born in 1594, became Master of Arts in 1614 and Doctor of Medicine in 1618. He died in 1638. His main work appeared in 1628 at Wittenberg. It is entitled: *Dissertatio de vita foetus in utero* and promises ample proof that the fetus is alive in the womb, not through the vital principle transferred from the mother, but through a vital principle of its own. Hence it can be recovered safe and alive from the womb of the dead mother, and in no well governed state should any pregnant mother be allowed to be buried without ascertaining the survival or death of the fetus by dissection. So far the title of the book[123].

Nymman says that by general consensus the fetus is alive in the womb. What actually maintains its life, however, whether the maternal life or one of its own has remained uncertain. As it does not breathe in utero and thus does not import the material for the building up of vital spirit, most authors have concluded that it is devoid of autonomous life and not productive of vital functions. At best such functions as are of the lowest order had been conceded to it, i.e. those called natural, but not the vital and animal functions. The fetal heart had been regarded as too small and soft for the reception of blood on the one hand and the preparation of vital spirits on the other. From the evidence which he obtained by dissection Nymman found all this to be untrue. Thus far the preface[124].

Of all more recent authors only Guilelmus Fabricius Hildanus (1560–1634), the most expert surgeon, had observed in passing and without further reasoning that the life of the fetus in the womb is not necessarily extinguished simultaneously with that of the mother. With this would agree the reasons given by Joh. Riolanus and repeated by Spigelius demonstrating that the vital organs are not altogether idle in the fetus. However, Nymman finds fault with the main argument adduced by Riolan: namely that the heart in the fetus must move in order to distribute heat to the parts and thus obviates putrefaction owing to the collection of excrement. Nymman thinks that the heat and "virtue" immanent in the uterus would suffice to accomplish just this [125].

His own arguments are partly scholastic and partly observational. All generation, he says, occurs in a moment; it is one indivisible process that is productive of one substance complete in itself and not admitting of external impulses and emanations that would confer vital faculties upon it. Nor could this be due to a series of "accidental" alterations, as in this case the embryo would be alive now more and then less and his life something purely "accidental"[126]. Nor could it be the transference of spirits from the mother. For who does not know that spirits are neither alive themselves nor able to bestow life on others, but are simply instruments that serve the soul? Otherwise that which is spirituous in the blood of animals and is sometimes seen as a vapour exhaled from it would be the soul of the animal itself and could be kept in a vessel—which is simply ridiculous. On the contrary, it is the fetus which prepares spirits proper and specific to it as an individual endowed with a soul of his own[127]. It is known to everybody that vital spirits are carried by the arteries and animal ones by the nerves. As there is, however, no nervous communication between mother and fetus, no animal spirits can be communicated from the former to the latter, but it is the fetus itself which produces them in order to be capable of movement. Such functions are of higher dignity than those engendered by the vital spirits. This is shown for example by their persistence in those sick or dying who have long since lost the power of moving feet or hands. It follows that where the higher functions and spirits are present those of lower dignity must be likewise, and indeed without the

124 Witebergae, December 14th, 1627. sig. A 2 to A 4 recto.

125 Pp. 1–9; with reference to Riolanus, Joh. fil., *Anthropographia*, ed. Paris 1626, 638 where the autonomy of the foetus and its distinctiveness from the mother is emphasised: "certum est Foetum Humanum perfectum et absolutum esse animal, a matre distinctum, quod non est pars uteri, neque matris, ut integro libello sive Galenus, sive alius author, docte et cumulative probavit, nec ipse Galenus sub finem lib. Definitionum Medicarum ab ea opinione recessit. Illudque animal, nempe Foetum, instar alterius animalis vivere prodidit. Quod si Foetus agit vitam sensitivam, quis dubitat eum esse praeditum Animali Facultate. Est autem Animalis Facultas actio cerebri ad voluntarias functiones edendas..." The fetus owes its progress beyond the limits of plant life to the early development and function of its heart: "Foetum vitam vivere plantae, nec vitali facultate frui, nisi perfecto et optime conformato Corde, quod accidit cum incipit moveri". Ibid. p. 636.

126 Pp. 11 et seq. "omnis generatio, proprie dicta, in instanti fiat, nec terminetur ad accidens, sed substantiam et quidem completam..." p. 15.

127 P. 16: "spiritus nec vivere nec alteri per se vitam largiri posse, sed animae et eius operationibus dumtaxat inservire famularique...".

heart the brain is totally incapable of working, as is obvious in syncope and other affections of the cardio-vascular system. Hence since the fetus prepares the spirits for the animal functions without the help of the mother, it similarly perfects the vital spirits unaided. Moreover it is fully equipped for this, possesses its own blood and a heart with all the facilities to receive it[128]. This is further confirmed by the arterial pulse in the fetus which persists when the umbilical cord is ligatured or compressed in experimental animals, a fact known to Galen, but not exploited by him[129]. If the pulsating virtue were transferred from the mother to the fetus, the experiment would lead to the cessation of arterial pulsation in the fetus itself while it persists in the chorion. It is clearly shown by ocular inspection (*autopsia*) that the pulse of all arteries, those in the fetal body as well as in the chorion, depends upon the fetal heart, and not upon the mother[130]. A further argument is that the fetus can be found moving while the mother is asleep and vice versa[131], and how could a fetus ever die in the womb while the mother survived, were its life totally dependent upon the mother?[132] For the embryo is not an "organ" or "part" of the mother's body, neither an essential nor an integral part. This is particularly well shown by a bird's egg that develops and lives entirely and obviously by its own life (*sua vita propria*), separated as it is from the mother, the influence of its vital force, its "soul", blood and spirits and unconnected by any umbilical vessels. *Cor et in foetu pulsat*—this Nymman observed with his own eyes (*autoptes*) in fetuses removed quickly from the womb of an animal. When the chest was opened, the heart was seen to elevate itself and to quiver invariably and in each of the fetuses (*ibi ad oculum vidi*, *cor in quolibet foetu elevari et quasi micare*)[133]. This removed the last doubt in his mind that the fetus in the womb lives by its own life and not another's and can achieve its vital functions without communication with the mother's heart, hence being able to survive the mother in utero and to be recovered from it alive.

According to Nymman the conceptus, i.e. the product of the male and female "semen" develops its own life immediately it has received its soul. There are several possibilities as to how the soul is received: it may evolve from the forces potentially contained in the matter of the conceptus (*e potentia materiae educatur*), it may be transferred from the parents, it may be sent down from heaven and the stars or infused by God. The semen itself, however, is not animated *actu*, as it is man potentially only, and nothing can be at the same time *in actu* and *in potentia*. However, after an interval varying with the animal species the soul is received and in an in-

128 P.18: "si infans in utero praestare potest id quod magis est, etiam id praestabit, quod minus esse videtur. Atqui magis est actiones animales exercere, et totum corpus movere, quam vitales functiones edere et Spiritum vitalem producere...'-

129 On this compare: FRANKLIN, K.J., *A survey of the growth of knowledge about certain parts of the foetal cardio-vascular apparatus and about the foetal circulation, in man and some other mammals. Part I: Galen to Harvey. Ann. Sci.* 1941, 57–89 (p.61): Galen noted that the pulsation of the placental arteries ceases if the umbilical arteries are compressed within the cord (*De placitis Hippocr. et Platon.*, lib.VI, cap.6, ed. Kühn, vol.V, p. 558). However it was left for Spigelius to see the significance of this observation (Franklin p.80).

Nymman here obviously bases his argument on the observations of Spigelius. It was also the latter, who, following Arantius, denied any direct communication between the minute placental branches of the umbilical arteries and the corresponding branches of the maternal arteries in the uterus (Franklin, ibidem)—all findings supporting fetal independance.

130 P.20: "autopsia ... clareque ostendit omnem illarum arteriarum, etiam earum, quae in secundis existunt, pulsum a corde foetus dependere".

131 P.21.

132 P.22.

133 P.26: "si pullus vitalis in ovo ... suaque vita propria et ibi vivere potest ... quid obstabit, quo etiam infans in utero..., sua propria vita, ... suos Spiritus vitales producat, hosque per proprii cordis motum proprium, per universum corpus quoquoversum distribuat ac dispenset". – p.28: heart beating in the fetus.

stant makes man from not-man and creates a new subject distinct from the mother and alive by virtue of its own vital principle (*fitque in instanti ex non homine homo, et suppositum a matre distinctum jam vita sua propria vivens*)[134].

It has been objected, however, Nymman continues, that there can be no life where there is no air for breathing, the ventilation and motion of the heart and the production of spirits. Nymman replies that air does not make, but merely ventilates and preserves spirits. What little air is needed for this purpose by the fetus can easily be supplied from the arteries of the mother. This explains such rare events as the birth of a weeping or crying infant (*vagitus uteri*)[135].

But why should nature have taken the trouble of forming the umbilical vessels, if the fetus produces the vital force and spirit by itself? Nymman's answer to this is that maternal arteries do not reach the embryo, but that the vessels in the membranes enclosing the embryo and in the latter are all formed by the semen and merely adjoin the arteries of the womb.

There can be no concoction of anything without the expulsion of excrement, as Galen showed. As no excrement can possibly be discharged from the heart of the embryo, there can be no "coction" or ever-renewed elaboration of spirits. Nymman feels, however, that the small amount of "smoke" resulting from this can be stored in the fetal lower abdomen or by insensible transpiration be dispersed through pores of the skin or mouth or nose and stored in the amniotic sac[136].

That the fetus, though living by its own vital principle, is not viable before its time, is no valid objection. Just as the egg is in need of incubation for a certain period, the fetus must be kept warm until its organs have reached perfection through its own force. Even so aborted embryos have survived for hours and premature infants reached old age.

Nymman winds up with an eloquent plea for systematic performance of the Caesarian section in the deceased mother. This is based on a eulogy of anatomical and especially comparative anatomical studies and a rejection of the calumnies levelled against those who practised Caesarian section. "It is the duty of the true philosopher to think about the universe and all the working mechanisms (*naturas*) which it embraces and to consider them in scientific terms. Of all creatures, however, man is the most noble and indeed is a microcosm. He who lacks knowledge of the latter cannot have knowledge of objects of lesser dignity and pride himself on partaking in wisdom[137]."

134 P.35.

135 P.39.

136 P.48.

137 P.55.

Nymman's booklet soon became influential in forensic practice and legislation[138]. The firm stand taken by him in favour of the autonomy of the *conceptus* or *ovum* (in the wider—Harveian—sense) is of considerable interest in view of the same opinion defended by Harvey. It is one of the major points in which the latter deviates from Aristotle (see above, p. 272) and on which he was taken up by Marcus Marci (p. 319).

Harvey was acquainted with Nymman's book. It is cited by him because of the observations supporting the independence of the fetus and its active cooperation in its own birth. This, Harvey said, was evident from the occurrence of the birth of live infants after the death of the mother, as in one case known to Harvey personally and others collected by Nymman[139].

138 JUL. PAGEL in *Biographisches Lexikon* ed. Hirsch, vol. IV, Wien und Leipzig 1886, p. 395.

The influence of Nymman is recognisable for example in the work of J.C. LE COURVÉE, *De nutritione foetus in utero paradoxa*, Dantisci, sumpt. Geo Foersteri, 1655. Front. (illustrating two embryos with dorsal segmentation carried in a kind of chariot) XX, 254 pp. cap. III, p. 6–8: probatur fetum in utero propria virtute et innata vi sanguinem conficere, adeo ut non habeat opus maternum attrahere, quo alatur. cap. V, p. 12: foetus in utero ut extra uterum eandem eodemque modo haematosin peragit. p. 16: ita non vivit materno sanguine per vasa umbilicalia perducto, sic enim non esset animal, sed pars animalis. Le Courvée, though following Harvey whom he calls: *praemonstratorem nostrum* in many respects, issues a long refutation of Epigenesis and Harvey's distinction between epigenesis and metamorphosis (hic maxime D. Harveum, alias subtilem et argutissimum Virum, ita turpiter hallucinatum esse, ut duplicem fecerit animalium generationem, alteram per epigenesin, alteram per metamorphosin), Pars II, cap. 4, p. 82. – Le Courvée denies succession in organ development; everything is generated simultaneously (pp. 78 et seq.).

139 HARVEY, *De partu* (append. to *On generation*) ed. 1662, p. 345; tr. WILLIS p. 536. See also MEYER, A.W., *Analysis of De generat. animal.* Stanford and London 1936, p. 130: "Harvey regarded the fetus very much as a free agent and concluded that it decided for itself when it was to be born... As one contemplates these singular narrations and other similar statements, one is reminded that even great men cannot escape from all the things that shackle common men ... for Aristotle and Arantius had held that the fetuses of mammals were expelled by the contraction of the uterus, the abdominal muscles and the diaphragm. One scarcely can escape the conclusion that in this instance at least if not also in others, Harvey was misled by an opinion derived from a study of the chick and of insects."

Marcus Marci's "Idea of Operative Ideas" and Harvey's Embryological Speculation

Introduction

We have discussed the vitalistic theories of Severinus (p. 239). These had been inspired by the work of Paracelsus and closely approached the doctrine of *Epigenesis* as developed later by Harvey, the Aristotelian naturalist and thinker.

It is not surprising that even closer contacts emerge between Harvey and Johannes Marcus Marci of Kronland. The latter called his work on generation: *Idea of Operative Ideas*[1] thus immediately proclaiming the vitalistic keynote of his speculation; the emphasis is laid on spirit rather than matter.

Marcus Marci was interested in the first place in *light*, its physical behaviour, but also its occult power. In the course of his work he arrived at an anticipation of a *Field-theory* in Embryology (p. 306) and, a decade later, of such discoveries as the colour of thin plates and diffraction through lattices[2]. He explained colour in terms of the refraction of light and seems to have foreshadowed Newton's *Experimentum crucis*[3]. At the same time Marci regarded light as a cosmic force charged with the task of translating the divine world of ideas and the spirit into visible reality. In this he was palpably influenced by Neoplatonism and the metaphysics of light. We shall return to these influences shortly (p. 291).

1 *Idearum Operatricium Idea sive Hypotyposis et Detectio illius Occultae Virtutis, quae Semina fecundat, et ex iisdem Corpora Organica producit. Authore Johanne Marco Marci Philosophiae et Medicinae Doctore et ordinario Professore eiusdem Medicae Facultatis in Universitate Pragensi, Physico Regni Boemiae.* Anno 1635. Colophon on sig. Tt 4 verso: Pragae. Typis Seminarii Archiepiscopalis. Anno 1635. *Dedication:* Serenissimo Hungariae et Bohemiae Regi etc. Ferdinando Tertio 2 pp. *Ad Lectorem:* the idea of writing the book came to him on a journey to Budweis where he was called in 1631 leaving his pregnant wife at home. 2 pp. *Defensio Idearum adversus adulterinas et supposititias Ideas.* 8 pp. III, IV, A1, A2, A3. On verso of A3 woodcut showing female figure with a lens mounted on a stand symbolising "optical" conception. Underneath: Errare nescit ratio quam farinat fides. Concepta mente libera ridet minas, Opinionum et te vel invita parit. Defence against the suspicion of impiety.

With reference to the history of the theory of generation Marci's work was first discussed by W. PAGEL, *Religious motives in the medical biology of the XVIIth century. Bullet. Hist. Medicine* 1935, III, 224–231 and with reference to Harvey in *William Harvey and the purpose of circulation, Isis* 1951, XLII, 22–38 (p. 32–33). See also Jos. NEEDHAM, *History of embryology*, Cambridge 1934, p. 63. (Early example of Field-Theory)

2 MAREK, JIRI, *Johannes Marcus Marci als erster Beobachter: Farben dünner Schichten. Arch. Int. Hist. Sci.* 1960, XIII, 79–85. Idem, *Observation in the year 1648 of Diffraction through a Lattice. Nature* 1961, p. 1092. With reference to Marci, *Thaumantias. Liber de Arcu Coelesti deque Colorum apparentium Natura, Ortu et Causis ... ducibus Geometria et Physica Hermetoperipatetica.* Prague 1648, p. 119: "in omni foramine, quantumvis exiguo, radiorum decussatio flat ... si reticulum opponas luminoso ... totidem irides, quot foramina..."—diffraction through a system of apertures. – p. 241 in soap bubbles "sequuntur colores mira elegantia et varietate ... post aliqualem moram ... tota superficies bullae ejusmodi coloribus variegatur ... in bulla aerem contineri crassum et vaporosum in quo refractio fiat ad perpendicularem, eo modo, quo in pila crystallina."—colour in thin plates. p. 103: "lamella in modum reticuli pertusa, aut filamenta convoluta totidem irides procreant, quot foramina, seu rimae luci perviae..."—spectral colours on the apertures formed by wire mashing. For detail see Marek, Jiri. *Pozorovani ohybu svetla a barev tenkych vrstev u Jana Marka Marci. Dejiny prirodnich ved a techniky* Praha VII, 1962, p. 62–78.

3 "Refractio superveniens radio colorato non mutat rationem (speciem) coloris" *Thaumantias* loc. cit. 1648, p. 100–101, Theorema XIX and XX: "sicuti vero refractio superveniens nihil officit radio colorato, ita praevia nihil eidem opitulatur."—"color sit quaedam imperfectio ... per quam virtus lucigena determinatur ad sphaeram novam sub illa imperfectione producendam". For detail: HOPPE, E.M., *Ein vergessener Physiker des XVII. Jahrhunderts. Arch. f. Gesch. Med. Naturwiss. Tech.* 1927, XXX, 1–2; restricting Marci's achievement: ROSENFELD, L.M., *Untersuchungen über das Prisma und ihr Verhältnis zu Newtons Farbenlehre. Isis* 1931, XVII, 325. On Marci in general: HELLER, A., *Geschichte der Physik* Stuttgart 1884, vol. II, p. 328; ROSENBERGER, F., *Geschichte der Physik* Braunschweig 1884, Teil II, p. 159. On Marci's achievements in mechanics (laws governing the impact of spherical bodies): MACH, E., *Die Mechanik in ihrer Entwickelung historisch-kritisch dargstellt.* Leipzig 1883. HOPPE loc. cit.

In Marci's work speculation on these lines was intimately blended with advanced insight in optics, in mechanics and in biology. He adhered to Aristotelian principles and to a certain extent incorporated spiritualistic Paracelsian ideas, but freely expressed his original and critical mind.

The life of Marci and his meeting with Harvey (pl. 42 and 44)

Marci was born on June 13th 1595 at Landskron in Bohemia, studied theology and subsequently medicine at Prague, became a professor in 1627 and physician to the Emperor Ferdinand III. and senior physician of Bohemia in 1647. In 1654 he was raised to the peerage with the title of "Von Kronland". In 1662 he officiated as Rector of Prague University and died five years later 1667)[4].

A discussion of Marci's ideas in biology and notably his theory of generation appears to be particularly pertinent, as we know that *Harvey met him personally in Prague*[5].

The meeting took place in 1636. Harvey then served as physician to Thomas Howard, Earl of Arundel who headed a large and stately embassy sent by Charles Ist to negotiate with Emperor Ferdinand on behalf of Prince Charles Louis, nephew of Charles I[st] and heir to the ill-fated Frederic of Bohemia. Having travelled through Germany stricken by the misery and terrors of the Thirty Years War and after preliminary meetings with the Emperor at Linz the embassy arrived at Prague on July 6th 1636.

Marci, the "Bohemian Plato" or as he was also known the "Hippocrates of Prague" had only in the preceding year published his treatise on generation. Though largely speculative it had offered one new approach to the perennial problem concerning the formation of a variety of tissues and organs from what appeared to be a simple and homogeneous "monad" uniting in itself the body and the idea of an individual. Marci was in his forty-first year and though almost twenty years Harvey's junior at that time the most promising natural philosopher and physician in the Empire.

The English embassy was a goodwill mission as well as a negotiating body, and was entertained by meetings with notable men as well as by visits to the best known collections, buildings and institutions. Harvey stayed at Prague for at least a week. It seems highly likely that Harvey and Marci would have met[6]. Despite its plausibility, however, up to a short time ago no proof had been given that such a meeting did indeed take place—al-

4 JUL. PAGEL in *Biograph. Lexikon d. hervorr. Ärzte*. Gurlt-Hirsch, vol. IV, 1886, p. 129; NOACK, LUDW., *Philosophie-geschichtliches Lexikon*. Leipzig 1879, p. 582 with ref. to GUHRAUER, G. E., *Marcus Marci und seine philosophischen Schriften, Zeit. f. Philos. Kritik* 1852, XXI, 241–259. – Of older biographical accounts that of his pupil J. J. Wenc. Dobrcensky de Nigroponte in Marci's *Liturgia mentis s. disceptatio medica, philosophica et optica de natura epilepsiae* Ratisb. 1678 should be consulted. See also: HASNER in *Prager Zeitschr. f. Heilkunde* 1883, IV, 170 and E. M. LEHMANN, *Gesundheitsbüchlein, Anhang zur Otosophie*, Landskron 1928.

5 PAGEL, W. and RATTANSI, P., *Harvey meets the "Hippocrates of Prague" (Johannes Marcus Marci of Kronland)*. *Med. Hist.* 1964, VIII, 78–84.

6 This had been postulated by KRUTA, V., *Harvey in Bohemia. Physiologia Bohemoslovenica*, 1957, VI, 433–439. In this paper an account has been given of the Bohemian landmarks and scenes of the time which should have impressed Harvey's party.

7 PAGEL and RATTANSI, loc. cit. 1964, in note [5] with reference to B.M. Add. MSS. 15970, f. 49; JOHN AUBREY, *Lives* 1813, II, 384; SIR GEOFFREY KEYNES, *Lancet* 1958, II, 859, loc. cit. p. 17 note [2].

Harvey's journey to Prague has been discussed in some detail in two accounts: SIR D'ARCY POWER, *A revised chapter in the life of Dr. William Harvey, 1636, Proc. roy. Soc. Med., Sect. Hist. Med. 10*, 1897, 35–59, and MARY S. HERVEY, *The Life, Correspondence and Collections of Thomas Howard, Earl of Arundel, London*, 1921. The primary sources were:

CROWNE, WILLIAM, *A True Relation of all the Remarkable Places and Passages Observed in the Travels of the right honourable Thomas Lord Howard, Earle of Arundell and Surrey, Primer Earle, and Earle Marshall of England and Ambassador Extraordinary to his sacred Majesty Ferdinando the second, Emperour of Germanie Anno Domini 1636*, London, 1637.

Historical Manuscripts Commission, Report (on MSS of the Earl of Denbigh), London, 1911. JOHN AUBREY, *Lives* 1813, loc. cit.

Earl of Clarendon, *State Papers* vol. I, London 1767 (containing letters from Arundel to the Secretary of State Windebank). B.M. Add. MSS. 15970 (containing letters from Arundel to the Rev. William Petty at Venice). Public Records Office, *State Papers, Foreign, Germany*, 1646. (Windebank-Arundel correspondence.)

A check through these sources shows that Mary Hervey has used and reproduced all the letters contained in them which have references to Harvey's visit, with two ex-

though the visit to Prague is mentioned in the Harvey-Feilding correspondence, as well as in the correspondence between Arundel, Windebanke and Petty[7].

Here we find "little Doctor Hervey" and "the little perpetual movement called Dr Herveye" who "would still be making of excursions into the woods, making observations of strange trees, and plants, earths etc and sometimes like to be lost. So that my Lord Ambassador would be really angry with him, for there was not only danger of thieves, but also of wild beasts."

The *proof* that the meeting between Harvey and Marcus Marci really occurred is provided by the latter himself and embedded in a critical discussion of Harvey's *De generatione animalium* of 1651 (see below p. 318). This is found in Marci's work *Philosophia vetus restituta* of 1662[8]. Here Marci expresses regret and disappointment at the omission on Harvey's part of any reference to his, Marci's, book, the *Idea* of 1635, on generation. As Marci says, Harvey could not have remained ignorant about it. "For I gave the book into his hands, here at Prague talking to him familiarly" (*neque ignotum id*—sc. Marci's hypothesis—*Harveyo. Cui librum hic Praguae in manus dedi familiariter cum eodem conversatus*[9].

To the present-day observer Marci's feeling of disappointment does not seem altogether unjustified. For there are not a few essential points in which Harvey's embryological theories conform with those published by Marci sixteen years before his own work. It is true, however, that Harvey did not avail himself of Marci's main approach to the problem which rested on an application of geometrical optics, notably the laws of refraction, to the unfolding of the many parts out of the simple germ. On the other hand Marci complains that he himself had offered a workable hypothesis, whereas Harvey ultimately lost himself in improbable assumptions and idealistic speculations.

It should be noted that Marci had been one of the earlier supporters of Harvey's discovery. Copies of *De motu* were extant in the Prague University Library[10]. What is more, Jacob Forberger, a pupil of Marci, defended under his presidency a thesis entitled: *De pulsu et eius usu* in 1642[11]. It contained a good précis of Harvey's work, although Harvey's name was not quoted even once—a phenomenon not unknown in the early history of the reception of *De motu* (p. 61).

Marci and the English Scene

Evidently Marci was instrumental in making Harvey's discovery and further work known and discussed in Eastern Europe. In

ceptions: (1) P.R.O., S.R. 80, vol. IX, fol. 205. The remarks about Harvey in this letter are of interest, since they cast further light on the circumstances in which he decided to visit Italy, and, while there, was asked to undertake a commission for buying paintings. Arundel writes from Ratisbon, 30/20 July 1636 to Mr Secretary Windebank: "Honest little Doctor Hervey, havinge a greate desire to see some partes of Italy, I thought fitte to let him take these days of vacancy, to rather satisfye his curiosity there, than in Hungary where he might have... hazarded his health more, for wante of necessaries."

(2) From B.M. Add. MSS. 15970, Lord Maltravers to the Rev. William Petty, 21 August 1636: "Wee were all heare extremely troubled to heare out of Germany that Doctor Harvey, went by Sienna and left you there sicke, but I hope in God there was no danger..."

To these may be added another reference to Harvey which does not seem to have been quoted before. It occurs in *The Calendar of State Papers, Domestic*, 1636/37 (London 1867) in a letter from Sir Thomas Roe to Elizabeth, Queen of Bohemia, 1 August 1636, p. 83: "... he heard also that Dr. Harvey assured his private friends of great hopes of justice and equity from the Emperor, but he believes, the doctor judges by symptoms, like a physician, and the Ambassador is so wise or so warned as not to show discontent, nor what he hopes or fears."

8 Pagel and Rattansi, 1964, loc. cit. in note [5], p. 79.

9 *Joh. Marci a Kronland Philosophia vetus restituta partibus V comprehensa*, Praguae 1662. Edition used: Francof. et Lipsiae sumpt. Christ. Weidmann, 1676 (the second ed.: XI, 580 pp), p. 352 in Pars III, subsectio 2 (n). See below p. 318.

10 A census of the copies of Harvey's works extant at Prague, made at my request and placed at my disposal by Dr. Marek, reveals a remarkable number including one of the first edition of *De Motu*. In detail: *De Motu* 1628 Keynes, G., (*A Bibliography of the Writings of Dr. William Harvey*. 2nd ed. Cambridge 1953) 1; National Lib. 18 H 191. – 1639 Keynes 3; Nat. Lib. 18 G 216. – 18 H 177. – Lib. Francisc. convent Vd 83. – 1643 Keynes 4; August. convent EE VII 40. – 1660 Keynes 9; Lib. Strahov CSV 40. – 1671 Keynes 11; August. conv. JJ IX 75. – *Exerc. de Generat. Animal.* 1651 Keynes 37; Lib. Strahov EK VIII 13. – Cruciati (Krizovníci) conv. XXIX C 3. – Augustinian conv. JJ IX 81. – 1662 Keynes 39 Nat. Lib. 16 L 32.

turn Marci was not unknown in England. Indeed his name occurs in the literature of the Puritan Revolution.

Thus Thomas Vaughan, the mystical philosopher, alchemist and naturalist referred to Marci's embryological theory. Indeed Marci's work was regarded by Vaughan as a principal source of support for "Natural Magic"—the interpretation of certain phenomena as "natural" (although still inexplicable) as against their rejection as develish or demonic illusions.

Vaughan deals with the ideal world of creative divine ideas which foreshadows the material world with its concrete and individual creatures. Owing to this ideal—"sophic"—world the sudden emergence, disappearance and revivification (*Palingenesis*) of things as it were from their ashes find its explanation with many other phenomena of natural magic. It has been Marci who had defended the possibility of such phenomena.

Vaughan says:

"... no sooner had the Divine Light pierced the bosom of the Matter, but the Idea or Pattern of the whole material world appeared in those primitive waters like an image in a glasse ... This mystery or appearance of the Idea is excellently manifested in the magical analysis of bodies; for he that knows how to imitate the protochymistry of the spirit by the separation of the principles wherein the life is imprisoned may see the impresse of it experimentally in the outward natural vestiments. But lest you should think this my invention and no practicall truth, I will give you another man's testimony. 'I inquire (saith one) what such great philosophers would say, if they beheld the plant as born in a moment in the glass vial, with its colours as in life, and then again die, and reborn, and that daily, and whenever they choose? But the power to deceive human senses I believe they include in the art magic of the demons.' They are the words of Doctor Marci in his *Defensio Idearum Operatricium*[12]."

Vaughan who lived from 1622 to 1665 (or 1666) thus wrote in 1650. Not long afterwards—in 1654—John Webster, a sectarian author who wished to introduce revolutionary changes in the teaching of the natural sciences at Oxford and Cambridge, wrote:

"What shall I say of *Staticks*, *Architecture*, *Pneumatithmie*, *Stratarithmetrie* ... the least of which is of more use ... to the life of man than almost all that learning that the Universities boast of ... and yet by them utterly neglected ... but what huge stupendous effects these can bring to pass, let our learned Countreyman Roger Bacon, let Cardinal Cusan, let Galalaeus, let Ubaldus, let *Marcus Marci*, let Baptista Benedictus, and many others speak,

11 KRUTA, loc.cit. in note [6], 1957, with reproduction of the title page of Forberger's thesis. See above p. 61, note [3].

12 VAUGHAN, THOMAS, *Anthroposophia Theomagica* (published under the pseudonym "Eugenius Philalethes"), London 1650, p. 9–10; ed. A.E.WAITE, *The Magical Writings of Thomas Vaughan* London 1888, p. 13. – The passage alluded to is found in Marci's *Idea* loc.cit. 1635, sig. A 2 recto and runs as follows: "Quid quaeso dicerent hi tanti Philosophi, si plantam quasi momento nasci in vitreo vase viderent, cum suis ad vivum coloribus, et rursum interire, et renasci, idque quoties et quando luberet? Credo daemonium arte magica inclusum dicerent illudere sensibus humanis. Pro falso enim et diabolico opera naturae habent, quae nequeunt resolvi in illorum principia, et falsas hypothese "

who remain a Cloud of Witnesses against the supine negligence of the Schools ...[13]"

These two quotations from somewhat unorthodox and elusive authors may be followed up by one from Boyle's *Examination* of a work of Hobbes:

"To omit antienter authors, such great personages as *Galileo*, *Mersennus*, *Verulam*, *Des Cartes*, *Gassendus*, *Balianus*, *Johannes Marcus Marci*, *Honoratus Fabri* (not to mention other moderns, nor those of our own assembly, as the eminently-learned *Sir Kenelm Digby*, and the others, whom their modesty forbids me here to name) had not most of them learnedly, and some copiously, written of local motion before Mr Hobbes's books, where he treats of it, came abroad into the world[14]."

Finally Marcus is listed among the "most eminent astronomers ancient and modern" by Sir Edward Sherburne in 1675 as follows: "1650 Johannes Marcus Marci Counsellor and Physician to the Emperor *Ferdinand* the Third, and primary Professor of Physick in the *University* of Prague, wrote, among other Physico-Mathematical Tractates, a Particular Treatise, *De Longitudine, seu Differentiis inter duos Meridianos, una cum Motu vero Lunae inveniendo ad tempus datae Observationis*, Printed at Prague in the year 1650[15]."

Marci and the Royal Society

The prestige that Marci enjoyed not only in sectarian but also truly scientific circles in England is reflected in the efforts made by Oldenburg, the Secretary of the Royal Society, in 1667 to establish a correspondence with him, which would probably have led to a Fellowship as with Leeuwenhoek and Malpighi. Alas, Marci had died in the same year, on April 10th, at the age of 72, and nothing came of it[16]. The documentary evidence for these efforts to take up contact with Marci is of great interest. Edward Browne (1644–1708), the eldest son of Sir Thomas Browne (1605–1682), writes to Oldenburg from Vienna, between 4 and 14 February 1668/69: "I cannot heare of Marcus Marci, so as I must desire a more particular addresse to him that I may know who he is and where he lives, as also a more particular information where *Herrngrundt* is, which you mention in your tenth inquiry[17]." Oldenburg answers (his only reply to Browne preserved at the Royal Society): "As for Marcus Marci, I believe you'll hear that he is at Prague, where by a Latin letter of yours to him he might doubtlesse be engaged to a correspondency with us which being but once by you begun, I shall be able enough to continue afterwards[18]." This is followed by a

13 Webster, John, *Academiarum examen, or the Examination of the Academies* London 1654, p. 52.

14 Boyle, Robert, *An Examen of Mr. Hobbes's Dialogus Physicus de Natura Aeris.* quoted from *Works*, ed. Thomas Birch, 1744, vol. I, p. 233.

15 Sherburne, Edward, *The Sphere of Manilius, translated*, London 1675, *Appendix: A catalogue of the most eminent astronomers ancient and modern*, p. 98. – The author is indebted for these passages to Dr. P. Rattansi, as also for a reference to Samuel Hartlib's *Ephemerides* 1658 (an unpublished manuscript preserved at Sheffield University Library and analysed by C. Webster —to be published). In this "An earnest enquiry made after a rare booke called Marcus Marci *De linea sphygmica*, printed at Prague, 1636 in 4° by Dr. Worthington for a nobleman..."

16 The present author is indebted to Dr. J. Marek for drawing first his attention to Marci's prospective contacts with the Royal Society. He referred to the book by W.E. Newbold, *The cipher of Roger Bacon*, Philadelphia (University of California Press) 1928, in ch. II, p. 32 (also printed in *Tr. Coll. Phys. Philadelphia* 1921, 415–430). Here it is also mentioned that Marci had studied under Athanasius Kircher in Rome and written a letter to Kircher concerning a cipher-manuscript of Roger Bacon.

For the documentary evidence concerning the intended invitation in detail see Pagel and Rattansi, loc. cit. 1964, p. 81–84.

17 Royal Society, marked: Read March 4, 1668/69, entered letter-book 200.

18 Oldenburg to Browne, London March 1st, 1668/69.

letter from Browne to Oldenburg, dated Norwich, 26 November 1669: "I forgot not to enquire after Marcus Marci in Prague, but I understoode he dyed 2 years since.[19]" As a corollary to this we read in Browne's travel account: "During my stay here, I had a great desire to have saluted *Johannes Marcus Marci*, a famous Physician, and Philosopher of *Prague*, and also to have induced him to a Correspondence with the *Royal Society*, but I understood that he had left this World, to the great grief of Learned Men in these and other parts[20]."

We may *conclude:*

Marci formed a well known figure in Puritan English Literature, as an empirical naturalist and physicist who would follow the light of observation and experience rather than preconceived ideas and systems such as notably Aristotelian Scholasticism. He was thus bracketed with such well known opponents to "Peripatetick Philosophy" as Van Helmont and that "profoundly learned man Dr *Fludd* and his work than which for all the particulars ... the world never had a more rare, experimental and perfect piece[21]."

Inevitably along with these Marci was held up as an example of the fruitfulness of the Paracelsian tradition—"the most admirable and soul-ravishing knowledge of the three great principles of nature, salt, sulphur and mercury ... clearly and evidently manifested by that miracle of industry and pains Theophrastus Paracelsus. Which however the *Schools* (as hating any liquor that is not drawn out of their own Cask, and despising all things that come by toil and labour) may slight and contemn it, and please themselves with their ayery *Chimaera* of an abstracted and scarce intelligible *materia prima* ...[22]"

It was also Marci's truly scientific achievement in optics and mechanics which had aroused the attention of members of the Royal Society and made contact with him desirable.

However, this appraisal of Marci, though justified in many respects, ignored his deep-seated affiliation to Aristotelian doctrine, especially in his theory of generation.

It is this field which we have to examine closely, as it is bound to be productive of parallels and contacts with Harvey, if only for the basic adherence to Aristotelian doctrine which they have in common.

Marci against Credulity and Charlatanism

It should also be remembered that Marci kept aloof from the unbounded and uncritical credulity shown by some of the Em-

19 Marked: read Feb. 3rd, 1669, entered Letter-book 200.

20 Browne, Edward, *An account of several travels through a great part of Germany: in four journeys*, London 1677, p. 125. – Browne visited Holland in 1668 and ended this journey at Cologne on October 10th 1668. His next journeys were one to Vienna, Hungary and Thessaly and one to Tyrol and Carinthia—from which he returned to England in 1669. – The correspondence of Sir Thomas Browne with his eldest son Edward during the latter's travels in 1668 and 1669 contains a reference to Oldenburg's efforts to secure a correspondent for the Royal Society in the Habsburg lands (*The Works of Sir Thomas Browne*, ed. G. Keynes, vol. VI, letters, London 1931—letter of March 1st 1668–1669). – Birch, in his *History of the Royal Society*, quotes the minutes of the Society's meetings in 1668/9 which mention that Oldenburg brought Browne's letters to the attention of members, but there is no direct reference to Marci. – On Browne's travels: Poynter, F. N. L., *Dr Edward Browne's visit to Vienna in 1668/9*, *Festschr. z. 80. Geburtst. v. Max Neuburger*, Vienna 1948, p. 381–385.

21 Webster, loc. cit. in note [13], p. 105—followed by the admonition: "Instead of Aristotelian learning, some Physical learning might be introduced into the Schools that is grounded upon sensible, rational, experimental and Scripture principles".

22 Webster, ibidem, p. 76 et seq.

pirics of the Paracelsian persuasion. This is shown in the sceptical attitude adopted by him towards microcosmic symbolism in general and the supposed *mineral semina* in particular. He displays similar scepticism in relating "stories" concerning malformations, giants, pygmees, hermaphrodites, satyrs, nymphs, kynokephaloi, sirens, tritons and harpys[23]. He expressly rejected Paracelsus' *homunculus* as "deliramenta" and "nugae", because there is a fundamental difference between the test-tube of the chemist and the human uterus whose warmth "*nulla ars, nulla industria ea ratione temperare potest, ut vitalem animalium calorem aemuletur*". It cannot be reproduced by any artifice, as it is not heat as such (a fiery quality) that sustains the fetus, but a heat-substance (*calor substantialis*) and vivifying spirit[24]. In a similar vein Marci doubts the stories about the missing heart in sacrificial animals and related tales[25].

Marci does not seem to have had patience with charlatans and their miracle cures. Thus the story has it that he came to blows with Thomas Grünberger over the latter's reputed cure of the wife of Count Burka who was dying of uterine carcinoma (*Mutterfraiss*). We are told that of all the doctors who had been invited to see the patient cured only Doctor Marcus Marci, *Decanus Facultatis Medicae*, appeared and challenged the quack for not having treated the patient who should have died methodically. In the subsequent row Marci is said to have thrown a glass of wine into Grünberger's face who retaliated with a blow which made Marci fall backwards in his chair to the ground, "whereupon the count himself rushed to the scene and tried to reconciliate the contestants, whilst the countess remained alive for a long time[26]." Grünberger is said to have accomplished many other cures by means of his "tincture" which, however, could not effect the transmutation of metals.

Marci's Theory of Generation

Introduction: The Physics and Metaphysics of Light as applied to Life before Marci

Marci's speculations on generation were informed by his deep interest and experience in optics. In this he was prompted by empirical—scientific—as well as metaphysical—non-scientific—considerations.

The latter belong to an ancient tradition connected with Platonism—a doctrine which regarded the rays of light as the bearers and distributors of those characteristics which are specific

23 *Idearum operat. idea*, loc. cit. in note [1] in the concluding chapters: cap. IV, sig. S 3 et seq. malformations; cap. VI, sig. Bb 4 et seq. giants and pygmees; cap. VII, sig. Ee 4 verso et seq. hermaphrodites; cap. VIII, sig. Ii 4 verso et seq. satyrs, nymphs etc.

24 Ibidem, Kk 3 verso to Kk 4 recto.

25 Ibidem, T 4 recto et verso.

26 *Catalogus manuscriptorum chemico-alchemico-magico-cabalistico-medico-physico-curiosorum* Wien 1788, p. 241 with reference to *Wahre Beschreibung meines ... magischen Kalenders*, dated Prague 25th of August 1655 (no 261 of the alchemical manuscripts listed).

to the individual and the species. Indeed light was looked upon as the individualising principle in nature, the vector of specificity[27].

In the Middle Ages this doctrine was prominent in the philosophies of Robert Grosseteste (d. 1253), Roger Bacon (1214–1294) and Petrus Hispanus (1226–1277).

The ultimate unity of all things as well as all multiplicity and individuation are explicable in terms of optics, the dispersion and concentration of light, says Grosseteste. "All is one by virtue of the perfection of the unique light and what is manifold is such by virtue of the diversity and multiplication of this very light." It is thus that "species" and "similitudo" are transmitted from one object to another—the result varying with the state and translucency of the surface by which the rays are absorbed or reflected. The shorter the distance between the object and the agent the shorter the rays and the more intense the effect. Rough surfaces with unequal parts destroy the rays or diminish their power[28].

In Roger Bacon's view rays and the lines, angles and figures formed by them achieve "the wonderful power of multiplying virtues" and of transmitting harmful effects such as the deadly heat of the sun, of contagion and the corrupting vapours emanating from a menstruating woman[29].

Petrus Hispanus, physician and pope (John XXI), based his metaphysics of light on the idea that the body *is* light and is thus bound to the higher world that transcends our sensual sphere, for light is the "celestial nature" in man. It makes the cooperation of the organs with each other possible in the same way as it brings about the harmony of the cosmic forces. There is "consensus" of all "sensibilia" in the world through their communication with light, the *Light of Nature*. The light when gaining access to an organ finds in it something akin to itself and is thus enabled to change it[30]. Light is understood not as an element like air or fire, but as a spiritual *form*, the first and noblest *form* in nature. Hence the soul is called *First Form*. Nothing composite can exist or operate without it[31].

In the Renaissance the idea of Light providing the driving force in the cosmos at large as well as in the microcosm of the living organism had been forcibly expressed by Paracelsus and his followers, by Servetus and perhaps most explicitly in the *Panaugia* of Patrizzi.

In the world of Paracelsus (1493–1541) nature is everywhere conditioned and determined by Light. Physical objects reach their perfection and destination by virtue of the *Light of Nature*.

27 On the underlying general—Platonic—principles see: MÜLLER, H. F., *Dionysios, Proklos, Plotinos. Ein historischer Beitrag zur Neuplatonischen Philosophie* (*Beitr. z. Gesch. d. Philos. d. Mittelalters* ed. C. Baeumker, vol. XX, 3–4), Münster 1918, p. 40–48, espec. p. 46. – The use of optical analogies, notably those connected with the mirror, was followed up through mediaeval and subsequent Christian mysticism in the important paper by HANS LEISEGANG, *La connaissance de Dieu au miroir de l'âme et de la nature. Rev. de l'Hist. et de Philos. Rélig.* 1937, vol. XVII, 145–171.

28 "Omnia esse unum ab unius lucis perfectione. Ea quae sunt multa esse multa ab ipsius lucis diversa multiplicatione" ROBERT GROSSETESTE, *De luce s. de inchoatione formarum*, BAUR, L., *Die philosophischen Werke des Robert Grosseteste. Beitr. z. Gesch. d. Philos. im Mittelalter* vol. IX, Münster 1912, p. 51 et seq. – All activity in Nature depends upon raylike lines, angles and figures and their reception by the surface of a substratum, i.e. upon reflection or refraction: *Libellus Linconiensis de phisicis angulis et figuris per quas omnes acciones naturales complentur.* Norinbergae 1503. See PAGEL, W., *Religious Motives in the Medical Biology of the XVIIth century. Bullet. Inst. Hist. Med.* 1935, III, 221. – For a comprehensive account of Grosseteste and his position in the History of Science: CROMBIE, A. C., *Robert Grosseteste and the Origins of Experimental Science 1100–1700.* Oxford 1953. DALES, R.C., *Robert Grosseteste's Scientific Works. Isis* 1961, LII, 381–402.

29 ROGER BACON, *Perspectiva* ed. Joh. Combach Francof. 1614: *Spec. Mathem.* p. 16, p. 49; cap. 6, p. 61. See PAGEL, W., *Religious Motives* loc. cit. 1935, p. 212, also with reference to ALFREDUS ANGLICUS, *De Motu Cordis* cap. XI, ed. BAEUMKER, *Beitr. z. Gesch. d. Philos. d. Mittelalters* vol. XXIII, Münster 1923, p. 46: "Quod spiritus vitae non movetur, sed fit ab irradiatione virtutis"; "generatione fit spiritus et sine tempore ... Aperto enim orificio simul fit emicatio ad totum, ut sol oriens aut fulgur sine tempore in quantumlibet remota radios jacit ... simul enim in extremis et medio pulsum sensus comprehendit, nullo temporis interventu. Quod si fluat spiritus, impossibile fit. Siquidem igitur sine tempore est generatio spiritus simulque per totum spargitur, simul fit in toto; neque fluere possibile". (ibid. 10–13, p. 49–51); p. 94, cap. XVI, 17: "... ad cerebrum fiat irradiatio virtutis vivificae spiritusque generativae". Generation and action of the spirit in the heart is instantaneous and "without time". Hence it does not flow, but emits the beams of its virtue into

Illuminated by it, an object achieves that internal "knowledge" that enables it to follow its specific life task and to produce its specific "fruit". It is through its guidance that the pear tree brings forth pears and no other fruit[32]. This is not external learning or wisdom from books or through rational thinking. It is an internal awareness that enlightens the "quintessential" kernel of the individual, its *Astral Body*. This light that makes nature work is the *World-Soul*—a gift of the *Holy Ghost*[33].

We discussed Servetus, his philosophy and his contribution to the pre-history of blood circulation above (p. 136). In the present context his ideas on light and its creative power should be mentioned. He said that each seed contains the properties of the individual to be formed by virtue of its immanent idea and light. Not only all generation and coming into being is thus brought about by light and ideas, but also all knowledge and mental activity. This operates by means of light-images which leave an imprint in the soul or rather raise and awaken the images or ideas which God through the light of His *logos* has conferred upon the soul in a germinal form[34].

J.B. Van Helmont (1579–1644) continued in the Paracelsian tradition. In his speculation Light assumed a central position. For he identified *Light* with *Form*—the *Form* that is given to each individual object by the Creator, the *Father of Lights*[35]. By virtue of the *Form* contained in it the semen becomes *luminous* and thus acts as the main instrument of the *Form*, comparable to a Master-Workman who "disposes" things under its guidance, as its *Architectus disponens*.

Illumination of the semen thus means *organisation*—the urge to equip a body with organs and members that are suitable receptacles for the Light. This was created as the beginning of all life on the first day[36]. Hence there is no life without light. It is this light that creates an harmonious organism by unifying the properties and diversities of a multitude of organs and members[37]. It follows that there are as many individuals and species as there are species of *Formal Light*[38].

It is seminal light that makes a drug efficacious and "grades" it. In warm-blooded animals the seminal light is "solar" in character, in cold-blooded "lunar"[39].

The Light of the *Forms* is divine and thus different from a natural "fireable" light which springs from the "lap of nature". In this we recognise the residue of an ancient tradition. In Stoicism a bright divine and productive fire had been distinguished from a "dark" (black), natural and destructive fire[40]. In the wake

the arteries and the pulse is felt everywhere in the body at the same time. This is comparable to the sudden breaking through of Light and the Sun after driving away the clouds. – On Alfred and his work see above p. 90 seq.

30 "Lux igitur ... adveniens ipsi organo, quia reperit in ipso organo aliquid simile et eiusdem naturae cum ipsa quia ultima completio organi, immutat ipsum organum, ipsi representans speciem sensibilis receptam." *Expos. in librum De Anima* quoted from SCHIPPERGES, H., *Makrobiotik bei Petrus Hispanus. Arch. f. Gesch. d. Med.* 1960, XLIV, 129–155 (p. 152). See also: Idem, *Medizinischer Unterricht im Mittelalter. Deut. Med. Wochschr.* 1960, LXXXV, 856–861; Idem, *Der Stufenbau der Natur im Weltbild des Petrus Hispanus. Gesnerus* 1960, XVII, 14–29 (p. 25); Idem, *Zur Psychologie und Psychiatrie des Petrus Hispanus. Confin. Psychiat.* 1961, IV, 137–157 with ref. to *Expos. in lib. De Anima* 279, 20: "... omnia sensibilia communicant in natura lucis ... per quod omnia immutent sensus proprios". (p. 151 and 157); Idem, *Arzt im Purpur. Leben und Werk des P.H. Materia Med. Nordmark* 1961, XIII, 591–600.

31 *Expos. in lib. de Anima* 278, 23–26: "omne corpus compositum habet in se naturam caelestem ut lucem incorporatam, qua mediante conservatur et est forma ejus particularis in sua materia ipsam perficiens ... sine hac natura conservante non potest conservari compositum, similiter nec potest in aliquam operationem exire nisi per absolutionem huiusmodi virtutis." *Quaestiones* 169, 28: "Et sic lux est forma prima, quae in genere naturae est nobilissima et ad quem omnes aliae ordinantur et propter quam sunt. Et sic anima dicitur esse forma prima." Quoted from SCHIPPERGES, *Arch. f. Gesch. d. Med.* 1960 loc. cit. p. 152.

32 *Philos. Sagax* Lib. I, 1 ed. Sudhoff vol. XII, p. 23–24. – PAGEL, W., *Paracelsus Introduction to Philosophical Medicine in the Era of the Renaissance* Basle and New York 1958, p. 75. – On Light of Nature and Time: *Die Erste Defension* (1537/38) ed. Sudhoff, vol. XI, p. 127–128.

K. GOLDAMMER, *Lichtsymbolik in philosophischer Weltanschauung, Mystik und Theosophie vom 15.–17. Jahrhundert. Stud. Generale* 1960, XIII, 670–682, rightly pointed out that the *Light of Nature* is not a light produced *by* Nature, but "ein die Natur konstituierendes, sie durchdringendes Prinzip; keine von ihr ausgehende Erhellung, sondern ein sie erhellendes ... Prinzip *hinter* der Natur ... die in den Dingen wirkende Kraft". See also ibidem for light symbolism in the philosophies of Nicolaus Cusanus,

of this tradition Paracelsus had separated an invisible, *essential* fire—the internal virtue of objects—from visible, dark, *material* fire. Consequently he had called the Life of Man a "celestial and invisible Fire[41]."

The Rosicrucian Julius Sperber who wrote at the turn of the sixteenth century elaborated on this speculation. God, he said, is the *Ignis Maximus*, the Father of Light and hence the source of life (*Fons Vitae*). He acts by virtue of a shining light and a "fiery Word". This is the "Spiraculum Vitae" or soul which he infused into man after he had formed him. In the latter it is kept burning by the "astral spirit" which works like oil in a candle. Generation is through "sparks" emitted by the soul (*Seelenfunken*). These together with astral spirit constitute the semen. In it the sparks "dispose", whilst the astral spirits engender the body and make it grow. Just as the spark hidden in flint needs air and a body to become visible, the spark hidden in semen is nourished into a visible flame by the womb which acts as a tinder. The divine sparks are enshrined in the heart of the embryo and hence carried around by the blood that envelops them. For it is said that all soul of flesh is in the blood[42].

Francesco Patrizzi (1529–1597) devoted his *Panaugia* to the omnipresence and total power of Light. He said: "Light animates all things, contains all things, supports all things, brings all things together, unites all things; it separates all things, it draws all things to itself ... it purifies whatever it has transformed; it perfects all things, it renews all things, it preserves all things and protects them from annihilation. It is the number and measure of all things. It is the image of the deity whilst the world is its coal[43]."

The nature of Semen

Quid semen—what is the seed, how and by whom is it produced—this is the main subject of Marci's *Idea*. Obviously, Marci argues, its purpose is the perpetuation and preservation of the world. It is the divine force in things liable to corruption that enables them to bring forth an offspring similar to themselves. It is a substance that is similar to the parent not as such, but by virtue of its inherent tendency (*potestate, non actu similis*)[44].

In addition to possessing the generative power (*vis opifex*) each semen also consists of some matter. This is indivisible. At no time are there any parts, neither such as are active, nor others that are passive. The substance is one and the same and is matter as well as operative virtue at the same time.

Pico, Ficinus (*Liber de Lumine, De Sole*), Agrippa of Nettesheym, Weigel, Böhme, Locke, Thomasius.

33 *Frag. de Fundament. Sap.* ed. Sudhoff vol. XIII, p. 325. – Pagel, W., *Das Medizinische Weltbild des Paracelsus. Seine Zusammenhänge mit Neuplatonismus und Gnosis.* Wiesbaden 1692, p. 54; see also ibid. p. 58; 101–102; 121; 125 (with reference to [Pseudo-]Weigel, *Studium Universale* [1618] cap. I, ed. 1695 [Sam. Müller s. l.] A 2 verso to A 3 recto.)

34 See Trechsel, F., *Michael Servetus und seine Vorgänger.* Heidelberg 1839, p. 128, with reference to: *De Trin. div.* L. IV, p. 145–147: "Non solum in luce omnia repraesentantur, sed in luce omnia consistunt... ejusdem lucis et ideae ratione continet semen quodvis quandam nasciturae rei formalem proprietatem ... et ea ipsa essentialis animae lux habet earum imaginum originale seminarium ex symbolo deitatis et verbi lucis, in qua est omnium exemplaris imago."

35 Van Helmont, *Formarum Ortus* 2. *Ortus Medicinae*, Amsterod. 1648, p. 130.

36 Ibidem 38, p. 139.

37 Ibidem 65, p. 144.

38 Ibidem 71, p. 145.

39 Ibidem 88, p. 148.

40 On the *Pyr noeron* of the Stoics: Kroll, J., *Die Lehre des Hermes Trismegistus.* Münster 1914, p. 266; 285; 301. – Lippmann, E.O. von, *Entstehung und Ausbreitung der Alchemie*, Berlin 1919, p. 197. – Pagel, W., *Das medizinische Weltbild des Paracelsus. Seine Zusammenhänge mit Neuplatonismus und Gnosis.* Wiesbaden 1962, p. 45; to the pertinent loci here quoted should be added: Jamblichus, *De mysteriis* lib. II, cap. 4, ed. Parthey, Berolini 1857, p. 77—dealing with the pure, the turbid and the mixed fire. Gods, archangels and angels are represented by splendor and light in purity, demons by "turbid fire" (*tholodes pyr*), heroes by "mixed fire". The impurities of the fire are particularly obvious in the souls owing to the many admixtures to which they are subject in the process of generation. The closer the relations to matter the less the purity of light, owing to mixture with "dissimilar" and "contrary" elements. See above p. 148, note [24].

41 Paracelsus, *Liber de renovatione et restauratione*, ed. Sudhoff, vol. III, p. 209; *De natura rerum* IV, ed. Sudhoff vol. XI, p. 330. To this: Pagel, loc. cit. 1962, p. 70 seq.

Nor is a distinction permissible between male—active—and female—passive—semen. Both are active and passive at the same time, and both are necessary for the work.[45]

Ex ovo omnia

All generation takes its origin from an ovum-like body. Plants as well as animals emerge from eggs (*non minus plantarum, quam animalium genus, ex ovo nasci*)[46]. For substance analogous to albumen, yolk and chalazae in the animal ovum can be found in the seeds of plants, although not even all animals show a differentiation between albumen and yolk.

Magnetic attraction of the semen by the uterus

The male semen is attracted by the uterus as though by a magnet, and the female semen is attracted in turn by the male seed[47]. Here Marci follows Paracelsus who had said: "In the matrix there is an attractive power which is like a lodestone and magnet that attracts to itself the semen[48]." And: "the matrix was ordained by God to have magnetic and lodestone nature and property to attract to itself male semen[49]."

Semen and Epigenesis

Again, and this time in detail Marci returns to his point that the matter of the semen is simple, homogeneous and without parts. The semen contains the whole of the organism to be formed at once "*confusa specie*". Hence there are no dissimilar parts, there is no "fabric" in it, only the "idea", the "power" and the "work" which cannot but obey the idea and power by which it is regulated (*semen ... substantia nimirum confusa specie corporis inde constituendi insignita ... nulla species distincta illi inest ita quoque nulla partium dissimilitudo, nulla fabrica eidem insit. Opus enim nequit recedere a sua idea a qua regulatur*)[50].

Semen therefore is correctly defined as a simple substance that is devoid of organs and contains the impulse inherent to its substance and the idea of an organic body as a formal, i.e. not material, seal. There is no distinct figure, there are no organs in it other than potentially, i.e. by a tendency to form them (*itaque semen recte definiri videtur, Substantia inorganica et simplex, in qua actus substantiae, et confusa idea corporis organici formaliter inest. Species autem distincta, atque ipsa organa solum potestate*)[51].

Indeed this is the *epigenetic* point of view, clearly expressed and given the rank of keynote of Marci's work as a whole. Consequently *Marci opposed preformation.* The parts are formed

42 SPERBER, JUL., *Mysterium Magnum, das ist das allergrosseste Geheimnuss 1. von Gott 2. von seinem Sohne und 3. von der Seele und dem Menschen.* Amsterdam 1660, p. 27; 30–31; 45–47 (with ref. to Plotinus, *Ennead.* I, 6, 3).

43 PATRITIUS, FR., *Nova de universis philosophia ... in qua Aristotelica methodo non per motum sed per lucem et lumina ad primam causam ascenditur* ... Venet. 1593, I: *Panaugia de luce, de diaphano, de radiis, de lumine, de opaco.* See: PAGEL, W., *Religious Motives* loc. cit. 1935, p. 221.

44 "Vim itaque indidit (sc. Deus) rebus corruptioni subjectis, sibi simile, priusquam deficiant, producendi, ut continuata hac similium productione, idem ex se ipso veluti renasceretur, et perpetuitas mundi ea ratione conservaretur ... substantia quae dicitur potestate, non actu similis, vim inditam habet a progenitore seipsam perficiendi, et sensim ad perfectam similitudinem perducendi. Haec autem substantia semen appellatur" Cap. 1, lib. I sig. Bl.

45 "Imprimis falso fundamento niti, qui Semen viri ac mulieris distinguunt, in ratione agendi et patiendi ... demum ex eo quod asserimus virile semen vim efficientis et materiae simul possidere, negamus propterea Semen alterius sexus inutile aut superfluum esse, cum absque eo nequeat constitui ille Sexus..." ibid. sig. B3 and B1.

46 Ibid. B4 verso.

47 Ibid. B4 recto.

48 PARACELSUS, *Buch von der Gebärung der empfintlichen Dinge in der Vernunfft* Tract. II, cap. 5, ed. Sudhoff vol. I, p. 621.

49 PARACELSUS, *Liber de Generatione Hominis*, ed. Sudhoff, vol. I, p. 295.

50 MARCI, *Idea*, C 1 verso.

51 Ibidem.

in a certain order, one part developing from the other until finally there is nothing that needs developing (*non quod simul omnes perficiantur, sed ordine quodam, parte una speciei ex alia evoluta, dum ad extremum nihil sit, quod evolui debeat*)[52].

The "circular" character of semen

As we have seen (p. 242) it was in the train of the idea of *Epigenesis* that Severinus had introduced the *circular* property of the semina. The seed goes through a series of motions that effect its conversion into an organism which perishes, but leaves behind a seed which again grows into an organism similar to its parent. Marci develops the same theme in the same setting of Epigenesis. The circularity of generations resembles the motion of the stars, for these too move back to the same point from which they started (*cum igitur generationes veluti circulo quodam se excipiant, astrorum motibus in eo similes, quod ad idem principium, unde oriebatur motus, terminentur*)[53]. In the world of living creatures this starting point is the seed. Although no rudiments of the future plant or animal are visible, there is in the seed a linking together of potential parts—a *mutua colligatio*—which is evident when parts of the seed are removed. With the bud ("oculus", "gemma") branches, leaves and flowers disappear, for they are *connexa et convoluta* with it, though not recognisable in it. It follows that these are essential to the seed whereas other structures are not. Such are the placenta and membranes enveloping the fetus—adventitial instruments that are formed by the uterus for the protection and growth of the embryo. Similarly the ova are not products of the semen, but comparable to fruit which acts as receptacle of the semina. Equally nutriment is derived from outside: humours contained in the earth for the seed of plants and menstrual blood for animal semen[54].

Again there are no composing parts in the semen (*semina nullam admittere compositionem*)[55]. To see in the semen a composite product of all or some parts of the parent means to convert a most orderly *cosmos* into *chaos*. Indeed Aristotle was right in emphasising the spiritual nature of the semen and in likening what makes it fertile to the element of the stars[56].

Marci stipulates the emergence of parts in succession *ex novo principio*, as against a conversion of preformed matter into something else. This principle holds good both in true generation and in *accretion* which takes place when parts of one plant are grafted to another. For in the grafted part the *tota species* of the plant is contained[57]. What is therefore essential in the seed is its tendency

52 Ibidem.

53 Marci, Idea, ibidem C 1 verso; see also S 3 recto.

54 Ibidem C 2 recto.

55 Ibidem, C 3 verso.

56 Ibidem, D 1 verso; spiritus, qui in semine spumosoque corpore continetur et natura, quae in eo spiritu est, proportione respondet elemento stellarum—with reference to Aristotle, *De gener. animal.* II.

57 Marci, *Idea*, D4 recto.

enshrined in its simple homogeneous structure (*idea seminalis*) and not the dissimilarity of parts (*partium dissimilitudo: non consistere in differentia essentiali*), the latter being an accidental feature.

The main task of the seed is the equal distribution of growth whereby the organism as a whole is maintained in its appropriate structure (*necesse illud—sc. incrementum—undique et in omnes partes aequaliter distribui, quo omnibus ex aequo adauctis, eadem ratio figurae in omnibus conservetur*). This "necessity" follows from the small size of the seeds.

Seeds and semina are thus visualised each as a *species intermedia*, an intermediary which is needed for the translation of an *idea exemplaris* into the reality of the visible material world[58].

Semina in the inorganic world

Should we assume the presence of semina thus defined in the realm of *minerals* and *metals* as well as in organic bodies? Severinus had answered this question in the affirmative (p. 242). Marci decides against it.

The search for semina in metals, Marci says, is linked with the hope of obtaining gold when an appropriate "semen" is projected on to an auriferous substance such as mercury. The gold-producing virtue was supposed to be liberated from the seed through the action of a liquor—those who described it under such names as *argentum vivum*, *menstruum*, *dragon's blood*, *acetum*, *infantile urine*, *lee* and others have been misleading rather than instructive (*non tam instruere quam illudere videntur*)[59]. Indeed the whole idea of alchemy is in conflict with the principle of specificity—the overriding principle in generation: if we want to produce apples we use the seed of the apple tree and not of a related plant. We know what to expect from this seed, but in the case of gold we have still to find it[60]. Paracelsus searched for the germs of minerals and metals in water—an *aqua mineralis* that was perfected in the bowels of the earth where it formed a tree-like structure, the latter being taken as an indication of its emergence from a seed. This tree was said to develop the varieties of metals somewhat as a tree develops its trunk, branches, bark, pith, leaves, flowers and fruit. Each metal was thus supposed to correspond to one part of an organic body. However, Marci objects, if the metals derive from one plant, they should all occur in the same mine, and gold and silver should not be missing anywhere[61]. Or else there should be a certain order of distribution of metals. Of this no trace can be found—in fact metals mix *nulla lege, nexu vel ordine*[62]. They do not seem to be comparable to fruit and flower,

58 Ibidem, E 2 recto.

59 MARCI, *Idea*, E 1 recto.

60 Ibidem, E 1 recto and verso.

61 E 2 verso. For the Paracelsian theories here alluded to (*Aqua mineralis* and *Mineral Tree in the Earth*) see PAGEL, W., *Das Medizinische Weltbild des Paracelsus. Seine Zusammenhänge mit Neuplatonismus und Gnosis.* Wiesbaden 1962, p. 76 with ref. to PARACELSUS, *De Natura Rerum* Lib. I ed. Sudhoff vol. XI, p. 318 and *Das Buch de Mineralibus* ed. Sudhoff vol. III, p. 37; see also: *Philos. Paracels. de Gener. et Fruct. quattuor Elementor.* Tract. III, cap. 10, ed. Sudhoff vol. XIII, p. 105.

62 E 3 recto.

but to earthy excrements or fungi that grow on plants, or to exuding liquids such as rubber, resin, pitch or oil, or to products of putrefaction—a particularly apt comparison for alum, salts and vitriols into which metals may be converted by dissolution[63]. Moreover, if metals are the organs of one and the same "plant", this in itself would refute alchemy which professes to transmute base metals into noble ones. For the seed supposed to produce one metal, namely gold, should by definition contain the virtue of producing all the other organs of the "plant" and not only one of them[64]. Nor is there any organic whole in the sphere of minerals and metals—when some are removed the others are in no way affected. Nor finally is there any organic structure in minerals which would allow of a gradual development from the centre by a gradual consumption of nutriment towards the periphery as it were in concentric circles, for metals are compact and devoid of anything comparable to veins and arteries. Even pores would not be sufficient to achieve this and nobody has ever seen a gradual transformation of substances added as "nutriment" (*amalgama*) to a metal into gold. Nor could mercury enter through such pores for it will not even enter wood with much larger pores than those found in metal.

Marci *concludes:* minerals and metals are not generated from a semen nor is the metaphor of a mineral plant in any way applicable to them[65].

Marci regarded this metaphor of the "mineral plant" as an example of the suppositious *parallelism between macrocosm and microcosm*, so widely exploited by Paracelsus and his followers, and opposed by himself. There is no real identity between man and the greater world or its constituents—it is the product of mere assertion (*mera opinione*) and deceptive similitude (*falsa similitudo*), Marci says[66]. Nor do the serial colour changes, supposed to accompany the transmutation of metals in the alchemical "work", indicate the activity of semina and "species". For these are immutable and do not admit of mutual inhibition or replacement, i.e. of transmutation. By contrast such colours as are shown by the "soul" of a metal, its "tinctura physica" or "Quinta Essentia", are unstable and, like all colour, are a product of the refraction of internal light (*has mutationes ex refractione lucis internae, unde omnes colores generantur*). Variations in refraction are due in turn to the presence of dense and subtle areas in the matter treated. At first dense parts prevail—hence the colour is black. Later, owing to sublimation, the coarse parts are attenuated and mixed with the subtle ones in such a way that a series of colour changes

63 Ibid. E 3 recto.

64 E 2 verso to E 3 recto.

65 Marci, *Idea*, F 4 verso to G 1 verso.

66 Ibidem, G 1 verso.

takes place[67]. Nor is the crystalline structure of minerals in any way comparable to organic structure. Unlike the latter it is perceptibly influenced by temperature. Moreover nothing is generated *de novo*, but when crystals form diffluent particles are merely recollected and thereby crystallised. This cannot be explained merely in terms of the evaporation of water by heat, for there is a special driving force which binds the particles—a force that is magnetic in character (*constat ergo salia, alumina, vitriola et quae horum natura participant magneticae assimili vi in crystallos colligi*[68]). Here again a fundamental difference from organic structures emerges: the latter being directed from one centre, the crystalline structures from two, i.e. the magnetic poles.

What is true of salts, however, also holds good for metals—no doubt the latter are of the nature of salt, as they can be completely dissolved into vitriol which is a kind of salt. The same can be shown for gems and precious stones which are not limited in size—as believed by those who find their origin in a seed—and can be produced artificially[69].

Semen, soul and formative virtue

Does the semen contain soul and is there only one soul in man? Aristotle defined soul as the "act"—the realising principle and impetus—of the organic body that is potentially alive. As the semen constitutes such a body, its "act" should be soul. Since everything is what it is by virtue of its "act", "form" or immanent principle, the semen of man *is* man, as that of the plant *is* plant. A semen which produces an insect from plant material through spontaneous generation is plant as well as animal[70].

Semen, then, is a substance "informed" by a "substantial form" i.e. a plastic virtue that is inseparable from it and specific to it (*forma substantialis, cuius proprietas sit illa plastica virtus, quae nulli alteri potest convenire ac proinde ab ea est inseparabilis*)[71]. Its effect is the fetus, its first formation and subsequent growth. Hence it must remain in the fetus as the vital "form" of its organised body, i.e. its soul.

In other words soul is not something supervening or entering the fetus later, but is immanent to it, from the very first. The semen manifests neither nutrition nor autogenic motion, but is shown to be alive and animated by its ability to produce the organic body and the instruments which maintain it. Its condition is no argument against its animation—just as in the case of blood which nobody doubts to be possessed of soul[72].

Consequently the essential vitality of the individual does not

67 Ibidem, G 1 verso to G 2 recto.

68 Marci, *Idea*, H 1 recto.

69 "Quis autem dubitat metalla de natura salis esse, quae in vitriolum salis speciem ex toto resolvuntur?" I 1 recto.

70 I 2 recto and verso.

71 I 3 recto.

72 Marci, *Idea*, K 2 recto to K 3 recto.

depend upon the presence of this or that soul, e.g. a rational, vegetative or sensitive soul, but simply upon the formation of the organism as a whole. This is not altered, but only perfected by the rational soul[73].

How does the formative virtue work?

It works from a material that is homogeneous, unformed and devoid of any recognisable dissimilar parts or particles. In other words *there is no preformation.*

It is particularly absurd to look in the semen for traces of bony or glutinous substance—the precursor of bone, tendon and fibres, as bricklayers look for earth, stone or sand as building materials—forgetting that fluid can be condensed at any time and that, on their own showing, elements can be transformed into one another[74]. Moreover, considering the wide variety of colours and shapes to be formed, is it really surprising that of the same material some should become soft, some hard and some remain fluid? In vain therefore the variety of parts that emerges in the formation of the fetus is referred, not to the activity of the building force, but to the slothful and inert material mass (*frustra profecto aget, qui hanc in formatione fetus conspicuam varietatem, non ad plasticam vim, verum ignavam inertemque materiae molem referre enitetur*). Indeed chaos would prevail, were there any preformation of parts. For the most intricate movements in opposite directions would be required to accomplish the segregation and shaping of parts at the same time, each part attracting material appropriate to itself and thereby mangling the semen[75].

If, then, it is not in matter that we are to look for an explanation of the diversity of parts, but the virtue of the creative form (*opifex forma*)[76], how does the latter work and what is its nature?

The Formative Virtue obeys the Laws of Light

First of all we must consider that the creative form is equally distributed throughout the semen, for even a particle of the latter, however minute, is capable of producing a whole fetus or even several fetuses. Nor are malformations due to the removal of portions of the semen[77]. Yet there is no pure simplicity, for the semen is productive of diverse parts[78]. To illustrate this paradox we must turn to the laws and effects of light, to optics[79].

A magnifying lens causes a uniform object to split up into a diversity of rays—diverse in composition and particularly in direction. Individual points of the object are drawn apart and owing to the oblique angle of their incidence the rays are re-

73 N 1 recto: "essentialia praedicata, ut esse animal ... neque ab una neque a pluribus animabus (sc. rationali et sensitiva), sed a toto composito desumi, quod utramque animam et simul materiam includit".

74 N 2 verso: "Divinus opifex, qui in imo corporis recessu operatur ... opusque producit admiratione dignum, tanta rerum dissimilium varietate et elegantia refertum, idque ex rudi et informi materia, in qua nulla dissimilitudo, nulla varietas sensibus occurrit. Non enim existimandum in semine praeextitisse illam soliditatem et duritiem pene lapideam, quae inest ossibus, aut illum viscidum lentorem, qui membranis et articulorum vinculis praestat firmitatem roburque. Absurde enim facere videntur, qui velut Cementarii ipsis utuntur Elementis in rebus a natura constituendis, ut si soliditate ... opus habeant, necesse sit ex Elemento terrae ... plurimum assumere... quasi vero fluidum nequeat solidari ... Sed et adversari sibi videntur ita sentientes, siquidem transmutari dicunt unumquodque elementum, et ex aqua rarescente aerem ex eadem densata terram fieri."

75 N 3 recto.

76 "Non ergo partium diversitas ex principiis materialibus petenda, verum ex virtute formae opificis, quae et figuram et soliditatem et magnitudinem et ordinem et nexum, singulis a se formatis membris tribuit". N 4 verso.

77 "Plastica virtus aequaliter diffundi per totam seminis massam—totam in toto et totam in qualibet parte ... et non minus ex una aliqua parte quam ex toto foetus integre perficiatur." O 3 recto.

78 "Verum tametsi in ordine ad subjectum, non habeat partes diversae rationis, in se tamen considerata, non est omnino simplex, sed veluti composita ex multis, siquidem illa virtutis portio, ut ita dicam, quae cerebrum conformavit, nequaquam cor aut hepar est effectura; et quae ossibus dedit figuram nequaquam membranas extendet aut intestinorum spiras convolvet..." O 3 verso.

79 "Non repugnare vero eiusmodi compositionem, tum ratione tum exemplis ostendere licet. nam in vitrea, aut crystallina lente ita se habent picturae rerum objectarum, quae in superficiem expansae, singula objecti puncta in illam planitiem diducunt, et ad quodlibet eiusdem punctum, totam speciem contrahunt. unde fit ut licet subjectum uniformiter se habeat ad partes omnes, magna tamen sit dissimilitudo partium formae, non modo quoad compositionem, verum etiam directionem, ad singula puncta differentem". O 3 verso.

fracted in various ways. Inspite of a confusion and diversity of rays the object as a whole, its *idea*, *form* or *species* remain the same and effective although it has been split up into a variety of parts. The same applies to the semen: although its plastic virtue is contained in it "confusedly", it has the power of unfolding itself methodically from this "confusion", just as the rays of the sun are methodically arranged by virtue of refraction through a lens[80].

The development of parts is thus seen as the emergence of a *form* that is "confuse" and inactive because it is indeterminate into activity and reality. It is through its splitting up, i.e. through the determination of parts that the *form* proceeds from potentiality into actuality, from involution into evolution.

In this process of sketching the organs in outline rays are instrumental. Diversity of form and function thus depends upon the length of these rays and the nature of the surface on which they fall. Some are long and strike the surface of the figure, others stop short soon after having started, some meet with a plane, others with a spherical surface, others end in a different way. It is thus that all variety is conferred upon the fetus, and the ratio between the sizes and mutual distances of the various organs is maintained ("saved"). Each point of the developing body is determined by the direction and behaviour of the ray to which it belongs, and in this way outer and inner borderlines and surfaces are drawn and finally the organism is fully developed[81].

The semen mirrors all parts of the parent body; these are concentrated and collected into each of its particles. Just as the intact mirror reflects one picture, the semen as a whole will produce one individual and so will each of its particles, just as a broken mirror reflects as many pictures as there are fragments. Each of these seminal particles forms a new centre—just as do the pieces of a magnet in which a rearrangement of axis and poles takes place, when a "Herculean stone" is divided[82]. The development of the whole from a centre can be visualised as progressing in *concentric circles*. However, there is no idea of a beginning with a small circle and apposition of circles of ever increasing size, comparable to those formed when a stone is thrown into water, but there is an equal ratio of growth inside where the circles are small and outside where they are big (*verum aequaliter intro et foras augentur*).

In other words the *fetus as a whole exists in outline at the very beginning*, though nothing appears to be clearly determined at this time. However, as soon as any development has started there

80 "Tametsi enim in semine confusa sit virtus plastica: habet tamen potestatem se evolvendi ex illa confusione quemadmodum radii solis e crystallina lente virtute refractionis evolvuntur." O 4 recto.

81 "Eo itaque modo quo est confusa, quia indeterminata, nihil operatur quemamodum species simili modo affecta nihil omnino representat. At cum illius potestas fit actu, et quod erat involutum, incipit evolvi, quia tum partes differunt per huiusmodi ideas et rationes seminales, mox et membra incipiunt distingui et a se differre. radii enim alii, quia longiores, ad extimam superficiem figurae pertingunt, alii subito ab exortu finiuntur. et alii quidem superficie sphaerica, alii plana, alii aliter terminantur, ex quo omnis varietas in faetum derivatur." O 4 recto.

82 "Cum itaque ... in unaquaque seminis particula, quantumvis exigua et insensibilis aestimetur a sensu, tota virtus, eaque indivisa colligatur, non mirum videri debet, si quandoque ex pusillo semine plures, et quandoque valde numerosi faetus nascantur, quemadmodum in piscium genere, et quibusdam insectis fieri videmus." O 4 recto. – "Tametsi illa virtus in totum semen sit diffusa, non tamen ex omnibus punctis, sed illius centro evolvi, quousque semen retinet partes inter se unitas: quemadmodum in speculo contingit, ut tametsi mole ingens, non nisi unum simulachrum remittat: diffractum vero, totidem referat idola, quot fragmenta. Simili modo res habet in semine, indivisum enim unam ex centro facit evolutionem: at si in plures partes distrahatur, unaquaeque sibi sufficit ad novam evolutionem. Et sicuti magnetica vis in lapide Herculeo, ad singulas divisiones se recolligit ad novam diametrum, sive axem: ita virtus formativa ad novum centrum." P 3 verso and P 4 recto.

is progressively less of that "confusion" that prevails at the "centre" as long as it was quiescent. From the equal distribution of the impetus for growth throughout the fetus to be formed, it follows that the movements in the smaller inner circles are slower than in the larger more peripheral ones. Although there is succession in the formation of individual organs, there is co-existence and co-extension of the *original* fields of developmental activity, fields that are visualised as concentric circles (*non enim circuli ita explicantur, ut alii aliis succedant*). The movement is a slow "promotion" of each inner and smaller circle into the space by which it is separated from its next outer and bigger neighbour. This movement is stimulated by nourishment that is ever newly accumulated in the inter-circular space. Hence the fetus, though still smaller than a flea, is already equipped with its channels which act as aqueducts through which nourishment is circulated to the individual parts. It is for this reason that those members which either generate or distribute the vital fluid become visible first[83].

The Source of the Plastic Force

The Singleness of the Idea and the Centre of Evolution

What is the source of the plastic virtue? This question is closely bound up with two other questions: first as to whether one and the same *idea* or *species* covers not only the development of forms and outlines, but also properties of the organism and its members such as colour, odour and taste; and secondly whether there is one sole centre of evolution. Both these questions Marci answers in the affirmative. All qualities, external and internal, are in fact coherent and the same formative virtue comprises them all. This co-existence of diverse faculties is comparable with our imagination in which impressions from different sensual spheres are united. Thus in a dream we may taste all sorts of dishes, hear the splash of wine being decanted and see at the same time various people displaying various gestures. Colours may be visible or not: as they merely indicate a certain affection of light and depend upon a suitable medium for its internal refraction, they have nothing to do with a permanent *species*. This is borne out by the ready change of colours through nutrition and temperature, e.g. those of leaves and flowers in different seasons and regions. Such changes are comparable to the change in taste which meat assumes when the animal is fed on fish for example[84].

As to the second question Marci has no doubt: there is only *one centre of evolution* and, closely related to this answer, there is no

83 "Etenim figura jam inchoata, non perficitur eo modo, quo circuli in aqua ex jactu lapidis excitati, qui a minimis facto principio, ita sensim se impellunt, ut demum ingentes orbes colligant: verum aequaliter intro et foras augentur." Q 1 recto. – "Haec autem successio non in ordine ad tempus, sed in ordine ad subjectum desumi debet." Q 2 recto. – "protinus incipere totius figuram et singulas partes jam tum in ea distingui; neque circellum in tam arctum cogi, quin omnes reliqui in eo distinguantur". Q 1 recto.

"Itaque faetus tametsi pulice minor, habet tamen jam tum suos canales et veluti aquaeductus, quibus ad singulas partes adducatur illius nutrimentum. unde etiam illa membra, quae vel generant, vel genitum distribuunt vitalem succum, primitus facta ex semine conspiciuntur." Q 1 recto and verso.

84 MARCI, *Idea*, Q 4 recto to R 2 recto.

simultaneous formation of the parts. For experience shows that on the second or third day of incubation the bird's egg will reveal the presence of the heart looking like a drop of congealed blood which moves in some miraculous way and sends out sanguineous fibres everywhere. It is only then that the brain is being outlined and seen to develop its continuation into the spinal cord. At this time no limb, or sense organ is seen or even outlined in traces. This stage corresponds to that of a human fetus that has reached the size of an ant. Yet all the organs formed or not yet formed are coherent with each other, as the fetal "field" as a whole is mapped out from the very beginning (p. 301). This field is full of invisible rays just as air is filled with pictures and rays intersecting in innumerable ways when an image is formed by a lens[85].

Malformations

How then are we to explain malformations? Here again Marci resorts to analogies taken from the refraction of light.

If the rays are allowed to convey the impulses from the *species* in straight lines to their normal destinations no malformation will occur. This in turn depends upon their passing through a homogeneous medium. If the latter contains areas of different rarity or density some rays will be deflected, travel in oblique direction and thereby convey the part of the *species* of which they are in charge to a wrong destination.

When a ray is totally absorbed by an opaque part of the surface a member or organ will remain unformed; when one part of the ray runs its normal course, but the other part is deflected, the member will be duplicated, as each part of the ray contains the *species* of the member or the organ as a whole. Or else a ray may be deflected from its course and thus be prevented from entering where it should and locate the *species* which it carries nearer the centre from which it started. Finally an uneven and rough surface may distort the *species* so much that mere chaos follows its reflection[86].

The centre from which all development takes its origin is the *heart*. Hence if there is more than one fetus forming, there must be more than one heart. Nor is the formation of the heart dependent on the refraction of rays, their normal or impeded course. It is otherwise with the brain, which is separated from the centre by a certain interval. Owing to faulty refraction of the rays which bear its "species" it can thus be found in the chest or the lower abdomen, or there may be several brains—as many "heads" as there were "ideas", i.e. species-bearing rays. Duplication of the

85 "Non nisi unum esse centrum evolutionis"; "demum non omnia simul fieri... non omnes partes speciei simul et aequaliter evolvi, tametsi cohaereant omnes: verum celeritate et tarditate plurimum differre: et quae celeritate praestant, ante alias perfici, tametsi forte a centro longius absint ... Itaque cor centro maxime vicinum, ob celerem evolutionis motum omnium primo perficitur: inde cerebrum tametsi remotum, non minus tamen cito, et ante alias consistit. Partes vero interjectae quia illarum species ob tarditatem motus, serius explicantur informes persistunt tantisper; quousque enim manet confusa idea, nihil omnino perfici potest. Porro speciem inaequaliter evolvi, ita ut alia parte subjecti distincte, alia magis minusve confuse insit, liquet exemplo specierum, quae lente crystallina transmissae in locis obscuris, ad certam distantiam recolliguntur, in vivacissimam picturam: ultra vero citraque magna inaequalitas perturbat: quod partes aliae distincte, aliae obscure, et veluti per nebulam, aliae omnino non discernantur... quemadmodum aer plenus eiusmodi picturis, in quo radii, mille modis se intersecantes, vario incursu simul confundunt et explicant non una ratione figuram." R 4 recto to S 1 recto.

86 S 3 recto et seq.

heart, however, always means duplication of the whole organism[87].

Any excess formation is thus due to gemination or further division of the "species" ("idea") of the organ in question and this is best explained in terms of refraction. These mechanisms are operative in such malformations as the duplication of the head of the humerus, the quadruplication of legs or the attachment of a second head to the abdomen. All such deformities, however, of necessity belong to an early phase of development, for as soon as the division of the species into parts has taken place, no new or duplicated parts can be formed. Malformations through intra- or extra-uterine trauma or a deficiency in nutriment or vital spirit are, of course, different in origin and make[88].

Whatever happens, the heart is not indispensable for life—as the experiments of Coiter and Marci's own observations in fishes have shown. We are told that on occasion no heart was found in a sacrificial animal. However, this cannot happen in sanguineous animals, for as the centre of evolution the heart is the first to emit the rays which are responsible for the formation of the animal and there is nothing that could impede its formation—as long as a fetus is developed at all. The story of the heartless sacrificial animal is more than doubtful, Marci observes. Perhaps the heart was not found because a demon had concealed it or whisked it away—for why was nothing like it ever seen by a butcher? There is no reason, however, why an animal could not live without a head—for this seems to be formed for utility rather than necessity. If in the embryo the heart is seen to live and move before the head is even formed in first outline, why should an animal not be fully formed and live without a head[89]?

The Power of Maternal Imagination

There is *no inheritance of acquired characteristics*. Errors in the fully developed form (*species*) are transient, accidental and not transmitted by the semen. The lame, the maimed, the night-blind and the mutilated are productive of perfect fetuses, for such deficiencies are not of the *species*[90]. Nor are all congenital errors due to the semen of either parent: for example those which are derived from a strong and lasting imagination of the pregnant mother. How can we account for them? To explain them in terms of stimulated humoral afflux means invoking uncertain causes for certain effects—comparable to suspecting as the author of a beautiful picture a child that has mixed paint in a bottle and poured the mixture on a plate. Indeed the efficient cause lies outside the sphere of humours

87 Marci, *Idea*, T 1 recto and verso.

88 Ibidem, T 1 verso.

89 Ibidem, T 4 recto and verso. Based on Aristotle, *De gen. anim.* IV, 4; 771 a 1 (no animal ever born without a heart) and 773 a 5 (one heart—one individual).

90 Marci, *Idea* Z 1 verso.

which are in fact directed by it. Marci finds it in a "foreign idea" which takes possession of the original *idea* or *species* that governs the formation of the fetus. This process is comparable to the distorted representation which the species experiences owing to faulty refraction of the rays which carry the images of its parts. Thus the similarity of parts of the body with animals of which the centaur and the Minotaur are classical examples should be due to the accession of an equine or bovine *idea* to the original human *idea*. In the same way strong imagination may add a "foreign idea" that disfigures, distorts or modifies the picture of the original *species*. Imagination, however, is a product of the brain. How is it to find its way to the semen?

Marci thinks that fetus and mother form an intimate union and that therefore all action due to imagination and all motion due to sensual inclination (*appetitus sensitivi*) are just as much present in the fetus as they are in the mother. For the former is a part of the maternal organism, just as a finger or any other organ, and like these takes part in the activity of the maternal soul, though not in its rational thinking. Passions of the mother should elicit in the fetus similar movements such as trembling or rolling of the eyes in wrath or pallor in fear.

It is unlikely, however, that such emotional transmission from mother to fetus travels by rays. The "species" which is the subject of the imagination in question is contained as a whole in the mother and again as a whole in each of her parts (*tota in toto et tota in qualibet parte subjecti*). Although there is only one soul in mother and fetus, the maternal soul, as far as its relationship with the fetus is concerned, acts as its own ape, imitating itself as pupils at a dancing lesson imitate the rhythmic movements performed by the dancing master. The head of a beast, bird or insect imagined by the pregnant mother will form the centre of a "species" represented in the head of the fetus. Similarly that part of the latter will be affected which corresponds to the maternal part injured or touched at the time when her imagination opened the door to a "foreign species". Touch, especially when combined with fright, has a localising effect, for example on any morbid eruption in the skin. It is the touched or injured part of the mother which determines her soul to "insert the root of the foreign species into the corresponding part of the fetus[91]."

Only a particularly strong insistent imagination is strong enough to overrule the plastic force of the embryo and to inflict on the latter an abnormal *species*. Otherwise such effects would be much more common. Moreover a great deal depends upon the

91 Marci, *Idea*, Z 2 verso to Aa 3 verso.

softness and immaturity of the fetal tissues: in the earlier stages maternal imagination has a greater power of expressing itself in errors of fetal configuration than later.

Marci's Field-Theory

It is Marci's conviction that the outlines of the individual to be formed, his configuration, are determined from the early beginning. The underlying figure is there as a whole and the detail is filled in by successive formation of parts. The figure, as "inducted" in the beginning, remains as such in the fetus and in the post-fetal stages of the individual. Not so, however, its size which is subject to great change from day to day. Yet there are limits to this as well—limits that seem to be determined in a characteristic fashion for each species. Which are the factors that determine size?

This obviously depends in the first place on the quantity of nutriment that is incorporated. This in turn is limited by those factors from which the "ratio of measure" must be derived. There is the influence of age: size diminishes with age. This could not happen if it simply depended on a linear progress in the deposition of nutriment. Indeed the decisive factors are not to be found in the sphere of matter and anything external—neither in "prime matter" which merely indicates capability of coming into being ("potentia") and lacks determination, nor in the four elements or humours of the ancients, nor finally in the three principles (Salt, Sulphur, Mercury) of the Chemists. For none of these has anything to do with configuration. The same holds good for the innate heat and the hardness and softness of the tissues which have been supposed to be significant for size. If they were, the biggest should be the warmest, i.e. adults hotter than children—which is obviously not so. Nor does hardness of texture impede the deposition of nutriment and hence growth and size, for fruits as hard as iron and bones grow and deposit nutriment steadily and progressively. There is no perfection in mere apposition of bodily mass—as shown in the giants of myth and pre-history[92].

Obviously it is the "virtue" contained in the "species"—the internal plan of form and function, a derivative of the soul—which delineates the figure and delimits its size. It is the species which by its unfolding induces the first increment and hence also the last. In fact size is closely correlated with shape—the latter is sketched in outline from the centre. It is here that the *species* by its organising action converts a state of "confusion" into one of determination, a potential whole into a commonwealth of parts, each with a function of its own. This organising action is a mo-

92 "Tametsi enim figura, quae primo fuit inducta, deinceps in faetu manet, magnitudo tamen in dies insignem habet mutationem." Bb 4 recto; "Sicuti enim figura determinatur, ita quoque illius magnitudo..." "Incipit cum motu ... accrescit cum motu". "Simili modo res habet in crystallina lente, in cuius singulis punctis confunditur imago totius objecti, ita ut non modo figura, sed etiam quantitas certa et determinata virtute insit, quae radiis evolutis, et non quomodocumque, sed ad certam distantiam productis, suam distinctionem, et debitam molem sortitur." Cc 4 recto.

tion which leads to configuration and at the same time to increase. There is no figure without size—the one being determined with the other.

Here again the optical lens illustrates what happens: it develops not only the distinctiveness of the pictured object, but also its dimensions, its due volume (*debita moles*)—in other words some quantity. This is strictly determined through the maintenance of certain distances between the rays that are produced and developed by the lens. The more oblique the direction of the rays the greater the size of the picture. It is in the same way, through slanting of the rays that convey the species to the various areas on the surface of the germ, that the larger types of animals such as the elephant, rhinocerus, whale and gryphon are formed and vice versa.

For the growth of the animal body, pores are of great significance. These absorb nutritive fluid like a sponge and are thereby dilated like bags. The absorbed fluid solidifies through drying and causes sub-pores to form by contraction. Thus part after part is developed, each when sufficient nutritive material has accumulated at its proper site. If the whole of the embryo is supposed to consist of concentric developmental areas, the movements of the developing plastic "species" must be quicker on the periphery than in the centre where smaller distances have to be covered. Consequently nutriment will be absorbed by the peripheral parts first so that lacunae develop in which further nutriment will collect for the central parts to form. Each part that has developed is thus connected with parts that are still undeveloped and waiting for new material to collect which will then "entice" their plastic virtue into the proper place[93].

It is thus the "species" which acts as the "rule and measure" through which the mass finds its limits and these bear a certain relationship to the perfection of the species. In fact it is through the mass and its limitation within certain ratios that the perfection of the "form" and its translation into the reality of the individual object are made possible. Thus the average size of the human body and its parts seems to have remained the same throughout the centuries—as shown by the Egyptian mummies. The hands which built the pyramids were no bigger than ours, and the giants of old and their huge weapons were exceptional. Samson was no giant, but a big and strong man. Pygmies do seem to exist, however. To account for such deviations from the average we have to assume changes in the species itself. Or else a supervening "foreign species", which may be conceived

93 MARCI, *Idea* Cc 4 et seq.

by imagination, may impede the normal unfolding of the original *species*. Here female imagination has an important part to play, and it is this which confers the average human figure upon the fetus. Hence certain racial differences in human size. All such changes should be explained in terms of the refraction of rays through a lens: if through diminished density of the plane the rays fall more obliquely than normal, the size of the body is increased and vice versa[94].

94 MARCI, *Idea* Ee 1 et seq.

Air and the "Lamp of Life"

Of the concluding chapters of Marci's book those on the role of air in the formation of animal spirits deserve an analysis within our present scope.

Marci refers to Adrianus Spigelius who denied that air has any nutritive function with regard to the animal spirits. Many sanguineous animals including fishes are endowed with vital spirit, although not taking in air. Moreover, why should Nature have formed most of the vital organs at a distance from the source of the air and why so inconveniently used the same passages for the intake of nutriment as for excretion? According to Spigel respiration was not made for the intake of the substance of air; it is largely a cooling mechanism. This had been Aristotle's doctrine. Galen too had subscribed to the cooling action of the air for the preservation of innate heat; in addition he had believed in its nutritive function for animal spirits.

Marci sees the human organism composed of the elementary body, the principal balsamic and oily fluid and the innate heat. These three components form a kind of burning lamp—an invisible fire which is the seat of the soul and through its movement up and down infuses life and order everywhere. Its upward movement is inhibited when too much heat is engendered—through the sun, bathing or drugs—and the comparatively small flame of life is absorbed by the great heat caused artificially. Or else heat cannot go upwards owing to extreme cold of the ambient air or immoderate ventilation or finally too much soot that accumulates when transpiration is impeded. In which way does the "lamp of life" depend upon the supply of air? Marci is sure that this is not through a material conversion of air into animal spirit, for if this were so, air would have to be converted first into the principal fluid and oily substance—the material by which innate heat and vital flame are maintained. Air, therefore, is not essential for the material substratum of vital flame and heat, but for its mobility. Air, itself mobile, acts as an accessory that constantly removes what may impede the free movement of the vital flame. It is air that prevents too much of the ascending spirit from accumulating at one place and thereby consuming the radical humour and it is also air that disperses the sooty products of the vital flame.

Innate heat enlivens all parts of the body, but remains longest and strongest at its focus in the heart, where it can be rekindled after having been extinguished in all other parts of the body, for example through frost[95].

95 MARCI, *Idea*, Pp 3 verso et seq.

Marci's Theory and Harvey's Views on Generation: Contacts and Parallels

Looking back on Marci's speculative Embryology we have no difficulties in tracing his contacts and parallels with Harvey's ideas and doctrines.

Epigenesis

First of all Marci was a determined Epigenesist. He vigorously opposed any preformationist ideas. The *semen*, and with this he means the same as Harvey's *conceptus*, the fertile germ, is to him simple, homogeneous and without parts.

Nothing in it is distinct and therefore nothing preformed—it is entirely "confused". The formative faculty does not work like a bricklayer looking out for suitable building material. Indeed there is no need for special material, since fluid substance can be condensed and one elemental component converted into another, as the Schoolmen who think on preformationist lines themselves assert. The variety of organs and tissues formed, then, is not due to a variety of materials used, but to the virtue of the creative form.

In all this Marci is informed by his anti-materialist, his truly vitalist convictions and thus fits well into the group of epigeneticist thinkers which we have already considered. We are strongly reminded of what Harvey has to say against those who supposed "that different parts of the body require different kinds of matter for their nourishment ... But Aristotle, with the greatest propriety, observes: Distinction of parts is not effected, as some think, by like being carried by its nature to like; for, besides innumerable difficulties belonging to this opinion in itself, it will follow that each similar part is separately created; for example the bones by themselves, the nerves, the flesh etc. But the nourishment of all parts is common and homogeneous, such as we see the albumen to be in the egg, not heterogeneous and composed of different parts. Wherefore all we have said of the matter from which parts are made, is to be stated of that by which they increase: all derive nourishment from that in which they exist in potentia, though not in act. Precisely as from the same rain plants of every kind increase and grow; because the moisture which was a like power in reference to all, becomes actually like to each when it is changed into their substances: then does it acquire bitterness in rue, sharpness in mustard, sweetness in liquorice, and so on".[96]

Generation, growth and nutrition

The passage just quoted from Harvey expresses a principle which he inculcates with emphasis in several places: growth *is* generation as generation *is* growth and the reception of nourishment (*quippe generatio et accretio non fiunt absque nutritione; nec nutritio et augmentatio sine generatione*)[97].

In other words there are not several different faculties—one that works by transformation of elemental components, another that is really formative and works by divine impulse and finally one that merely promotes the growth of parts, as Fabricius thought[98].

Field-Theory and Succession in Organ Development

Marci's reasoning is very close to this: nutrition, growth and generation are indissolubly interlocked. This follows for Marci from the fact that there is no figure without size. The outlining of a figure, however, is according to him the beginning of all generation—its basic phenomenon. In fact Marci anticipated in his own way modern *Field-Theory*[98a]. As far as a basic field is concerned he would not admit of succession: it is there ready with all its parts—*in potentia*. This, however, cannot mean a denial of succession in the formation of the various parts—*in actu*. With this we find Marci subscribing to Epigenesis, not only by virtue of his opposition to preformation, but also by emphasising a successive order in the formation of actual parts.

In Marci's opinion the *heart* is the *first organ* to exist; it is the heart from which the *conceptus* as a whole is directed and outlined —if there are two hearts there will be two fetuses. With this alone Marci reveals his adherence to the principle of succession.

Marci emphasises the presence of the *Field* from the first. This idea is not altogether foreign to Harvey who says: nature "like a potter first divides her material, and then indicates the head and trunk and extremities; like a painter she first sketches the parts in outline, and then fills them in with colours; or like the shipbuilder, who first lays down his keel by way of foundation, and upon this

96 "Plurimum vero hallucinantur, qui diversas corporis partes diversa pariter materia nutriri autumant. Quasi nutritio nil aliud esset, quam alimenti idonei selectio et attractio: nulla autem requireretur in partibus singulis nutriendis concoctio, alimentatio, appositio et transmutatio ... Verissima.... Aristoteles: Distinctio partium non... quia ad simile suapte natura simile fertur (with reference to ARISTOTLE *De Generatione Animal.* II, 4; 740b)... At vero, alimentum omnium partium commune est, et similare, quale in ovo albumen cernitur; non autem heterogeneum et ex diversis partibus compositum. Ideoque quod diximus de materia partium, ex qua fiunt; idem quoque de illa statuendum est, ex qua augentur..." HARVEY, *On Generation* tr. WILLIS Exerc. LV, p. 409 (modified above), *Exercit. De Gener. Anim.* Amstelaed. 1662, p. 223.

See also: ibid. Exerc. LVI, ed. 1662, p. 231–232; p. 417, tr. WILLIS: "actions of the formative faculty ... following each other in regular order ... all arising from the same mucilaginous and similar matter. Not indeed in the manner ... that like is carried to its like".

97 Exerc. LIV, p. 399 (tr. WILLIS), p. 214 (1662). Also: "Animal quod per epigenesin procreatur materiam simul attrahit, parat, concoquit et eadem utitur: formatur simul et augetur ... dum augetur formari et augeri dum formatur" Exerc. XLV, tr. WILLIS p. 335; 336 and 338 (1662, p. 155). "Ex eadem materia fiunt, nutriuntur et augentur omnia Exerc. XLV, p. 339 (tr. WILLIS), p. 159 (1662).

98 Ex. LIV, p. 397 seq. (tr. WILLIS).

98a NEEDHAM, J., *History of Embryology*, Cambridge 1934, p. 63.

raises the ribs and roof or deck[99]". Obviously with this he again follows Aristotle who has it almost verbatim: "All the parts are first marked out in their outlines and acquire later on their colour and softness or hardness, exactly as if nature were a painter producing a work of art, for painters, too, first sketch in the animal with lines and only afterwards put in the colours[100]."

In Marci's view the centre from which the *Field* is constructed is the heart. Harvey likewise sees in the heart "or at all events its rudimentary parts, namely, the vesicle and the pulsating point" the organ that constructs "the rest of the body as their future dwelling-place; when erected it enters and conceals itself within its habitation which it vivifies and governs, and applying the ribs and sternum as a defence, it walls itself about. And there it abides, the household divinity, first seat of the soul, prime receptacle of the innate heat, perennial centre of animal action; source and origin of all the faculties; for each a solace in adversity[101]." Or as he expresses it at another place: "the punctum pulsans and the blood, in the course of their growth attach (*asciscere*) round themselves the rest of the body, and all the other members of the chick, just as the yolk in the uterus, after being evolved from the ovary, surrounds itself with the white; and this not without concoction and nutrition[102]."

In observational detail Harvey can show that the "first concretion of the future body (*primum futuri corporis concrementum*)"—an outline, a *nebula*—soon follows the first appearance of the principal organ, the *punctum sanguineum pulsans*, the "foundation of the future structure (*futuri aedificii fundamentum*)" which "directs" all further development. The structure as a whole is gradually divided and distinguished into parts which appear in succession, one after the other, and each in its proper order (*non simul omnes, sed alias post alias natas et ordine quasque suo emergentes*)[103].

The early emergence of the *Field*, then, does not preclude a successive appearance of individual organs in the later stages. This latter point is a postulate of *Epigenesis* to which both Marci and Harvey adhered. Perhaps Marci valued the concept of Field more highly than that of successive development of parts; by contrast Harvey laid emphasis on the latter. However, like Marci, Harvey limited succession to the organs. He denied, against Fabricius, a sequence of similar and organic tissues. Although the head and the rest of the body first consist of a mucus or soft jelly, i. e. all are of *similar* constitution, organ materials are "simultaneously" produced in virtue of the same processes directed by the same agent; and in the same proportion as the matter resembling

99 Exerc. LVI, p. 418 (tr. WILLIS); ed. 1662, p. 232.

100 ARISTOTLE, *De Gener. animal.* II, 6; 743 b.

101 Ex. XLVI, p. 341 (WILLIS), p. 160 (1662): "Cor ... reliquum corpus ... fabricat: jamque exstructum ingreditur, in eo se recondit, vivificat illud et gubernat ... estque veluti *lar quidam familiaris*, prima animae sedes ... facultatum omnium fons et origo, unicuique in adversis solatium".

102 Ex. XLIII, p. 327 (WILLIS), p. 147 (1662): "punctum pulsans ... sibi reliquum corpus atque omnia pulli membra asciscere..." Ex. XLV, p. 334 (WILLIS), p. 154 (1662): "Horum fabrica a parte aliqua, tanquam ab origine, incipit: ejusque ope reliqua membra adsciscuntur: atque haec per epigenesin fieri dicimus".

103 Ex. XLV, p. 337 (WILLIS), p. 156 (1662).

jelly increases, in like measure are the parts distinguished; for they are engendered, transmuted and formed simultaneously; similar and dissimilar parts exist together, and from a small similar organ a larger one is produced (*eadem ... opera, atque ab eodem opifice, fiunt simul et augentur; et prout creverit illud glutini simile, partes pariter distinguntur. Simul nempe generantur, immutantur et formantur; similares una existunt, et dissimilares; et ex parvo similari, fit organum magnum*)[104].

In the early stages, therefore, the only succession admitted by Harvey as well as Marci is the priority of the *sanguineous point* which becomes the heart. Fabricius was in error when he stated that the heart was formed simultaneously with the liver or any other organ of the chest or abdomen.

Indeed the basic view of development as a whole is common to Marci and Harvey: the directional centre, the heart (blood) is first. This is followed by the *Field*, the outline of the future edifice. It is after this that the principle of succession materialises: the carina antedating the eye, whilst eyes, beak and sides come before the abdominal organs, and stomach and gut before liver and lungs. Priority in *time* may be conceded to the vegetative part of the vital principle (*anima*) as against the sensitive and motive element, for without the former, i. e. without the organs, the sensitive principle cannot exist *in actu*—the sensitive soul being the actualisation of an organic body. However, Nature "aimed first and foremost at that which was the principal and most noble; wherefore the vegetative force is by nature posterior in point of *order*, as subordinate and ministrative to the sensitive and motive faculties[105]".

The Circularity of the Field and of Generation (pl. 15 and 16)

Marci's basic scheme shows the *Field* to consist of *concentric circles*. Harvey says that the central "spot dilates from the very commencement of incubation, and *expands in circles*, in the centre of which a minute white speck is displayed, like the shining point in the pupil of the eye; and here anon is discovered the punctum saliens rubrum, with the ramifications of the sanguiferous vessels, and this as soon as the fluid which we have called the colliquament has been produced[106]."

Already Volcherus Coiter (1572) had described a "white circle of moderate size with a point or miniature orb of the same colour in its centre" which he had seen in the ovum on the first day of incubation[107].

Fabricius ab Aquapendente (1604) speaks of the small circle (*exiguus circulus*) that represents the cicatricula and small cavity in

104 Exercit. LIV, ed. 1662, p. 215; tr. WILLIS, p. 400.

105 Exercit. LIV, ed. 1662, p. 221; tr. WILLIS, p. 406. ARISTOTLE, *Anima* 414b 28.

106 Macula ... in *circulos* dispertitur; in quorum centro punctum exiguum album (instar cicatriculae, in pupilla oculi) sese exerit; ubi mox punctum rubrum pulsans cernitur" Ex. LV, p. 407 (WILLIS), p. 222 (1662).

See also: Ex. XII, p. 215 (WILLIS), p. 44 (1662): "*Circulus* albus et perexiguus, vitelli tunicae (tanquam cicatricula quaedam inusta) adnascitur". – Ex. XV, p. 230 (WILLIS) and Ex. XVI, p. 232 (WILLIS), p. 59–60 (1662): "Secundo incubationis .... die ... macula dilatatur ad pisi, vel lentis, magnitudinem, et in *circulos* (ceu circino circumdatos) dispertitur, qui punctum album perexiguum habent pro centro". "cicatriculae *circuli* ... intra hos *circulos* ... liquor continetur." According to MEYER, A.W., *Analysis of De generatione animalium of William Harvey*, Standford and London 1936, p. 89 the "circles" seen by Harvey on the third day of incubation may have been suggested "by the headfold, the border of the foregut, and possibly the inner border of the area opaca beyond the proamnion, or the border of the advancing mesenchyme. That the white spot which he said was at the center of the circles probably was the rudiment of the heart is suggested by subsequent statements ... At the beginning of the third day the circles of the cicatricula were said (Willis tr. p. 232) to have become large and more conspicuous, and may now be the size of the nail of the ring-finger, sometimes even that of the middle finger. In the absence of instruments for accurate measurement, this statement is good evidence of the fact that Harvey scrutinized the details of development very carefully indeed ... he apparently recognised the area opaca and pellucida and compared them to the cornea of the eye with a white speck at the center for pupil ... On this account he called the entire object the oculum ovi, the eye of the egg".

107 *De ovorum gallinaceorum generationis primo exordio progressuque et pulli gallinacei creationis ordine*. In: *Externarum et internarum principalium humani corporis partium tabulae*. Noribergae 1573, p. 33.

Coiter and the progress achieved by his observations on eggs opened every day after incubation were praised by HARVEY. These observations, Harvey said, were nearer the truth (*veriora multo et autopsiae magis consona*) than those of his predecessors (Exerc. XIV, p. 55 [1662]; p. 226–227 [tr. WILLIS]). Although his story of the "three

the obtuse part of the ovum. It conforms to a circle (*circulum refert*) in chickens and many other, though not all, species. Being coin-shaped—*perexiguus nummulus vulgo soldino appellato*—it does not exceed the size of the nail of the little finger, to begin with, but gradually grows. Accordingly the circular pattern of the *Anlage* is outlined in Fabricius' illustrations[108].

However, neither Coiter nor Fabricius seem to have attached any importance to the circular shape of the embryo at its earliest visible stage. This is different in the works of Marci and Harvey. The latter's book is not adorned with illustrations, but we can assume that the basic scheme of the concentric circles of the *Field* would have been one of them, for it is prominently shown in the figures of Langley which were drawn to illustrate Harvey's text[109]. The same scheme was then depicted in the classical work of Malpighi and before by Highmore (1651)[110].

The "circular" scheme recalls the idea of "*circularity*" which we traced above in the work of Severinus and which also forms one of the stock patterns in the embryological speculation of Marci as well as of Harvey. Marci sees in the cycles of generation a circular movement which repeats the movement of the stars. As Harvey has it: "And this is the *round* that makes the race of the common fowl eternal; now pullet, now egg, the series is continued in perpetuity; from frail and perishing individuals an immortal species is engendered. By these, and means like to these do we see many inferior or terrestrial things brought to emulate the perpetuity of superior or celestial things.

And whether we say or do not say that the vital principle inheres in the egg, it still plainly appears, from the *circuit* indicated, that there must be some principle directing this revolution from the fowl to the egg and from the egg back to the fowl, which gives them perpetuity. Now this, according to Aristotle's views, is analogous to the element of the stars[111]."

It is with the concentric circular pattern of the germ that Marci associated the relationship between generation, growth and nutrition. This, according to him, is of the greatest intimacy and he thus sees it in the same way as Harvey did. The concentric circles in Marci's view form a basic pattern in the *Field;* they act as a guide with the help of which the formative virtue locates and outlines the parts to be and also as a structure that regulates the conversion of nutriment into parts by the plastic activity which progresses in the intercircular spaces at varying though determined time rates.

globules" is a fable and he did not correctly describe the point where the fetus originates in the egg, he rightly stated to have seen the beak and eyes from the seventh day of incubation, but yet nothing of the viscera—as it befits an expert dissector (*ut peritum dissectorem decuit*): Exercit. XVIII, p. 73 (1662); p. 246 (tr. WILLIS).

108 *De formatione ovi pennatorum; pennati uterorum historia. Opera omnia anatomica et physiologica* ed. B.S. Albini. Lugd. Batavor. 1738, p. 13 and 30. – For illustration plate III, fig. 1 following p. 32. See also ADELMANN, 1942, loc. cit. (p. 317, note [130]), p. 715.

109 LANGLY, WILHELM, *Observationes et Historiae e Harveyi libello de Generatione Animalium excerptae.* Amstelod. 1674, fig. I, p. 137, see fig. 44.

110 MALPIGHI, *Dissertatio Epistolica, De Formatione Pulli in Ovo* (1673). Fig. I, quoted from: *Bibliotheca Anatomica* ed. Le Clerc and Manget vol. I, 577, Tab. XXVII, 1687, see fig. 45. – HIGHMORE, N., *History of gener.* Lond. 1651, p. 66–71.

111 "Facit ... hic *circuitus* gallinaceum genus sempiternum ... Atque ad hunc similem modum multa inferiora superiorum perpetuitatem aemulari cernimus ... ex hoc ... *circuitu* patet, aliquod principium esse istius revolutionis a gallina ad ovum, et ab ovo denuo ad gallinam. quod sempiternitatem iis impertiat. Estque id ipsum (autore Aristotele) *analogum elemento stellarum;* facitque ut parentes generent, eorumque semina, sive ova foecunda sint ... ita pariter in genere gallinaceo, *vis enthea*, sive principium divinum, modo virtus plastica, modo nutritiva, modo auctiva dicitur; conservativa autem, et vegetativa semper habetur; modo etiam gallinae, modo ovi formam refert: permanet tamen eadem illa virtus in aevum." Ex. XXVIII, p. 285 (WILLIS), p. 109 (1662). – "Protei instar" ibid.

Blood, Soul and Generation

Harvey states that the ovum is possessed of its own operative soul "which is all in the whole and all in each individual part[112]". This is the well known formulation of the Aristotelian concept by Plotinus. It is also found in Marci in a similar context[113]. It should be remembered, however, that Harvey emphasises the independence of the soul in the ovum of the parental soul, whereas according to Marci it is shared by the embryo.

Like Harvey, Marci regards the blood as a *part* of the body which is animated. It is a *pars vaga*—a part that is movable like spirit, warming and invigorating the parts to which it has access, but causing them to fail and to die when it retires to the source of life, the heart. In Harvey's view blood is the part that is instrumental in causing the vital principle which it contains to come to "be all in all, and all in each particular part"—using Plotinian parlance again[114]. It is a real part, although this has been denied by some in view of the insensibility of blood. Harvey denies the blood to be without sensation, nor does it follow that it should not form "a part and even the foremost part of a body endowed with sensibility" (*corporis sensitivi partem, eamque praecipuam*)[115]. At all events the argument is meaningless: as everybody knows, such organs as the brain, cord or the crystalline and the vitreous humour of the eye are insensitive, "though by the common consent of all, philosophers and physicians alike, these are parts of the body". Thus Aristotle and Hippocrates regarded the blood as a *part*, the former as one of the tissues (*partes similares*), the latter as one of the *parts contained*, as the "animal body according to him is made up of containing, contained and impelling parts[116]."

Ex ovo omnia

Harvey's famous epigram: *ex ovo omnia* is found not in the text, but on the frontispiece of his book *On generation*. The text has: *ovum esse primordium commune*. This too was anticipated by Marci.

In the first chapter of his book *On generation* Harvey generalises the statement of Fabricius that *many* animals hail from an *ovum*. "We, however, maintain", Harvey says, "that *all* animals, even the viviparous, and even man himself, emerge *ex ovo;* that their first conceptions, from which the fetuses are made, are *ova* of a certain kind." He then extends the analogy to the realm of the plants—"as well as the seeds of all plants. Hence it is said by Empedocles not inappropriately: the *egg bearing race of trees*. Therefore the natural history of the *ovum* has a rather wide significance, because through it the modus of every kind of generation is illuminated[117]".

112 "Habet igitur ovum, procul omni dubio, animam suam opificem, quae tota in toto, et tota in unaqualibet parte insit." Ex. XLIII, p. 327 (Willis), p. 147 (1662). Also: Ex. LI, p. 378, p. 194 (1662): with reference to the blood as carrier of the soul (see note [114]).

113 "hoti hole en pasi kai en hotooun autou hole" Plotinus, *Enneades* IV, 2, 1 ed. H.F. Mueller Berol. 1880, vol. II, p. 6. To this: Kirchner, C.H., *Die Philosophie des Plotin* Halle 1854, p. 66 with further references. – Aristotle, *De Anima* I, 5; 411b: "en hekatero ton morion hapant' enhyparchei ta moria tes psyches kai homoeide eisin allelois kai te hole, allelon men hos ou chorista onta, tes d'holes psyches hos diairetes ouses"—in each of the bodily parts there are present all the parts of the soul, and the souls so present are homogeneous with one another and with the whole; this means that the several parts of the soul are indisseverable from one another, although the whole soul is divisible. Ed. Im. Bekker Oxonii 1837, p. 182; tr. J.A. Smith Oxford 1931.

On Marci's use of the phrase see above p. 305.

114 "Illius (sc. sanguinis) gratia (sc. anima) *tota in toto, et tota in qualibet parte* (ut vulgo dicitur) inesse, merito censeatur. Ex. LI, p. 378 (Willis), p. 194 (1662).

115 Ex. LII, p. 382 (Willis), p. 198 (1662). – Accordingly the fifty-second Exercise of Harvey's book bears the title: *De Sanguine, prout est pars principalis*. See also: "Sanguinem esse primam particulam genitalem: et cor ipsius organum circumlationi ejus destinatum" Ex. LI, p. 374 (Willis), p. 191 (1662).

116 Ibidem, Exercit. LII, ed. 1662, p. 198; tr. Willis, p. 382.

See also the reference from alchemical literature above, p. 257 and the work of Temkin on Glisson (1964), p. 256. Before this: Needham, J., on Harvey establishing tissue irritability 25 years before Glisson (loc. cit. in note [98a], p. 123).

117 Ex. I, p. 170 (tr. Willis modified above), p. 2 (1662) with reference to Arist. *De Gen. Animal.* I, 23; 731a.

We find the same analogy with the seed of plants in Marci: "the genus of plants no less than that of animals is born from the *ovum*, for parts analogous to albumen and yolk and even to the treads can equally be distinguished in the seed (*semen*) of plants, although the white and the yellow are not differentiated in all animal ova[118].

In the same vein Marci attributes to the ovum a position of independence and high dignity. The *ovum* is not a direct product of the semen, but forms the fruit of each animal[119]. The female "semen" is thus also credited by Marci with much more significance than it enjoyed in the teaching of Aristotle. In the latter it had been regarded as a product of the menstrual blood that provides the merely passive material on which the male semen works. Those err, Marci says, who distinguish between the male and the female semen, *in ratione agendi et patiendi*[120]. The male semen not only contains the active principle, but also provides matter for the germ—this, however, in no way detracts from the essential part played by the female. The former is attracted by the uterus as if by a magnet and the female part in turn by the male semen.[121]

Marci here again deviates from Aristotle. According to the latter the semen enters the ovum, but merely provides the stimulus of fertilisation without contributing matter to the conceptus. Marci also shows himself remote from Harvey's ideas in which no more than the role of *contagium* is accorded to the semen which acts on the ovum from the distance[122]. There are further essential differences concerning the position of the ovum which we discuss elsewhere (p. 318 seq.).

Yet already Marci had pointed out, against Aristotle, the activity of the female in the production of ova.

He had also insisted on the possession by the *ovum* of a vital principle (soul). Similarly Harvey denies that the male seed is "the efficient of the chick, neither as an instrument capable of forming the chick by its motion, as Aristotle would have it, nor as an animate substance transferring its vitality (anima) to the chick. For in the egg there is no semen, neither does any touch it, nor has ever done so ... and therefore the vitality of the semen ought not to be said to exist in it; and although the vital principle may be the efficient in the egg, yet it would not appear to result more from the cock or his semen than from the hen[123]." Harvey was driven to these conclusions largely because he failed to find any trace of semen in the female after coition. "For in no part of the hen is the semen to be found ... it is nowise present and conjunct either in the egg or in the uterus; neither in the matter from which the chick is

118 "Non minus plantarum, quam animalium genus, ex ovo nasci, cum non minus in plantarum Semine distinguere liceat partes, albumini et vitello, aut etiam grandini analogas: siquidem neque in omnibus animalium ovis inest differentia albi et lutei" Marci, *Idea* B 4 verso to C 1 recto.

119 "Ova secundum externarum speciem atque partes in eo contentas non produci a semine, sed esse veluti fructus ipsius animalis" Marci, *Idea* C 3 recto.

120 "Falso fundamento niti, qui Semen viri ac mulieris distinguunt, in ratione agendi et patiendi ... idem agere in se, et a se ipso pati" Marci, *Idea* B 3 recto. To this Harvey, Ex. XXXV, p. 300 (Willis); p. 123 (1662): against Aristotle's teaching that the one is active and confers form, whereas the other is merely passive and supplies matter.

121 "Ex eo quod asserimus virile Semen vim efficientis et materiae simul possidere, negamus propterea Semen alterius sexus inutile, aut superfluum esse, cum absque eo nequeat constitui ille Sexus ... ab utero veluti magnete attrahitur genitura viri, ab hac vero Semen mulieris" Marci, *Idea* B 4 recto.

To this: Harvey, Ex. XXIX, p. 287 (Willis), p. 111 (1662)—the egg is a true generative seed analogous to the seed of a plant; Ex. XL, p. 315 (Willis), p. 137 (1662)—the male is no more the first principle ... than is the female which creates an egg without his assistance.

122 Ex. XL, p. 315 (Willis), p. 137 (1662); Ex. XLI, p. 321 (Willis), p. 143 (1662); Ex. XLIX, p. 358 (Willis), p. 175; Ex L, p. 364 and 372 (Willis), p. 180 and 188 (1662); Harvey's letter to Nardi, November 30th 1653, tr. Willis p. 610–611.

123 Ex. XLVII, p. 348–349 (Willis); p. 167 (1662).

fashioned, nor yet in the chick itself already begun, and as responsible either for its formation or perfection[124]." Harvey declares the male—semen—and the female—egg—to be the efficient instruments of a superior power[125]. Hence the designation *semen* should be reserved not for what is emitted by the male in coition, but for the fertile germ which takes its origin from both male and female and thus compares with the seed of plants. Indeed it is from this *semen* or *conceptus* or *ovum* and not from the *geniture* emitted by the male that the foetus—the fruit—originates[126]. As we have seen Marci, too, uses the word *semen* in a similar way, comprising the male and female part after fertilisation and comparing it with the seed of a plant[127].

In *conclusion:* The common ground between Marci and Harvey is *Epigenesis*. Marci subscribed to it in all its aspects, notably in his opposition to preformation. He also recognised the successive development of parts—in the later stages. For the earlier stages he insisted upon co-existence of the potential and future parts in the *Field*. This is outlined as soon as the heart, the directional centre, has started work. Harvey in turn emphasised succession of parts, but also admitted the *Field* and the early co-existence of potential parts therein.

Nor does it seem to be an accident that both Marci and Harvey prominently use the *circle* as the basic pattern characteristic of the *Field* and the cyclical renovation of successive individuals as the signature of the divine purpose in generation.

There are other minor points in which agreement between Marci and Harvey is obvious, for example the animation and high dignity accorded to the blood, the independent position of the ovum and the *Omnia ex ovo*.

On the other hand Marci's main view—the interpretation of development and the differentiation of parts, of distinctiveness emerging from "confusion", in terms of optics—was not discussed by Harvey, let alone adopted.

It may be mentioned in passing, however, that the idea of spiritual action by radiation was not entirely alien to Harvey. He had toyed with it in the Lumleian lectures where he gives it as his own opinion that "the spirits do not simply flow (*progredi*) in the nerves, but irradiate and thus sense, perception and motion are the result of an action that is comparable to that of light on air or perhaps to the flux and reflux of the sea[128]."

In the same vein Harvey ventilates the question of the nervous action on muscle in terms of electric impulse such as imparted by torpedo, the electric ray, and of irradiating and illuminating light.

124 Ex. XLVII, p. 349 (WILLIS), p. 167 (1662); Ex. XLIX, p. 357 (WILLIS), p. 175 (1662). See also on absence of any trace of semen after intercourse: Ex. XXXII, p. 295 (WILLIS), p. 118 (1662); Ex XLIV, p. 331 (WILLIS) p. 151; Ex XLVII, p. 346 (WILLIS), p. 165. – On the semen not being "attracted" into the uterus: Ex. XL, p. 317 (WILLIS), p. 139 (1662).

125 Ex. XXXV, p. 300 (WILLIS), p. 123 (1662); Ex. L, p. 366 (WILLIS), p. 183 (1662)—on the divine power see Ex. XL, p. 315 (WILLIS), p. 136 (1662) "maris genituram non ideo esse prolis opificem, quia primus conceptus ex illa corporatur, sed quia spiritosa est, et effervescens, tanquam foecundo spiritu, et *numine* turgescens"—Ex. L, p. 370 (WILLIS), p. 186 (1662); Ex. LIV, p. 402 (WILLIS), p. 217 (1662).

126 Ex. XLII, p. 324 (WILLIS), p. 145 (1662)—with reference to Aristotle, *De Gen. Anim.* I, 18; 724b—: "id quod a mare in coitu provenit, non vere et proprie *semen* dicitur, sed genitura potius ... semen autem est, quod ex ambobus coeuntibus illis originem trahit, quale semen plantarum omnium est ... quasi conceptus promiscuus quidam; et quale ovum esse, supra in historia declaravimus, quod tum fructus, tum semen dicitur."

127 MARCI, *Idea* B 4 recto: "Semen esse materiam et opificem corporis formam", comparison with plant seed: ibid. et seq.

"Ostensum fuit in praecedenti tractatu, ex *semine* veluti materia, faetum et singulas in eo partes constitui: formam vero, et reliquum apparatum esse ab anima, quae in semine habitatur, et in cujus potestate omnes dicti effectus continentur." Z 3 verso.

128 *Praelectiones anatomiae univers.*, fol. 94 verso. See, however, above p. 253, note [11], Harvey supporting CREMONINUS against ALBERTUS MAGNUS and the introduction of light as a celestial component of the body.

He does so in his work *on the local movement of animals* (1627), referring to Fabricius, *De musculi utilitatibus*[129]. It should be mentioned that the latter associated a similar irradiating effect with the semen and its spiritual substance. This explains the swiftness and wide range of its action which affects the whole uterus and all the yolks in reach. It is as frothy as it is airy and volatile (*spirituosus*); being of a cold complexion it can hold much of the native heat and thus prevent its digestion and dissipation. In this way it manifests its superior—divine—virtue and property[130].

A further point in which Harvey distinctly differs from Marci is the role attributed to the male semen as actually entering and directly working on the female matter and thus becoming part of the fetal body—a point asserted by Marci (following the Aristotelian lead) and denied by Harvey. We return below (p. 319) to Marci's sustained criticism of Harvey's idea of the distance action of the male semen by a kind of contagion, and also to the differences in the dignity and position accorded to the ovum which separate their ideas by a distinct gulf.

There was also the fundamental difference between Marci and Harvey as personalities and in their approach to biological problems: Harvey is primarily biologist, observer and collector of scientific data which are blended with biological speculation on Aristotelian lines, the latter being subject to correction by the former. Marci was primarily interested in physics and given to speculation and reasoning on Aristotelian and Neoplatonic lines interwoven with sound observations, largely culled from the work of others.

Marci finally develops ideas that have a Paracelsian ring—for example in the broad elaboration of the effects of maternal imagination on the fetus and such minor points as the magnetic attraction of the semen by the womb. However Paracelsian ideas are not missing in Harvey's speculations, as we have seen (p. 270).

Marci and Harvey met personally in 1636 and exchanged their views on embryology. Marci's book should at that time have been in the news. Later it became well known in England of which we have proof for just the time of the publication of Harvey's *De generatione* (1651).

At all events Marci deserves a place in the first rank of the advocates of *Epigenesis* between Aristotle and Harvey. It is for this reason that his work has been examined and assessed here in comparison with Harvey's ideas. Marci's work illuminates certain aspects of the latter and may well form one of the sources that has hitherto been neglected.

129 *William Harvey, De motu locali animalium.* Edited, tr. and introduced by G. WHITTERIDGE. Cambridge 1959, cap. XVI p. 108–109.

130 Fabricius ab Aquapendente, De *formatione ovi et pulli*, cap. II *Opera omnia anat. et physiol.* ed. Albinus, Lngd. Batav. 1738, p. 20; p. 30.

Fabricius' idea was associated with a "battery-fertilisation" of eggs by seminal storage in the "*Bursa*". The whole idea was rejected by Harvey (Ex. XLVIII, ed. 1662, p. 171; tr. WILLIS, p. 353), and—for different reasons, namely in an argument against Harvey—by NATH. HIGHMORE, *The History of Generation*, London 1651, p. 99. Highmore seems to have known of Harvey's work through personal contact as well as through Sir Kenelm Digby whose ideas he criticised from an atomistic point of view. Harvey probably had Highmore in mind when rejecting atomistic ideas in generation (p. 234 and note [7]).

On the Fabrician side of the matter see: ADELMANN, H.B., *The embryological treatises of Hieron. Fabricius ab Aquapendente*, Ithaca 1942, p. 724.

Marcus Marci's Criticism of Harvey's Ideas on Generation (pl. 43)

The emphasis laid by Harvey on the generating idea, the *conceptus* that is not unlike imagination produced in the brain by sensory impression, seemed to place his speculation close to Marci's *Idea of Operative Ideas*.

Yet it was Marci who criticised Harvey in his work: *Philosophia Vetus Restituta* of 1662[131]. Nearly thirty years before, in 1635, Marci had published his ideas on embryology. One year later he met Harvey at Prague, and, as he tells us, gave him a copy of his work[132]. Harvey's book *On generation* was finally printed in 1651, i. e. fifteen years after his meeting with Marci, and only six years before Harvey's death in 1657 at the age of 79. It was eleven years after the publication of Harvey's book and five years after his death that Marci, then at the hight of his career and—at 67—having achieved European renown as the *Philosophus huius seculi acutissimus*[133], reviewed in a cross section through all parts of Natural Philosophy the current opinions of his time against the background of ancient wisdom.

In the chapter in which he examines Harvey's speculation on the mystery of conception he comes to the conclusion that "neither the reasons nor the factual data advanced by Harvey compel us to diverge from the line taken by Aristotle and the Medical Schools[134]".

How can this be reconciled with the obvious kinship that we have found between the ideas of Marci and those of Harvey?

First of all there is the note of disappointment sounded in Marci's discourse. Harvey, who could not have remained ignorant of Marci's attempt to explain the formation of the fetus in terms of optics, not only failed to adopt this, but did not even bother to mention Marci's theory and to define his own position with respect to it. His theory, Marci says, can indeed serve as an explanation of the mystery, whereas none of Harvey's theories can. Harvey may have disapproved of Marci's book, because he thought it to be based on the Aristotelian and School doctrine that generation is brought about by male and female semen. However, as Marci himself has shown, his theory holds good even if the truth of Harvey's theory were admitted[135].

Marci's criticism pivots around Harvey's denial that the male semen becomes part of the fetal body and even that it finds access to the uterus. To this Harvey had been led by his failure to see anything in the female genital organs opened shortly after coition. Marci in no way doubts the truth of this observation as such. He

131 *Johannis Marci Marci a Kronland Philosophia Vetus Restituta partibus V comprehensa: I de Mutationibus quae in universo fiunt II De Partium Universi Constitutione III De Statu Hominis secundum Naturam IV De Statu Hominis praeter Naturam V De Curatione Morborum.* Praguae 1662. Edition used: Francof. et Lipsiae sumpt. Christ. Wiedmann 1676. XI, 580 pp.

132 *Philos. Vetus Rest.* Pars III, subsectio II (n). ed. 1676, p. 352.

133 Thus called on the title page of the *Phil. Vetus Rest.* ed. cit. in note [131].

134 Ibid. p. 361.

135 p. 352.

finds, however, that Harvey based on this a system of conclusions which lead from one absurdity to another and provide no platform from which to refute the classical doctrine, as was Harvey's intention.

It is generally agreed that the female receives the fertilising principle from the male during coition. Any similarity with the father shown by the offspring must derive from the semen and the latter's plastic force must have been transferred to the fetus. Indeed there can be nothing in the fetus that did not previously exist in the semen potentially. If, however, the same faculty is found in both, their matter from which the faculty is inseparable must be the same and hence the semen is matter as well as the fashioner of the fetus[136].

Admittedly Harvey found no visible semen in the female shortly after coition—but does this prove that nothing of the semen was there at all? On Harvey's own showing the "essential" semen—i.e. that which is fertile—is spirituous and effervescent. If, then, the foamy body of the semen is merely the envelope of an essential spirit, should the uterus also be inaccessible to the latter, simply because no gross semen is seen? Or if the latter escapes after coition would this necessarily apply to the spirit as well? Why, then, should the corporeal semen before perishing have communicated to the uterus another energy (*vim*) that stands for it vicariously and act on the fetus merely from outside? Therefore the opinion of Aristotle and the Schools is more correct: not only the plastic energy, but also the matter out of which the fetal body develops is propagated and inserted into the uterus, just as the plant develops from the seed. There is no need for quantities that are visible to the naked eye—as Hippocrates already said: there must be powerful forces in the semen when, through the loss of so little of it, we are perceptibly weakened. And what end is served by the complicated apparatus involved in the formation of semen if it has to perish or to be discharged immediately it has "touched"? If the plastic force were mere "phantasma" short of any material substratum received by the uterus, there would be no hereditary transmission of disease, nor could man be said to generate man any more so than fire to set alight another fire if he did not participate in constituting the substance of the fetus.

Harvey believed that there was no female seminal matter in the uterus simply because he too easily accepted the stories of women who maintained to have conceived without emitting seminal fluid after coition and without orgasm[137]. In fact many admit to

136 p. 349.

137 With reference to *On generation*, Exerc. XXIV, ed. 1662, p. 121; tr. WILLIS, p. 299; Exerc. XL, ed. 1662, p. 139; tr. WILLIS, p. 316–317.

emission of female seminal matter and to prevention of conception if it was made to occur after emission of the male semen.

Although a minimal quantity of the semen contains the idea of the whole chick, not any quantity is sufficient. Hence the need for repeated coition to ensure the fertility of a multitude of *ova*. Though imperceptible, the small quantity of semen is not nothing, but something material in which the germ of the fetus is ideally contained. It works from inside the *ovum*—unlike the artisan who fashions a piece of wood. Relying too much on ocular inspection and failing to see any way in which the semen could reach the *ovum*, Harvey denied its material participation in the fetal body—as if there were no access to the body for a spiritual *aura*, because none could be demonstrated for its coarse envelope. Basil Valentine tells us that mines productive of gold and metal can die out suddenly when the mineral spirit chooses to leave them and to build up new mines in a remote area. Should it be easier for mineral spirits to pervade rocks than for animal spirits to penetrate spongy flesh? All the more so as the parts of the body down to the smallest particles are in harmonious cooperation owing to their all pervading spirit (*totum corpus conspirabile et confluxile*)[138].

Being at a loss in his search for natural agents, Harvey compared generation with the creation of the world and invoked God as its efficient agent. But, how, Marci asks, could monsters be reconciled with this, whereas he—Marci—himself had explained their formation plausibly in terms of natural philosophy and without the necessity of finding an error in the prime cause of everything.

According to Harvey the action of the male is comparable to the heat of the sun in summer which effects the ripening of fruit. However, it is the *vis opifica*—the power of the maker—and not the ripening of something already present which is conferred by the male to the *ovum*.

Harvey's comparison of the uterus with the brain is a mere metaphor. It provides neither reason nor *modus operandi* for generation, and in particular does not explain the "limitation" of the plastic virtue in such a way that a diversity of parts results from one and the same indivisible "Idea". Indeed the *conceptus* of a painter who draws a face is different from the *conceptus naturalis*. For the former works with particular ideas each of which "limits" a single action—drawing circular and straight lines first in his mind which are then imitated by hand and brush. The idea which Harvey believes to be impressed on the uterus, however, is an indivisible whole and the mere analogy with the mental concept

138 Et licet illa pars seminis sit imperceptibilis, non tamen est nihil; sed quid corporeum: in quo primordia foetus idealiter continentur: ex reliquo vero ovo eiusdem incrementum p. 357. Nimirum vero sensibus subjectus fuit Harveus p. 358.

of an immaterial idea does not teach us what it is that "stirs up the virtue here and restrains it there[139]."

Nor is the mental concept localised in the brain in the same way as conception is in the uterus. For the former belongs to the soul which is as a whole in the organism and as a whole in each individual part. Nor is it any less absurd to attribute the efficient force through which the fetus is formed to the uterus—as if the latter fashions the fetus in the same way as an artist does his work. For it is through the vital principle in the fetus itself that it is formed.

It is therefore the confluence of *ovum* and male semen which brings about generation, a process comparable to the sprouting of a grain of wheat that is putrefying in the earth by virtue of its ferment.

Harvey freely admitted his difficulties in the tract On conception: the male "contagium", he says, – be it atoms, odorous particles, fermentation or anything else—is not of the nature of any corporeal substance; it is therefore incorporeal. On the other hand it can be shown to be neither spirit, nor demon, nor soul, nor any part of soul, nor anything having a soul. Hence, Harvey continues, I am unable to conjecture anything besides, nor has anyone imagined aught else even in his dreams, and I have to confess myself at a stand-still[140]. To this Marci retorts on a note of personal disappointment: What I have said in my book on the *Ideas* therefore has to Harvey not even the value of dreams and those who approve of it are even inferior to dreamers. If he is at a complete loss how is he to get farther than we in our credulity—he who on his own admission introduced ideas that at first sight appear as fiction and fable?[141]

In a subsequent chapter Marci expresses his feeling that Harvey contradicted himself. For he denied that the fetus has its life from the mother and yet assumed that the *oviform primordium* of the fetus was a product of the uterus in the same way as the egg was a product of the hen. From this it would follow that there is life in the *primordium* of the fetus before the *salient point*—the precursor of the heart—is observable, and this life must have been borrowed from the mother (*non ergo vitam a corde, quod necdum est, sed aliunde, nimirum a matre obtinet*)[142]. This should have been Harvey's conclusion all the more so because in his opinion nothing of the fetus is made by the semen. It was Harvey who rejected the latter's union with the female "semen" (*geniture*) and merely made provision for a distance action comparable to the transference of a magnetic stimulus.

At the same time Marci has no intention of contesting the points

139 p.350.

140 HARVEY, *On conception* in *De generatione animal.*, ed. 1662, p.384; tr. WILLIS, p.581. – Marci's text contains in the quotation of the Harveian passage a bad mistake: *corporeum, instead of incorporeum.*

141 MARCI, 1662, p.358–359.

142 Ibidem, p.373.

adduced by Harvey in favour of fetal independence. Indeed the fetus is autonomous: it enjoys a *vita propria* as manifest in its pulsating arteries that are full of blood and spirit long before an attachment to the uterus can be demonstrated. Moreover the embryonic vessels are not worked (*agitari*) by the heart of the mother, but by that of the fetus itself (*virtute cordis proprii*). Maternal and fetal pulse are neither synchronous nor equal. Nor can any anastomoses between maternal and fetal vessels be made evident. Fetuses recovered from the dead mother by Caesarian section can be viable. Finally, the placenta, the "uterine liver", is kept alive by the fetus and not by the mother—it quickly decays when left in the mother after removal of the fetus.

However, whilst admitting these points Marci differs from Harvey in the conclusions which he felt should be drawn. The evidence adduced by Harvey in favour of fetal independence applies to its motion, but not necessarily to its life as such. Phenomena of motion may be derived from one source, life itself from another. In Marci's opinion the latter is received from the mother, whilst motion is directed by a vascular system different from that of the mother and following its own course.

Life may persist long after motion has stopped. The inequality between the arterial motion in the embryo and the mother merely indicates diverse principles directing vital action—not, however, different life (*vita essentialis*) as such. The light of a candle and the light of the sun are essentially the same—yet they appear in different shape and intensity. Nor is the absence of a union between *ovum* and uterus in the early stages (which Harvey adduced) a valid argument against the dependence of the life of one upon the life of the other[143]. This is borne out by the communication of life (*communio vitae*) which the organs owe to the blood that assiduously circulates through them without entering into any close anatomical union with them (*alioquin communio vitae non esset inter sanguinem et partes corporis in quibus assidue circulatur*)[144]. Detachment and separability do not exclude *nexus*. Indeed before the heart develops the primordial fetus (*conceptus oviformis*) has been endowed with life by the mother with whom it shares the rational soul until it receives one of its own when it is eventually separated from her. For the new *idea* of the fetus is neither part nor appendix of the maternal *idea*, but evolved from the paternal sphere (*ex chao paterno evoluta*) where it finds the other soul that is ordained for the new individual. In its very early stages, however, the fetus is the fruit of the mother (*fructum maternum*) and a product of an ovum (*ex ovo nasci*), *as Harvey has eruditely and anatomically demon-*

143 p. 381.

144 Ibidem.

strated (*erudite et anatomice demonstrat Harveus*). It is then that fetus and mother form a unified composite natural object (*unum compositum substantiale physicum*). In this the fetus is "irradiated" by the soul of the mother, in the same way as the set of yolks by the soul of the hen and fruit by the soul of the tree[145].

145 p. 370

146 p. 370.

In conclusion, then, Marci's first and foremost objection concerns Harvey's denial of an actual union of the semen with the *ovum* and the seminal contribution to the "body" of the ovum and the fetus that develops from it. Marci's second main argument is that Harvey, in his opinion, had proved the independence of the fetus of the mother in certain vital actions, but not in its life as such.

Obviously Marci had little understanding for Harvey's appraisal of the *ovum* and its unfertilised *primordium* as the embodiment of the cyclical nature of generation—the claim of the species to eternal regeneration and life. In this view the potentially immortal *ovum* assumed a rank of higher dignity and responsibility than the ephemeral body of the mother (p. 274 seq.).

On the whole, however, it is not the facts and points adduced by Harvey to which Marci is opposed, but their interpretation. To the modern observer this would not separate Marci from Harvey by a wide gulf, considering the many observations, theories and opinions which they have in common (p. 309). These include those which Harvey expressed in 1651 and had been anticipated by Marci in 1635 as well as those of Harvey's points with which Marci agreed in 1662. Indeed Marci remained conscious of his agreement with Harvey on many scores and he made no secret of his deep admiration of Harvey—not only of his great discovery (p. 287), but also of his book *On generation*. It is this work to which he refers an adversary in the most appreciative terms: had you read, he addresses him, Harvey's book on the generation of animals which saw the light of day before your book, his—Marci's—own opinion would not have impressed you as so absurd, in the light of Harvey's erudite and anatomical demonstration[146].

Final Assessment and Epilogue

Harvey and his two great works

Harvey—unius libri; Harvey of the single book. His *Anatomical Exercise on the Motion of the Heart and Blood in Animals* is the unique and single work which made Harvey what he is to-day: the founder of modern biology and medicine as based on the scientific method which he introduced into these disciplines. It is in this book that, as Sir Henry Dale said, he "created and displayed for all times the method by which discoveries of profound and permanent significance may be attained and made secure[1]."

Harvey *is* this single book, he is *of* it and *in* it. So at least it seems. He published *De motu* in 1628, when he was fifty years of age, a man in full youthful vigour of mind and body who was soon to reach the climax of social status and authority. His book was revolutionary and therefore was not to achieve success without opposition. Indeed *De motu* solved the problem of circulation and the truth of the matter was established and acclaimed during the lifetime of the discoverer. The book was slim in volume, but filled from cover to cover with an array of observations, experiments and arguments, each more brilliant and cogent than the one preceding it.

Twenty three years later—in 1651—Harvey's second book was published—the *Anatomical Exercises on the Generation of Animals*. It is a sizable volume comprising seventy two large chapters and supplementary essays, *On Parturition*, *On the Membranes and Fluids of the Uterus* and *On Conception*, *apart* from the *Epistle Dedicatory* of George Ent, the editor, and four introductory essays by the author. Harvey in the meantime had become an old man of 73, suffering from gout and harassed and distracted by what must have impressed him as the downfall of his own world at the hands of an ignorant and wilful mob.

His big book *On generation*, so it would seem, was a discursive and somewhat ill-assorted collection, the product of an ageing mind. Indeed it has been called a "great failure"—in comparison with *De motu*, one of the greatest achievements in the literary history of science and medicine[1a]. By contrast with the latter, the much larger treatise, we are told, failed to solve its problem, that of fertilisation and generation. Accordingly—so it has also been said—it failed to exert any influence on the progress of the subject. Moreover it contains factual errors and reveals its author's credulity.

And yet it is the same Harvey who wrote both these books. Nor is the work *On generation* really the product of his old age. We have

1 *The Harveian Oration on Some Epochs in Medical Research*, London 1935, p.6.
1a MEYER, A.W., *An analysis of the De generatione animalium of William Harvey*. Stanford Univ. Press and London 1936, p.138 et seq.

evidence that the problems here dealt with agitated Harvey's mind at the time when he compiled his lecture notes on anatomy, i.e. from 1615 onwards, and there are references to this in *De motu* as well as in the work that appeared "late", in Harvey's old age. It is true, it was at this time in Harvey's career that it appeared, but it was conceived, composed and partly written much earlier, not very long after *De motu*[2].

Nor is the union of the two books merely a personal one, lying in the identity of the author. Nor are they the completely unequal children of the same parent. For we can clearly recognise the same mind, the same type of man at work in both books. Indeed there is the same array of observation, experiment and argument in both, the same keen concern with the problem, the same acute reasoning. There is admittedly much speculation and symbolism in the work *On generation*, but these elements are by no means missing in *De motu*. What *is* different is the result: the spectacular discovery which altered history in one and a collection of data and conclusions which do not seem to have so influenced history in the other.

It is, then, not the fault of the author, nor any personal factor such as old age, which accounts for the difference in results. Nor is it a tendency on Harvey's part to lose himself in speculation in the "late" work. The main error which marred its success may be said to lie in his principal conclusions: 1. that nothing passed from the female testis (ovary) into the uterus in mammals and 2. that the uterus did not receive the sperm from the male. Yet "they were reached by the most brilliant experimenter of his age, using a perfectly sound method upon unrivalled material[3]". The backwardness of the optical equipment available at his time explains much, and so does the royal munificence which provided him with a wealth of objects of that species which seems to be least suitable for the research in which Harvey was engaged[4]—to wit the deer that were available in the royal parks and freely placed at his disposal.

The perennial success of circulation lets us forget only too easily the erroneous ideas that were bound up with it. It can be seen as a breakaway from the two-centre doctrine of Galen and a return to the uni-central idea of Aristotle: the latter had made the heart the sole source of all vessels and of all blood, and subordinated to it the liver, Galen's second—venous—centre. This, in turn, led to Harvey's neglect of the basic differences between arterial and venous blood which had been clearly recognised by Galen. It may even be said that his discovery was bought at this

2 Such references include for example the communications of the air spaces of the lung with the chest cavity (Lumleian *lecture notes* fol. 83 verso and *On generation*, Exerc. III, tr. Willis p. 174), the priority of the blood (*lecture notes* fol. 73 recto and *On generation* Exerc. XVII, tr. Willis p. 237). Blood retaining pulsation in the right auricle after the signs of life have disappeared from the heart substance (*De motu*, cap. IV, tr. Willis p. 28) and nature coming full circle in animal generation from homogeneous matter (non-ens) via the fully developed individual back to homogeneous matter (male and female geniture) (*De motu*, cap. IV, tr. Willis p. 29 and *On generation*, Exerc. XXVIII, tr. Willis p. 284 et seq.: the circuit described by the ovum from fowl to egg and back from egg to fowl; Exerc. XLIII, tr. Willis p. 326: the sequence—egg—colliquation—blood—chick—egg; Exerc. LV, tr. Willis p. 414: the primogenate part must contain both the beginning and the end). – All this is of course, based on Aristotle, *De generat. animal.* lib. II, cap. 6; 741 b: what comes into being last fails first, and the first last. Nature running a double course, so to say, and turning back to the point from whence she started. For the process of becoming is from the non-existent to the existent, and that of perishing is back again from the existent to the non-existent (tr. Platt. Oxford 1910). See: Pagel, W., *Harvey and the purpose of circulation. Isis* 1951, XLII, p. 33. See above p. 84.

3 Punnett, R. C., *Ovists and Animalculists. The American Naturalist* 1928, LXII, 481–507, p. 483–485.

4 Meyer, A. W., loc. cit. 1936 in footnote [1a], p. 109 et seq. with ref. to Th. Lud. Wilh. Bischoff, *Entwickelungsgeschichte des Rehes*. Giessen 1854, and Keibel, F., *Zur Entwickelungsgesch. d. Rehes. Verhand. d. Anatom. Ges.* XIII. Versalg. 1899, vol. XVI, suppl., pp. 64–66 and ibid. vol. XIX, 1901, pp. 184–191.

price, and it has been rightly inferred that this neglect played a leading role in the process of Harvey's "invention[5]". We mentioned the shortcomings of his quantification elsewhere in the present book (p. 73).

On Generation and its merits

With the same ease which makes us overlook the fortunate one-sidedness of the discoverer of circulation, we give prominence to the apparent failures of the student of the mystery of generation and are only too prone to forget the wealth of sound and advanced observations and basic new insights that history owes to the author of the book *On generation.*

These may be briefly presented under the following headings[6]:

1. All animals derive from primordia with the shape and properties of *ova*—the famous *omne vivum ex ovo*—. Under *ovum* Harvey bracketed the true ovum of the oviparous animals, notably the chick and the *conceptus of* mammals, i.e. the fertilised product of the male and female *genitures*, i.e. of spermatozoon and true ovum. He was ignorant of the latter as well as of the ovarian follicles. Yet his idea of the ovoid "primordium" common to all animals marked a substantial advance and implied some doubt on spontaneous generation. Harvey did not deny its existence, but reduced its importance to a minimum, excluding generation from excrement or mud.

2. Harvey traced the site of origin of the fetus in the *cicatricula* and thereby superseded the erroneous ideas of his predecessors, notably Fabricius.

3. Harvey decided for *Epigenesis*, stipulating that the things formed derived from things unformed in chronological sequence of organ development. It is true that Harvey was guided in this by unaided observation without any knowledge of cells, germ-layers or the folding, splitting and unequal growth of the latter. He may thus not have added to the knowledge or opinions of Aristotle in this matter, but he certainly held a sounder view than his preformationist successors from Swamerdam to Haller and kept open the line of ideas to be eventually substantiated by Caspar Fried. Wolff (1759)[7].

4. Harvey recognised the independent position of the female "geniture", the primordial *ovum*, refuting the Aristotelian view of its passive, merely material, and "excremental"—*katamenial*— nature. This applied to all animals, although Harvey failed to recognise the significance of the ovary in mammals. He was fully

5 Lord Cohen of Birkenhead, *The germ of an idea, or What put Harvey on the scent?* J. Hist. Med. 1957, XII, p. 102–105.

6 The present author here largely follows Needham, Jos., *History of Embryology* Cambridge 1934, p. 129–130; see also Meyer, loc. cit. 1936 in note [1a], p. 131–132.

7 Wolff, Casp. Fred., *Theoria generationis.* Halae 1759; Idem, *Theorie von der Generation.* Berlin 1764; idem, *De formatione intestinorum. Novi comment. Acad. Sci. Imp. Petropo.* 1768, XII; 1769, XIII. (tr. by J.F. Meckel, *Über die Bildung des Darmkanals im befruchteten Hühnchen.* Halle 1812); Idem, *Von der eigenthümlichen und wesentlichen Kraft der vegetabilischen als auch der animalischen Substanz* in: Blumenbach and Born, *Zwo Abhandlungen über d. Nutritionskraft* St. Petersburg 1789. See also: Herrlinger, R., *C.F. Wolffs Theoria generationis (1759). Die Geschichte einer epochemachenden Dissertation. Zeit. Anat. Entwickgesch.* 1959, CXXI, 245–270. – Aulie, R.P., *Casp. Fried. Wolff and his Theoria Generationis, 1759. J. Hist. Med.* 1961, XVI, 124–144.

aware of it in birds, however, and consciously generalized his observations in the latter as applying to the whole animal kingdom.

5. Harvey observed peristalsis in the uterus and tubes.

6. Harvey stipulated the independence of fetal and maternal circulations. He established tissue irritability (J. Needham).[8a]

7. Harvey rightly concluded that amniotic fluid is not sweat or urine, but that it served nutritional purposes.

8. Harvey above all methodically employed time-series which led to one of the most accurate descriptions of the developing chick in the history of embryology.

This list could be substantially enlarged by going into more detail, but there is no point in doing so. The moral we have to learn from what has been said is simple enough: Through no fault of his methods or of the soundness of his reasoning, Harvey followed up not a few blind alleys, and it is these which are much more conspicuous in his work *On generation* than in *De motu*. Inspite of the secular advance achieved by him he remained short of the standard reached by following generations in many questions of principle and detail. Why should it be otherwise? It was the same Harvey who against heavy odds unravelled the mysteries of the movement of the heart and blood and who denied the actual *amphimixis* of male and female geniture, but believed in distance action by the male comparable to contagion, just as he believed in a kinship between conception by the womb and the brain, or for that matter in the emergence of Persian mice fetuses in a pregnant condition from the mother, the tonguelessness of the cassowary and the inability of children to walk until the length of the legs and thighs exceeds that of the rest of the body[8].

To-day we have difficulties in understanding the co-existence of sound and spectacularly successful scientific methods with stubborn adherence to Aristotle, a tendency to speculate and a belief in what appear to us to be old wives' tales.

However, below the surface, *On generation* with all its "faults" teaches us as much about the historical Harvey as does *De motu* in all its impeccable and perennial freshness. Obviously it behoves the historian to find the link which is bound to exist between the two rather than to resign his main task—the understanding of a historical figure and the world that was his own.

Harvey as an Exponent of his Era

Indeed the two aspects which we found united in the personality of Harvey seem to mark him as a typical exponent of his age, the period of *Baroque*. This is often presented as the matrix from which

8 MEYER, 1936, loc.cit. in note [1a], p. 136–137.

8a Already ALBERTUS MAGNUS used pricking of the embryo with a needle to demonstrate fetal irritability at an early age, as did later Harvey (*De animalibus*, lib.IX, 3; ed. Venet. 1495, fol. 105 verso). PAGEL, W., *William Harvey, fetal irritability —and Albertus Magnus, Med. Hist.* 1966, X, *in press*.

science sprang. In this view the light of day took the place of mediaeval darkness with a surprising speed that seems to defy historical continuity.

When the savants of the period are more carefully examined, however, it will soon be evident that the scientific achievements due to them are often embedded in settings that are thoroughly speculative, religious, cosmological or metaphysical, in short non-scientific. To present them as the achievements as which they appear to-day it is necessary to ignore the setting in which they were originally offered and out of which they were born. Only then will it be found possible to fit them into the chain of factual progress which a particular scientific subject seems to have followed in straight lines from antiquity to modern times.

The savant of the past is therefore not comparable to the modern scientist, but presents an organic whole in which scientific tendencies and activities form one of many other components. This whole may be called *Philosophia naturalis* or *Pansophia naturalis* and compared with the play of light and shade, the chiaroscuro which enabled the artist of the *Baroque* period to conjure up the perspective of infinity and dynamic motion. It is the latter which forms the theme of Harvey's *Anatomia animata*. It took the place—or so it seems—of dead anatomy, the description and drawing up of an inventory of the parts of the human body. This, so it is said, had been a typical concern of the Renaissance, whereas the new-dynamic—outlook stands for the typical ideals of the *Baroque*. This may pass as a fair summing up of the situation created through Harvey's entry into the history of European thought. It may do so, however, only if it is realised that the origin and results of this situation are far more complex than its appreciation as the hour of birth of modern science pure and simple would convey.

Harvey displays all the marks of the modern scientist, but there are in addition many other traits which are decidedly non-scientific, and, what is more important, are indissolubly bound up with the former. Harvey's most intimate concern would seem to lie in the question of purpose: what are the ends which Nature pursues in making blood circulate or causing individuals to take part in a seemingly eternal cycle of generation from structureless material through the formed individual and back to its structureless origin.

Harvey's Biological Speculation, Symbolism and Aristotelianism

Harvey's speculative leanings are closely associated with 1. his adherence to Aristotle and 2. the use of symbolism, notably the search for microcosmic analogy in the world at large.

1. Aristotle, the unsurpassed master of biology, the thinker on the method to be followed in scientific invention and the role of empiricism and reasoning therein, had to give Harvey everything —so at all events Harvey must have felt. This also provides the key to our understanding of his lack of sympathy with Bacon. It is not only the professed antagonism of the latter to Aristotle, but also the whole world of ideas and their presentation which is different from Harvey's world. There is, therefore, no place in history for a Harvey who, inspite of anything that he may himself have said and felt, practised the Baconian principles, however easily pieces may be dissected out of his work which seem to show him up as a Baconian. This similarly applies to the supposed influence of Galileo on Harvey.

Against this there is Harvey's genuine adherence and loyalty to Aristotle in which he maintained remarkable consistency.

However, it is not this or that doctrine of Aristotle that matters here. What does matter is the vitalist point of view which Harvey kept up throughout and in which he surpassed the Philosopher. One such point is Harvey's view of the blood as the seat of the vital principle, the sensitive soul, in preference to the Aristotelian heart. Seen from the surface, any identification of a bodily substance such as blood with soul would seem to bespeak materialism and it was for this reason that Aristotle had rejected it. In Harvey's case closer examination shows that, on the contrary, the Aristotelian vitalist lead had been decisive.

Aristotle does not speak here of the immortal soul, but of the vegetative and sensitive soul, the vital principle, and so does Harvey. It would appear that neither the former nor the latter had raised, let alone answered, the question of immortality or for that matter the seat of the immortal soul[9]. To Aristotle "soul" is the "first grade of actuality" (*prote entelecheia*), the *form* of a natural body (e.g. the eye) that has life (e.g. vision) potentially within it.

It is something functional, the plan of form and function that follows from the *perfection* of a given individual that develops and displays in actuality what slumbers in it potentially. In other words, soul is not something incorporeal—a "spirit"—that is added to a body, but it is the body itself to the extent that it functions, is alive and accomplishes the purposes inherent in its plan. Form and function constitute an idea or "spirit" that is "given" with the body and inseparable from it.

It was precisely this that Harvey predicated of the blood in preference to the heart. In this, then, he was more Aristotelian than Aristotle himself, for he followed the latter's vitalist lead to its

9 See below, p. 344 and note [26].

logical conclusion. Nor did he ever mean to erect a barrier between the heart and the blood or to decide in favour of either one or the other. On the contrary, even where he extols the virtues and priority of the life-giving and life-maintaining blood he says: the heart, with the veins and arteries and the blood they contain, is to be regarded as the beginning and author, the fountain and original of all the things in the body, the primary cause of life—just as the brain with all its sensory nerves, organs and the spinal medulla is the one adequate organ of sensation. If, however, by the term "heart" its body made up of auricles and ventricles alone is understood, then I do not believe that the heart is the maker of the blood. Nor do I believe that the blood owes its power, virtue, conduct (*ratio*), motion or heat to a gift from the heart[10]. In other words heart and blood form a functional unit. They are complementary and indispensable to each other. There is, however, no transference of vital power from the heart as a monopolised life-centre to the blood—as if the latter were merely something passive and corporeal to which spiritual force has to be added. This view of the blood as active working-matter with inherent spiritual impetus indeed follows from Harvey's intransigent vitalism. His point of view is informed by the Aristotelian concept of the *Connate Pneuma* and thus remains essentially Aristotelian even where he seems to diverge from the Master.

Like the blood the semen with its generative—creative—power displays the action of a spirit (*pneuma*) that is immanent and not superadded to matter and transcendent. Like the semen blood *is* spirit because of its extraordinary powers and virtues. Indeed it is celestial and analogous to the essence of the stars. Hence its simplicity. There is nothing composite about it, no elementary conglomerate or mixture.

Harvey would go farther than this. His objection is to the appraisal of any individual thing in terms of material composition or mixture—indeed he visualises the object as "prior" to its material components. It is therefore not this or that matter—the elements of the ancients or the three principles of the Chymists—which he has in mind, but matter in general. The factor that determines form and function, i. e. all that makes an object what it really is and maintains it as such is its vital principle, a plan or idea or purpose—the Aristotelian *telos* or *arche*. It is a divine principle to which Harvey ascribes a numinous character, for example with reference to the semen and its effervescent fertilising spirit.

Harvey's adherence to Aristotle was not an attitude of blind admiration and worship. He went against principles that were

10 *Exercit. II de circulat. sang. ad Riolanum*, ed. Roterod. 1649, p. 127–128; tr. WILLIS, p. 137. – In a similar vein heart and blood are bracketed as the primogenate parts which contain beginning as well as end, in *De generat.*, Exercit. LV, ed. 1662, p. 228; tr. WILLIS, p. 414. See also: Exerc. XLVI, ed. 1662, p. 160, tr. WILLIS, p. 341; and above, p. 311, note [101].

essential to Aristotelianism such as the principality of the heart (as against that of the blood) and the excremental—katamenial—nature of the female geniture (as against the independence and "primordial" character of the *ovum* and its predecessor in the body of the female).

Why, then, should Harvey have turned to Aristotle at all? Was it perhaps a sign of ingrained reaction or intellectual backwardness which prevented him from joining the anti-Aristotelian trend that emerged at his time and found its main spokesman in Bacon? Or, for that matter, would such a policy have taken him further in his endeavour to solve the problem of generation or would it have allowed him a broader view of the nature of arterial and venous blood?

All these questions should, in the present author's opinion, be answered in the negative. Aristotle's work was at Harvey's time a biological source and authority that was very much alive; it is by no means extinct to-day. It is firmly built in the framework of Harvey's personal development as a biologist and thinker on matters of natural philosophy, at least since his Paduan days.

Above all Harvey's was a synthetic mind thinking in terms of ideas and of plan and purpose. The wealth of observations and experiments which Harvey presented in *De motu* are all grouped around the magisterial idea of circulation and it would seem that this idea was the first one. It occurred to him when reflecting on the quantity and source of the blood that passes from the right heart to the left. Significantly this reflection was associated with analogy: the analogy, that is, between the return to the heart of the blood from the lungs and that from the periphery through veins. The further analogies that are found in close vicinity betray the Aristotelian scholar expounding the new idea that was to start the new era in biology and medicine. For this the truly scientific elements, observations, experiment and in particular quantification, are indispensable. They were, however, employed as instruments in the service of the idea in the same way as were analogy and circular symbolism. Taken all together they form the unique and unified world of Harvey. This is deeply rooted in Aristotelianism.

It is the latter which explains the preference given to the heart as the centre of blood formation and regeneration, the source from which the blood goes out and to which it has to return in a perpetual circular motion. The heart is the Aristotelian *arche* which cannot allow of a second blood centre such as the Galenic liver—Aristotelian thoughts that for Harvey implied the unity of arterial and venous blood, denied by the anti-Aristotelians. Moving in the world of Paduan Aristotelianism would therefore appear to have been more conducive to Harvey's discovery than a breakaway from it. Nor is it easy to see why the latter would have helped him to overcome the difficulties placed in his way by insufficient instruments of magnification or the unsuitability of his animal material in following up the early stages of generation in mammals. The view that it was opposition to Aristotle which ushered in and was largely responsible for the rise of modern science in the late sixteenth and in the seventeenth centuries is one-sided and misleading. At all events it does not apply to biology and medicine. It may suffice to recall the foundation of modern systematical Botany by the Aristotelian Cesalpino and that of Zoology by Gesner, Aldrovandi, Rondeletus and Coiter who were all perceptibly influenced by Aristotle, and so were Fabricius, the teacher of Harvey, and Glisson who came after him.

In embryology it was Aristotelian methods, the following up of time series and the broad application of comparative anatomy, that led Harvey to many ingenious observations of detail. Aristotelian vitalism prompted him to take his advanced stand in the question of *epigenesis* versus *preformationism* and to refute crude mechanistic pseudo-explanations which had a vogue in his time and before. It is the same vitalism which was responsible for his views of structureless *primordia*, the embodiment of specific development-plans and ideas in all organisms, the *ova*—a view which greatly reduced the belief in spontaneous generation.

Influence of Stoicism and Neoplatonism

In Harvey's concept of acting and operating matter that owes its virtue not to a spirit which enters matter from outside, but to itself, the Aristotelian lead is essential. Nevertheless the monistic view of matter and spirit which this concept implies is reminiscent of the *seminal reasons* of ancient Stoicism. Among sources and parallels more contemporary with Harvey the *Sensus rerum* of Campanella, the *Liquor vitae* of Paracelsus and the *Gas* of Van Helmont should be mentioned. There is Harvey's idea of a kinship between conception by the womb and mental conception that takes place in the brain. Linking the former with imagination and magnetic action brings Harvey's speculation into proximity to Paracelsus and some of his followers, notably Van Helmont.

The *ovum* finally forms a *mean*—it is the beginning of the individual to be formed and the end by means of which the latter gives rise to new individuals. It is also plastic matter, i.e. it has a material and a spiritual aspect; it is the product of male and female and the bearer of the seal of eternity in that it maintains the everlasting generative series which preserves the species, endowing it with that eternal durability to which the individual as such cannot attain. It is neither fully equipped with life nor entirely without vitality. A closely similar statement was made by Harvey with reference to the blood *qua* bearer of the vital principle (*anima*): it is not entirely body, Harvey said, nor is it entirely without body, and as such not essentially different from soul.

All these formulations have a strong flavour of Renaissance Neoplatonism and the ideas of Ficinus and Agrippa concerning the subtle-material, "pneumatic" or "ethereal" carrier of the soul, the *astral body*, and also Van Helmont's concept of *Middle Life*. Some of Harvey's arguments in favour of the independence of the fetus from the mother derive from the position of primordiality ascribed to the *ovum* by Harvey and can be found in the work of Gregory Nymman with which Harvey was acquainted, and after Harvey in the less significant book by Le Courvée.

Peter Severinus and Marcus Marci as Sources of Biological Speculation

Harvey's vitalist and Aristotelian leanings culminate in his concept of *Epigenesis*. In this he had important predecessors in the Paracelsist Peter Severinus and in Marcus Marci of Kronland. He had seen the latter in Prague—not long after the publication of Marci's embryological theory. This was based on an early *Field-theory* in which the driving force was explained in terms of optics. Harvey did not adopt this theory, but contacts and parallels can be easily shown to exist.

Harvey knew his Aristotle from first hand perusal, just as he knew his Galen and for that matter the whole syllabus of ancient and contemporary medicine notably including anatomy and what physiological data had been emerging from it. What may be surprising is his acquaintance and patience with the work of Paracelsus—inspite of his dislike of the chemists of which we are apprised by Aubrey[11]. In this connexion we may remember that the chemical connotation of circulation, as first mooted by Cesalpino, was not foreign to him. The use of Neoplatonic terminology and ideas in Harvey's speculation on the independent position of the *ovum* and on *Epigenesis* may have been prompted by similar Neoplatonic

11 "He did not care for chymistrey, and was wont to speak against them with undervalue", *Lives*, London 1813, vol. II, p. 385; see above p. 192, note [79].

trends in the speculation of Marci and Van Helmont. Moreover it is reasonable to assume that Harvey had read Severinus whose work was available in Harvey's time in two editions and was to be re-published in a third edition not long after Harvey's death, supplemented by a voluminous commentary by the Scotsman William Davisson. In England attention had been drawn to Severinus and the soundness of his exposition by Bacon.

2. Harvey was not the first to apply circular symbolism to the movement of the blood. This goes back to Greek antiquity. We have, however, sources much nearer to Harvey from which it is likely to have come to him. A fertile almost contemporary source is Giordano Bruno who persistently emphasised the "circular" going out and return of blood from and to the heart, and also the rapidity and perpetuity of its motion. Still much closer to Harvey is Robert Fludd—a personal friend and colleague. What is more, Fludd had published his speculations on the "circularity" of the blood at the critical time, namely in the early twenties, when Harvey is likely to have conceived the idea. This seems to be missing from the Lumleian lecture notes which originate in the second half of the second decade of the century—the famous entry giving the gist of the discovery in a few lines bearing all the marks of a later addition. The pertinent ideas of Fludd are admittedly far off the mark—they are partly based on the chemical concept of circulation meaning distillation (a feature not altogether alien to Harvey and originating in Cesalpinus), and partly on phantastic ideas of a transference of macrocosmic "circularity" to the heart and the vital spirit (blood) through the air.

However, here was a work in which *circulatio* was conspicuously displayed with reference to the blood—written by a member of the very circles in which Harvey moved at the very time at which the idea must have struck him. That it was Fludd's *Mystical Anatomy of the Blood* that sensitised Harvey to the notion of circularity and thus contributed to the discovery which provided the scientific basis for modern biology and medicine is a reasonable suggestion, however unexpected and perhaps distasteful to the modern. Harvey made the macrocosmic analogy his own and prominently so. What is less well known is the patience he had with such expositions of the microcosmic theory as the work of the crypto-Paracelsian Stephan Roderic de Castro (appearing shortly before Fludd), and indeed with Paracelsus, the herald of this theory, himself.

The Predecessors of Harvey

Harvey, and Harvey alone, was the discoverer of Blood Circulation. There is little doubt about this and it is by now almost universally accepted. Before Harvey, however, the movements of the heart and blood had been studied and fundamental facts been found which provided the basis for his research. Indeed this tradition goes back to antiquity, and Aristotle, Erasistratus and Galen form the great landmarks therein. We have just explained the advantages which could have offered themselves to the discoverer by following the Aristotelian line and how this implied the neglect of a fundamental truth on the credit side of Galen. Understandably, the question as to how far Harvey's discovery had been prepared by the detailed fact-findings and ideas of his predecessors in cardio-vascular and blood physiology is not as firmly settled as the question as to who discovered circulation, and there appears to be considerable latitude in judgment and difference of opinion.

Harvey's work has often been presented as a concerted anti-Galenic effort, but nowadays a tendence has emerged to minimise the differences between Galen and Harvey. Indeed the former is seen as having been on the way to Harvey's discovery which—so it is said—he missed by a small margin of error. Modern tendencies in this direction have had the salutary effect of stimulating pertinent research and have again confirmed the high scientific standard of Galen's experimental method and observations; this had been rightly pointed out before and in connexion with Harvey by such a profound historian as J.F. Payne. However, these tendencies have gone far beyond the mark—as they had nearly one hundred and fifty years ago when J.F.C. Hecker ventured to raise more sweeping claims on behalf of Galen. In fact the points in which Harvey supersedes Galen mark a tremendous breakaway from the traditional view of the centrifugal flow of the venous blood from its reputed origin, the liver, in favour of its perpetual return to its origin, the heart. In this essentially anti-Galenic point lies the scientific revolution in biology due to Harvey. The unitary—Aristotelian—view taken by Harvey with reference to the heart and blood is a further important point.

Of the more immediate predecessors of Harvey the expositors of the pulmonary transit of venous blood such as Servetus and Columbus and the influence of Vesalius on them are less controversial topics than are the doctrines of Cesalpinus. As to the former it should be remembered that their merit lies in the denial of interventricular communications in the heart and the demonstration of the pulmonary transit of venous blood from the right ventricle to the left. This applies to that part of the venous blood which had been known, since before Galen, to be sent up from the liver, but by no means to the whole of the venous blood which was still believed to be distributed by the liver to the periphery. Hence there was no question of a return of the venous blood to the point of its departure, i.e. the right heart, and therefore no idea of a "lesser circulation". This was not discovered by Servetus, by Columbus or for that matter by Ibn an-Nafis. Indeed there is no lesser circulation without the systemic one and Harvey remains the discoverer of both, as Max Neuburger has shown. As a sideline, an influence of Vesalius on Servetus and Columbus and their anatomical ideas on the pulmonary transit deserves serious consideration.

The Role of Cesalpinus

The questions connected with Cesalpinus, his factual knowledge, what he intended to convey and the extent to which he anticipated Harvey are by no means settled. When all the relevant passages in his treatises are carefully read, interpreted and weighed up, it remains the fact that he almost literally repeated over more than thirty years the verdict that blood perpetually moves through the veins into the right heart, from this into the left and hence through the arteries into the periphery. With this he associated "*circulatio*" of the venous blood in the chemical sense of distillation and thereby of a continued and ever repeated "cyclical" process.

It was the *chemical* connotation of *circulatio* which played an important part in the ideas of Harvey's followers and indeed of Harvey himself. For this reason and because of the meaning of a cyclically repeated process implied in the chemical concept of circulation, this Cesalpinian idea can claim more attention in the history of the discovery than is usually accorded to it because of its chemical association.

Cesalpinus also appreciated the continuity of veins and arteries as maintained by *oscula*. Owing to this, he said, the whole of the blood can be evacuated through a venaesection opening, the dark venous blood emerging first to be followed by the brighter (*flavior*) arterial blood.

The most controversial point is Cesalpino's knowledge of the centripetal direction of the peripheral venous flow as evidenced by the tourniquet in venaesection and the linking of this observation with the general statement about the perpetual movement of blood to and from the heart. A careful weighing up of the evidence suggests that Cesalpinus regarded the centripetal venous flow, as revealed by the tourniquet, as the normal and not only as an exceptional event, occurring in sleep, impending suffocation and in venaesection. It is true, however, that he failed to draw the appropriate conclusion and declare the invalidity of his scheme of an arterio-venous shunt operative in suppyling blood to the organs and notably the brain.

For this reason ambiguous statements remained and there is no clear assurance in this matter on the part of Cesalpinus. Hence, although in possession of salient facts, he fell short of the decisive synthesis, i.e. the discovery. Nor had he any clear conception of the movements of the heart.

On the other hand his criticism of Galen and the refutation of such of the latter's theories as the subordination of cardiovascular function to respiration, the admission of air to the heart and vessels, the pulse-making force transmitted to the arteries and the expulsion of smoky waste—all this brings Cesalpinus into proximity to Harvey. In this the adherence to Aristotelian ideas provides an important common denominator. Harvey can hardly have failed to take notice of Cesalpinus, the leading Aristotelian of his time. Caspar Hofmann had based much of his work on Cesalpinus and was one of the contemporaries quoted in *De motu*. Indeed he forms an important figure in the life of Harvey who at one time was even suspected of being a follower of Hofmann, and nothing else.

The Date of Harvey's Discovery. The Role of Robert Fludd

When did Harvey discover the circulation of the blood? His own answer may be found in the *Dedicatio* of *De motu*. Here Harvey says that he had demonstrated his new ideas "on the motion and the use of the heart and the circuit of the blood" for "nine and more years"—which would bring the date back to 1619. Certainly at that time his research on the heart must have been in full progress and accordingly many original observations are found in the Lumleian *Lecture notes on the whole of Anatomy*, from 1616 onwards. However, these notes would appear to be disappointing in the search of information for the exact dating of the discovery of circulation. The famous isolated entry in which it is given as a short summary of the finished product bears all the marks of a late addition. The rest of the notes is reticent and possibly even suggests that Harvey was still ignorant of it when the bulk of the notes was written.

We are thus driven to conjecture. If it is true that Fludd's circular symbolism had a sensitising influence on Harvey (p. 117), the latter part of the first half of the 1620's may be accepted as the critical period.

The *Lecture notes* retain their eminent value for the history of Harvey. They form the basis on which the first part of *De motu* is founded—the first eight chapters that deal with the heart and precede those devoted to the circulation of the blood. They already reveal the clarity and accuracy of Harvey's insight into the true nature of systole and diastole and the definite progress which he thereby achieved over his predecessors, including Columbus. It is also from the *Lectures* that we obtain a true portrait of all aspects of Harvey's personality: his careful sifting and criticism of the literature, ancient and contemporary, his by no means uncritical leanings towards Aristotle, his interest in the blood and its principality (against Aristotle), his interest in Embryology, Pathology and general Medicine, his pursuit of blind alleys and many a biographical detail.

Harvey's supposed change of mind: Blood versus Heart

Too much may be made of this defection of Harvey from Aristotle and it is for this reason that we should examine it still further.

What were Harvey's motives in emphasising the blood as against the heart, especially in those of his writings which made their appearance in the last decade of his life, and when did the "defection" take place?

The question of motive can be answered simply: it was a scientific—observational—motive. Harvey had *seen* a drop of blood as the first detail that can be made out in the developing embryo. As Harvey puts it: "so far as my *observations* enable me to conclude the blood has seemed to go before the pulse[12]." This perfectly explains any change of emphasis that may have taken place between 1628, the year of publication of *De motu*, and 1651, the year in which *On generation* was published. Such change of emphasis is small when the wording of the seventeenth chapter of *De motu* (p. 57) is compared with the relevant passage in the forty sixth Exercise *On generation* (p. 311). In 1628 the emphasis naturally lay on the heart as the motor driving the blood round and conferring momentum to it. In 1651 what happens in the embryo was equally naturally the main concern, as was also the primordial nature of such working-matter with inherent autochthonous spi-

12 *On generation*, Exercit. XVII, ed. 1662, p. 64; tr. Willis, p. 237.

rit as the *ovum*, the semen—and the blood. *Qua* primordial, life-conferring and maintaining the eternity of species in the transient individual, these substances, endowed with a virtue analogous to that of the stars, were self-sufficient and did not need to beg or borrow vitality from elsewhere.

There is no need, then, to search for motives other than scientific observational conviction and the immediate vitalistic world of ideas that was Harvey's throughout his life.

This is confirmed by the time-table. When did the "defection" take place? It might be suggested that it was the ageing Harvey who was converted to the blood and depreciated the heart, thereby reflecting the change that had broken out from the Monarchy (comparable to the heart) to the Commonwealth (as symbolised by the *tiers état* of the—ubiquitous—blood).

On closer examination it will easily emerge that Harvey never "crossed the floor". He had made his basic observation of the priority of the blood in his early days when he compiled his notes for the lectures on anatomy[13]. It is repeated at a prominent place in *De motu:* the blood itself, Harvey here says, retains its inherent *impetus* for a certain time after the signs of life have departed from the heart substance—an event that is paralleled in the early development of the fetus. Within the first seven days of incubation a drop of blood makes its appearance and it is from the latter that the auricles of the heart are formed and finally the whole heart[14].

This is one of the examples of a process in which Harvey showed particular interest: Nature, retracing her steps so that what is formed first dies last, coming full circle. This incidentally reveals the significance of the circular pattern in her operations, notably in generation at large when progress is made from a homogeneous fleck of albumen, something not animal, to animal, from *non-ens* to *ens*—the latter conversely being rolled back from *ens* to *non-ens*[15].

It is at the same place in *De motu* that Harvey finds in the obscure inherent palpitations of the blood a factor that it has in common with the effervescent—palpitating—prolific spirit of the semen.

Finally in the work *On generation* Harvey states that according to his observations blood comes before pulse[16].

In other words what we should note is Harvey's *consistency in the matter of the priority of the blood.*

There was no basic change in the conclusion which he drew from his early embryological observation, throughout the thirty five years that lay between the *Lecture notes* and the work *On generation.* Against this the significance of the supremacy of the heart,

13 *Lectures on Anatomy* fol. 73 recto. Fol. 33r: sanguis author viscerum...anima est in sanguine.

14 *De motu,* cap. IV, tr. WILLIS p. 28; ed. 1628, p. 28.

15 Ibidem tr. WILLIS, p. 29; ed. 1628, p. 28.

16 *On generation* Exercit. XVII, tr. WILLIS, p. 237.

given in more generous terms in *De motu* than in the later work, loses much of the importance ascribed to it. It is fully explained in terms of a scientific regard to the different main subjects of the two books. This is further borne out by Harvey's consistency in his appreciation of the blood as manifestation of its innate and niseparable spirit.

In 1627 Harvey says that it is the spirit that is the principal organ of movement, that through it the heart beats, and that it is one with the blood[17].

In 1628, in *De motu*, Harvey again insists that blood and spirit are inseparable[18].

In 1649, in the *Second anatomical exercise to Riolan*, this is repeated almost verbally: the spirit is the act and power of the blood[19].

In 1651, in *De generatione*, we are given the final verdict: spirits are not found anywhere apart from the blood. Hence the latter is the immediate instrument of the soul[20].

Harvey and the Change of Wind in the Market Place

Indeed, then, Harvey remained faithful to his early conclusions.

Nor was the work *On generation* really a "late" work, however late in Harvey's life its appearance in print. There is no idea of a new light which Harvey might have seen in his old age and embodied in this work, prompted by the change of wind which had occurred in the market place.

The editor, Dr George Ent, tells us in the *Epistle dedicatory* that he wondered that "such a treasure should have lain so long concealed[21]." The book was to have included the account of Harvey's researches into the generation of insects, lost through the civil war as early as 1642[22]. Not only the primacy of the blood, but other points are made which already occur in the *Lecture notes on anatomy*, for example the pores by which the lung is supposed to communicate with the chest cavity[23]. It is true that some parts must have been composed after 1642, for it is in this very book that Harvey complains about the injury done to him by the republican mob which robbed him "of the fruits of many years of toil" with the resulting loss of his notes. This happened to him "whilst in attendance on His Majesty the King[24]". Harvey thus saw no reason to hide his allegiance and the place where he felt he belonged in a book that was published after the new order had secured power.

It was, therefore, not only his scientific opinions which remained basically unchanged, but also his feelings towards the Sovereign and the institution of monarchy. This is borne out by

17 HARVEY, *De motu locali animalium* ed. G.Whitteridge. Cambridge 1959, cap.XIV, p.94–95 with reference to "Dr Flud" (see the discussion of this point above p. 116). Also ibid., p.102: "W.H. spiritum esse organum motus ... unde cum omnis motus pulsus et tractus ... Spiritum per arterias influere motum ex corde: sanguis et spiritus una res, et musculus et spiritus motivus, unde nutriri spiritus et corpus." *Praelect. anat.* 85 v: spiritus et sanguis una res.

18 *De motu*, Prooemium ed. 1628, p.13; tr. WILLIS p.12: "Quod si, qui in arteriis est sanguis uberiori spirituum copia turgeat, tamen existimandum est hos spiritus a sanguine inseparabiles esse, sicut illi in venis, et quod sanguis et spiritus unum corpus constituant (ut serum, et butyrum in lacte, aut calor in aqua calida) quo corpore replentur arteria et cuius corporis distributionem a corde arteriae praestant, et hoc corpus nihil aliud, quam sanguis est."

19 *Second Exercit. to Riolan*, ed. Roterodami 1649, p.70; tr. WILLIS p.117: "spiritus, per venas aut arterias excurrentes, a sanguine non separantur, ut nec flamma a nidore inflammabili; sed sanguis et spiritus unum et idem significant..."

20 *On generation* Exercit.LXXI, ed. 1662, p.316; tr. WILLIS, p.504: "cum eadem omnia a sanguine praestari queant; nec spiritus ab illo vel latum unguem (citra interitum) recedant. Imo vero sine eo nuspiam (tanquam corpora separata) vagantur, aut penetrant..."

21 "tam ingentem thesaurum tandiu absconditum latuisse", sig.X 4, ed. 1662; tr. WILLIS, p.148.

22 *On generation*, Exercit.LXVIII, ed. 1662, p.294; tr. WILLIS, p.481–482; Aubrey, *Lives*, 1813, vol.II, p.379. See above, p. 18.

23 See above, note [2], and p.229, note [94].

24 See above, note [22].

the title-page of his *Anatomical Exercitation on the Circulation of the blood to Riolan*, appearing first at Cambridge in 1649, not long after the execution of the King. On this he is called: *Anglo, in Collegio Medicorum Londinensium Anatomes et Chirurgiae Professore;* serenissimaeque Majestati Regio Archiatro (*Englishman, Professor of Anatomy and Surgery in the College of Physicians of London and*Physician in ordinary to the most serene Majesty the King). This is repeated in the Rotterdam edition of the same year and even in the first English translation of *De motu* of 1653[25].

All this may be taken as a sign of the freedom and latitude still allowed by the Republic; but at the same time it removes any reason why Harvey should have altered his opinions in order to conform with the authority and power of the State.

The Charge of Heresy

Harvey, an Aristotelian savant and natural philosopher, had nothing to fear, for what he had to say was outside the religious field, nor had he anything to gain from an attempted concealment of heresy, for there was no case for heresy to answer in the subjects covered by his writings. Aristotelian philosophy, physics and biology ruled in his time at orthodox universities throughout Christendom, Catholic as well as Protestant. It may be that Harvey—like the Philosopher[26]—left the question of the immortality of the individual rational soul unanswered and possibly did so advisedly. We know nothing about this, since Harvey mentions this soul but on rare occasions[27]. When he does discuss soul, he speaks about the vegetative and sensitive soul, the vital principle. This is borne out by Harvey's use of Neoplatonic ideas and parlance with reference to that "soul" in which he is alone interested —the "pneumatic" or "ethereal" element that is "not entirely body—and yet not entirely without it"—in other words the *astral body* of ancient and Renaissance Platonists. Locating this in the blood Harvey has behind him the authority of Scriptures[28].

Beyond this mere conformity with Scriptures Harvey was praised for having, by his discovery of blood circulation," contributed more to the understanding of this and many other places of Scripture then all that ever undertook that Charge". Thus we read in the quaint book by John Smith (1630–1679) on *King Solomons Portraiture of Old Age*—a "sacred-anatomical" paraphrase on the 12th chapter of *Ecclesiastes*[29]. Smith, of course, believes that the true "Doctrine of the excellency and motion of the blood, and of the use of the Heart" was perfectly known to *Solomon*. "Yet it pleased the Lord that this knowledge should with the professor

25 Keynes, Sir Geoffrey, *A bibliography of the writings of Dr William Harvey*, 2nd ed. Cambridge 1953, No. 30–33, p. 40–43; No. 19, p. 24.

26 Aristotle's position in this matter is one of the stock problems discussed in the classical Histories of Philosophy. "Die Ursachen von dem auffallenden Phänomen, dass über die *Unsterblichkeit* der Seele ... Aristoteles so kalt hinweggeht, lassen sich entdecken, wenn man theils seine Denkungsart, theils den eigenen Charakter seiner Philosophie in Erwägung ziehet. Da die Betrachtung der Natur ... das Nachdenken dieses Philosophen in vorzüglichem Maasse beschäftigte, und aus diesem Gesichtspunkte auch die Seelenlehre bearbeitete, so konnte er in diesem Theile nicht wohl auf die Unsterblichkeit kommen ... Ja selbst die Naturbeschreibung, welche er von der Seele entwirft, musste eher dazu dienen, das Interesse, welches die Idee der Unsterblichkeit bei sich führt, zu schwächen als zu beleben. Denn das Resultat derselben führte darauf, daß die meisten der Seele beigelegten Kräfte von Bedingungen der Organisation abhängen..." Tennemann, W.G., *Geschichte der Philosophie*, vol. III, Leipzig 1801, p. 207.

"Es ist ein alter Streit, ob Aristoteles die Unsterblichkeit der Seele gelehrt oder geleugnet habe... Daher kann man nur aus dem Zusammenhange der Aristotelischen Lehre urteilen, und dieser beweist deutlich, dass Aristoteles an eine Unsterblichkeit des einzelnen vernünftigen Wesens nicht dachte, der allgemeinen Vernunft aber ein ewiges Sein und unsterbliches Wesen in Gott beilegte..." Ritter, Heinrich, *Geschichte der Philosophie alter Zeit*, vol. III, 2nd ed., Hamburg 1837, p. 298, note 2.

"Dass er eine persönliche und individuelle Fortdauer gelehrt habe, lässt sich... nicht sagen ... ja er hat die Frage allem Anschein nach gar nicht aufgeworfen." Zeller, Ed., *Die Philosophie der Griechen*, vol. II, 2; 2nd ed. Tübingen 1862, p. 467.

27 For example: *On generation*, Exercit. LXXI, *de calido innato*, ed. 1662, p. 322; tr. Willis, p. 509–510. Here nothing is said about mortality or immortality, but the power and "divinity" of generation are extolled as transcending those of the sensitive and vegetative soul and being beyond understanding (*captus*, apprehension) by the rational soul.

Harvey's possible sympathy with "mortalist" heresies has been ventilated by Hill, Ch., *William Harvey and the idea of monarchy. Past and Present*, 1964, No. 27, p. 54–72. To this: Whitteridge, G., *William Harvey, a Royalist and no Parliamentarian, ibidem*, 1965, No. 30 (April), p. 104–109, Hill, ibid. No. 31, p. 97.

of it, sink into dust and darkness ... till it was retreived thencefrom by the wisdome and industry of that incomparable, and for ever to be renouned Dr. *William Harvey*, the greatest honour of our Nation, and of all Societies of which he was a member, who stands, and ever will do, with the highest note of Honour in the Calendars both of Physicians and Philosophers, and it were but justice to put him with the same eminence into that of the Church..."

Nor was the location of the vital principle in the blood necessarily tantamount to a denial of the immortality of the individual soul. For Charleton who believed in it thought that the blood was the most suitable place where the incorporeal should join the body—"with the testimony of sundry admirable Experiments, both revived and asserted by our perspicacious Countryman, Dr Harvey in his *Exercitations* concerning the Generation of Animals[30]." This was printed in 1657, the year of Harvey's death. It was no *obiter dictum*, but a point of major interest for Charleton. For four years later he published a small separate volume entirely devoted to it, as seen from its title: *A letter-dissertation on the origin of the human soul derived naturally and on its own accord from the most famous Harvey's Historia Animalium to the most distinguished Dr. Henry Yerburie* (*Dissertatio Epistolica, de ortu animae humanae e clarissimi Harvaei Historia animalium genuine et quasi sua sponte deducta ad ornatissimum virum D. Henricum Yerburie, M.D.*). The book consisting of 24 leaves was published by R. Daniel in London in 1660 —the same year in which the same publisher brought out the first edition of Harvey's *De motu* to be printed in England. The date of Charleton's letter to Dr Henry Yerburie, Member of the Royal College of Physicians and Fellow of Magdalen College Oxford, is July 4th 1659.

We should also remember that Harvey was a "firm Christian" and the evidence that suggests personal acquaintance if not friendship and mutual inspiration between Harvey and John Donne—evidence that is due to the fine work of Poynter. "For the Royal physician not to have met the Royal chaplain, who could tell the Lumleian lecturer and the physician at St Bartholomew's his boyhood reminiscences of both College and hospital, would indeed be extraordinary. Especially when the chaplain was one so well read in medicine as Donne and one so fascinated by the problem of ... how the blood, which to the heart doth flow, doth from one ventricle to th'other goe[31]."

Even so, however, religion remained outside the scope of Harvey's speculation. This was biological and included the micro-

28 "For the life of the flesh is in the blood" (ki nephesh habassar baddam hi), Levitic. XVII, 11. – "for it is the life of all flesh, the blood of it is for the life thereof" (ki nephesh chol bassar damo b'naphsho hu); "for the life of all flesh is the blood thereof" (ki nephesh chol bassar damo hi), ibidem, v. 14. – R. SOLOMON B. ISAAC (Rashi) commenting on *damo b'naphsho hu* says: the soul, i.e. the vital spirit, is suspended in the blood—*she-hanephesh th'lujah bo*. On Deuter. XII, 23: the prohibition of eating blood is because it is regarded as the *living part* of the animal. See above, p. 145 note [12].

It is never *ruach* (*spirit*, *Geist*), but always *nephesh*, the vegetative and sensitive soul, of which in biblical parlance the essence (*ousia*) is blood: DELITZSCH, F., *System der biblischen Psychologie*, 2nd. ed. Leipzig 1861, p. 244. – The soul as such is more comprehensive and not identical with the blood. On the other hand blood is visualised as the original matter (*chaos*) out of which God has peopled the earth (*ex henos haimatos*—Acts, XVII, 26). Blood is "soul" not only *qua* vital, but also *qua* generating principle (p. 246–247).

29 *Gerokomia basilike ... wherein is contained a Sacred Anatomy both of Soul and Body and a perfect account of the infirmities of old age incident to them both. And all those Mystical and Aenigmatical Symptomes, expressed in the six former Verses of the 12th chapter of Ecclesiastes are here Paraphrased upon, and made plain and easie to a mean Capacity.* London, J. Hayes for S. Thomson, 1666, p. 233–234.

A similar interpretation to the relevant topic was given by the 18th century Orientalist JOH. HEINR. MICHAELIS, as J.O. LEIBOWITZ pointed out in: *The Old Age description in Ecclesiastes*, *J. Hist. Med.* 1963, XVIII, 283–284.

30 CHARLETON, W., *The Immortality of the Human Soul Demonstrated by the Light of Nature*, London 1657, p. 184. – See on this work and its tendencies: PAGEL, W., *The reaction to Aristotle in XVIIth century biological thought. Science, Medicine and History* Oxford 1953, vol. I, p. 489–509, p. 496–497.

See also Noah Biggs who wrote in 1651 that "the soul or vital strength, resides in the chariot of the bloud". Hence bloodletting led to a "fall or losse to the whole ocean of strength" (incidentally a Helmontian motive in combatting Galenic venaesection and its misuse in contemporary—humoralistic—medicine). BIGGS, N., *Mataeotechnia medicinae praxeos*, London 1651, p. 137. – Similarly, again inspired by Van Helmont, G. Starkey wrote that "the life is in the bloud". *Natures explication and Helmont's vindication*, London 1657, p. 265.

cosmic symbolism which was basically Aristotelian and with its Stoic and Neoplatonic embellishments akin to theories which enjoyed the widest tolerance and respectability during the Renaissance and the following period. Consequently his adversaries were not the theologians, or politicians, but the Galenic physicians.

Alexander Ross, Clergyman, Aristotelian and Critic of Harvey

Indeed, even when Harvey was attacked by a theologian, it was not on points of theology or a charge of heresy, but on questions of biology and embryology that opposition was expressed. This is borne out by the criticism levelled against Harvey by such a representative divine as Alexander Ross (1591–1654). The latter is mainly concerned with the activity of the female geniture, as stipulated by Harvey and at variance with Aristotle who was zealously defended by Ross. Nor is the argument brought forward by Ross against Harvey's idea that the blood forms the "immediate instrument of the soul" religious in character. It is simply based on the lack of blood in some animals and in the spermatic parts of all. Yet bloodless animals are endowed with spirit and the spermatic parts with formative faculties. Were blood (*qua* lodgement of the soul) celestial, the whole body should be likewise. It follows that spirit is nearer to the nature of soul than blood which merely acts as a "material cause".

Following the same Aristotelian lead Ross opposes on the other hand Harvey's spiritualist view of conception, notably the comparison used by Harvey with the distance action of a magnet. A corporeal agent should be responsible for conception. Otherwise, Ross argues, what need was there for a male, why laws against adultery and why the appreciation of virginal conception as a miracle? Man, the noblest of creatures, cannot be the result of "accidental causes", the Aristotelian *symbebekota*, but there must be something "essential", a "substance" or "subject" which conveys his "cause" to the womb. If, as Harvey says, the womb in conception resembles brain, it does not follow that its function is similar to that of the brain—the stomach and gut though very much alike in structure are quite different in function. The brain is endowed with "phantasms", the heart with "appetite", neither of which reside in the womb[32].

It is not religion, then, but on orthodox Aristotelianism that this "refutation of Dr Harvey's book *De generatione*" is based. Ross singled out for criticism just those points in which Harvey

To this compare: Debus, A.G., *Paracelsian Doctrine in English Medicine.* In: *Chemistry in the Service of Medicine*, ed. F.N.L. Poynter, London. Pitman. 1962, p. 17.

31 Poynter, F.N.L., *John Donne and William Harvey. J. Hist. Med.* 1960, XV, 233–246. – Donne was six years Harvey's senior. He was less than three years old when his father, a prosperous London merchant, died in January 1576. In the same year John Syminges, a wealthy physician who was President of the College of Physicians for at least six and possibly nine years, became the poet's stepfather. In 1584/4 Syminges took a house in the precincts of St Bartholomew's Hospital.

32 Ross, Alexander, *Arcana Microcosmi, or The hid secrets of Man's Body discovered in anatomical duel between Aristotle and Galen concerning the parts thereof ... with a refutation of Dr Brown's Vulgar Errors, the Lord Bacons Natural History, and Dr Harvey's Book De Generatione, Comenius and others* ... London, Th. Newcomb, 1652. 2nd Edition, Appendix, cap. III, pp. 224–235.

33 In: *Commentum de terrae motu circulari*, 1634, Ross criticises the Copernican theory and compares the heart with the sun, on Aristotelian lines. – In 1645 appeared his: *Medicus Medicatus: or the physicians religion cured, by a lenitive or gentle potion. With some Animadversions upon Sir Kenelm Digbies Observations on Religio Medici.* London, printed by James Young, sold by Charles Green. Here he defends on p. 21 et seq. Aristotelian physics against Sir Thomas Brown. He says: "but is not Nature a principle of motion and rest. No, say you: What then? (A straight line, a settled course, Gods hand and instrument). Is not this obscurum per obscurius? Nature is not a line, for it is no quantity ... and why is Nature rather a straight then a circular line? We see the world is round, the motion of the heavens and starres are circular, the generation and corruption of sublunary bodies is also circular: the corruption of one being still the generation of another: snow begets water, and water snow; the rivers returne to the sea, from whence they flow: Redit labor actus in orbem. *And what say you to the circulation of the bloud in our bodies? Is not Nature then a circular, rather than a straight line?*

Againe, Nature is not a settled course, but in the workes of Nature there is a settled and constant course; if you will speak properly, and like a philosopher, which you love not to doe..."

Thorndike, Lynn, *History of Magic and Experimental Science*, vol. VII, New York, 1958, p. 511 in note 85, says: "Ross also had written against Harvey on the circula-

deviated from Aristotle, such as the concession of activity to the female geniture, the absence of corporeal contact between the latter and its male counterpart and blood as the immediate instrument of the soul. It is true that Ross mentions spiritual agents such as angels or demons to which fertilisation would have to be ascribed in the absence of any corporeal factor—an assumption open to the suspicion of heresy. This, however, is merely said in passing and quite unrelated to the hub of the argument which is factual and Aristotelian, and not religious or Christian.

Significantly Ross did not criticise Harvey's discovery—the circulation of the blood. On the contrary, he seems to have accepted it and from the context in which he mentions it he did so as a faithful Aristotelian[33].

The position taken by Alexander Ross reveals a further point of great interest in our discussion. Ross is not only a *staunch defender of Aristotle*, but also and *at the same time a zealous believer in the immortality of the soul.* This symbiosis of Aristotelianism and immortalism is well shown on the title page of his *Philosophical touchstone*, the treatise which he wrote against *Sir Kenelm Digbie's Discourses of the Nature of Bodies, and of the reasonable Soule ... in which the Truth and Aristotelian Philosophy (are) vindicated, the immortality of mans Soule (is) briefly, but sufficiently proved*[34].

This work provides ample proof that Aristotelianism in itself had nothing in common with "mortalism", but on the contrary served as a secure philosophical platform for upholding the immortality of the rational soul.

Ross, the Aristotelian, here challenges Digby for his leanings towards atomism and such strange results as his belief in the "weapon-salve" and its "magic" action at a distance. Ross would not deny that "strange things" can be done by *naturall magic* such as "anticipating the time prefixed by nature in producing of divers effects, by applying *activa passivis*" such as the production of a rose in winter or the raising of parsley out of the ground within a few hours after the seed is sown. There is also *mathematicall magic*—Archytas causing "that woodden Pigeon to flie; and that brasen head which Albertus Magnus made to speak. That worthy man Boethius was very skilful in this way." There is, however, also *diabolicall magic* "in working strange things by the power of *Sathan*, by a contract which Witches make with them, God permitting, in his secret judgement, the affectors of such evill things to be deluded and abused by the evill *Angels*." We should therefore "not practise such things as have no cause or ratio in nature: as to cure diseases by *spells* or *words*, *characters* and *knots*, which,

tion of the blood, and in 1634 against the Copernican hypothesis." There is no reference for this and we believe that the above passage from the *Medicus Medicatus* implies acceptance of circulation by Ross, although the latter believed in spirits as the driving force of the blood.

34 London, J. Young, 1645.

being artificiall, and quantities, cannot naturally operate ... Paracelsus, the inventor of the weapon salve, is ill reported of, to wit, to be a Magician ... for if it be not magicall, it is suspicious, considering the author..." Healing effects thus brought about and reported may be due to imagination and "sometime *Sathan* may concurre, for his own ends, videlicet, to confirme superstition and errour[35]."

Speaking here against the weapon salve in the same terms as the Jesuits and other Aristotelians at the time[36], Ross indeed brings a charge of heresy against practising and believing in certain magic effects. This, however, is basically different from the criticism levelled against Harvey's modifications of Aristotelian biological doctrine.

Ross is a sharp controversialist whose arguments are mainly derived from Aristotelian logic and epistemology. In biological matters his wish to contradict seems sometimes to get the better of his Aristotelian loyalties. He thus confesses uncertainty as to such a fundamental Aristotelian position as the principate of the heart in generation which his adversary Digby had confirmed. He merely concedes this to be probable, but adds that Galen had good reason to deny it and thinks that the opinion of Hippocrates is most likely to be true "that all the parts are formed at the same time by the *spirits* in the seed[37]."

Nevertheless Ross is a first rate source for the atmosphere in which the work of Harvey was received in clerical circles of his own time and country. The yardstick by which it was judged by churchmen was not heresy which they still all too easily "smelt" in natural philosophers and notably those of the Paracelsian persuasion, but Aristotelian doctrine and tradition. Unlike these natural philosophers Harvey was not suspected of heresy or traffic with "spirits" or demons, but censured for deviation from well established Aristotelian biological theory.

The Dates and Places of Harvey's Publications

Why were Harvey's books published at the times and places that they were? Again there is no need to resort to any circumstances other than ordinary ones. On Harvey's own showing, he wanted to wait until he was sure of the truth of his discovery. From all the evidence we have (p. 211) it would appear that the period of waiting was not as protracted as formerly assumed. In other words if we ask: Why did Harvey not publish his discovery much earlier, the answer should be: because he had not made it. The "more than

35 *Philosophical Touchstone*, p. 29–31.

36 See PAGEL, W., *J.B. Van Helmont. Einführung in die Philosophische Medizin des Barock*, Berlin 1930, p. 96–100 and DEBUS, A.G., *Robert Fludd and the use of Gilbert's De magnete in the Weapon-Salve controversy*, *J.Hist. Med.* 1964, XIX, 389–417, p. 416–417.

37 *Philosophical Touchstone*, p. 40. – See to this: JOS. NEEDHAM, *History of Embryology*, Cambridge, 1934, p. 108.

nine years" of which Harvey speaks, seem to a large extent to apply to what he has to offer in original insight into the movement of the heart, as laid down in the *Prooemium* and the first seven chapters of *De motu*, rather than to the discovery of circulation which follows from chapter VIII onwards. Nevertheless, several years must have elapsed before he finally published the wole work. There was nothing in it that might have been interpreted as religious heresy. For nothing had been said in the book about the soul.

So reasons of this kind are not applicable to the long incubation of the work. Nor do they apply for the publication of *De motu* on the Continent. The true reasons, as we have suggested (p. 115), were possibly of a much more prosaic nature: the author knew that his friend Fludd's continental publisher not only did not ask for a subsidy, but even paid royalties—by contrast with his British colleagues. What Harvey had to anticipate was not religious persecution, but the hostility of the medical profession, at home as much as on the Continent.

The Reception of Harvey's work—The adversaries

This is borne out by the reception of Harvey in Catholic Italy. The second edition of *De motu* appeared in 1635—in Venice[38]. It had the adverse criticism of Parisanus intercalated—but so had the third edition of 1639 which did not appear in Italy, but in free and Protestant Holland[39]. Again, the fourth edition is a product of Catholic Italy—appearing in 1643 at Padua. This time already there were no adverse notes, but instead the two letters of Joh. Walaeus of Leyden, *quibus Harveji doctrina roboratur*[40].

In Holland Harvey's discovery was remarkably slow to penetrate into academic circles. It was coldshouldered by the two Leyden professors Valckenburg and Heurnius, and it remained to a practitioner, Johan van Beverwyck of Dordrecht (1594–1647), to express agreement and appreciation at an early date. When young de le Boe (Sylvius) defended Harvey at Leyden University he found nothing but opposition and even frank mockery. However, he succeeded by his experiments and demonstrations to convince Johan de Wale (Walaeus, 1604–1649) of the truth and it is the work of the latter which greatly promoted the general recognition of Harvey[41]. As late as 1641—the year in which de Wale published his two *letters on the motion of the chyle and blood to Thomas Bartholinus*—Gerard John Vossius (1577–1649), Professor at Leyden and Amsterdam and prebendary in the Cathe-

38 KEYNES, loc.cit. in note [25], No. 2, p. 8.

39 KEYNES, No. 3, p. 9.

40 KEYNES, No. 4, p. 10.

41 LINDEBOOM, G.A., *The reception in Holland of Harvey's theory of the circulation of the blood. Janus* 1957, XLVI, 183–200.

dral of Canterbury, said that there are two ways open to the blood from the liver: into the heart and brain for the generation of vital and psychic spirit and the other through the veins of the whole body to accomplish the last stage of digestion (*alterum per venas totius corporis, ut tertia perficiatur concoctio*)[42]. Though largely relying on ancient sources and intent on a revival of Stoicism Vossius must have been conversant with contemporary medical literature, for not far from the locus quoted he mentions Columbus with reference to the blood flow from the right heart through the lungs and at another place Cardanus, Scaliger, Fernel and again Columbus who dissented from the Galenic Laurentius in favour of Erasistratus[43].

Who were Harvey's early adversaries, who his early supporters? Among the former James Primrose, Ole Worm (a protestant Dane), Alexander Read, Parisano, Gassendi and Caspar Hofmann (of the Protestant university of Altdorf) are well known *dramatis personae*[44]. Among his early supporters two Italians are outstanding: Giovanni Trullius—physician to Pope Urban VIII—who defended circulation publicly in 1642[45], and Andreas Argoli. The latter had done so already in 1639. In his book, published at Padua, circulation is presented in the microcosmic symbolical setting; but five years later, in 1644, Argoli published one of the best short factual accounts of the new theory (p. 59). A year before another Italian, Claudio Berigardo, had referred to it fairly extensively and favourably in the context of Aristotelian physics and philosophy[46]. Indeed Harvey's Aristotelian leanings should have recommended his work in Italy.

It would appear that there were roughly as many supporters as there were adversaries in each of the European countries, and no preference in dates or numbers can be given to any one of them. Resistance seems to have lasted longest in France, the country of Patin and Riolan.

Concerning the work *On generation* we have dealt with the absence from it of any case for heresy: it just did not arise, any more than in any other piece of Aristotelian biology, or for that matter in any discussion taking its vitalistic interpretation to its logical, if overstretched conclusion. We have also discussed the discursive nature of the work, which must have taken two decades or even more to compile. Unlike *De motu*, it had not led to a solution of the major biological problem with which it was concerned: that of fertilisation. Harvey may have entertained hopes of reaching such a solution, and therefore kept the manuscript unpublished, for a long time. Nor were the upheavals in the wake of the Civil

42 *De theologia gentili et physiologia Christiana s. de origine ac progressu idololatriae ... deque naturae mirandis quibus homo adducitur ad Deum.* Amsterdami 1641, Lib. III, p. 826 (cap. 21).

43 Loc. cit. in note [42], p. 922 (cap. 39) on the simultaneous motion of heart and arteries. – On the revival of Stoicism and Vossius' role therein: DILTHEY, W., *Weltanschauung und Analyse des Menschen seit Renaissance und Reformation.* Leipz. Berlin 1923, p. 443 and 446.

44 WEIL, E., *The echo of Harvey's De motu Cordis 1628–1657. J. Hist. Med.* 1957, XII, 167–174; p. 168.

45 PAGEL, W. and POYNTER, F.N.L., *Harvey's doctrine in Italy: Argoli (1644) and Bonaccorsi (1647) on the circulation of the blood.* Bullet. Hist. Med. 1960, XXXIV, 419–429; p. 420.

46 See above, p. 60, in a previous chapter, note [29].

War conducive to the continuation of Harvey's researches, which had flourished in the peaceful and sheltered conditions he had enjoyed under the *ancien régime*. He finally decided to give in to Ent's entreaties to have the book published in the form in which it had probably remained for several years, as he could then not anticipate any further enlightenment on the subject—in view of his age, infirmities and the change in the whole situation. These reasons perfectly explain the long incubation of the work—it had been waiting for further experimental and observational results, and hardly for any greater freedom that the Republic might have been expected to extend to the *Archiatro Regio Serenissimae Maiestatis*.

Epilogue

We have tried to present the world of Harvey as a unified whole. The modern scientist who finds much to praise, but equally much to blame in Harvey will hardly see this world as an organic whole in which the scientific and non-scientific elements support rather than impede each other. To him Harvey at best becomes comprehensible as a "dweller in two worlds". To Harvey himself, however, there could be only one world—the world of Harvey. The same is true of the historian who sets out to understand his hero as the centre of a world that is unique and at the same time unified in this central figure. Taken in its entirety it has no predecessors or successors—such only emerge where parts and facets are selected from a complex whole and examined by themselves in isolation. The historian can afford no such selective practices. The only authority to which he is answerable is historical truth and this can only be the whole truth. He cannot accept directions or dictates from tribunals foreign to history itself such as science and the standards which it has developed through its own history up to the modern climax. Nor can he ignore or soften the facts of history in the interest of ephemeral simplification.

Hence the historian of Harvey and for that matter of any savant will do well to remember the incomparable words of the Lord Chancellor: "Historians should not be like critics who spend their time praising or blaming; but the facts themselves should be represented plainly and descriptively, with not more than sparse insertion of opinions. The material should be drawn not from the works and opinions of others, but all the main sources which are extant from a certain period should be consulted; not, however, merely read, but digested and understood in the peculiarity of their propositions, style and methods whereby the literary genius of that age as if by a magic formula should be raised from the dead[47]".

47 SIR FRANCIS BACON, *De augmentis scientiarum* lib. II, cap. 4. Amstelod. Henr. Wetsten., 1694, p. 105. To this: CROMBIE, A.C., *Scientific change*, London (1961), p. 2.

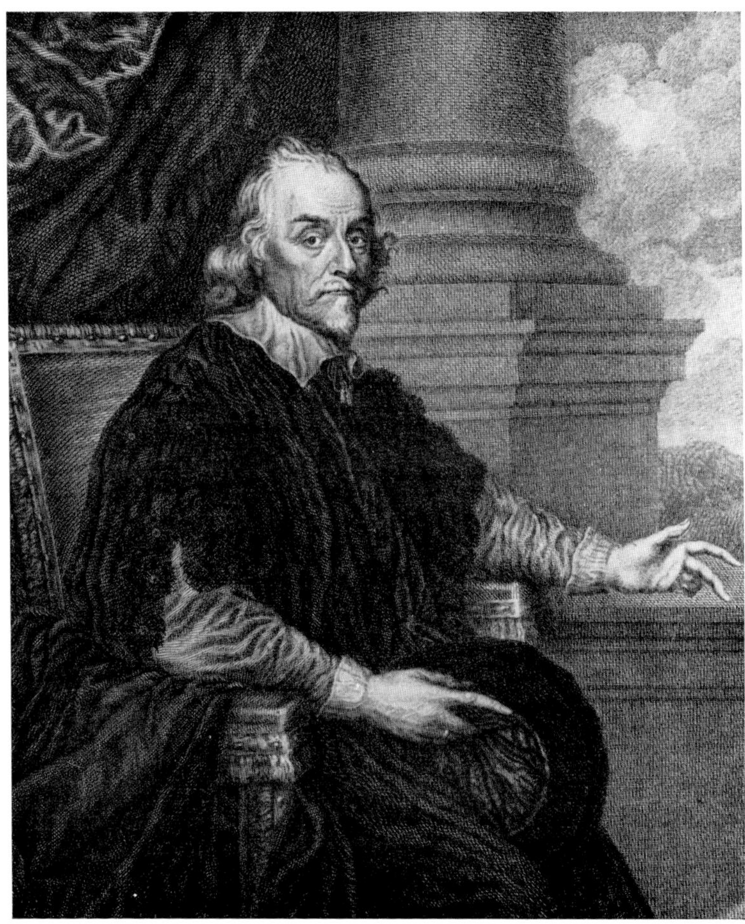

Fig. 1 (to p. 18)
William Harvey (1578–1657). From the line engraving by J. Hall after the picture in the Royal College of Physicians London. Impression in the Wellcome Collections. By courtesy of the Wellcome Trustees. See: *Guilelmi Harveii Opera Omnia a Collegio Medicorum Londonensi edita*. London 1766; the portrait facing the title. – For the original painting: KEYNES, Sir Geoffrey, *The Portraiture of William Harvey*, London 1949, p. 8 and plate V.

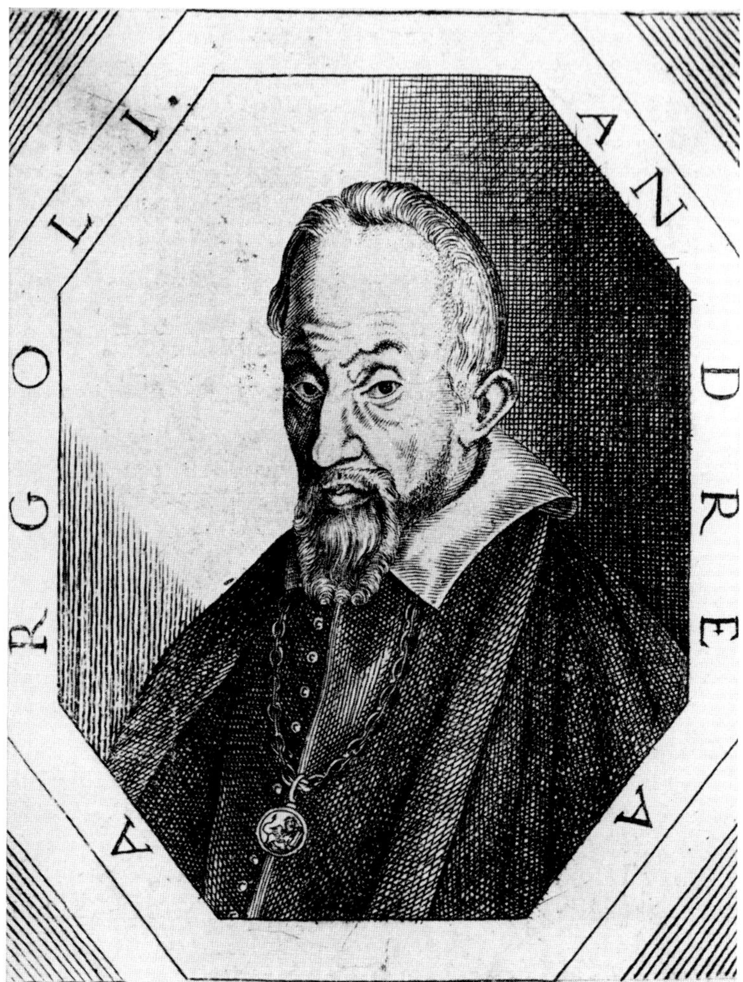

Fig. 2 (to p. 59)
Portrait of Andrea Argoli (From an engraving in the Wellcome Collection). By courtesy of the Wellcome Trustees.

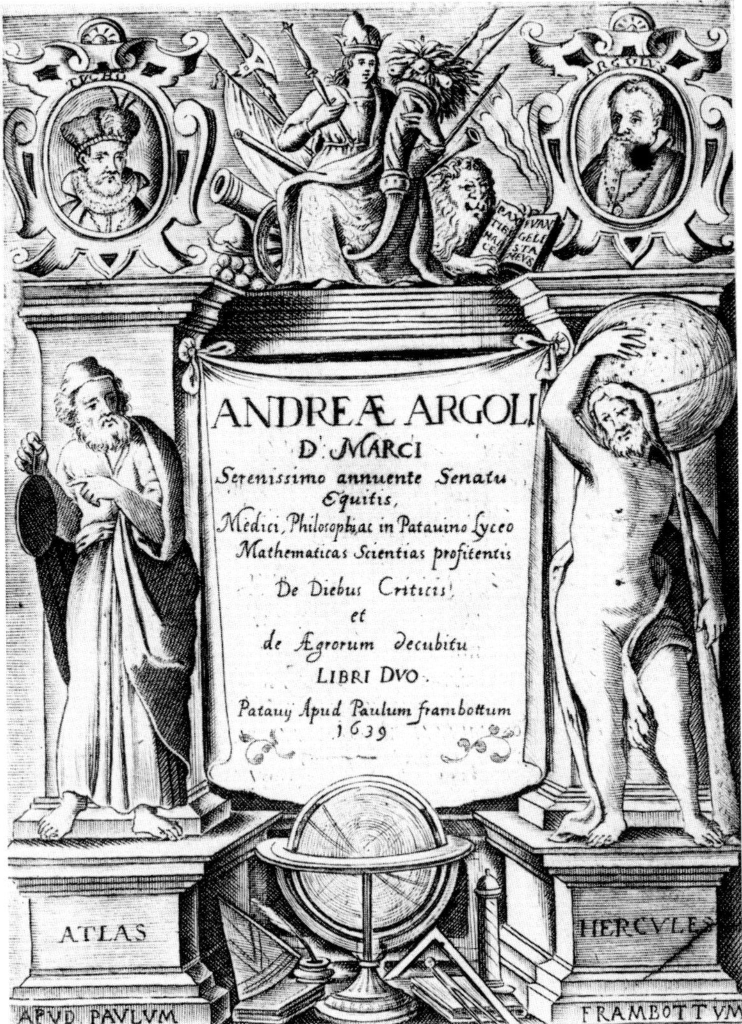

ANDREÆ ARGOLI
D. MARCI
Serenissimo annuente Senatu
Equitis,
Medici, Philosophiae in Patauino Lyceo
Mathematicas Scientias profitentis
De Diebus Criticis
et
de Ægrorum decubitu
LIBRI DVO.
Patauij Apud Paulum frambottum
1639

ATLAS
HERCVLES
APVD PAVLVM
FRAMBOTTVM

Fig. 3 (to p. 60)
Argoli, *De diebus criticis*, Padua 1639.
Title-page. By courtesy of the Wellcome Trustees.

ANDREÆ ARGOLI
SERENISSIMI SENATVS VENETI
EQVITIS,
Et in Patauino Lyceo Mathematicas
profitentis
PANDOSION SPHÆRICVM.
In quo ſingula in Elementaribus regionibus, atque
Ætherea, mathematicè pertractantur.

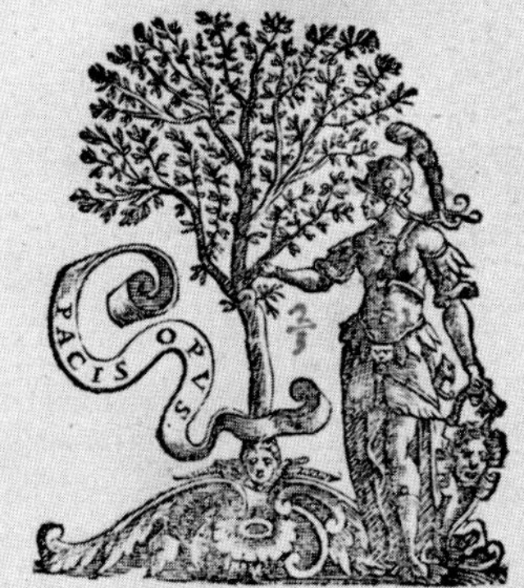

PATAVII, M.DC.XLIV.

Typis Pauli Frambotti Bibliopolæ.
Superiorum permiſſu.

Fig. 4 (to p. 61)
Argoli, *Pandosion sphaericum*, Padua 1644.
Title page. By courtesy of the Wellcome Trustees.

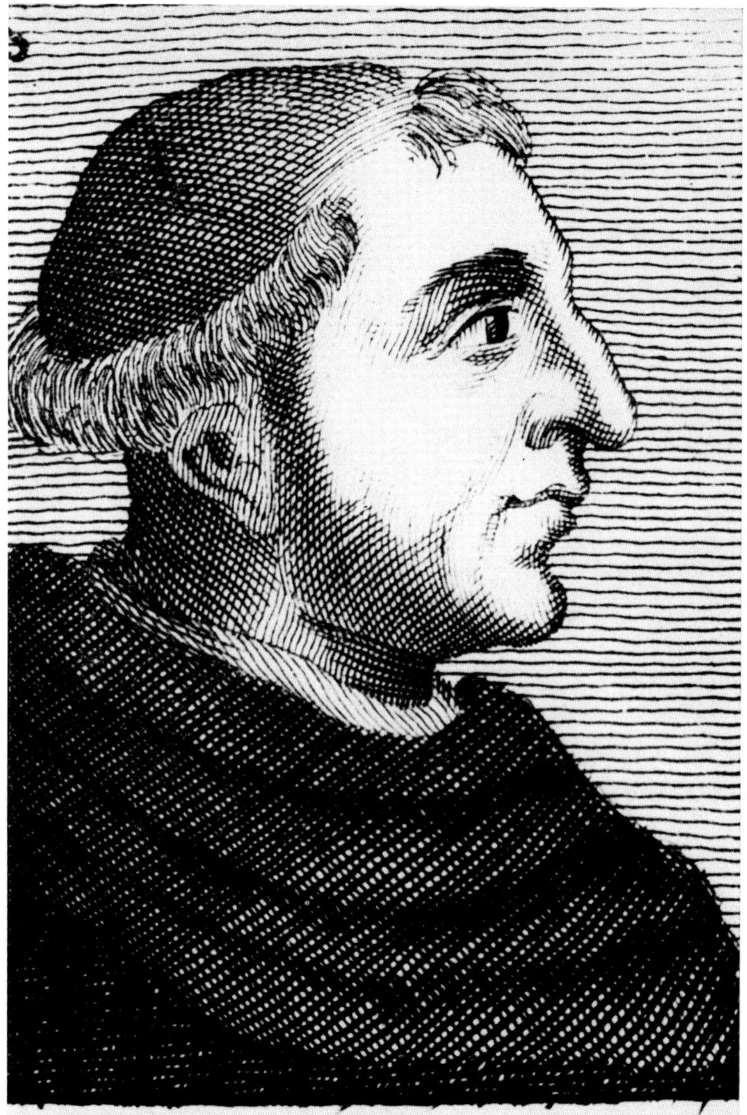

Fig. 5 (to p. 90)
St Thomas Aquinas, Portrait. From: P. Freher, *Theatrum virorum eruditione clarorum*. Nuremberg. J. Hofmann 1688, fac. p. 1418. Copy in the Wellcome Collections. By courtesy of the Wellcome Trustees.

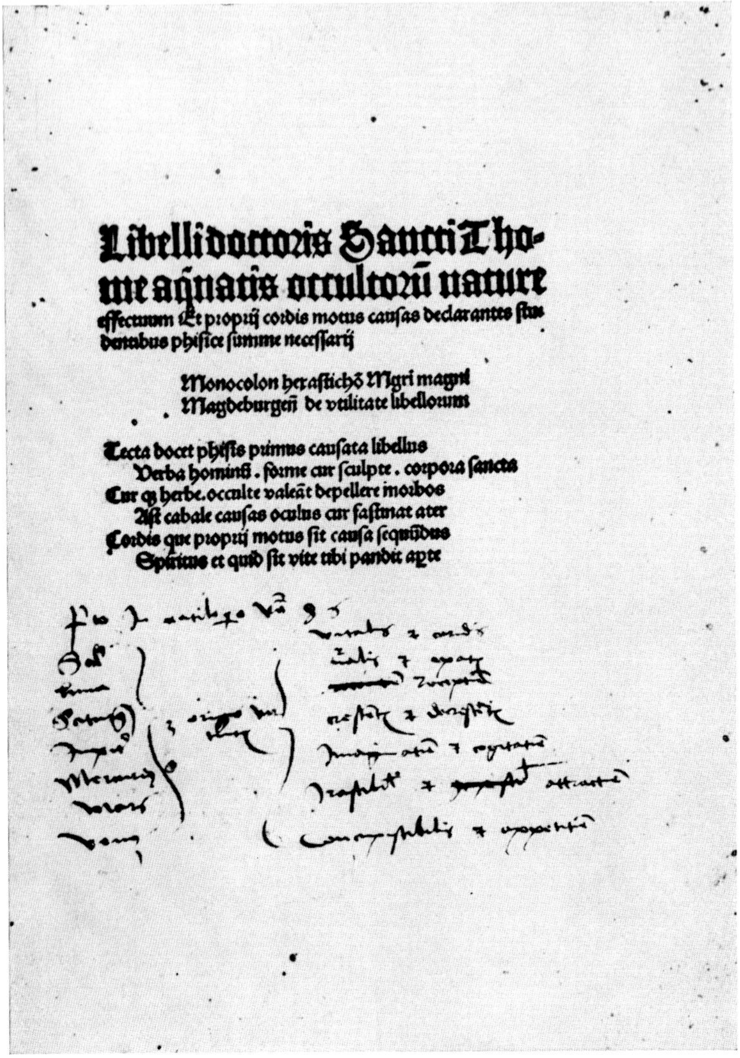

Libelli doctoris Sancti Tho-
me aq̄natis occultorũ nature
effectuum Et proprij cordis motus causas declarantes studentibus phisice summe necessarij

Monocolon hexastichō Mgri magni
Magdeburgeñ de vtilitate libellorum

Lecta docet phisis primus causata libellus
Verba hominū . forme cur sculpte . corpora sancta
Cur qȝ herbe . occulte valeāt depellere morbos
Ast cabale causas oculus cur fascinat ater
Cordis que proprij motus sit causa sequūdus
Spiritus et quid sit vite tibi pandit apte

Fig. 6 (to p. 90)
St Thomas Aquinas, *De motu cordis*.
Leipzig 1499. Title-page.

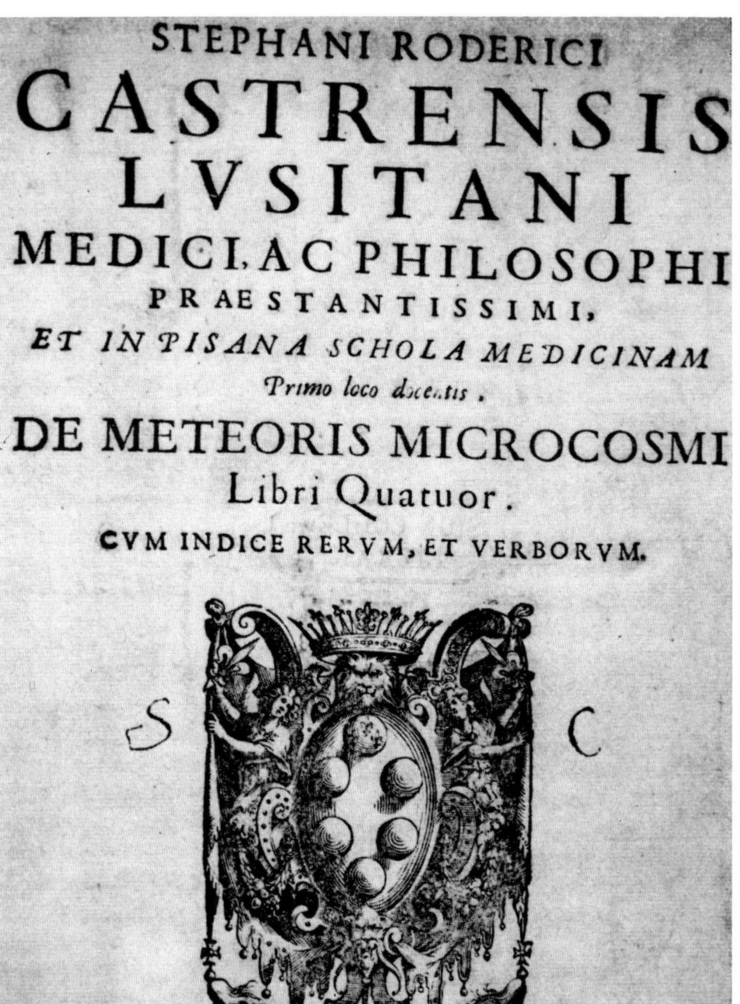

STEPHANI RODERICI
CASTRENSIS
LVSITANI
MEDICI, AC PHILOSOPHI
PRAESTANTISSIMI,
ET IN PISANA SCHOLA MEDICINAM
Primo loco docentis.
DE METEORIS MICROCOSMI
Libri Quatuor.
CVM INDICE RERVM, ET VERBORVM.

S C

FLORENTIAE, M.DC.XXI.
Apud Iunctas.

SVPERIORVM PERMISSV.

Fig. 7 (to p. 94)
Castro, Steph. Roderic.,
De meteoris microcosmi, Florence 1621.
Title-page.

Æt. XLIX.
M.D.C.XLIII.
Sculp
Ἰητὴρ ἀγαθὸς, βȣληφόρος ἠδὲ δίκαιος,
οὗτος ΙΩΑΝΝΗΣ εἰμὶ ΒΕΒΕΡΒΙΚΙΟΣ.
Arte bonus Medica, juſtus patriæque Senator,
Talis IOHANNES ſum BEVEROVICIVS.

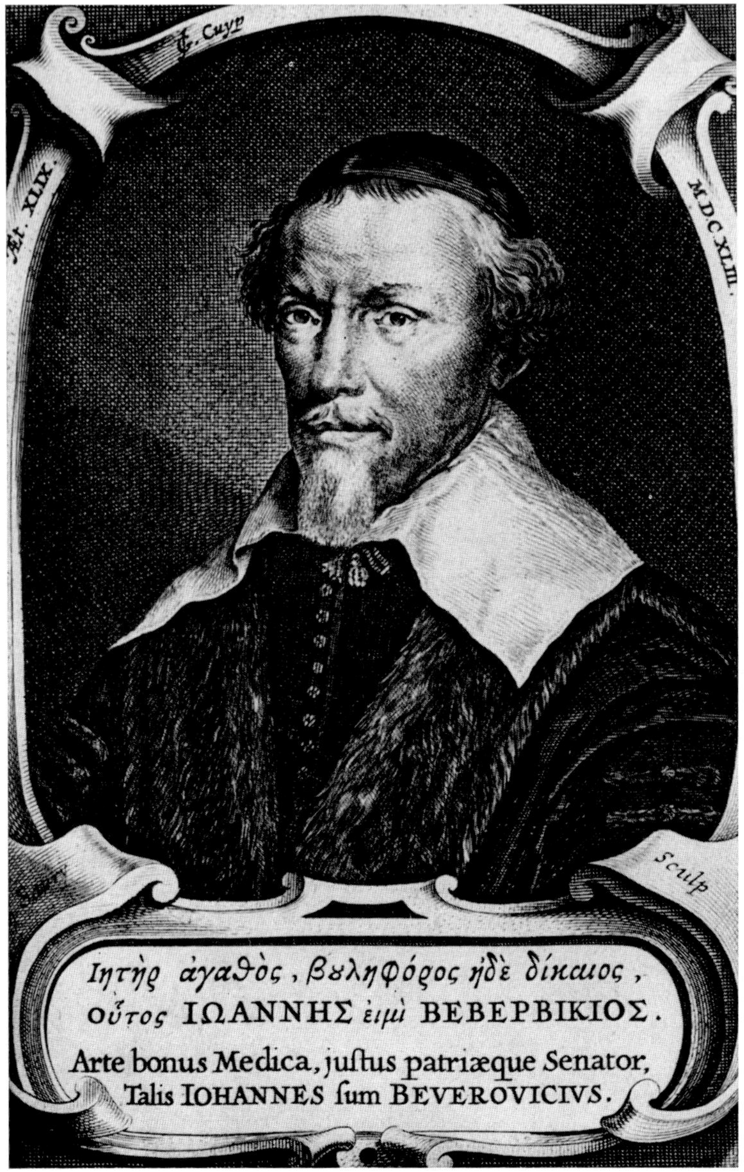

Fig. 8 (to p. 99)
Jan van Beverwyck (1594–1647). Portrait from an Engraving by Savery after J. G. Cuyp. From the Wellcome Collections (WHML 2747). By courtesy of the Wellcome Trustees.

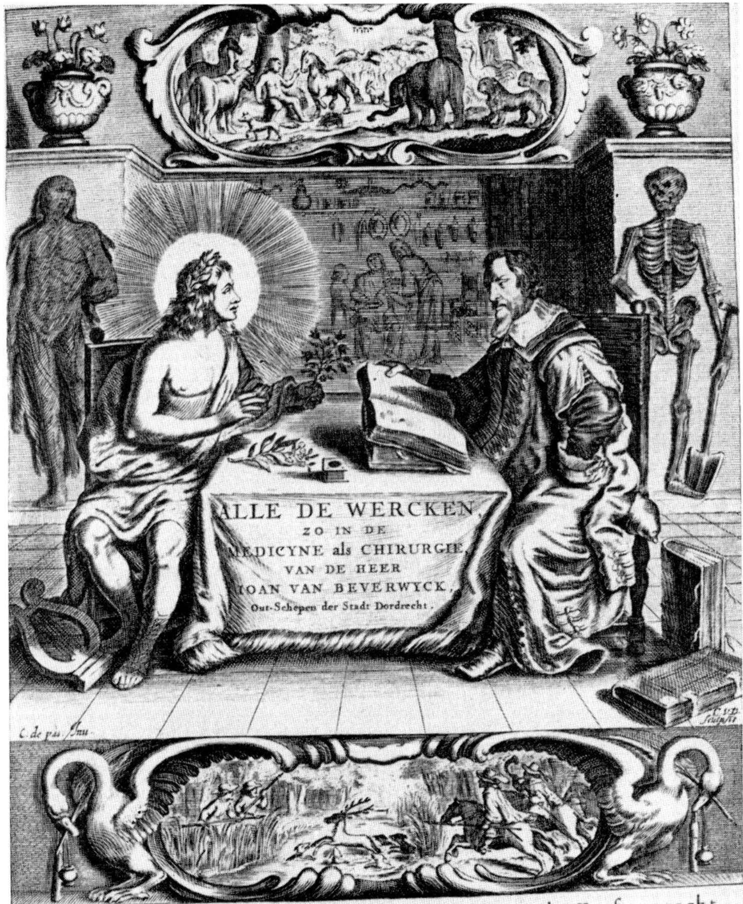

Fig. 9 (to p. 99)
Apollo imparting his knowledge of herbs and plants to Jan van Beverwyck. Frontispiece to the latter's *Alle de Wercken zo in de Medicyne als Chirurgie*. Amsterdam. J. J. Schipper. 1660. From the Wellcome Collections (WHML 2748). By courtesy of the Wellcome Trustees.

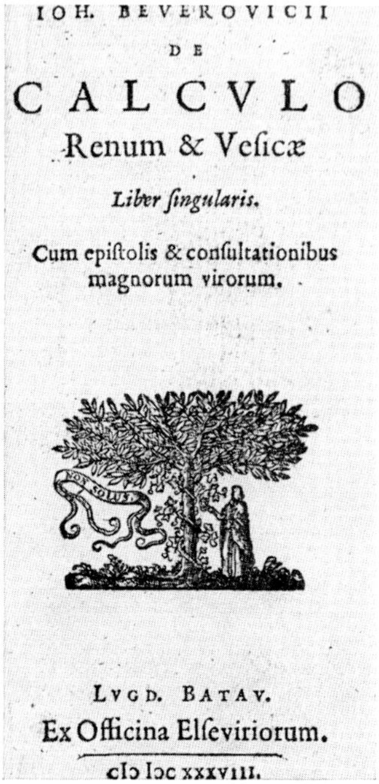

IOH. BEVEROVICII
DE
CALCVLO
Renum & Vesicæ
Liber singularis.
Cum epistolis & consultationibus magnorum virorum.

LVGD. BATAV.
Ex Officina Elseviriorum.
cIↃ IↃc XXXVIII.

Fig. 10 (to p. 99)
Beverwijck, Jan van, *De calculo renum*, Leyden 1638. Title page. By courtesy of the Wellcome Trustees.

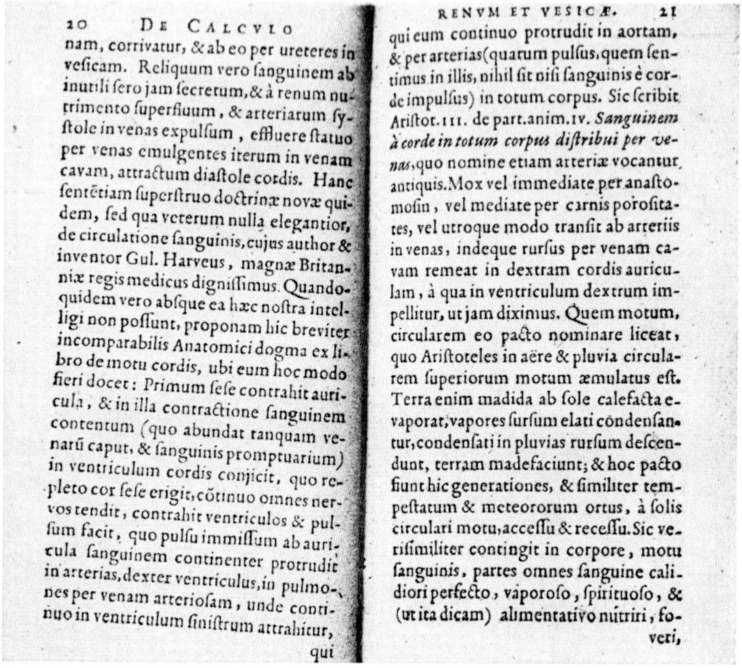

20 DE CALCVLO

nam, corrivatur, & ab eo per ureteres in vesicam. Reliquum vero sanguinem ab inutili sero jam secretum, & à renum nutrimento superfluum, & arteriarum systole in venas expulsum, effluere statuo per venas emulgentes iterum in venam cavam, attractum diastole cordis. Hanc sentẽtiam superstruo doctrinæ novæ quidem, sed qua veterum nulla elegantior, de circulatione sanguinis, cujus author & inventor Gul. Harveus, magnæ Britanniæ regis medicus dignissimus. Quandoquidem vero absque ea hæc nostra intelligi non possunt, proponam hic breviter incomparabilis Anatomici dogma ex libro de motu cordis, ubi eum hoc modo fieri docet: Primum sese contrahit auricula, & in illa contractione sanguinem contentum (quo abundat tanquam venarũ caput, & sanguinis promptuarium) in ventriculum cordis conjicit, quo repleto cor sese erigit, cõtinuo omnes nervos tendit, contrahit ventriculos & pulsum facit, quo pulsu immissum ab auricula sanguinem continenter protrudit in arterias, dexter ventriculus, in pulmones per venam arteriosam, unde continuo in ventriculum sinistrum attrahitur, qui

RENVM ET VESICÆ. 21

qui eum continuo protrudit in aortam, & per arterias (quarum pulsus, quem sentimus in illis, nihil sit nisi sanguinis è corde impulsus) in totum corpus. Sic scribit Aristot. III. de part. anim. IV. *Sanguinem à corde in totum corpus distribui per venas*, quo nomine etiam arteriæ vocantur antiquis. Mox vel immediate per anastomosin, vel mediate per carnis porositates, vel utroque modo transit ab arteriis in venas, indeque rursus per venam cavam remeat in dextram cordis auriculam, à qua in ventriculum dextrum impellitur, ut jam diximus. Quem motum, circularem eo pacto nominare liceat, quo Aristoteles in aëre & pluvia circularem superiorum motum æmulatus est. Terra enim madida ab sole calefacta evaporat, vapores sursum elati condensantur, condensati in pluvias rursum descendunt, terram madefaciunt; & hoc pacto fiunt hic generationes, & similiter tempestatum & meteororum ortus, à solis circulari motu, accessu & recessu. Sic verisimiliter contingit in corpore, motu sanguinis, partes omnes sanguine calidiori perfecto, vaporoso, spirituoso, & (ut ita dicam) alimentativo nutriri, foveri,

Fig. 11 (to p. 99)
First endorsement of Harvey's discovery in a medical treatise: Beverwijck, *De calculo renum*, 1638, p. 20–21. By courtesy of the Wellcome Trustees.

IOH. BEVEROVICII

EXERCITATIO

IN

HIPPOCRATIS

APHORISMVM

de Calculo

AD N.V.

CLAVDIVM SALMASIVM

Equitem, & Conſ. Regium.

Accedunt ejuſdem argumenti Doctorum Epiſtolæ.

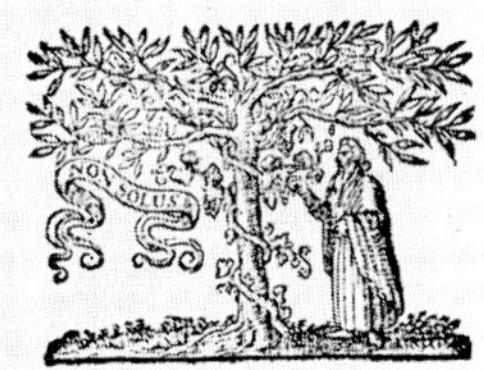

LVGD. BATAVORVM,

Ex Officinâ Elſeviriorum.

cIↄ Iↄ c XLI.

Fig. 12 (to p. 99)
Beverwijck, *In Hippocratis aphorismum de calculo*, Leyden 1641. By courtesy of the Wellcome Trustees.

SPICIL. DE CALCVLO. 191

Ex Hippocratis, Galeni, & aliorum ſententia glutinoſum requiri ad Calculi generationem: neque ſtuporem renum eo videri neceſſarium.

IOHANNI BEVEROVICIO,
Senatori, & Medico Dordrechtano,

GVL. HARVEVS S.D.

QVod in itinere Germanico pridem à me ſuſcepto, Vir præſtantiſſime, te, patriæ artiſque Medicæ decus, vidiſſe non contigerit, pariter uti te, tuæ literæ gratiſſimæ mihi (quas cum libello, præterita ſeptimana, accepimus) dolore non mediocri affectum ſignificarunt; ita quoque doleam, ſcire poteris, ubi noveris quo ſim animo in viros cordatos, ſagaceſque rerum naturalium indagatores tui ſimiles Quod ſanguinis circulatio inventa, tam docto capiti non diſpliceat, eo quidem nomine mihi jam nunc demum magis placere cœpit, animumque dabit plura & multo majora meditanti, cum conatus noſtros, eruditis placere intellexerim. Pergratus mihi doctus & elegans, vereque ſingularis liber tuus de Calculo renum & veſicæ, in quo firma ſolidaque nominis famæque jeciſti

192 IOH. BEVEROVICII

jeciſti fundamenta; quin pergas porro indies ſuperſtruere, ſplendidumque ingenii tui monumentum exædificare. Ego calculum haud illubens adjiciam meum, nec ſuos opinor tibi denegabunt alii, iique, quos præſens ætas fert melioris notæ, Medici.

Stephanus Rodericus Caſtrenſis magni Hetruriæ ducis Medicus, & Sennertus veſter, quam parum à ſententia tua abſint, is judicabit optime, qui hujus Inſtitutiones, illius de Microcoſmi meteoris libros perſpectos habet. Paracelſo, ejuſque ſequacibus ea certe gemma placere debet, quam ex illius minera erutam, magis tamen authoritate antiquorum politam & optimis obſervationibus & argumentis illuſtrem & ornatam in omnium manus tradidiſti. Nec Hippocrati quidem, nec Galeno, ſi jam poſtliminio revocari poſſint, eam diſplicere poſſe putem. ea cum reverentia ſententias eorum tractas, ac ſi priſcorum Medicinæ procerum ſcita placitaque non tam refellenda, quam candide explicita, in meliorem ſenſum accipienda judices. Si quis denique libertatis philoſophicæ aſſertor, è rebus ipſis, & naturæ ſinu, quam è libris, ſapere, quam diſcere malit, ſcire quam credere, habes quod etiam

Fig. 13–14 (to p. 99)
Harvey's letter to Beverwijck, from *In Hippocratis aphorismum de calculo*, p. 191 and 192, with the citation of Castro and Paracelsus. By courtesy of the Wellcome Trustees.

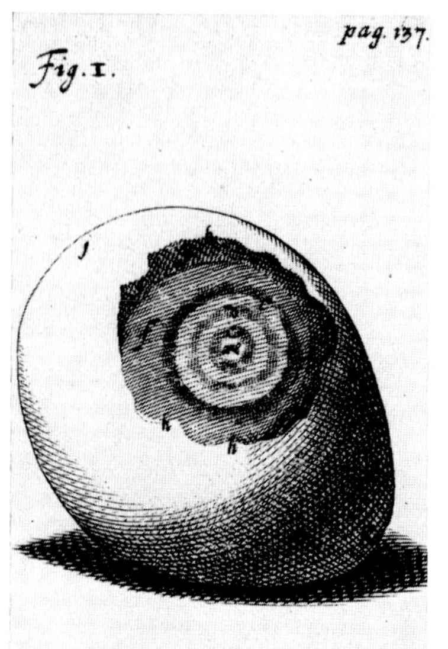

Fig. 15 (to p. 313)
The circular pattern of the early embryonic *field*, from Willem Langly, *Observationes de generatione animalium*, 1674, fig. 1, p. 137. By Courtesy of the Wellcome Trust.

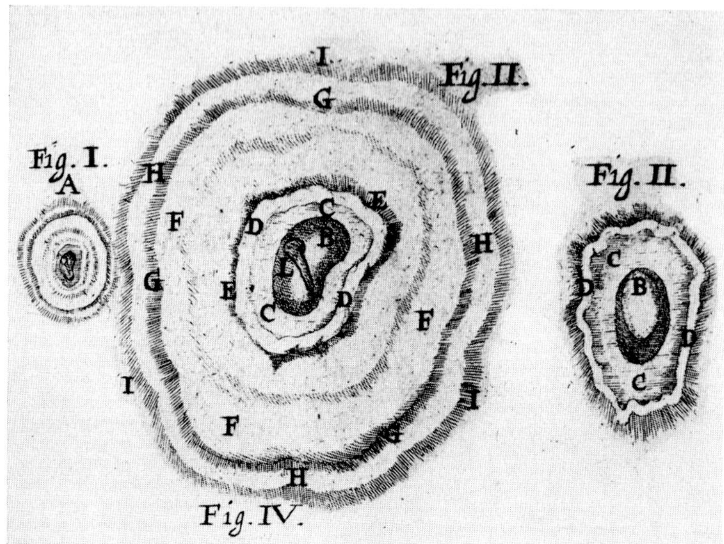

Fig. 16 (to p. 313)
The circular pattern of the early embryonic *field*, from Marcello Malpighi, *De formatione pulli in ovo*, London, J. Martyn, 1673, Tab. Ia, figgs. I and II. From the Wellcome Collection. By courtesy of the Wellcome Trust.

In the same year in which Harvey's book appeared Nathan. HIGHMORE gave a detailed and illustrated description of the *circles* in the *cicatricula* of the egg: *The history of Generation*, London 1651, p. 66–71, mentioning the use of the *microscope*.

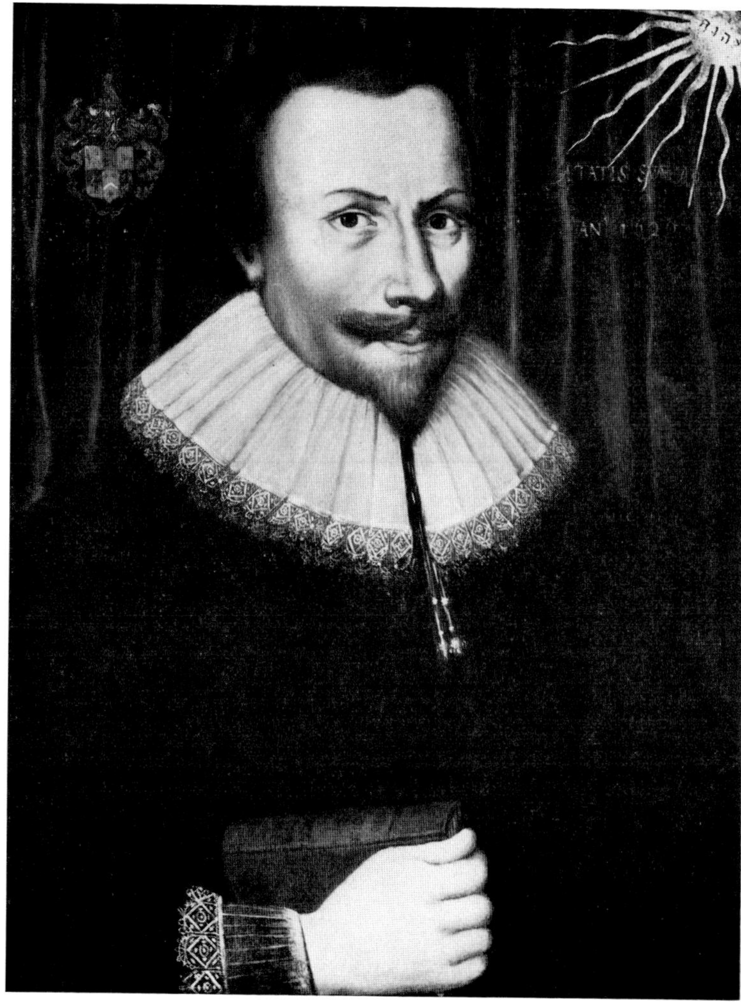

Fig. 17 (to p. 113)
Robert Fludd. From a painting attributed to Frans Pourbus, the younger. Flemish School. In the Wellcome Collection. By courtesy of the Wellcome Trust.

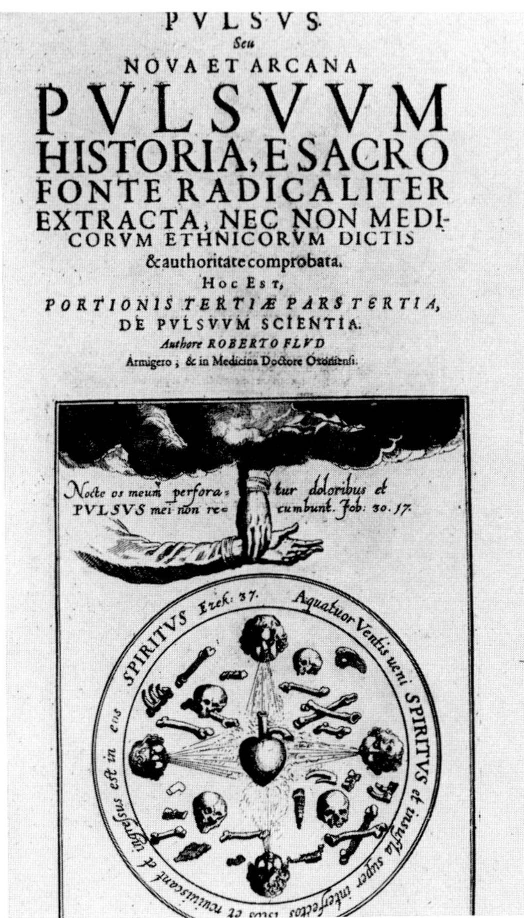

PVLSVS.
Seu
NOVA ET ARCANA
PVLSVVM
HISTORIA, E SACRO
FONTE RADICALITER
EXTRACTA, NEC NON MEDICORVM ETHNICORVM DICTIS
&authoritate comprobata.
Hoc Est,
PORTIONIS TERTIÆ PARS TERTIA,
DE PVLSVVM SCIENTIA.
Authore ROBERTO FLVD
Armigero ; & in Medicina Doctore Oxoniensi.

Nocte os meum perforatur doloribus et
PVLSVS mei non recumbunt. Job: 30. 17.
SPIRITVS Ezek: 37.
A quatuor Ventis ueni SPIRITVS et insuffla super interfectos istos et reuiuiscant

Fig. 18 (to p. 114)
Robert Fludd, *On the Pulse*, in *Integrum morborum mysterium*, Francof., W. Hofmann for G. Fitzer, 1631. From the Wellcome Collection. By courtesy of the Wellcome Trust.

De Pulsuum mysterio. 11

quo consistit humidum illud radicale, & calidum occultum diuinum, in quo cuncta viuunt, crescunt & multiplicantur. De quo diuino spiritu verbi dixit Euangelista vitã tam immortalium quàm mortalium fuisse: atque istam vitam vocauit lucem hominum: de quo spiritu etiam ista Propheta Ezekiel: *Quocunq, ibat spiritus, illuc eunte spiritu rota pariter euehebantur sequentes eum: spiritus enim vitæ erat in rotis; & vnumquodque animalium quatuor vbicunque erat impetus spiritus illuc gradiebatur*, &c. In quo Prophetæ sermone per quatuor animalia ignea quatuor mundi intelligentias ventorum præsides intendit; de quibus Angelus ad Zachariam. Isti sunt quatuor venti cœli, seu quatuor ventorum intelligentiæ quæ egrediuntur & stant coram Domino totius terræ, &c. Et per rotas ipsos ventos arguit. Denique spiritum vitæ in medio earum intendit diuinam essentiam seu emanationem centraliter & essentialiter in Angelis & ventis mouentem. Quòd etiam iste spiritus vnicus, habeat in se proprietatem quatuor ventorum, & quòd vitæ afflatus sit spiritualis quidam effluxus de occultis quatuor ventorum proprietatibus emissus mediante isto spiritu supremo ventorum domino & rectore, nos expressis verbis sic docet Propheta: *Veni spiritus à quatuor ventis, & insuffla vel inspira interfectos istos vt reuiuiscant.* Ioan. 1. Ezech. 1. Ezech. 37. 9

Quo quidem sermone innuere videtur, quòd spiritus iste (quem loco præcedenti vocat vitæ spiritum in quatuor rotis) est catholicus vitæ inspirator & vitæ spiritus dator, & quòd vitæ creaturarum spiritus sit ex quatuor spirituum cardinalium naturis more abstrusissimo conflatus: nam humidum radicale per se de spiraculo Septentrionali & Occidentali commune quid habet, vnde fit; vt naturali sua genitura sit de proprietate contractiua particeps, vnde & ad naturam quietis est procliue. Verùm quatenus illud de spiritu illo igneo, quẽ à spiraculo Orientali accepit, est particeps, eatenus in vaporem Meridionalem dilatatur; atque hac ratione ex parte Septentrionis contractiuam proprietatem sibi vendicat spiraculũ vitæ, & ad consistentiam madoris Occidentalis in sua contractione tendit: verùm ab Orientali iterum dilatatur in naturam madoris vaporosi & Meridionalis, atque ita more circuli mundani rotatur in suis vasculis arterialibus in diastole & systole, hoc est se dilatando ratione portionis Orientalis in spiritum Meridionalem, ac subitò more fluxus & refluxus maris se iterum contrahendo ratione portionis quam accepit de afflatu Septentrionali in consistentiam Occidentalẽ. Vnde vt videmus, quòd vnica chorda cũ suo pondere quasi actu catholico minutas horæ in horologio motione vnius circuli siue rotæ modo motu illius antrorsum, & immediatè postea retrorsum faciat, idq; partim agendo, partimq; resistendo: ita quidem catholico spiritus vnius actu mouetur in vitæ officio, idq; circulo quasi ventoso vitalis in suis vasculis spiritus.

Hoc exactè illam viri grauissimi Gulielmi Haruei, Medicinæ Doctoris peritissimi, arte Anatomica quàm clarissimi, necnon in profundis Philosophiæ mysteriis versatissimi, compatriota mihi charissimi, & collegæ fidelissimi, sententiam atq; opinionem confirmare videtur; qua, idq; consultè & prudenter satis mundum in *libello quodam suo, cui titulus est: Exercitatio Anatomica, De cordis sanguinisq; in animalibus motu*; instruit, insigniterq; cùm rationibus à Philosophiæ arca deprompris, tum multiformi demonstratione oculari declarat motum ipsius sanguinis esse circularem. Et quid ni (ô vos Cynici, quorum est faciliùs rem aliquam sine ratione negare, quàm probatam veris Philosophiæ & experientiæ telis redarguere atq; refellere,) quidni (inquam) cùm certum sit quòd vitæ spiritus respectu cœlestium spiritualẽ Zodiaci circuli impressionem in se retineat, vtpote in quo & per quem Luna periphericum suum quolibet mense iter perficiat, ad cuius motum proculdubio eius astra imperceptibilia sanguinis spiritui perfusa, spiritum etiam sanguinis, & consequenter ipsum sanguinem arterialem secum circulari suo motu rapit? Nonne etiam videmus ipsum spiritum mundanum; imò verò & ipsum mare in fluxu & refluxu Solis & Lunæ virtutibus obedire? Ait Salomon: *Sol lustrans vniuersa in circuitu pergit spiritus, & in circulos suos reuertitur.* Qualem etiam habet Luna in mari & aëre potestatem neminem in rebus marinis versatum latere potest. Nonne ergo homo microcosmus ob ipsius ad macrocosmũ relationem? Quidni igitur virtute Lunæ & Solis non taliter circumrotetur, sanguis vitæ qualiter tam aëra quàm æthera ab ipsis (centraliter mouente ipso qui dat motum & vitam omnibus) motu certo circulari moueri testatur experientia? Porrò in regione sublunari spiritum catholicum secundùm ventorum prædominantium flatum gradatim à natura in naturam à consistentia in consistentiã rotari, videlicet à natura Boreali in Occidentalẽ, ab Occidẽtali in Meridionalẽ, ac deniq; à Meridionali in Orientalẽ nõ aliter quàm à grosso semper in subtilius gradibus quaternis tenditur. Si ergo spiritus humanus ab illo mundano, si vitæ præsides ab illis cœlestibus dependeant, vti hi faciunt, necesse est vt illi etiam hoc idem ad motum & inst[illegible] eorũ agant: nam cùm quod facit tale sit magis tale, necesse habemus credere vt illud q; fecit tale reddat hoc q; factum est tale in suo motu & proprietate tale quale ipse erat author. Sed ad propositũ. Eccles. 1. 6.

Flud. de Pulsibus. BB Dicitur

Fig. 19 (to p. 115)
Endorsement of Harvey's discovery on the grounds of microcosmic symbolism by Robert Fludd issued at an early date, probably the first literary record of the discovery. From Fludd, *Pulsus … historia* in *Integrum morborum mysterium*, Francof. 1631 (as incorporated in Fludd's *Medicina catholica* of 1629). p. 11. From the Wellcome Collections. By courtesy of the Wellcome Trustees.

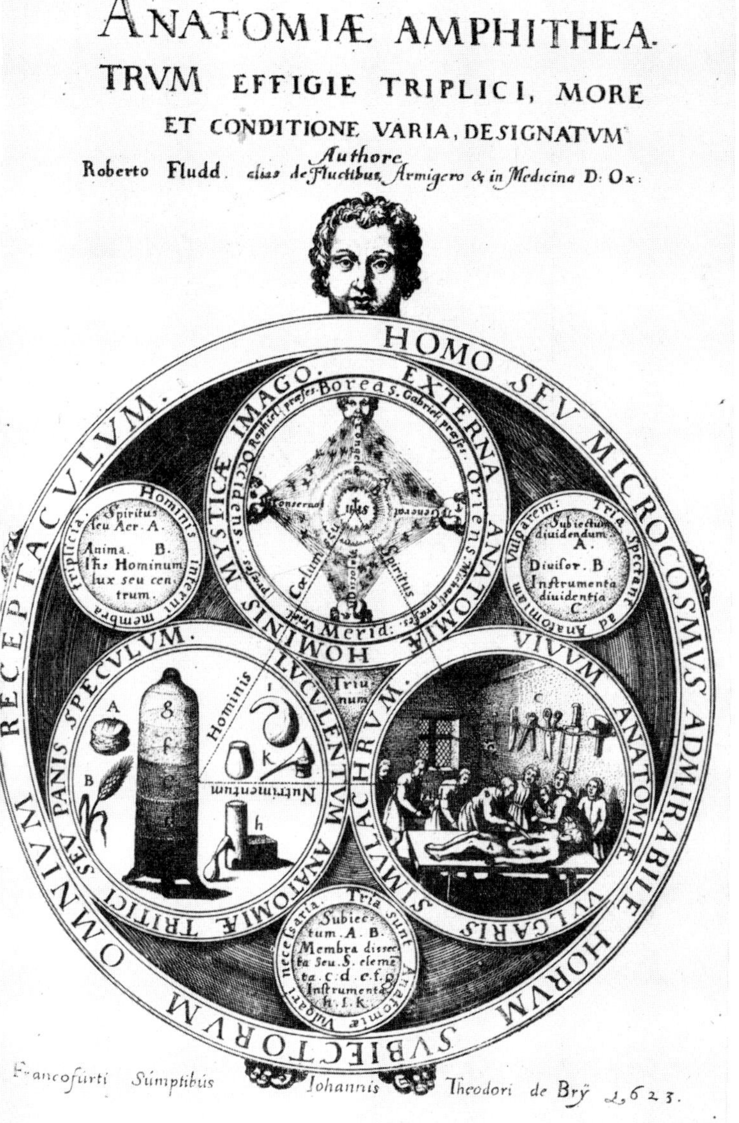

Fig. 20 (to p. 112)
Fludd's *Anatomiae Amphitheatrum*, Francof. E. Kempffer for J.T. de Bry, 1623. Title-page. From the Wellcome Collections. By courtesy of the Wellcome Trustees.

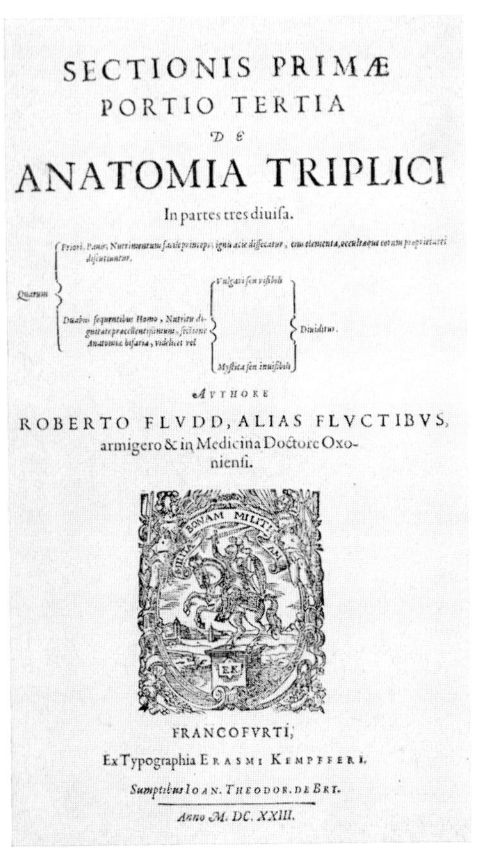

SECTIONIS PRIMÆ
PORTIO TERTIA
DE
ANATOMIA TRIPLICI
In partes tres diuisa.

Quarum { Priori, Panis, Nutrimentum facile princeps, ignis acie dissecatur, cum elementa, occultaque eorum proprietates discutiuntur. Duabus sequentibus Homo, Nutritu dignitate praecellentissimum, sectione Anatomica bifaria, videlicet vel { Vulgari seu visibili / Mystica seu inuisibili } Diuiditur.

AVTHORE
ROBERTO FLVDD, ALIAS FLVCTIBVS, armigero & in Medicina Doctore Oxoniensi.

FRANCOFVRTI,
Ex Typographia ERASMI KEMPFFERI.
Sumptibus IOAN. THEODOR. DE BRY.
Anno M. DC. XXIII.

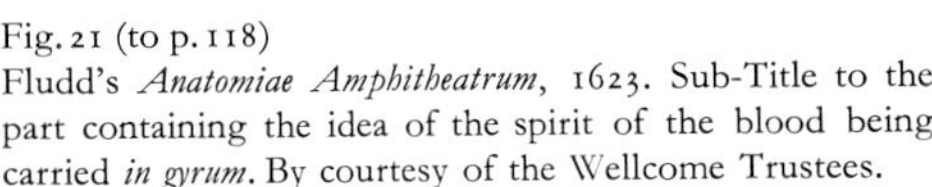

Fig. 21 (to p. 118)
Fludd's *Anatomiae Amphitheatrum*, 1623. Sub-Title to the part containing the idea of the spirit of the blood being carried *in gyrum*. By courtesy of the Wellcome Trustees.

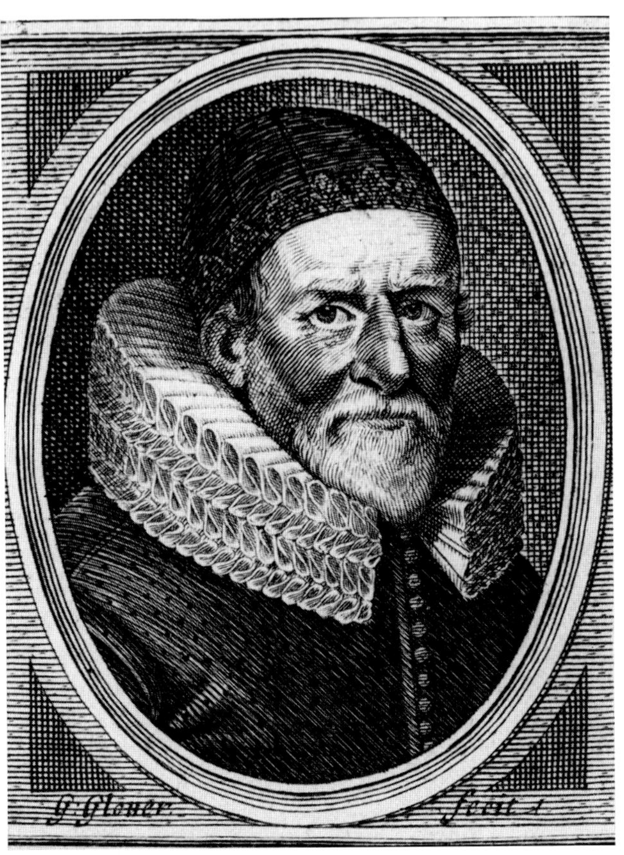

Fig. 22 (to p. 116)
John Woodall (1556?–1643). Portrait from the *Surgeons Mate*. London 1639 (bottom centre of engraved title-page). By courtesy of the Wellcome Trustees.

IORDANI
BRVNI NOLANI
DE MONADE NVMERO ET
Figura liber Conſequens Quin-
que DE MINIMO MAGNO
& Menſura.
Item
DE INNVMERABILIBVS, IM-
menſo, & Inſigurabili; ſeu De Vniuerſô
& Mundis libri octo.
AD ILLVSTRISSIMVM ET RE-
uerendiſs. Principem HENRICVM IV-
LIVM Brunſuicenſium & Lunebur-
genſium ducem, Halberſtaden-
ſium Epiſcopum, &c.

FRANCOFVRTI,
Apud IOAN. Vvechelum & PETRVM
Fiſcherum conſortes. 1591.

Fig. 23 (to p. 106)
Giordano Bruno, *De monade*, 1591.
Title-page.

266 Sect. I. Port. III. Part. III. Liber III.

quatur priuatio seu nocturna quies, hoc est cessatio à formæ actionibus; at vero superante forma, iterum
informationis dies & sol informans resurgit. Sed & hoc à sapiente luculenter in his verbis confirmari videtur, *Generatio*, (inquit ille) *vna abit. & altera aduenit, quamuis terra in seculum permaneat, ortusq; sol postquam occi-*
derit Sol iterum ad locum suum aspirat, vbi oriatur, quo quidem innuere videtur, quod generatio & corruptio
relationem habeant ad ortum & occasum solis. A solis igitur seu cordis mundani ortu seu vita succedit vita hominis, vtpote qui est filius mundi, & vt in primordio mundi Sol ab Astrologis dicitur motum suum
fecisse ab ortu, tanquam à termino à quo, quemadmodum etiam & Sol spiritualis dicitur ab ortu die vltimo
venturus, sic etiam probabile est, quod vita humana suum ortum habuerit à plaga microcosmi Orientali
ad imitationem principij vitæ macrocosmicæ, quæ ab angulo Orientali occipit, &, consequenter quod cor
sit angulus seu cardo ille Orientalis, quippe à quo vitæ lux primum in embrione effulsit.

CAPVT III.

Quod vitæ flatus procedat ab oriente tam in macro quam microcosmo, & de metaphysica vitæ & animarum vtriusque mundi ratione.

CVm igitur cor sit microcosmo plaga orientalis non aliter quam locus ortus solis, angulus orientalis,
horoscopus dictus, sequitur, quod ventus similis ab huiusmodi cardine in homine spiret: Atq; hic ventus spirat vitæ animam vniuerso spiritui humano, non aliter quam ille macrocosmicus vitã dicitur dare &
motum spiritui, seu aeri, seu vento humano. Vnde dicit Sapiens, *quod postquam occiderit Sol, iterum ad locum*
suum aspiret, vbi oriatur, properet ad meridiem, & circumeat Aquilonem; Ex quibus verbis liquet, *quod Sol, in quo*, (iu-
xta Platonicos) *est mundi anima sita* (ac etiam Psalmist. dicit, *quod Deus posuerit Tabernaculum suum in Sole*) sit
principalis ventorum motor atque incitator, atq; hinc pergit Sapiens subnectendo istiusmodi sermonem
præcedenti; *Conuersione sua circumiens properet aer.* (vel. vt Hieronym. interpretatur, *spiritus*) *& secundum circui-*
Eccl. 1. 4. *tus suos reuertatur aer*, quod Pagninus sic interpretatur, *subinde circumeundo pergit ventus, & ad circuitus suos reuer-*
titur ventus. Hieronymus ait: *Lustrans in circuitu suo pergit spiritus, & in circulos suos reuertitur*: quo quidem sermone sat luculenter arguit Sapiens. quod aeris dispositio à motu solari dependeat, vtpote cuius radij sunt
quasi anima ad eum. Vnde non aliter mouetur aer naturaliter, quam ad motum solis, cuius actione agitatur motu circulari. Hinc igitur est quod venti dicantur infantes Titanis, Astreæ, & Aurora, quatenus à calore Solis geniti, vt ait Aristot. qui aerem reddunt subtilem & rarum, hocq; præcipue in Aurora: At vero
dicuntur mandatis Iunonis obedire quatenus non flant nisi in aere qui dicitur Iuno. Pari ratione videmus
spiritum vitæ ab oriente microcosmi, hoc est à cordis Thalamo tanquam Æoli microcosmici, capsula spirare, atque afflatu suo omnem sanguinis spiritum aereum secum in gyrum quasi rapere, mediantibus cuius
radiis viuit ille spiritus, & motu viuifico venti tam aquilonares & meridionales, hoc est lienales & hepa-
tici, quam occidentales in microcosmo excitantur; nam vt in superiori Sapientis sermone dictum est: *Or-*
Eccl. 1. 4. *tus Sol postquam occiderit iterum ad locum suum aspirat vbi oriatur, properat ad meridiem & circumit aquilonem, con-*
uersione sua properat aer, &c. Sic etiam in microcosmo ad imitationem macrocosmi dicere possumus, Ortus
solis viuifici seu caloris vitalis postquam occiderit, in vasa spermatica, & tum postea subtus in vuluam seu
terræ meridiem descenderit, iterum ad nouum quasi ortum aspirat, & properat per ramos aortæ, ad meridiem hepaticam, & septentrionem lienalem, & in iis flatus varios excitat: Nam cum cordis flamma sit
solis propago, & verus filius (vnde dicitur *cor sedes animæ humanæ, vt Sol est sedes animæ mundi* & illa anima in
corde à Zenone *ignis naturalis* nuncupatur, & à Prometheo *ignis cælestis, vitæ hominum datus*) sequitur, q; ipsa
moueatur ad motum solis, vtpote quæ est radius eiusdem, quæ ab eo separari nequit, vnde fit vt pars ad totius motũ moueatur. Atq; hinc erat quod Merc. Trismeg. *hominem mundi filium*, & per consequens eius cor
Solis filium, vt cordis calorẽ lucis internæ Solis, seu mundi animę filium dictitauerit. Vnde vt à Solis mundani centro eiaculantur vitæ & lucis viuificæ spermata in spiritum mundanum (quæ etiam à corde hauri-
untur, mediante inspiratione) sic etiam à solis microcosmi centro seu cordis anima calor vitalis vndique in
spiritu microcosmico (qui etiam ab aere mundano deriuatur) disseminatur atque dispergitur, quod etiam
Psal. 4. 23. verbis expressis fatetur propheta regius hoc modo: *Cor tuum custodi supra omnem obseruationem, quia ab eo prode-*
unt actiones vitæ.

Sed vt ad venti Orientalis tam macro quam microcosmi animam internam seu metaphysicam, atque
naturam eiusdem tam in sole quam in corde accedamus: diximus Deum vitam in creaturas suas originali-
ter per spiritum suum inspirasse, hocque mediantibus angelis suis, qui sunt ministri eius ignei, cuius exte-
rius seu manifestum est aer seu ventus, interius vero ignis diuinus, vnde scriptum est, *nomen Iehouæ in angelo*
quem misit Deus ante Israelitas, fuisse. Hinc ergo (inquid Dauid) *qui facis angelos tuos ventos, & ministros tuos ignem*
Exod. 23. *vrentem, facientes placitum tuum*; declarauimus etiam alibi, quod alij angeli habeant curam vitæ, alij corpo-
Psal. 103. 4 ris, &c. At vero quia omnibus est notum, solem mundi, esse vitæ fontem atq; originem, videamus obsecro,
quis angelus ei præsit, quænam sit eius natura, & an sit spiritus Princeps habens dominium in flatus, an
vitæ

Fig. 24 (to p. 118)
The passage from Fludd, *Anatomiae Amphitheatrum*, p. 266 relating to the circular movement of the spirit in the blood. From the Wellcome Collection. By courtesy of the Wellcome Trustees.

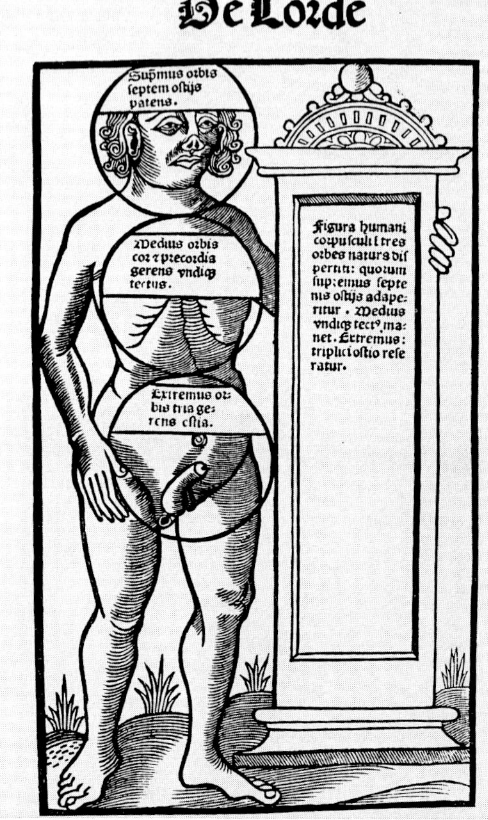

Fig. 25 (to p. 111)
The heart as a "closed circle". From: Carol. Bovillus (Charles de Bouelles). In hoc opere contenta... Liber cordis... Paris. J. Badius Ascensius, 1523, fol. xiii verso. By courtesy of the Wellcome Trustees.

Fig. 26 (to p. 106)
Bruno, on the heart as microcosmic centre.
From: *De monade*, p. 23.

DE MONA. NVM. ET FIGV. 23

in Megacosmo solónia illuminãs, & viuifico calore irradians, uelutq; in medio residẽs Nympharũ Apollo. Vnũ Tẽplũ seu Area ubi tot Numina admirabilẽ sine intermissione choreã celebrãt. Aër unus oĩa circũtẽperans. Vnus humor omnia suffundens. Vna Lex omnia coordinans.

II. ¶ Vestam in centro & meditullio Telluris collocatam ex intentione Pythagoræ definiunt &, eiusdem numen, animam, atq; vitam esse intelligunt: unde significanter in Prytaneo iguis ad aram inextinctus seruabatur. Vnũ in quocunq; globo centrũ est & quasi pũctum, ad qd' omnis circũstãs virtus directa peruadẽdo penetrat; quẽadmodũ ad centrũ usq; Telluris sydcrũ omniũ radios influere existimant Platonici; ibidẽq; tanquã uno in medio fortissimas esse & efficacissimas oẽs impressiones. Ob idq; ipsum diuitias totã p mũdi regionẽ circõferentialẽ sparsas ibi congregatas unitasq;. Ex indeq; illum Pluto, Ditiq; diuitiarum Deo locum adsignarũt.

TERTIVS ORDO.

Vnũ in Microcosmo centrũ est cor, â quo p totũ animal spiritus vitales egrediuntur, in quo arbor uniuersa vitæ figitur & radicatur, & ad cuius primitiuam custodiam & conseruationem referuntur. Vnũ cerebrũ omnis motus principiũ atq; sensus. Vnũ os uniuersalis attractatiõis organũ. Vnũ Epar nutriminis amphitrites.

II. ¶ Vno in medio vehementior est omnis efficacia, tum qa recti undiq; stant ad cẽtrũ radij: tũ quia in angustũ & indiuiduũ oẽs colliguntur: hoc est unũ in quacũq; figura, atq; figurato medium. Monadẽ verò istã in omni perfectè cõposito inuenimus, & agnoscimus. Hãc secretioris philosophię cõteplatores agnoscunt, & operando pro uirib. persequũtur: Vbi qppe nõ punctũ attingere posse datur, ibi ad minimũ, vel circulũ, uel sphærã tamquã ad unitatem contendendo respiciunt, ubi de unitate desperãt, unionẽ moliũtur. Isti verò sicubi cõtrarietas obsistit, cũ uni⁹ uno symmetriæ ordine cõtẽperãt.

Fig. 27 (to p. 107)
Giordano Bruno, on the blood running about in a circle, *ibidem*, p. 524.

524 IORD. BRVN. NOLAN.

Arteriis ſuſos tendentibus undiq; ramos?
Spiritus humenti hinc verſum ſe quaq; refundat
Virtute. Atque frui qui poſſent munere uitæ
Ni ſedes animæ ſanguis ſubſtantiaq; humens
Inſita ſit cunctis atomorumq; ordia nectat?
Sic non conſtarent aſtrorum corpora quæ ſunt
Numina, ſunt mundi, ſunt uere animantia prima,
Quorum ſunt uita reliqua omnia uiua ſubinde.
Viſcera Telluris referunt ita uiſcera noſtra, &
Reptãtum, & nãtum, ſerpentumq;, & uolitantum,
Plantarumq;, & eorum quæ ſunt prompta minæris,
Atq; horum tenuis quorum ſubſtantia fallit
Senſum, aut eſt oculis prorſus non peruia noſtris.
Sic & compoſita eſt nitidi ſubſtantia ſolis,
Subiectum ut lucis conſtans ſiet atq; caloris.
Quin & concretum proprijs de partibus eſſe
Hoc magis id corpus conſtanti humore petitis
Debet, quo tantam firmet lucem, atq; calorem.

CAPVT VIII.

Vt in noſtro corpore ſanguis & humores omnes virtute ſpiritus per totum circũcurſant & recurſant, ſic in toto mundo, aſtro, Tellure; quid enim in noſtro corpore dices deorſum? pedes? tibias? cur non illic omnia diſtant grauia?

Qua-

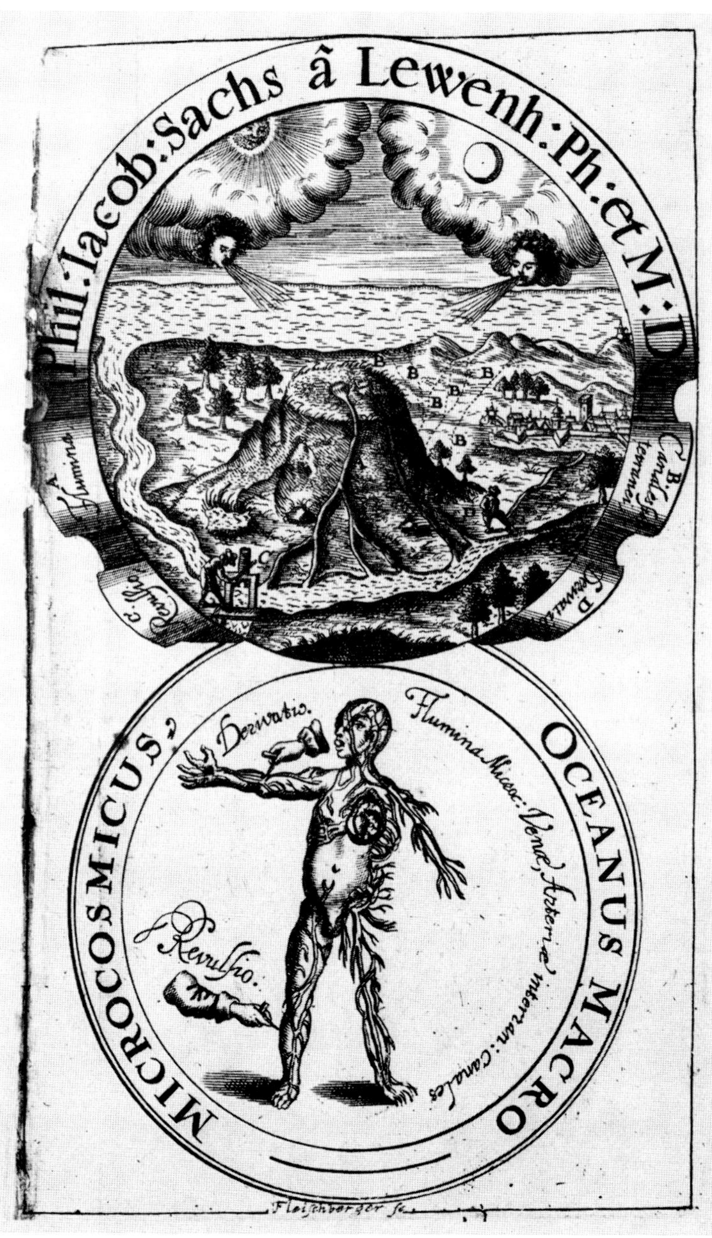

Fig. 28 (to p. 121)
Sachs a Loewnheimb, Frontispiece to *Oceanus macro-microcosmicus*, Breslau 1664. Allegorical representation of the cardiovascular system in the greater and lesser world. By courtesy of the Wellcome Trustees.

DISSERTATIO
ANATOMICO-MEDICA
DE
MOTU BILIS
CIRCULARI
EJUSQUE MORBIS.
Quam publicè olim habuit.
MAURITIUS van REVERHORST,
MEDIC. CAND. Lugd. Batav.
Nunc Professor Anatomicus
Hagæ-Comitis.

LUGDUNI BATAVORUM,
Apud JORD. LUCHTMANS, 1696.

Fig. 29 (to p. 121)
M. van Reverhorst, *On the circular motion of the bile*, 1696. Title-page. By courtesy of the Wellcome Trustees.

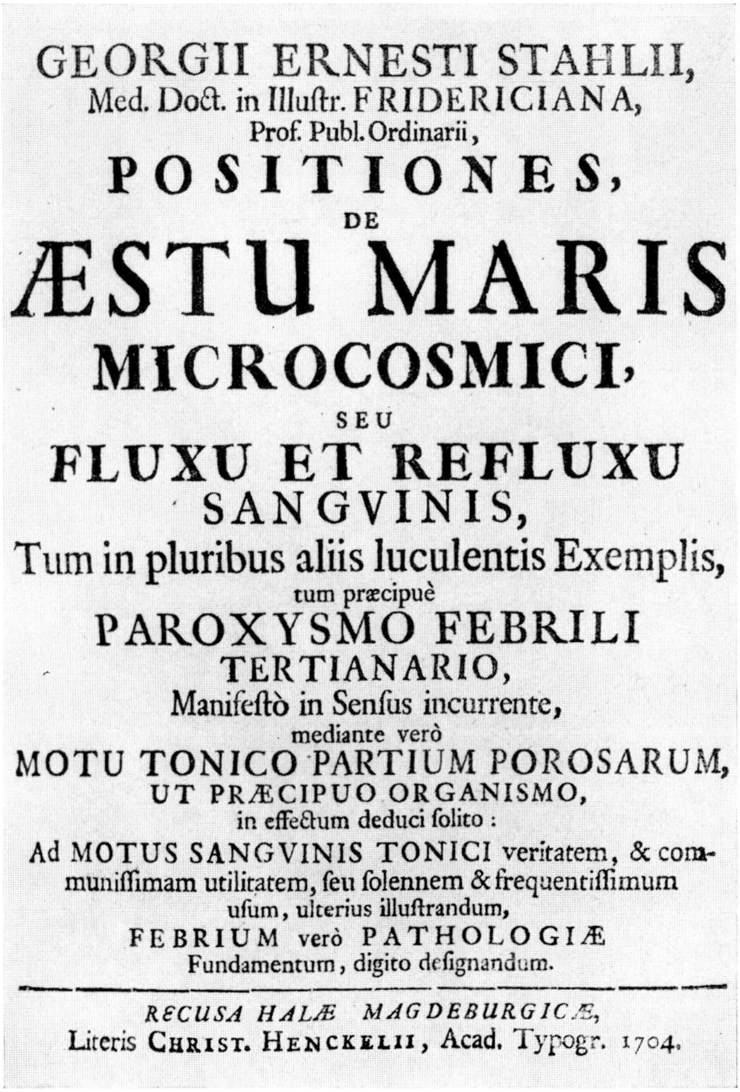

GEORGII ERNESTI STAHLII,
Med. Doct. in Illuſtr. FRIDERICIANA,
Prof. Publ. Ordinarii,

POSITIONES,
DE
ÆSTU MARIS
MICROCOSMICI,
SEU
FLUXU ET REFLUXU
SANGVINIS,

Tum in pluribus aliis luculentis Exemplis,
tum præcipuè
PAROXYSMO FEBRILI
TERTIANARIO,
Manifeſtò in Senſus incurrente,
mediante verò
MOTU TONICO PARTIUM POROSARUM,
UT PRÆCIPUO ORGANISMO,
in effectum deduci ſolito:
Ad MOTUS SANGVINIS TONICI veritatem, & communiſſimam utilitatem, ſeu ſolennem & frequentiſſimum uſum, ulterius illuſtrandum,
FEBRIUM verò PATHOLOGIÆ
Fundamentum, digito deſignandum.

RECUSA HALÆ MAGDEBURGICÆ,
Literis CHRIST. HENCKELII, Acad. Typogr. 1704.

Fig. 30 (to p. 122)
G. E. Stahl, *On the tide of the microcosmic sea or the flux and reflux of the blood*, 1704. Title-page. By courtesy of the Wellcome Trustees.

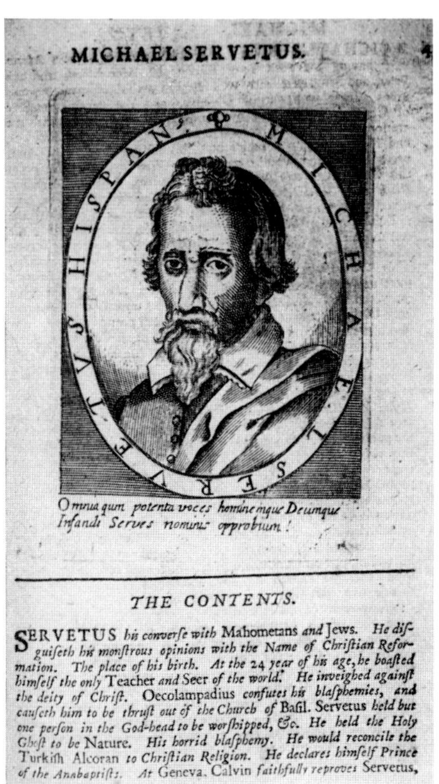
MICHAEL SERVETUS.

Omnia quum potenta voces hominemque Deumque
Infandi Serves nominis opprobium!

THE CONTENTS.

SERVETUS *his converse with* Mahometans *and* Jews. *He disguiseth his monstrous opinions with the Name of Christian Reformation. The place of his birth. At the 24 year of his age, he boasted himself the only* Teacher *and* Seer *of the world. He inveighed against the deity of Christ.* Oecolampadius *confutes his blasphemies, and causeth him to be thrust out of the Church of* Basil. Servetus *held but one person in the God-head to be worshipped, &c. He held the Holy Ghost to be* Nature. *His horrid blasphemy. He would reconcile the* Turkish Alcoran *to Christian Religion. He declares himself Prince of the Anabaptists. At* Geneva. Calvin *faithfully reproves* Servetus,

Fig. 31 (to p. 136)
Portrait of Servetus. From: Alexander Ross, *Viewof all Religions*, p. 43.

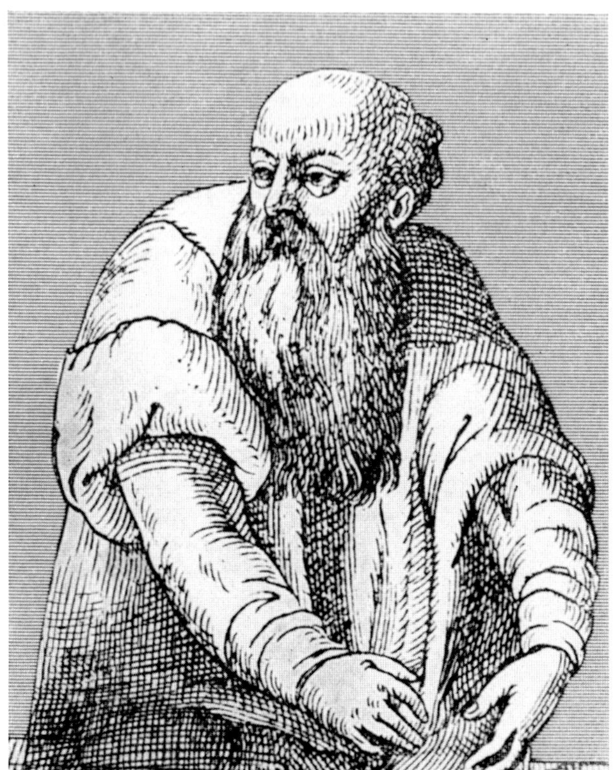

Fig. 32 (to p. 154)
Matthaeus Realdus Columbus. Portrait from Frontispiece to the first edition De re anatomica libri XV, Venet. 1559.

ANDREA CESALPINI ARETINO, DOTTISSIMO
FILOSOFO, E BOTANICO INSIGNE, ARCHIATRO
DI CLEM.TE VIII, PRIMO DISCUOPRIT.RE DELLA
CIRCOLAZ.NE DEL SANGUE NEL CORPO UMANO.
nato nel MDXIX. morto in ROMA il dì 23. Feb.° MDCIII.
Dedicato all' Ill.mo e Rev.mo Mons.re Diodato Andrea de Conti
di Bivignano Patrizio. Aretino Vescovo di S. Sepolcro &c.
Preso da un Ritratto antico esistente nel Museo del Giardino Botanico di Pisa

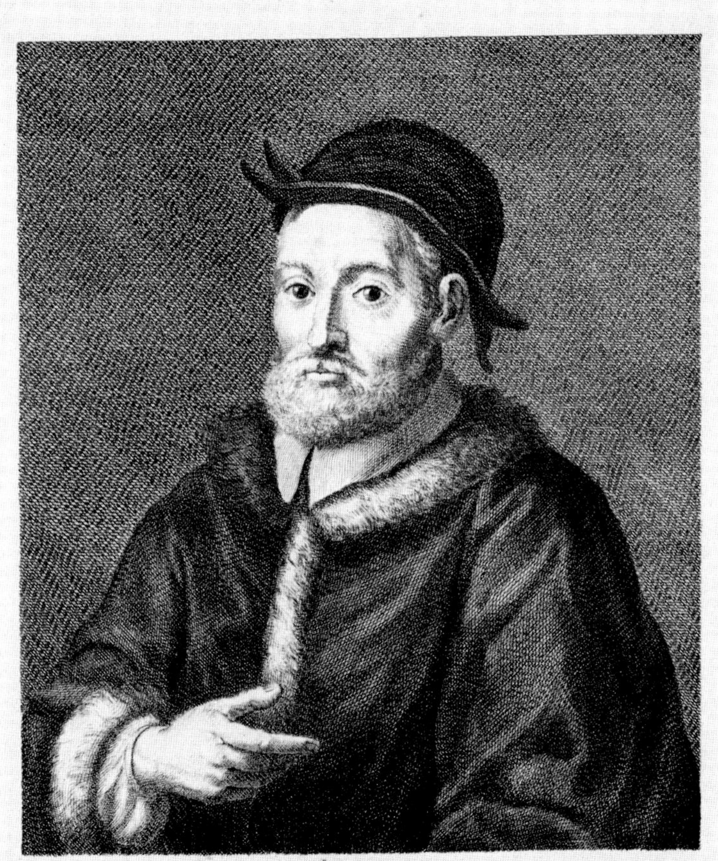

Fig. 33 (to p. 169)
Andreas Cesalpinus. Line engraving by F. Allegrini after G. Zocchi. From the Wellcome Collection. By courtesy of the Wellcome Trust.

Motus enim ſit ex uenis in cor caliditate alimentum trahente, ſimul autem ex corde in arterias, quia hac ſolum patet iter propter membranarum poſitionem: idem enim motus utraque oſcula aperit uenæ ſcilicet in cor, cordis autem in arterias.

1. Peripateticarum quaestionum lib. V, 1571.

QVA autem ratione fiat alimenti attractio, & nutritio in plantis, conſideremus. Nam in animalibus videmus alimentum per venas duci ad cor tanquam ad officinam caloris inſiti, & adepta inibi vltima perfectione per arterias in vniuerſum corpus diſtribui agente ſpiritu, qui ex eodem alimento in corde gignitur.

2. De plantis lib. XVI, 1583.

Motus enim fit ex venis in cor caliditate alimentum trahente, ſimul autem ex corde in arterias, quia hac ſolum patet iter propter membranarum poſitionem: idem enim motus vtraque oſcula aperit venæ ſcilicet in cor, cordis autem in arterias.

3. Quaestionum peripateticarum lib. V, 1593.

Hæc Ariſtoteles. Pro cuius loci explicatione illud ſciendum eſt: Cordis meatus ita à natura paratos eſſe, vt ex vena caua intromiſsio fiat in Cordis ventriculum dextrum, vnde patet exitus in pulmonem: Ex pulmone præterea aliũ ingreſſum eſſe in cordis ventriculum ſiniſtrum, ex quo tandem patet exitus in arteriam Aortam, membranis quibuſdam ad oſtia vaſorum appoſitis, vt impediant retroceſſum: ſic enim perpetuus quidam motus eſt ex vena caua per cor & pulmones in arteriam Aortam: vt in quæſtionibus peripateticis explicauimus.

4. Quaestionum peripateticarum lib. V, 1593.

ad venam cauam eſt, educens autem arteria eſt in pulmonem ducens ad locũ refrigerii. In ſiniſtro venæ oſculum eſt introducens ex pulmone, educens autem eſt arteriæ aortæ principium. Singulis oſculis mẽbranæ quædam appoſita ſunt, quæ intromittentibus aperiuntur ad ingreſſum ſanguinis, clauduntur autẽ ad egreſſum. Oppoſito modo in educentib. patent ad egreſſum, clauduntur ad ingreſſum, vt continuus quidam motus fieret ex venis in cor, & ex corde in arterias.

5. Catoptrum, 1605.

In dextro oſculum introducens ad venam cauam eſt: Educens autem arteria eſt in Pulmonem ducens ad locum refrigerij. In ſiniſtro venæ oſculum eſt introducens ex Pulmone: Educens autem eſt Arteriæ Aortæ principium. Singulis oſculis membranæ quędam appoſitæ ſunt, quę intromittentibus aperiuntur ad ingreſſum ſanguinis, clauduntur autem ad egreſſum. Oppoſito modo in educentibus, patent ad egreſſum, clauduntur ad ingreſſum: vt continuus quidam motus fieret ex venis in Cor, & ex Corde in Arterias.

6. Praxis universae artis medicae, 1606.

Fig. 34 (to p. 170)
Cesalpinus' basic statement on the blood flow, repeated with slight modification between 1571 and 1603. Composite reproduction of the relevant passages from the works of Cesalpinus. Passage (4) is from the *Medical Questions*, lib. II, quaest. 17, fol. 234 recto (as issued together with the second edition of the *Peripatetic Questions*). By courtesy of the Wellcome Trust.

LIBER SECVNDVS. 234

A Neceſſe enim eſt ex ea apprehenſione virtutem cordis non commu-
nicari cerebro, ideo tolli ſenſum & motum voluntarium toti corpori:
at non eſt neceſſe oppleri adeo pulmonem, vt ſuffocetur. Sed illud
ſpeculatione dignum videtur, propter quid ex vinculo intumeſcunt
venæ vltra locum apprehenſum, non citra: quod experimento ſciunt,
qui uenam ſecant: vinculum enim adhibent citra locum ſectionis, nõ
vltra: quia tument venæ vltra vinculum non citra. Debuiſſet autem
oppoſito modo contingere, ſi motus ſanguinis & ſpiritus à viſceribus
fit in totum corpus: intercepto enim meatu non vltra datur progreſ-
ſus: tumor igitur venarum citra vinculum debuiſſet fieri. An ſolui-
tur dubitatio ex eo quod ſcribit Ariſtoteles de ſom. cap. 3. vbi inquit.
Neceſſe enim quod euaporatur aliquo uſque impelli, deinde cõuerti
& permutari ſicut Euripũ: calidum enim cuiuſque animalium ad ſuperiora natum eſt ferri: cum autem in ſuperioribus locis fuerit, multũ
B ſimul iterum reuertitur, ferturque deorſum: Hæc Ariſtoteles. Pro
cuius loci explicatione illud ſciendum eſt: Cordis meatus ita à natura paratos eſſe, vt ex vena caua intromiſsio fiat in Cordis ventriculum
dextrum, vnde patet exitus in pulmonem: Ex pulmone præterea aliũ
ingreſſum eſſe in cordis ventriculum ſiniſtrum, ex quo tandem patet
exitus in arteriam Aortam, membranis quibuſdam ad oſtia vaſorum
appoſitis, vt impediant retroceſſum: ſic enim perpetuus quidam motus eſt ex vena caua per cor & pulmones in arteriam Aortam: vt in
quæſtionibus peripateticis explicauimus. Cum autem in vigilia motus caloris natiui fiat extra ſcilicet ad ſenſoria: in ſomno autem intra,
ſcilicet ad cor: putandum eſt in vigilia multum ſpiritus & ſanguinis
ferri ad arterias, inde enim in neruos eſt iter. In ſomno autem eũdem
calorem per venas reuerti ad cor, non per arterias: ingreſſus enim naturalis per venam cauam datur in cor, non per arteriam. Indicio ſunt
C pulſus, qui expergiſcentibus fiunt magni, vehementes, celeres, & cre-
bri cum quadam vibratione: in ſomno autem parui, languidi, tardi,
& rari 3. de cau. pul. 9. & 10. Nam in ſomno calor natiuus minus vergit
in arterias: in eaſdem erumpit vehementius, cum expergiſcuntur. Venæ autem contrario modo ſe habent: nam in ſomno fiunt tumidio-
res, in vigilia exiliores, vt patet intuenti eas quæ in manu ſunt. Tranſit
enim in ſomno calor natiuus ex arterijs in venas per oſculorum communionem, quam Anaſtomoſin vocant, & inde ad cor. Vt autẽ ſanguinis exundatio ad ſuperiora, & retroceſſus ad inferiora inſtar Euripi
manifeſta eſt in ſomno & vigilia, ſic non obſcurus eſt huiuſmodi motus in quacumque parte corporis vinculum adhibeatur, aut alia ratione occludantur venæ. Cum enim tollitur permeatio, intumeſcunt ri-
uuli qua parte fluere ſolent. Forte recurrit eo tempore ſanguis ad prin
cipium, ne interciſus extinguatur. Non efficit autem ſuffocationem
Gg 2 quælibet

Fig. 35 (to p. 173)
Cesalpinus on the centripetal direction of the venous flow. From: *Quaest. Medicinales*, lib. II, quaest. 17, fol. 234 recto. By courtesy of the Wellcome Trust.

ÆT: LX 1632.
CASPAR HOFMAN MEDICINÆ DOCTOR ET PUBLICUS PROFESSOR IN ACADEMIA ALTORFINA.
Hortorum vitas qui in floribus excolit, Hoffma
Dicitur, et Medici quid magis ornat opus?

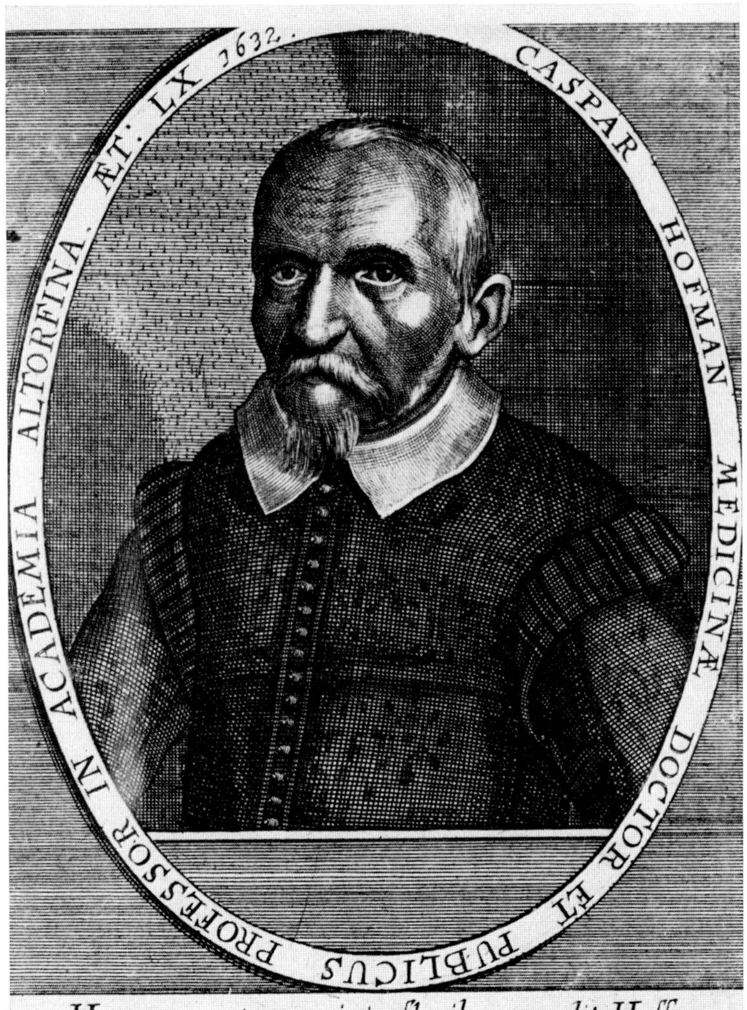

Fig. 36 (to p. 196)
Caspar Hofmann. Portrait from: Boissard, *Bibliotheca chalcographica*, 1650. By courtesy of the Wellcome Trust.

CASP. HOFMANNI
COMMENTARII
IN GALENI
DE
USU PARTIUM
CORPORIS HUMANI
LIB. XVII.
CVM VARIIS LECTIONIBVS IN VTRVMQ; Codicem, Græcum & Latinum, & Indice gemino.
OPVS, NON MEDICIS TANTVM, sed & Philosophis, nec minus Philologis paratum.

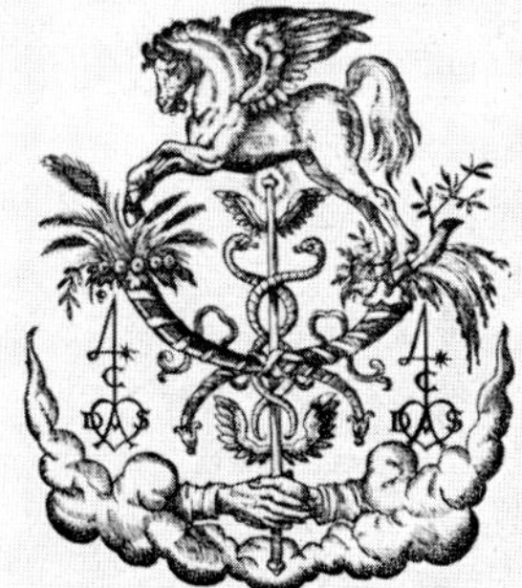

FRANCOFVRTI AD MOENVM,
Typis Wechelianis, Apud Danielem & Davidem Aubrios, & Clementem Schleichium.
ANNO MDCXXV.

Fig. 37 (to p. 196)
Title-page to Caspar Hofmann's *Commentaries on Galen on the use of the parts*, 1625, as quoted by Harvey. From the copy in the Wellcome Historical Medical Museum and Library. By courtesy of the Wellcome Trust.

CASP. HOFMANNI
DE
THORACE,
EJUSQUE PARTIBUS
COMMENTARIUS
TRIPARTITUS.
In quo discutiuntur præcipuè ea, quæ inter Aristotelem & Galenum controversa sunt.

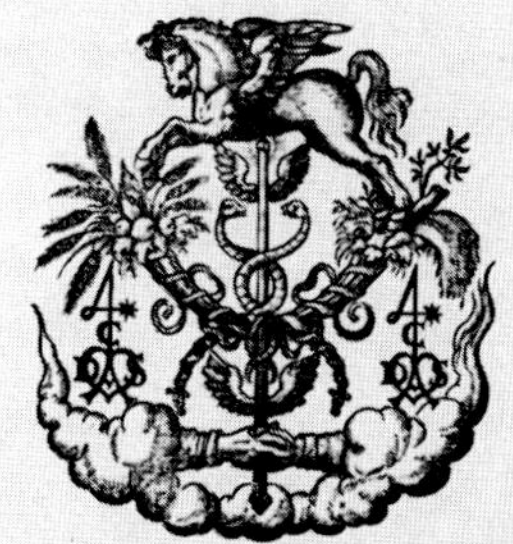

FRANCOFVRTI
Typis & Sumptibus Wechelianorum, apud Danielem & Davidem Aubrios & Clementem Schleichium.
ANNO M. DC. XXVII.

Fig. 38 (to p. 196)
Title-page to Caspar Hofmann, *On the chest*, 1627, containing important references to Aristotle and Cesalpinus. From the copy in the Wellcome Historical Medical Museum and Library. By courtesy of the Wellcome Trustees.

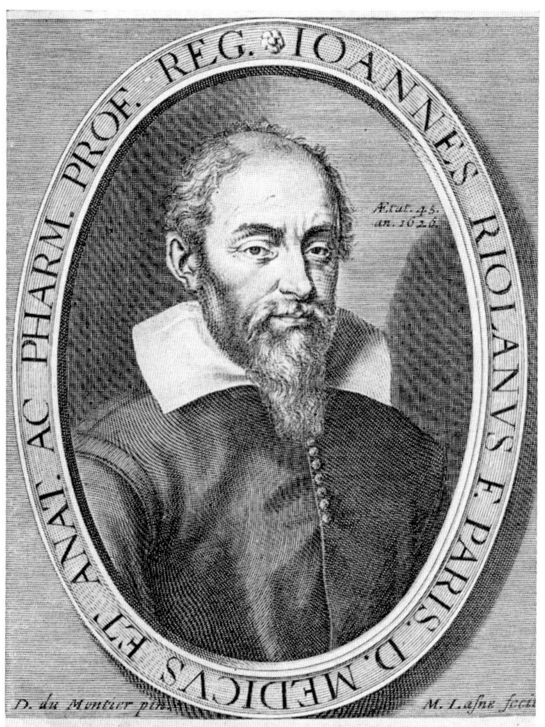

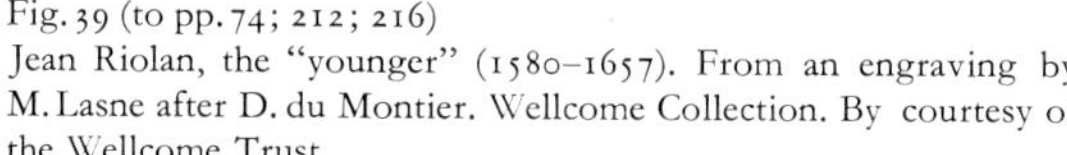

Fig. 39 (to pp. 74; 212; 216)
Jean Riolan, the "younger" (1580–1657). From an engraving by M. Lasne after D. du Montier. Wellcome Collection. By courtesy of the Wellcome Trust.

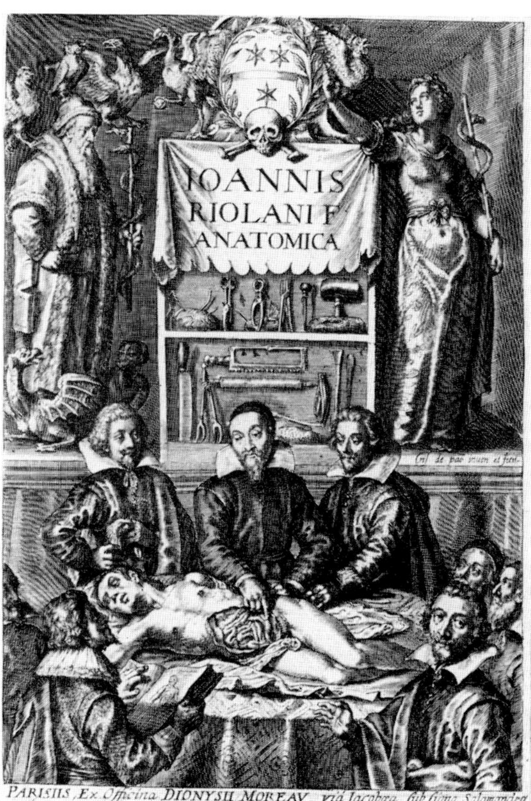

Fig. 40 (to pp. 212 and 216)
Jean Riolan, the "younger". Title-page to *Anthropographia et osteologia*. Paris 1626. By courtesy of the Wellcome Trust.

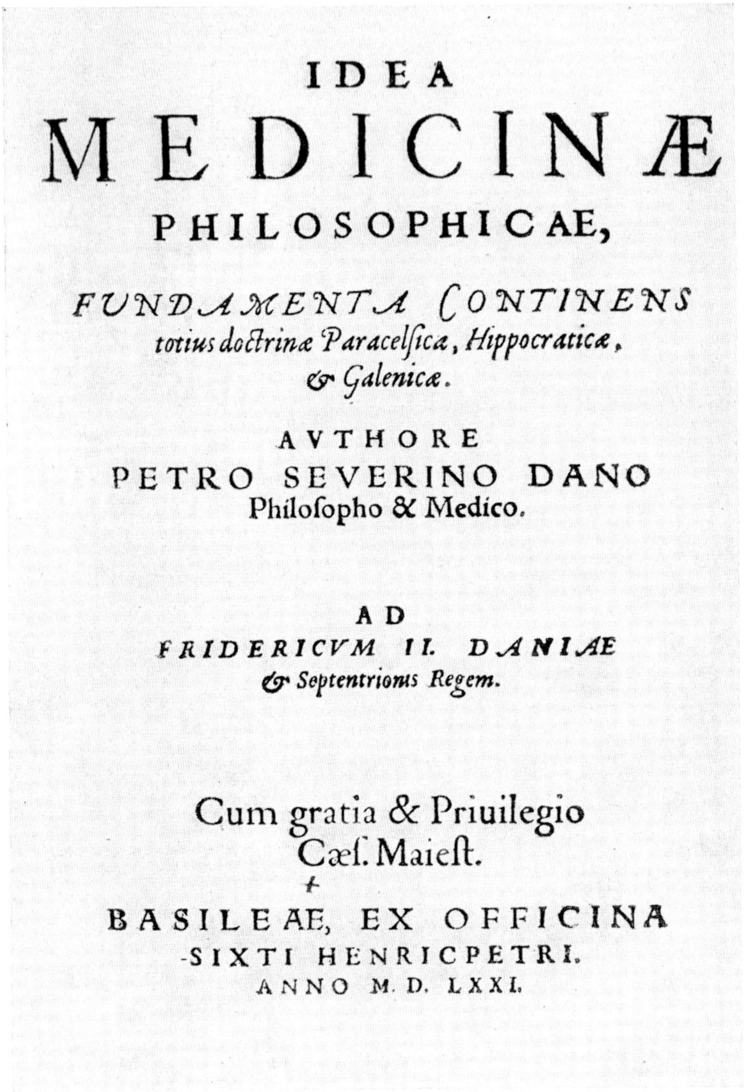

IDEA
MEDICINÆ
PHILOSOPHICAE,

FUNDAMENTA CONTINENS
totius doctrinæ Paracelsicæ, Hippocraticæ, & Galenicæ.

AVTHORE
PETRO SEVERINO DANO
Philoſopho & Medico.

AD
FRIDERICVM II. DANIAE
& Septentrionis Regem.

Cum gratia & Priuilegio
Cæſ. Maieſt.

BASILEAE, EX OFFICINA
SIXTI HENRICPETRI.
ANNO M. D. LXXI.

Fig. 41 (to p. 240)
Peter Severinus, *Idea of Philosophical Medicine*, 1571. Title-page.
By courtesy of the Wellcome Trust.

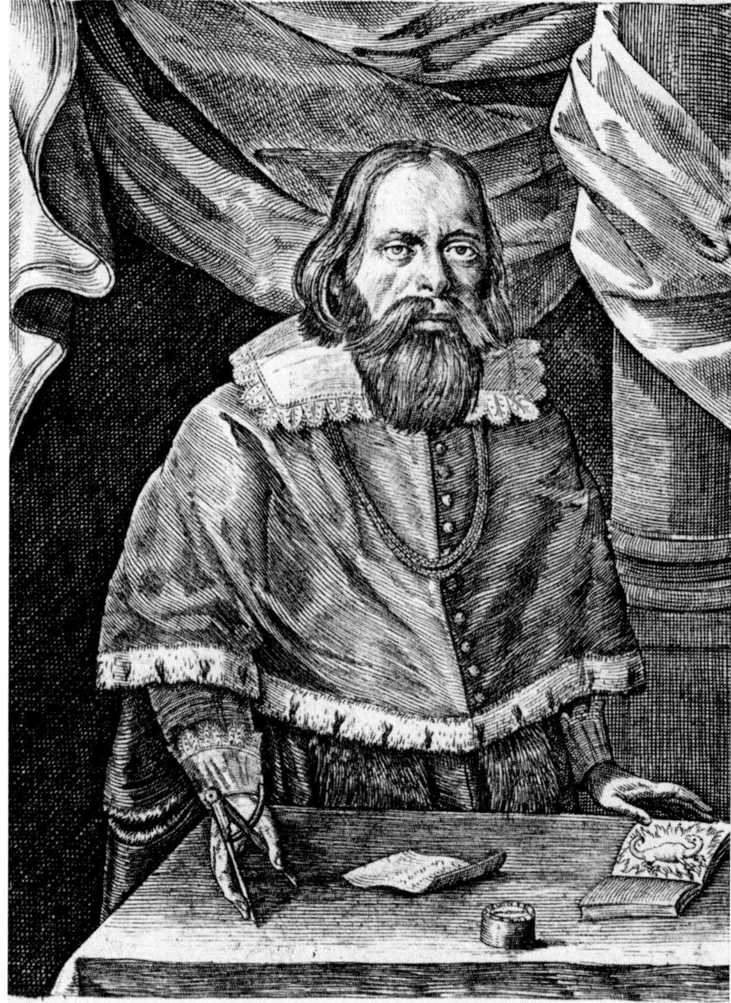

Fig. 42 (to p. 285)
Marcus Marci of Kronland.
From: *De proportione motus*, Prague 1639.
By courtesy of the Wellcome Trust.

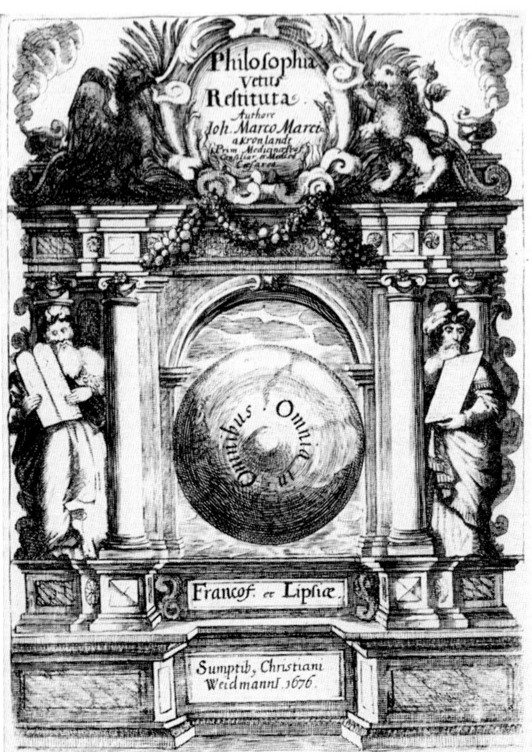

Fig. 43 (to pp. 287 and 318)
Marcus Marci, *Ancient Philosophy restored*, 1662. Frontispiece of the second edition. Francof. 1676. By courtesy of the Wellcome Trust.

352 *Philoſ. Vet. reſtit. Pars III.*

habet: cui alia determinatio in hac, alia in illa parte producenda convenit ob legem cui anima tum eſt ſubjecta. prout penicillum in manu pictoris eſt indifferens ad lineam rectam, vel circularem: at ubi directionem accepit ad lineam rectam, non poteſt ab eodem duci aut pingi linea circularis, Eadem ratione in utero, ſeu ovipara ſeu vivipara ſint, anima ineſt & ab eo ipſo in fœtu dependet; non tamen hujus efficientia utero, ſeu animæ quatenus utero ineſt, tribui poteſt: ſiquidem aliam legem in utero, aliam in fœtu ſequitur. *(l)* neque ex aliqua parte uteri fit fœtus aut ipſum ovum: unde ſuperflua eſt idea ſeu quævis alia virtus, aut phantaſma quod uterus ex tactu ſeminali recipere dicitur: ſiquidem anima non prout in utero eſt, ovum aut ex ovo pullum fabricat. & ſi utero ineſſet illa vis, oporteret partem illam uteri ex qua fit fœtus corrumpi. *(m)* Cùm verò uterus dicitur ovum aut ex eo fœtum procreare, eo modo intelligi debet quo caput dicitur videre, cujus pars ſunt oculi quibus propriè convenit viſio. Verùm ſive hoc ſive illo modo res habeat, eadem difficultas manet, qua nimirum ratione anima ex ſe indifferens ad hoc illudq; agendum determinetur ad unum quodque ex eadem materia conſtituendum tantâ elegantiâ & varietate, non aliter quàm ſi ab arte fieret; neq, tamen electione prout artifex operetur. faciunt ait Hippocrates quod neſciunt & ſcire ſibi videntur: omnia verò per Divinam neceſſitatem. *(n)* Hanc difficultatem agnovit & fatetur exerc. 49. *quamvis* inquiens *notum ſit omnesque fateantur prolem à mare & fœmina ortum ſuum ducere, & proinde ovum à gallo & gallina procreari & ex ovo pullum: modum tamen quo gallus aut ejus ſemen ex ovo pullum cudat, nec medicorum ſchola nos docuit, neq; Ariſtotelis ſagax ingenium aperuit.* Qua ratione formatio fœtûs fiat ſatis opinor à me explicatum in libro idearum; neque ignotum id Harveo: cui librum hic Pragæ in manus dedi familiariter cum eodem converſatus. verùm fortaſſe ex eo improbatū, quòd ſupponere videbatur cum Ariſtotele & ſchola Medicorum generationem fieri ex ſemine maris & fœminæ. quæ tamen ibidem à me demonſtrata non minorem vim habent etiam in ſententia Harvei, ſi veram hanc eſſe demus. *(o)* At in nulla hypotheſi ab eodem explicari poteſt, qua ratione formatio fœtus fiat. Itaque deſpe-

rata

Fig. 44 (to p. 287)
Harvey's visiting Marci at Prague—Marci's account in *Ancient Philosophy restored* (p. 352 in the second edition).

General Index